GASTROINTESTINAL AND LIVER

GASTROINTESTINAL AND LIVER

SECRETS

PETER R. McNALLY, DO, MSRF, MACG
Chief Gastroenterology
Evans Army Hospital
Colorado Springs, Colorado

ELSEVIER

Elsevier
1600 John F. Kennedy Blvd.
Ste 1800
Philadelphia, PA 19103-2899

GASTROINTESTINAL AND LIVER SECRETS, SIXTH EDITION   978-0-323-93637-8

Senior Content Strategist: Marybeth Thiel
Senior Content Development Specialist: Akanksha Marwah/Sneha Kashyap
Publishing Services Manager: Shereen Jameel
Senior Project Manager: Beula Christopher
Senior Designer: Renee Duenow

Printed in India

Last digit is the print number: 9   8   7   6   5   4   3   2   1

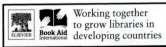

The editor dedicates this book to his wife, Cynthia;
to his children, Alex, Meghan, Amanda, Genevieve, and Bridgette;
and to his grandchildren Charlotte, Xavier, Adelaide, Benette, Greer, and Tatum.

CONTRIBUTORS

Mitali Agarwal, MD
Center for Inflammatory Bowel Disease
Cleveland Clinic
Cleveland, Ohio

Mohammed Eyad Alsabbagh, MD
Assistant Professor of Medicine
Department of Gastroenterology
Saint Louis University
St. Louis, Missouri

Ganesh Aswath, MD
Assistant Professor of Medicine
SUNY Upstate Medical University
Syracuse, New York

Bruce Raymond Bacon, MD
Emeritus Professor of Internal Medicine
Department of Internal Medicine, Division of
    Gastroenterology and Hepatology
Saint Louis University School of Medicine
St. Louis, Missouri

Geoffrey Bader, MD
Gastroenterology Faculty
Division of Gastroenterology
Brooke Army Medical Center
San Antonio, Texas

Ji Young Bang, MD, MPH
Director of Clinical Research
Digestive Health Institute
Orlando Health
Orlando, Florida

Kalyan Ram Bhamidimarri, MD, MPH, FACG, FAASLD
Professor of Clinical Medicine
Department of Medicine
University of Miami
Miami, Florida

Devina Bhasin, MD
Transplant Hepatologist
Piedmont Transplant Institute
Piedmont Hospital
Atlanta, Georgia

Jacqueline Birkness-Gartman, MD
Assistant Professor
Department of Gastrointestinal and Liver Pathology
Johns Hopkins University School of Medicine
Baltimore, Maryland

Gabriel A. Bolaños Guzmán, MD
Fellow
Department of Gastroenterology
University of South Alabama College of Medicine
Mobile, Alabama

Richard Bower, MD
Gastroenterologist
Department of Gastroenterology
Naval Medical Center San Diego
San Diego, California

Mathew J. Bradley, MD
Professor
Department of Surgery
Uniformed Services University of the Health Sciences
Bethesda, Maryland

Landon Brown, MD
Department of Gastroenterology
University of Texas Health Science at San Antonio
San Antonio, Texas

Roderick Seth Brown, DO
Fellow
Division of Gastroenterology
University of South Alabama
Mobile, Alabama

Cassandra Burger, BA
Senior Clinical Research Coordinator
Digestive Health Institute
Children's Hospital Colorado
Aurora, Colorado

Carol Ann Burke, MD
Director
Department of Gastroenterology and Hepatology
Center for Colon Polyp and Cancer Prevention
Cleveland Clinic
Cleveland, Ohio

Mitchell S. Cappell, MD, PhD
Senior Gastroenterologist
Department of Gastroenterology
Aleda E. Lutz Veterans Administration Hospital
Saginaw, Michigan;
Professor of Medicine
Oakland University William Beaumont
    School of Medicine
Royal Oak, Michigan

William Carey, MD, MACG, FAASLD
Professor of Medicine
Cleveland Clinic Lerner College of Medicine;
Staff Hepatologist
Cleveland Clinic
Cleveland, Ohio

Karen Chang, DO
GI Fellow
Department of Gastroenterology
University of California
Riverside, San Bernardino

Joseph G. Cheatham, MD
Associate Professor of Medicine
Uniformed Services University
Bethesda, Maryland;
Program Director,
Gastroenterology Fellowship
Naval Medical Center San Diego
San Diego, California

Bradford Jin Chong, MD
Fellow
Department of Gastroenterology
Oregon Health and Science University
Portland, Oregon

Steven Clayton, MD, FAAFP, FACP, FACG
Assistant Professor of Medicine
Department of Internal Medicine, Section of
  Gastroenterology
Wake Forest Baptist Medical Center
Winston Salem, North Carolina

David Cleaver, DO, FAOCD, FAAD
Assistant Professor
Department of Dermatology
Kirksville College of Osteopathic Medicine,
  A.T. Still University
Kirksville, Missouri

Gregory A. Coté, MD, MS
Head,
Professor of Medicine
Department of Medicine
Division of Gastroenterology and Hepatology
Oregon Health and Science University
Portland, Oregon

Anton Jordan De Witte, MD
Resident Physician
Department of Internal Medicine
Vanderbilt University Medical Center
Nashville, Tennessee

Amar R. Deshpande, MD
Professor of Medicine
University of Miami Miller School of Medicine
Miami, Florida

Jack A. Di Palma, MD
Professor of Medicine and Gastroenterology,
Fellowship Director
Division of Gastroenterology
Frederick P. Widdon College of Medicine at the
  University of South Alabama
Mobile, Alabama

Gerald Dryden, Jr., MD, PhD, MSPH
Professor of Medicine
University of Louisville
Louisville, Kentucky

David T. Dulaney, MD
Assistant Professor,
Staff Gastroenterologist
Division of Gastroenterology and Hepatology
Brooke Army Medical Center
San Antonio, Texas

Trevor Dunbar, DO
Physician
Department of Internal Medicine
Arrowhead Regional Medical Center
Colton, California

John E. Eaton, MD
Associate Professor of Medicine
Department of Internal Medicine, Division of
  Gastroenterology and Hepatology
Mayo Clinic
Rochester, Minnesota

Katherine Falloon, MD
Inflammatory Bowel Disease Fellow
Department of Gastroenterology, Hepatology,
  and Nutrition
Cleveland Clinic Foundation
Cleveland, Ohio

Francis A. Farraye, MS, MD, MACG
Director
Inflammatory Bowel Disease Center
Mayo Clinic
Jacksonville, Florida

Michael G. Fox, MD, MBA
Professor of Radiology
Department of Radiology
Mayo Clinic Arizona
Phoenix, Arizona

John Gancayco, MD
Gastroenterology Fellowship Program Director
Division of Gastroenterology
Brooke Army Medical Center
San Antonio, Texas;
Associate Professor
Uniformed Services University of the Health Sciences
Bethesda, Maryland

Adil Ghafoor, MD
Gastroenterology Fellow
Department of Gastroenterology
Advocate Aurora Health
Milwaukee, Wisconsin

John S. Goff, MD
Partner
Department of Gastroenterology
Rocky Mountain Gastroenterology
Lakewood, Colorado

Meghana Golla, MD
Resident
Department of Internal Medicine
Vanderbilt University
Nashville, Tennessee

Samuel Han, MD
Assistant Professor
Division of Gastroenterology, Hepatology, and Nutrition
The Ohio State University Wexner Medical Center
Columbus, Ohio

Stephen A. Harrison, MD
Visiting Professor of Hepatology
Radcliffe Department of Medicine
University of Oxford
Oxford, United Kingdom;
Chairman and Founder
Pinnacle Clinical Research,
Chairman and Co-Founder
Summit Clinical Research
San Antonio, Texas

William P. Hennrikus, MD
LT, MC, USN
General Surgery
Walter Reed National Military Medical Center
Bethesda, Maryland

Jorge L. Herrera, MD
Professor of Medicine
Division of Gastroenterology
University of South Alabama Whiddon College of Medicine
Mobile, Alabama

Brenda J. Hoffman, MD
Professor
Division of Gastroenterology and Hepatology
The Medical University of South Carolina
Charleston, South Carolina

Isabel A. Hujoel, MD
Clinical Assistant Professor
Department of Gastroenterology
University of Washington
Seattle, Washington

John W. Jacobs, MD
Associate Professor of Medicine
Division of Digestive Diseases and Nutrition
University of South Florida Morsani College of Medicine
Tampa, Florida

Savio John, MD
Chief of Gastroenterology
Department of Medicine
SUNY Upstate Medical University
Syracuse, New York

Zachary Johnston, MD
Gastroenterology Fellow
Department of Gastroenterology
Walter Reed National Military Medical Center
Bethesda, Maryland

Ryan Kaliney, MD
Musculoskeletal Radiology Section Chief
Bone and Joint Institute
Hartford Healthcare
Hartford, Connecticut

Zeid Kayali, MD, MBA
Department of Internal Medicine
University of California Riverside
Rialto, California

Jami A. Kinnucan, MD, FACG, AGAF
Senior Associate Consultant,
Chair, GI Clinical Practice
Department of Medicine, Division of Gastroenterology and
  Hepatology
Mayo Clinic
Jacksonville, Florida

Kimi L. Kondo, DO, FSIR
Associate Professor
Department of Radiology, Division of Interventional
  Radiology
University of Colorado School of Medicine
Aurora, Colorado

Heather Korus, MSN, APNP, FNP-BC
Nurse Practitioner
Urgent Care
Advocate Aurora
Greater Milwaukee, Wisconsin

Prashant Vasanth Krishnan, MD
Chief Medical Officer and Board Member
Peak Gastroenterology Associates and Gastro Care
  Partners;
Clinical Professor
University of Colorado
Denver, Colorado;
Rocky Vista University
Parker, Colorado;
Kansas City University
Kansas City, Missouri

Kristine A. Kuhn, MD, PhD, FACR
Associate Professor
Department of Medicine, Division of Rheumatology
University of Colorado Anschutz Medical Campus
Aurora, Colorado

Anand V. Kulkarni, MD, DM
Department of Hepatology
Asian Institute of Gastroenterology
Hyderabad, Telangana, India

Jeffrey Laczek, MD, FACP, FACG
Associate Professor
Department of Medicine
Uniformed Services University of the Health Services
Bethesda, Maryland

Samuel H. Lai, MD
General Surgery Resident
Section of Colorectal Surgery
Division of GI, Trauma, and Endocrine Surgery
Department of Surgery
University of Colorado School of Medicine
Denver, Colorado

Anthony J. LaPorta, MD, FACS
Professor of Surgery
Rocky Vista University
Parker, Colorado

Bret A. Lashner, MD
Professor of Medicine
Department of Gastroenterology, Hepatology,
   and Nutrition
Cleveland Clinic
Cleveland, Ohio

James Latanski, MD
Department of Radiology
Walter Reed National Capital Consortium
Bethesda, Maryland

John W. Lee, MD
Physician
Department of Gastroenterology
Walter Reed National Military Medical Center
Bethesda, Maryland

Linda S. Lee, MD
Medical Director of Endoscopy
Department of Gastroenterology
Brigham and Women's Hospital;
Associate Professor of Medicine
Harvard Medical School
Boston, Massachusetts

Mike H. Lee, MD
Chief
Department of Radiology
Walter Reed National Military Medical Center;
Vice Chair of Education
Department of Radiology and Radiological Sciences
Uniformed Services University of the Health Sciences
Bethesda, Maryland

Yoo Jin Lee, MD
Department of Medicine, Karsh Division of Digestive and
   Liver Diseases
Cedars-Sinai Medical Center
Los Angeles, California

Anthony Lembo, MD
Vice Chair of Research
Cleveland Clinic
Digestive Diseases and Surgery Institute
Cleveland, Ohio

Kenneth Leung, MD
Attending Physician
Department of Gastroenterology
Kaiser Permanente Baldwin Park
Baldwin Park, California

Carole Macaron, MD
The Cleveland Clinic
Department of Gastroenterology and Hepatology
Digestive Disease Institute
Cleveland, Ohio

Peter Mannon, MD, MPH
Professor of Medicine,
Chief
Division of Gastroenterology and Hepatology
University of Nebraska Medical Center
Omaha, Nebraska

Katherine S. Marchak, MD
Assistant Professor
Department of Interventional Radiology
University of Colorado
Aurora, Colorado

Martin D. McCarter, MD
Professor of Surgery
University of Colorado School of Medicine
Aurora, Colorado

Peter R. McNally, DO, MSRF, MACG
Chief Gastroenterology
Evans Army Hospital
Colorado Springs, Colorado

Gil Y. Melmed, MD, MS
Professor
Department of Medicine,
Director
Inflammatory Bowel Disease Clinical Research
Cedars-Sinai Medical Center
Los Angeles, California

Andrew T. Mertz, MD, MAJ, MC
Gastroenterology Fellow
Department of Gastroenterology
Walter Reed National Military Medical Center
Bethesda, Maryland

Alex D. Michaels, MD
Medical Instructor
Department of Surgery
Duke Health
Durham, North Carolina

Robert Moran, MD
Associate Professor of Medicine
Division of Gastroenterology and Hepatology
Medical University of South Carolina
Charleston, South Carolina

Amber M. Moyer, MD
Resident Physician
Department of Surgery
University of Colorado
Aurora, Colorado

Rupa Mukherjee, MD
Assistant Professor of Medicine
Harvard Medical School;
Medical Director of the Celiac Center at Lexington
Division of Gastroenterology
Beth Israel Deaconess Medical Center
Boston, Massachusetts

Nathalie Nguyen, MD
Assistant Professor of Pediatrics
Department Pediatric Gastroenterology, Hepatology and
    Nutrition
Children's Hospital Colorado
Aurora, Colorado

Kiyoko Oshima, MD, PhD
Associate Professor
Department of Pathology
Johns Hopkins University School of Medicine
Baltimore, Maryland

Theodore N. Pappas, MD
Professor of Surgery
Duke University
Durham, North Carolina

Anish Patel, DO
Director
IBD Center
Division of Gastroenterology
Brooke Army Medical Center
San Antonio, Texas

Dhyanesh A. Patel, MD
Assistant Professor of Medicine
Department of Gastroenterology
Vanderbilt University Medical Center
Nashville, Tennessee

Nathalie A. Pena Polanco, MD
Gastroenterologist
Department of Gastroenterology and Hepatology
Mercy Medical Center
Cedar Rapids, Iowa

Pranav Penninti, DO
Fellow
Department of Gastroenterology and Hepatology
University of Texas Health San Antonio
San Antonio, Texas

Shajan Peter, MD
Associate Professor
Division of Gastroenterology
University of Alabama at Birmingham
Birmingham, Alabama

Kevin D. Platt, MD
Clinical Instructor
Division of Gastroenterology and Hepatology
University of Michigan
Ann Arbor, Michigan

Siobhan Proksell, MD
Assistant Professor of Medicine
University of Miami Miller School of Medicine
Miami, Florida

Vikram Rangan, MD
Assistant Professor of Medicine
Department of Gastroenterology
Beth Israel Deaconess Medical Center
Boston, Massachusetts

Satish S.C. Rao, MD, PhD, FRCP
Professor of Medicine
Department of Medicine, Division of Gastroenterology and
    Hepatology
Augusta University
Augusta, Georgia

K. Rajender Reddy, MD, FACP, FACG, FRCP, FAASLD
Founders Professor of Medicine
Department of Internal Medicine, Division of
    Gastroenterology and Hepatology
University of Pennsylvania
Philadelphia, Pennsylvania

Michael D. Rice, MD
Associate Professor
Department of Internal Medicine
University of Michigan
Ann Arbor, Michigan

Mark D. Riddle, MD, DrPH, FISTM
Community (Adjunct) Faculty
Internal Medicine Associate Dean
Naval Medical Research Center
Silver Spring, Maryland

Carol Rouphael, MD
Associate Staff
Department of Gastroenterology
Cleveland Clinic
Cleveland, Ohio

Mark W. Russo, MD, MPH
Clinical Professor of Medicine
Atrium Health Wake Forest School of Medicine
Charlotte, North Carolina

Michael Saag, MD
Professor Emeritus
Department of Medicine
University of Alabama at Birmingham
Birmingham, Alabama

George Saffouri, MD
Assistant Clinical Professor
Department of Gastroenterology and Hepatology
UC Riverside School of Medicine
Riverside, California

Rebecca Salvo, DO
Fellow
Department of Gastroenterology
Valley Hospital Medical Center
Las Vegas, Nevada;
Physician
Department of Gastroenterology
Santa Barbara Cottage Hospital
Santa Barbara, California

Lawrence R. Schiller, MD
Chair
Institutional Review Board Administration
Baylor Scott and White Research Institute;
Adjunct Professor
Department of Medical Education
Texas A&M University College of Medicine
Dallas, Texas

Tomoki Sempokuya, MD
Fellow
Department of Gastroenterology and Hepatology
University of Nebraska Medical Center
Omaha, Nebraska

Raj J. Shah, MD, MASGE, AGAF, FACG
Professor of Medicine,
Director, Pancreas and Biliary Endoscopy
University of Colorado Hospital
Aurora, Colorado

Roshan Shrestha, MD
Medical Director of Liver Transplantation
Piedmont Hospital
Atlanta, Georgia;
Clinical Professor of Medicine
Mercer University School of Medicine
Savannah, Georgia

Andrew P. Sill, MD
Chief Resident
Mayo Clinic Arizona Diagnostic Radiology Residency
Phoenix, Arizona

Ashwani K. Singal, MD, MS, FACG, FAASLD, AGAF
Professor
Department of Gastroenterology and Hepatology
University of South Dakota;
Chief Clinical Research and Transplant Hepatologist
Department of Transplant Hepatology
Avera Transplant Institute;
Health Research Scientist
VA Medical Center;
Director, Hepatology Elective
Sanford School of Medicine
University of South Dakota
Sioux Falls, South Dakota

Chad M. Spencer, MD
Instructor of Medicine
Department of Gastroenterology
University of South Alabama
Mobile, Alabama

Holly V. Spitzer, DO
General Surgery
William Beaumont Army Medical Center
El Paso, Texas

Christina M. Surawicz, MD
Professor Emerita
Department of Gastroenterology
University of Washington
Seattle, Washington

Shalini Tayal, MD
Section-Chief, Anatomic Pathology
Department of Pathology
Veterans Affairs Eastern Regional Medical Center;
Associate Professor
Department of Pathology
University of Colorado School of Medicine
Aurora, Colorado

Zachary A. Taylor, DO, FACS
Assistant Professor
Norman M. Rich Department of Surgery
Uniformed Services University of the Health Sciences
Bethesda, Maryland

Camille S. Thélin, MD, MS
Assistant Professor of Medicine
Digestive Diseases and Nutrition
University of South Florida Morsani College of Medicine
Tampa, Florida

Dawn M. Torres, MD
Program Director GI Fellowship
Department of Medicine
Walter Reed National Military Medical Center;
Professor of Medicine
Department of Medicine
Uniformed Services University of the Health Sciences
Bethesda, Maryland

James F. Trotter, MD
Medical Director of Liver Transplant
Division of Transplant Hepatology
Baylor University Medical Center
Dallas, Texas

Nimish Vakil, MD, FACP, FACG, AGAF, FASGE
Clinical Professor of Medicine
Department of Medicine
University of Wisconsin School of Medicine and
    Public Health
Madison, Wisconsin

Shyam Varadarajulu, MD
President
Digestive Health Institute
Orlando Health
Orlando, Florida

Stephen M. Vindigni, MD, MPH
Clinical Assistant Professor
Department of Medicine
University of Washington
Seattle, Washington;
Gastroenterologist
The Oregon Clinic
Portland, Oregon

Jon D. Vogel, MD
Professor of Surgery
Division of Colorectal Surgery, Department of Surgery
University of Colorado School of Medicine
Aurora, Colorado

Lisa Walker, MD
Assistant Professor
Department of Radiology
University of Colorado
Aurora, Colorado

John Westhoff, MD, MPH, FACEP, FACOEM, FAWM
Interim Chair
Department of Internal Medicine
University of Nevada, Reno School of Medicine
Reno, Nevada

Clemence C. White, DO
Internal Medicine Physician
Department of Gastroenterology (Medicine)
Water Reed National Military Medical Center
Bethesda, Maryland

Gina A. Wideroff, MD
GI Fellow
University of Miami Miller School of Medicine
Miami, Florida

C. Mel Wilcox, MD, MSPH
Faculty
Digestive Health Institute
Orlando Health
Orlando, Florida

Tamara J. Worlton, MD, FACS, FASMBS
Associate Professor
Department of General Surgery
Uniformed Services University of the Health Sciences
Bethesda, Maryland

Patrick E. Young, MD, MACP, FACG, FASGE
Director
Division of Digestive Diseases, Department of Medicine
Uniformed Services University;
Interventional Gastroenterologist
Department of Medicine
Walter Reed National Military Medical Center
Bethesda, Maryland

Sarah Zimmer, MD
Intern
Department of Internal Medicine
Naval Medical Center Portsmouth
Portsmouth, Virginia

PREFACE

Peter R. McNally, DO, MSRF, MACG

To practice the art of medicine, one must learn the secrets of pathophysiology, diagnosis, and therapy. In this text, you will find the answers to many questions about hepatic and digestive diseases. We hope that medical students, residents, fellows, and, yes, even attending physicians will find the sixth edition of *Gastrointestinal and Liver Secrets* instructive and insightful.

As the editor, I wish to thank Marybeth Thiel, Akanksha Marwah and the staff at Elsevier for their wonderful support of this project and their courage and determination to make this book available on the web. I am most appreciative of all my contributing authors who have shared their invaluable secrets and made this book a treasure trove of clinical secrets.

CONTENTS

SECTION 4 PANCREATIC DISORDERS

SECTION 5 SMALL AND LARGE BOWEL DISORDERS

SECTION 6 COLON DISORDERS

SECTION 7 GENERAL SYMPTOMS AND CONDITIONS

SECTION 10 SURGERY AND THE GASTROINTESTINAL TRACT

VIDEO CONTENTS

TOP 100 SECRETS

Peter R. McNally, DO, MSRF, MACG

1. *Campylobacter jejuni* infection is the most common infection associated with Guillain-Barré syndrome (GBS). Molecular mimicry of the bacterial lipopolysaccharide and ganglioside moieties on peripheral nerves appears to be a dominant mechanism. In the developing world, it is estimated that one-third of all cases of acute flaccid paralysis are GBS caused by *Campylobacter*.
2. Patient-related risk factors for post–endoscopic retrograde cholangiopancreatography (ERCP) pancreatitis include female sex, age <50 years old, prior history of post-ERCP pancreatitis, and suspected Sphincter of Oddi dysfunction. A landmark randomized trial found that in patients at high risk for post-ERCP pancreatitis, the preadministration of rectal indomethacin was associated with a lower risk of pancreatitis (9.2% indomethacin vs. 16.9% placebo).
3. Liver transplantation (LT) remains the definitive treatment of choice for hepatocellular carcinoma (HCC) in patients with cirrhosis. The Milan criteria restrict LT in adults with HCC as follows: (1) single tumor diameter <5 cm; (2) not more than three foci of tumor, each <3 cm; (3) no angioinvasion; and (4) no extrahepatic involvement. Patients who meet the Milan criteria have a posttransplant survival rate of 75% at 4 years.
4. Always consider these potential complications of celiac disease: osteoporosis, infertility, hepatitis, arthritis, dermatitis, and hyposplenism. Test for HLA-DQ2/DQ8 in someone who is on a gluten-free diet but has suspected celiac disease. If present, proceed with a gluten challenge and serologic testing.
5. Tenofovir alafenamide (TAF) has not been extensively studied in pregnancy, so Tenofovir disoproxil fumarate remains the therapy of choice in pregnant patients. Additionally, TAF has not been thoroughly investigated in those with decompensated cirrhosis (Child-Pugh class B or C) and should be avoided in these patients until more data become available regarding its safety and efficacy.
6. Extraintestinal manifestations of inflammatory bowel disease (IBD) occur in approximately 50% of patients. They are more common in patients with Crohn's disease and include arthralgia, peripheral arthritis, axial arthritis, erythema nodosum, pyoderma gangrenosum, episcleritis, uveitis, and primary sclerosing cholangitis (PSC).
7. Live vaccines that are contraindicated in patients with IBD on immune suppressive therapies include attenuated influenza (intranasal), varicella vaccine, zoster live vaccine (no longer used in the United States), yellow fever, measles-mumps-rubella, typhoid live oral, Bacillus Calmette-Guerin (not given in the United States), polio live oral (no longer used in the United States), anthrax, monkeypox, and smallpox.
8. Patients with PSC have an increased risk for gallbladder cancer. Cholecystectomy should be considered for gallbladder polyps: size greater than 8 mm or interval growth; sessile/mass-like morphology; or an arterial signal on Doppler.
9. Since celiac disease can mimic autoimmune hepatitis (AIH), this diagnosis must be considered in seronegative patients that otherwise resemble AIH.
10. All patients with cirrhosis and positive hepatitis B surface antigen should be treated for hepatitis B, regardless of alanine aminotransferase (ALT) or hepatitis B virus (HBV) DNA levels.
11. Irritable bowel syndrome (IBS) symptoms develop in approximately 10% of healthy individuals with postinfectious (PI) gastroenteritis. PI-IBS is most commonly reported after a bacterial infection such as *Campylobacter*, *Salmonella*, and *Shigella* but has also been reported after viral, bacterial, protozoa, and nematode infections.
12. The Triangle of Calot is formed by the cystic duct, cystic artery, and common hepatic duct. The hepatocystic triangle is the area between the cystic duct, common hepatic duct, and the border of the liver. These areas should be familiar to all surgeons performing laparoscopic cholecystectomies as they are fundamental to safe cholecystectomy.
13. Patients presenting with oropharyngeal dysphagia (coughing immediately with swallows of solids or liquids), halitosis, regurgitation of undigested food, and neck gurgling—think of Zenker diverticulum.
14. A restrictive hemoglobin transfusion goal of 7 g/dL has superior clinical outcomes compared to higher hemoglobin goals, excluding patients in hemorrhagic shock or with cardiovascular disease.
15. In patients with acute pancreatitis (AP) and gastrointestinal (GI) hemorrhage—think of hemosuccus pancreaticus. It can be diagnosed with computed tomography (CT) angiography and treated mesenteric angiography with coil embolization.
16. Risk factors for developing PI-IBS in persons who have had gastroenteritis are (1) female sex, (2) age younger than 60 years, (3) absence of vomiting, and (4) prolonged diarrhea with the infection. Additionally, anxiety, neurosis, somatization, and stressful life events before or during the infection also appear to be risk factors for determining who will develop PI-IBS.

17. In patients with achalasia with shortened life expectancy or medical conditions that preclude surgery, consider endoscopic injection therapy with botulinum toxin. Botulinum toxin injections are a safe, minimally invasive, and effective initial treatment for achalasia that is best suited for patients who are not candidates for myotomy (laparoscopic Heller myotomy or peroral endoscopic myotomy) or pneumatic dilation.

18. Any bariatric patient with prolonged nausea and vomiting, which presents with a triad of confusion, double vision, and ataxia—think of thiamine deficiency. Urgent parenteral replacement is critically important.

19. Upper endoscopy should be performed within 24 hours of presentation for upper GI bleeding, with more urgent endoscopy (within 12 hours) considered for select high-risk patients including those with bright red hematemesis, persistent hemodynamical compromise after initial resuscitation, or suspected variceal hemorrhage. Endoscopy should not be delayed for correction of coagulopathy. Antibiotic prophylaxis is indicated for patients with cirrhosis and GI bleeding of any etiology.

20. Hepatic hydrothorax, a transudative pleural effusion secondary to portal hypertension, is present in 4%–12% of patients with cirrhosis, usually unilaterally and in more than 75% of cases confined to the right side. A serum-to-pleural fluid albumin gradient >1.1 g/dL is suggestive of hepatic hydrothorax.

21. Two novel biomarkers, cytolethal distending toxin B antibody and antivinculin antibody, have been proposed to discriminate postinfectious IBS. Studies have shown that patients with IBS-D are more likely to have elevated antibody levels compared to patients with IBD and celiac disease.

22. Patients with PSC should undergo a screening colonoscopy at the time of diagnosis, regardless of the presence of concurrent IBD. Chronic ulcerative colitis can develop even after an LT just as PSC can develop following a colectomy.

23. Pancreatic cancer can release enzymes, which cause fat necrosis resulting in a triad of lower extremity arthritis, tender skin nodules, and eosinophilia (Schmidt triad).

24. Celiac disease can be associated with arthritis, and the most frequent rheumatic manifestations including symmetric polyarthritis (~25%) involving predominantly large joints (knees and ankles > hips and shoulders) occurs. The arthritis may precede enteropathic symptoms in 50% of cases. The arthritis responds to a gluten-free diet in 46%–60% of cases.

25. Hemoglobin released from upper GI tract bleeding is digested and usually not immunologically reactive to fecal immunochemical test (FIT). Therefore upper GI tract bleeding usually does not produce a positive FIT test.

26. Liver biopsy is not needed to confirm the diagnosis of hereditary hemochromatosis (HH) or alpha-1 antitrypsin (α1-AT), but it may have a role in fibrosis staging in some patients with HH if they have elevated liver enzymes or ferritin >1000 ng/mL at the time of diagnosis.

27. Spider angiomas and palmar erythema are common and appear in approximately two-thirds of pregnant females without liver disease. Small esophageal varices are present in approximately 50% of healthy pregnant females without liver disease because of the increased venous flow in the azygous system.

28. As many as 30% of ulcerative colitis and 70% of patients with Crohn's disease will require surgery for their IBD. The PUCINNI study demonstrated that patients with IBD undergoing intra-abdominal surgery within 12 weeks of tumor necrosis factor inhibitor (TNFi) exposure had almost identical rates of infections compared with those who were not exposed to TNFi (18.1% vs. 20.2%, respectively). The conclusion is that preoperative TNFi exposure and drug levels are *not* associated with postoperative infections in these patients. However, preoperative corticosteroid use, current smoking, prior bowel resection, and diabetes are independent risk factors for postoperative infections in these patients.

29. An appendiceal neoplasm may be found incidentally, and it is estimated to be found in 0.7%–1.7% of appendectomy specimens. However, for patients who are over 40 years old with complicated appendicitis, the incidence of appendicular neoplasm ranges from 3% to 17%.

30. Up to 80% of patients with primary biliary cholangitis also have coexistent extrahepatic autoimmune diseases. The most common extrahepatic autoimmune disease is sicca (Sjögren) syndrome which includes autoimmune thyroiditis, scleroderma/CREST (calcinosis, Raynaud phenomenon, esophageal, telangiectasia), rheumatoid arthritis, dermatomyositis, mixed connective tissue disease, systemic lupus erythematosus, renal tubular acidosis, and idiopathic pulmonary fibrosis.

31. Evaluation for liver transplantation should be considered once a patient with cirrhosis has experienced a complication such as ascites, hepatic encephalopathy, variceal hemorrhage, or hepatocellular dysfunction that results in a Model for End-stage Liver Disease score ≥15 or is refractory to medical therapy.

32. Foreign bodies in the esophagus should be removed within 24 hours to maximize the chance of successful removal and minimize complications. Asymptomatic patients with objects in the stomach do not always require endoscopy. Objects in the stomach that are wider than 2.5 cm should be removed as these are less likely to pass the pylorus. Similarly, objects longer than 6 cm, such as pencils, pens, or toothbrushes, should be removed due to difficulty passing the duodenal sweep.

33. Symptoms of severe abdominal pain disproportionate to physical examination is a typical feature of intestinal ischemia. If ischemic bowel disease is suspected, first-line imaging is computed tomographic angiography.

34. Magnetic resonance imaging (MRI) is accurate in differentiating HCC from dysplastic nodule(s), with HCC usually having increased T2-w signal and dysplastic nodule(s) having decreased T2-w signal.
35. Chronic ulcerative colitis (CUC) and, less frequently, Crohn's colitis is present in at least 70%–80% of patients with PSC. In contrast, only 5%–8% of patients with IBD will have concurrent PSC.
36. Hallmarks of ischemic hepatitis (shock liver) include marked elevations in aspartate transferase, ALT (10 times upper limit of normal), bilirubin, prothrombin time (PT), and profound elevations in lactate dehydrogenase after an episode of systemic hypotension or decreased cardiac output.
37. Microbiota dysbiosis is an important contributing factor for the development of IBS. Fecal bacterial analysis using 16S ribosomal RNA polymerase chain reaction/DNA amplification of variable regions V3 and V9 (GA-map Dysbiosis Test) has become a promising tool to define and quantify a dysbiosis index (DI). A recent placebo-controlled trial demonstrated that fecal microbiota transplant (FMT) has a durable 3-year benefit in the majority of patients with IBS as measured by IBS severity scoring system (IBS-SSS) and DI. Further perfection of the FMT technique and confirmation of safety are needed before FMT is approved as a mainstream treatment for IBS.
38. Treatment of AIH with azathioprine can be continued throughout pregnancy, whereas the use of Mycophenolate mofetil is contraindicated in pregnancy.
39. Any patients with IBD who display a change in symptoms or concerns for flare should be tested for *Clostridioides difficile*. When positive, treatment in these patients should be with oral vancomycin (125 mg PO QID × 14 days); fidaxomicin and metronidazole are not recommended.
40. In patients from or living in Latin/South America with dysphagia, you should suspect Chagas, an infection caused by the vector-borne parasite *Trypanosoma cruzi*.
41. All patients with inflammatory small joint arthritis, positive rheumatoid factor, and elevated liver–associated transaminase levels should have hepatitis C infection ruled out before receiving the diagnosis of rheumatoid arthritis.
42. Patients with cirrhosis who consume raw oysters are 80 times more likely to develop *Vibrio vulnificus* infection and 200 times more likely to die of the infection.
43. Celiac disease (CD) evaluation is divided into diagnostic and confirmatory testing:

    Diagnostic Testing
    - Preferred test is immunoglobulin A (IgA) anti–tissue transglutaminase (TTG).
      - I5f IgA is normal: 95% sensitive and specific.
      - Poor test if IgA deficient (more common in celiac disease).
    - If IgA deficient: deaminated gliadin peptides.
      - Alternative test is IgG TTG.
    - HLA-DQ2 and -DQ8 testing is an excellent negative predictive test.
    - In children younger than 2 years, IgG TTG alone or with deamidated gliadin peptide.
    - All patients should be on a gluten-containing diet before antibody testing.

    Confirmatory Testing
    - Duodenal biopsy (≥2 duodenal bulb and ≥4 from the second and third portions of duodenum)
    - Histologic findings consistent with Marsh or Corazza criteria

44. Pancreatic cancer screening is indicated for patients with a strong family history of pancreatic cancer, hereditary pancreatitis, and certain genetic syndromes (i.e., Peutz-Jeghers or Lynch syndrome).
45. Patients with achalasia have a 28-fold increased risk of developing squamous cell carcinoma. Even though the relative risk is high, the absolute risk of developing esophageal cancer is still very low. Both the American College of Gastroenterology and the American Society of Gastroenterology recommend *against* routine endoscopic surveillance for esophageal cancer in patients with achalasia.
46. Almost all patients with hemochromatosis are homozygote for C282Y, but only a few patients who are compound heterozygote C282Y-H63D will have clinical disease.
47. Any patient with IBD presenting with cutaneous abscesses and nodules with sinus tracts, located in the axilla, mammary "milk line" and inguinal regions should be evaluated for hidradenitis suppurativa. It may precede or follow the onset of IBD disease activity and is treated with antibiotics, anti-TNFα, or surgery.
48. Microscopic colitis can be diffuse or can involve the colon discontinuously. Thus it is important to biopsy both the left and right colon for diagnosis. In one study the highest yield was from biopsies of transverse colon.
49. Lymphocytic colitis (LC) has been associated with the use of sertraline. Other potential medications associated with the development of microscopic colitis include aspirin, acarbose, clozapine, entacapone, flavonoid, proton pump inhibitors (especially lansoprazole), ranitidine, and ticlopidine. LC is more common among smokers and those with celiac disease.
50. Botulinum toxin should not be given to patients with an egg allergy.

51. Patients with IBD have an increased risk for cervical dysplasia and cancer-causing human papillomavirus (HPV) serotypes including cervical, vulvar, vaginal, penile, anal, and oropharyngeal cancers, particularly if on immunosuppression for greater than 6 months. Recombinant HPV 9-valent vaccine (Gardasil 9) is indicated for all females and males aged 9–45 years.

52. Recent studies have shown that uncomplicated appendicitis may be effectively managed nonoperatively with antibiotics. Predictors of antibiotic failure include abscess, fever exceeding 38°C, and appendiceal diameter ≥ 15 mm.

53. A prophylactic paraesophageal hernia repair in an asymptomatic patient is now rarely performed as the mortality rate after elective hernia repair in an asymptomatic patient ranges from 0.5% to 1.4%, whereas the probability of developing acute symptoms that will require emergent surgery is estimated to be 1.1%. However, all patients with symptoms or signs associated with the paraesophageal hernia should undergo repair in the absence of prohibitive surgical risk. Also, *all* patients with gastric volvulus, obstruction, strangulation, perforation, and bleeding should undergo emergent repair.

54. Azithromycin is the agent of choice for empiric treatment of febrile traveler's diarrhea, particularly when one notes blood, pus, or mucus in stool.

55. Suspected cystadenomas or cystadenocarcinomas should not be sampled, even with small, skinny needles to avoid the risk of needle-tract seeding, pseudomyxoma peritonei, or peritoneal carcinomatosis.

56. Suspected pheochromocytomas should not be sampled with fine needle aspiration, because of the risk of hypertensive crisis, while possible hepatic carcinoid metastases should not be sampled, because of the risk of profound hypotension.

57. Many with cirrhosis no longer need screening for varices by means of endoscopy if transient elastography by FibroScan is <20 kPa and the platelet count is 150k or higher.

58. Serrated polyps are the precursor lesions for approximately 30% of colorectal cancers.

59. If high-quality colonoscopy has not been done within a year of diagnosis of initial diverticulitis or complicated diverticulitis, colonoscopy should be done at least 6–8 weeks after the diagnosis or after the resolution of symptoms.

60. Post–transjugular intrahepatic portosystemic shunt portosystemic pressure gradient should be reduced to <12 mm Hg for variceal bleeding and <8 mm Hg for refractory ascites or hepatic hydrothorax.

61. For idiopathic AP, remember to consider medications and risk modifying mutations in certain genes such as *CFTR*—even in patients without cystic fibrosis or a family history of pancreatic disease.

62. Thiopurine drugs (azathioprine and 6-mercaptopurine) are metabolized and inactivated by the hepatic enzymes thiopurine methyltransferase (TPMT) and nudix hydrolase 15 (NUDT15). In Europeans and Africans, inherited TPMT deficiency is the primary genetic cause of thiopurine intolerance, whereas for Asians, risk alleles in NUDT15 explain most thiopurine-related myelosuppression. There is increasing evidence that DNA testing for NUDT15 and TPMT before initiating thiopurine therapy is clinically useful.

63. Tylosis is a rare autosomal dominant trait caused by a mutation in RHBDF2 located on the *17q25* gene. It is characterized by focal thickening of the skin of the hands and feet (hyperkeratosis palmaris et plantaris) and esophageal cancer.

64. Reiter syndrome consists of the triad of inflammatory arthritis, urethritis, and conjunctivitis/uveitis with or without mucocutaneous lesions that characterize reactive arthritis that may develop 2–4 weeks after an acute urethritis or diarrheal illness. The frequency of the triad varies with the causative enteric organism: *Shigella*, 85%, *Yersinia*, 10%, *Salmonella*, 10%–15%, and *Campylobacter*, 10%.

65. *Vibrio parahaemolyticus* and Norovirus are the most common pathogens acquired when one ingests raw oysters.

66. The ACCSENT study and DIABOLO trial suggest that Hinchey 1A diverticulitis with isolated pericolic air may undergo initial nonoperative therapy with intravenous antibiotic administration. However, clinical deterioration, such as the development of an acute abdomen or sepsis, may necessitate surgical intervention.

67. Persons considered for recombinant zoster vaccination should either have a documented history of chickenpox infection, varicella vaccination, or confirmed varicella antibodies.

68. Hepatitis E infection is fulminant in up to 20% of pregnant patients, compared with less than 1% of nonpregnant females.

69. Immune checkpoint inhibitors have been associated with immune-mediated liver injury and are frequently steroid-responsive, but the liver injury lacks autoantibodies and typical histological features of AIH.

70. In patients with mild gallstone pancreatitis, laparoscopic cholecystectomy is considered safe within the first week of the index hospitalization. Studies have shown that discharging the patient home to undergo an elective laparoscopic cholecystectomy results in 20% of those patients experiencing adverse events that require readmission before the scheduled surgery.

71. If you suspect Ménétrier disease, cold forceps biopsy is insufficient for diagnosis. Snare or band/cap-assisted biopsies are required.

72. Lower GI (LGI) bleed patients with Oakland score (<8) have a 95% probability of safe discharge.

73. *Helicobacter pylori*–negative mucosa–associated lymphoid tissue lymphomas may still respond to antibiotic therapy, likely due to the presence of other helicobacter species.

74. Natural history of LGI bleeding (LGIB) from diverticulosis: 17% of all LGIB is due to colonic diverticular disease; ~80% of these patients stop bleeding spontaneously; ~70% will not rebleed; and ~30% will rebleed and may require treatment.

75. Barrett's esophagus is a precancerous lesion diagnosed in about 7%–10% of individuals with chronic gastroesophageal reflux disease (GERD). About 0.3% of patients with Barrett's esophagus will go on to develop esophageal adenocarcinoma every year. New screening guideline for Barrett's esophagus excludes the mandatory requirement of GERD symptoms!

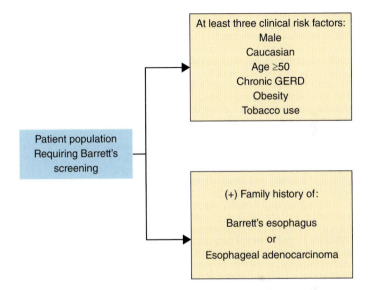

At least three clinical risk factors:
Male
Caucasian
Age ≥50
Chronic GERD
Obesity
Tobacco use

Patient population
Requiring Barrett's
screening

(+) Family history of:

Barrett's esophagus
or
Esophageal adenocarcinoma

76. Consider cystic fibrosis in a young patient with chronic pancreatitis with infertility and/or pulmonary complaints.

77. The Appendicitis Inflammatory Response score based on vomiting, rebound tenderness, right iliac fossa pain, fever, polymorphonuclear leukocytosis, and elevated C-reactive protein has supplanted the Alvarado score for clinical diagnosis of appendicitis.

78. A trial of antibiotics alone is a reasonable option for smaller intra-abdominal abscesses, less than 4–5 cm. For larger abscesses, patients may undergo percutaneous drainage, typically via CT guidance along with antibiotic treatment. Surgical intervention may be necessary if the external approach is too challenging or if a deteriorating clinical status suggests advancing infection despite percutaneous drainage.

79. Acute-onset diarrhea during hospitalization is most likely due to *C. difficile*.

80. Think of left-sided portal hypertension (sinistral portal hypertension) secondary to splenic vein thrombosis, in a patient with chronic pancreatitis presenting with upper GI bleed and splenomegaly.

81. Small intestinal bacterial overgrowth is common and should be considered in any case of chronic diarrhea.

82. Evaluate for HCC in any patients with cirrhosis with a new diagnosis of portal vein thrombosis.

83. Chronic pancreatitis may lead to splenic vein thrombosis in approximately 12% of cases.

84. Up to 10% of all patients with polyarteritis nodosa have positive hepatitis B serologies and evidence of viral replication (hepatitis B e-antigen or HBV DNA). They may present with a combination of fever, arthritis, mononeuritis multiplex, abdominal pain, renal disease, or cardiac disease.

85. Colorectal cancer (CRC) surveillance endoscopy is offered to patients with Peutz-Jeghers syndrome (PJS) because the lifetime risk of CRC is 39%. The lifetime risk of gastric cancer (29%) and small bowel cancer (13%) are also significantly increased in patients with PJS. Colonoscopy, upper endoscopy, and small bowel screening (wireless capsule endoscopy or CT/MR enterography) should start at the age of 8–10 years.

86. Herpes simplex hepatitis can be fulminant in pregnancy and associated with high mortality rates. Patients present in the third trimester with fever, systemic symptoms, and possibly vesicular cutaneous rash. Associated pneumonitis or encephalitis may be present. Response to acyclovir therapy is prompt; there is no need for immediate delivery of the baby.

87. Pyogenic liver abscesses arising from a biliary source tend to be multiple and of small size involving both lobes of the liver. Septic emboli from the portal vein may be solitary and tend to be more common in the right lobe of the liver because most of the portal vein flow goes to the right lobe. Abscesses arising from a contiguous source tend to be solitary and localized to one lobe only.

88. Postembolization syndrome after transarterial embolization, transarterial chemoembolization, or selective internal radiotherapy occurs in up to 90% of patients and is characterized by fever, abdominal pain, anorexia, nausea, vomiting, and fatigue. Symptoms usually arise 24–48 hours after the procedure, last for 1–2 weeks, self-limited, and usually managed supportively.

89. Portal and or splenic vein thrombosis is a contraindication to balloon-occluded retrograde transvenous obliteration procedure, due to the risk of occluding portal system outflow, which may result in mesenteric or splenic infarction.

90. Minocycline and nitrofurantoin account for 90% of all drug-induced autoimmune-like hepatitis.

91. Patients with limited gastric intestinal metaplasia on high-quality surveillance endoscopy (Sydney protocol, multiple 5-site biopsies) do not need to repeat the esophagogastroduodenoscopy, unless they have other established risk factors for gastric cancer.

92. Drug-induced AP (DIAP) is the cause of up to 2% of patients with AP. Drugs confirmed by rechallenge to cause DIAP include mesalamine, trimethoprim/sulfamethoxazole, furosemide, anabolic steroids, estrogen, tetracycline, thiopurines, and valproic acid.

93. Focal nodular hyperplasia (FNH) is a round, nonencapsulated liver mass, usually exhibiting a vascular central scar. FNH is the second most common benign liver tumor. Over 90% occur in females and usually are diagnosed between 20 and 60 years of age. Oral contraceptives are not directly linked as a causative agent of FNH and do not need to be discontinued in patients with FNH.

94. Chronic hepatitis B and C are associated with an increased risk of drug-induced liver injury (DILI) with highly active antiretroviral therapy, azithromycin, and isoniazid. Otherwise, preexisting chronic liver disease (CLD) is not a risk factor for DILI. However, patients who develop DILI in the background of CLD have increased mortality (threefold) compared to those who do not have underlying CLD.

95. Up to 75% of patients with HH have noninflammatory degenerative arthritis, most commonly involving the second and third metacarpophalangeal joints, proximal interphalangeal joints, wrists, hips, knees, and ankles. Of importance, this arthropathy may be the presenting complaint (30%–50%) of patients with hemochromatosis and is frequently misdiagnosed in young males as seronegative RA.

96. CA 19-9 is a tumor marker used in the diagnosis of cholangiocarcinoma: levels >100 U/mL are found in over 50% of patients with cholangiocarcinoma and values >1000 suggest unresectability.

97. Kasabach-Merritt syndrome is a rare condition often associated with giant hepatic hemangioma, consumption coagulopathy, and thrombocytopenia that can be treated surgically.

98. Hepatic adenomas are well-demarcated, fleshy tumors with prominent surface vasculature. Microscopically, they consist of monotonous sheets of normal or small hepatocytes with no bile ducts, portal tracts, or central veins. MRI is the imaging modality of choice to determine if a liver mass is a hepatic adenoma because the contrast agent gadoxetate disodium (Eovist) is excreted by the biliary system. Because adenomas do not have bile ducts gadoxetate disodium will not uptake the contrast and adenomas will not enhance the biliary phase of imaging. This is particularly useful in differentiating adenomas from FNH.

99. Amebic liver abscesses tend to be solitary and large. Most commonly, they are located in the right lobe of the liver. The right lobe receives a major part of the venous drainage from the cecum and ascending colon, which are the parts of the bowel most commonly affected by amebiasis. Abscesses located in the dome of the liver or complicated by a bronchopleural fistula are typically amebic in origin.

100. If traveling within 4 weeks to an endemic area for hepatitis A virus, one should receive immunoprophylaxis with anti–human immunodeficiency virus Ig as it takes 4 weeks after vaccination to develop adequate antibodies.

GASTROESOPHAGEAL REFLUX DISEASE

CHAPTER 1

Camille S. Thélin, MD, MS and John W. Jacobs, MD

 Additional content available online.

1. What is gastroesophageal reflux disease (GERD)?

The retrograde passage of gastroduodenal contents into the esophagus is a normal physiologic event. However, GERD is a condition during which this refluxate becomes pathologic, leading to chronic clinical symptoms or histopathologic macroscopic injury and/or complications (e.g., esophagitis, Barrett esophagus [BE], and strictures).

2. What are the most typical symptoms of GERD?

Heartburn (pyrosis) and regurgitation are the most typical symptoms and are often enough to make a clinical diagnosis. Pyrosis usually occurs within 30–60 minutes after ingesting the largest meal of the day and is defined as a burning sensation in the retrosternal area. Unfortunately, it is often misunderstood and often described as indigestion, sour stomach, and bitter belching. Regurgitation is defined as the reflux of bitter or salty gastric contents or the return of food or bilious material.

3. What are some of the atypical symptoms and signs of GERD?

GERD-related chest pain, unexplained nausea, water brash (hypersalivation), globus sensation, dysphagia, or odynophagia can be associated with GERD, but these are not usually enough to make a clinical diagnosis. A good clinical history must be taken with each patient.

4. Are there extraesophageal symptoms of GERD?

Often controversial, extraesophageal symptoms include chronic cough, chronic laryngitis, dysphonia, sore throat, wheezing, hoarseness, postnasal drip, throat clearing, sinusitis, otitis media, halitosis, dental erosions, and recurrent aspiration pneumonia. In these patients, GERD is usually overestimated in its role as the causal diagnosis, as the etiology is often multifactorial. Furthermore, coexisting pathophysiologies such as mechanical defects, physiologic abnormalities, heightened nociception, hypersensitivity, hypervigilance, and behavioral disorders (such as supragastric belching or rumination) can confound the presentation. Thus it is recommended that other disorders are excluded before attributing these symptoms to GERD.

5. What should be included in the differential of GERD?

The differential can be broad, including esophageal motor disorders (e.g., achalasia), types of esophagitis (e.g., infectious, eosinophilic, or pill), mechanical obstructions (e.g., esophageal webs, rings, diverticula, and esophageal or gastric neoplasm), peptic ulcer disease, dyspepsia, gastroparesis, rumination syndrome, coronary artery disease, and biliary tract diseases.

6. What is the epidemiology of GERD?

The prevalence of symptomatic GERD is rising in the Western world (with more than 30% of US adults reporting weekly symptoms), while it is less than 5% in Asia. The prevalence differs from country to country due to awareness and understanding of the condition. While the distribution of GERD is equal among the sexes, males experience more complications (primarily esophagitis and BE). Increasing prevalence is also related to the increase in obesity in Western countries. In the United States, GERD contributes to the health care burden given the significant workup (clinic visits, endoscopic and/or surgical procedures) and medicines prescribed required to make a diagnosis and treat it.

7. What are the risk factors for GERD?

An increase in intra-abdominal pressures (e.g., obesity or pregnancy) and anatomic factors (such as the presence of a hiatal hernia, which contributes to decreased lower esophageal sphincter [LES] tone) are associated with GERD. Modifiable factors such as medicines and foods, which change the LES pressure, can also be risk factors. Lifestyle risk factors, such as excessive body weight, moderate/high consumption of alcohol, smoking, postprandial physical activity, lack of physical activity, and eating habits (such as irregular meal patterns, voluminous meals, and postprandial supination), also may contribute to GERD symptoms.

8. **What is the pathophysiology of GERD?**
Different intrinsic and structural mechanisms may lead to the disruption of the esophagogastric junction (EGJ) barrier, consequentially leading to esophageal exposure to acidic gastroduodenal contents. For example, esophageal dysmotility or ineffective peristalsis can lead to impaired clearance of this content, while abnormalities in the tone of the LES, increased reflux during transient LES relaxations (TLESRs), and even impaired gastric emptying and increased intragastric pressure are believed to be key etiologic factors. Esophageal hypersensitivity—a condition in which there is increased nociceptor stimulus—may also contribute to symptoms.

9. **What are the components of the EGJ?**
The EGJ is an antireflux high-pressure barrier that consists of three components: the LES, the crural diaphragm, and the anatomic flap valve. The anatomic flap valve is a musculo-mucosal fold opposite to the lesser curvature of the stomach (best seen on retroflexion), which functions to keep the distal part of the LES in the abdomen and to maintain the angle of His. At rest, the LES is a major component of the antireflux barrier.

10. **How does LES impairment lead to GERD?**
At rest, the LES (also known as the cardiac sphincter) is a tonically contracted smooth muscle segment, involving the distal 3–4 cm of the esophagus. While normal resting pressures are in the range of 10–35 mm Hg, only pressures of 5–10 mm Hg are needed to prevent GERD. Dysfunction in this resting tone can cause GERD and, if frequent enough, can lead to damage to the esophageal mucosa. Different medicines, food, and hormones can affect the basal resting tone of the LES (see Questions 12,13,14).

11. **How are increased TLESRs thought to contribute to GERD?**
In healthy individuals, TLESR occurs to facilitate the passage of food into the stomach. In those with GERD, it is believed that frequent (or excessive) TLESRs are not triggered by swallowing with ingestion of food. This leads to increased intragastric pressure that overcomes LES basal pressures and allows a pathologic amount of acidic gastroduodenal contents into the esophagus. Obesity can also increase the number of TSLERs.

12. **What types of medicines affect the resting pressure of LES?**
Medications that increase the LES pressure include cholinergic agonists, antacids, metoclopramide, and domperidone. Conversely, cholinergic antagonists, secretin, glucagon, oral contraceptive pills, calcium channel blockers, morphine, nitroglycerin, benzodiazepines, nonsteroidal anti-inflammatory drugs, and antidepressants decrease LES pressure. Psychoactive drugs such as tobacco and alcohol also decrease LES pressures.

13. **What types of hormones affect the resting pressure of the LES?**
Gastrin and motilin increase LES pressure, while secretin and glucagon decrease LES pressure. Interestingly, estrogen and progesterone also decrease LES pressure, thereby contributing to the pathophysiology and increase in GERD symptoms that are commonly experienced during pregnancy.

14. **What types of foods affect the resting pressure of the LES?**
Protein increases LES pressure, while fatty foods, peppermint, and chocolate may decrease LES pressure. While these foods can decrease the LES pressure, they do not always correlate with GERD symptom presentation.

15. **How is a hiatal hernia associated with GERD?**
A hiatal hernia acts as a reservoir for refluxed acidic contents. It weakens the high-pressure zone of the EGJ by displacing the LES from the diaphragmatic crura and thus hindering its function. It can even increase the size of the diaphragmatic hiatus. A hiatal hernia can exist independently without causing symptoms of GERD.

16. **How do impaired esophageal mucosal defenses lead to GERD?**
The squamous mucosa of the esophagus provides a mucosal barrier to gastroduodenal contents, which are comprised of acidic contents (hydrochloric acid and pepsin) and alkaline contents (bile salts and pancreatic enzymes). With prolonged exposure to refluxate, the defense barrier is weakened, resulting in inflammation, basal cell hyperplasia, papilla elongation, and dilation of intercellular spaces that are seen on microscopy. These histopathologic findings are not specific to GERD and can be seen with other types of injury to the esophagus.

17. **How can impaired esophageal peristalsis impact GERD?**
With impaired esophageal peristalsis comes decreased activity of salivary bicarbonate clearance of the gastroduodenal contents that reach the esophagus. Impaired peristalsis is seen in conditions such as scleroderma, mixed connective tissue diseases, esophageal motor diseases, and oropharyngeal dysphagia.

18. **How important are dietary and lifestyle modifications?**
While there are limited studies showing the efficacy of dietary modifications, individualized treatment plans for the removal of "triggers" (e.g., alcohol, fatty foods, chocolate, caffeine, spicy foods, peppermint, and acidic foods such as citrus or tomatoes, or carbonated beverages) are rational in those that have improvement with avoidance.

In contrast, studies have shown efficacy in the following lifestyle modifications: weight loss in overweight or obese patients, smoking cessation, circumventing nocturnal right-sided recumbency, discontinuation of eating meals within 2–3 hours of bedtime, and elevation of the head of the bed in those with nighttime reflux.

19. What type of medical therapy is used for GERD?

Medical therapy focuses on neutralizing or reducing gastric acid. These therapies include antacids, histamine-2-receptor antagonists (H2RAs), and proton pump inhibitors (PPIs). PPIs should be used as treatment, over H2RAs, in patients with erosive esophagitis (EE) and BE. PPI therapy is recommended indefinitely in those with severe EE (Los Angeles [LA] grade C or D) and BE. The addition of medical therapies (alginates and baclofen) in PPI nonresponders is recommended, while therapies such as prokinetics (metoclopramide or domperidone) are not due to their significant adverse events profile. All these therapies should be tapered to the lowest effective dose.

20. What type of medical therapy is used for GERD during pregnancy (and lactation)?

Gestational reflux, which can occur at any trimester, is diagnosed solely on symptoms and requires no imaging, endoscopic, or pH studies. It is usually self-limiting once pregnancy is complete. The management of heartburn during pregnancy and lactation begins with lifestyle modifications. In situations where disease severity increases, medical providers must discuss the risks and benefits of these medicines with the patient in detail. Antacids (aluminum-, calcium-, or magnesium-containing), alginates, and sucralfate are the first-line medical agents. Magnesium trisilicates are avoided at high doses and as a long-term therapy. Sodium bicarbonate is not safe for use in pregnancy as it can cause fluid overload and metabolic alkalosis. If symptoms persist, any of the H2RAs can be used except for ranitidine or nizatidine (due to safety concerns related to N-nitrosodimethylamine). PPIs are reserved for females with intractable symptoms or complicated GERD. All PPIs are US Food and Drug Administration category B drugs, except for omeprazole, which is a category C drug.

21. What enzyme systems are involved with PPIs?

PPIs act by irreversibly blocking the hydrogen/potassium adenosine triphosphatase enzyme system ($H^{++}+/K^+$ ATPase), known as the "gastric proton pump," of gastric parietal cells. PPIs only act on active proton pumps—those that are actively secreting acid—and thus timing is crucial, with medicine being recommended 30–60 minutes prior to meals, and not at bedtime. PPIs are metabolized to a degree by several cytochrome P450 (CYP) isoenzymes—namely, CYP2C19 and CYP3A4. CYP polymorphisms could explain the wide variation in individual intragastric pH control between PPIs, as genetic differences could affect PPI response, and thus explain why changing PPIs may work. At this time, genetic testing is not recommended.

22. How safe are PPIs?

PPIs are very safe. Some medical studies have suggested an association between long-term use of PPI and the development of numerous adverse conditions including pneumonia, stomach cancer, osteoporosis-related bone fracture, chronic kidney disease, deficiencies of vitamins and minerals, heart attacks, strokes, dementia, and early death. Per ACG Guideline on GERD-2022: "high-quality studies have found that PPIs do **not** significantly increase the risk of any of these conditions except intestinal infections." Although adverse effects have been reported, the absolute risk is overall low, and these medicines remain the gold standard for safe and effective treatment of GERD. It is recommended to administer PPIs in patients who will gain substantial clinical benefit and then taper when appropriate.

23. What is the management algorithm for patients with GERD?

Patients with typical reflux symptoms without alarm symptoms can be offered a 4- to 8-week trial of once-daily PPI therapy. Responders can then be weaned to the lowest effective dose. If symptoms remain controlled, on-demand therapy can even be possible. Those needing chronic PPI therapy can be offered reflux testing at a 1-year time point to determine the need for long-term therapy. For nonresponders or partial responders, dosing twice a day or switching to a more efficacious PPI can be offered. If they remain refractory, esophageal testing (see Question 35) is suggested. In those with extraesophageal symptoms, we recommend esophageal testing prior to empiric PPI trial (Fig. 1.1).

24. What is refractory GERD?

Approximately two-thirds of patients have recurrent symptoms despite the use of medical therapy. Refractory symptoms are defined as those with continued symptoms despite having taken as-directed PPI therapy (twice a day, for at least 8–12 weeks). Of course, nonadherence or incorrect timing of the use of medicines needs to be excluded from this group. Given the multiphenotypic presentation of GERD, it is also necessary to rule out alternative diagnoses prior to recommending surgical or endoscopic therapeutic measures.

25. What are the surgical and endoscopic options for GERD?

Surgical and endoscopic treatments can be considered in those with refractory GERD symptoms despite medical optimization, those that have had serious PPI-related adverse events, those that are hesitant to be on lifelong PPI therapy, or those with anatomic defects (e.g., large hiatal hernias). Surgical options include laparoscopic Nissen

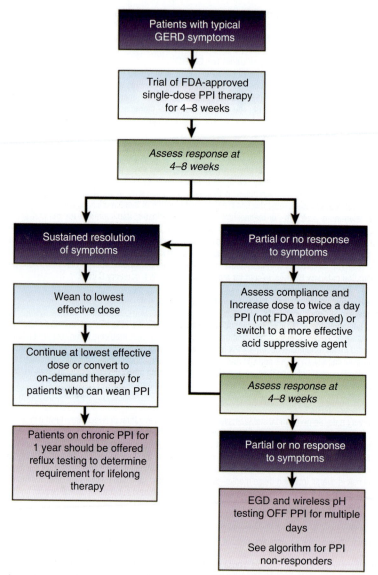

Fig. 1.1 American Gastroenterological Association Clinical Practice Update on management algorithm of empiric PPI therapy in suspected GERD. *EGD*, Esophagogastroduodenoscopy; *FDA*, US Food and Drug Administration; *GERD*, gastroesophageal reflux disease; *PPI*, proton pump inhibitor. (From Yadlapati R, Prakash Gyawali C, Pandolfino JE, on behalf of the CGIT GERD Consensus Conference Participants. AGA clinical practice update on the personalized approach to the evaluation and management of GERD: expert review. Clin Gastroenterol Hepatol. 2022;20(5):984-994. doi: 10.1016/j.cgh.2022.01.025. Copyright © 2022 AGA Institute.)

fundoplication (the gold standard), laparoscopic anterior 180-degree fundoplication, or bariatric surgery in obese patients. Risks of antireflux procedures must be discussed prior to recommending this avenue of treatment. Currently, there are also minimally invasive endoscopic therapies that are available, including magnetic sphincter augmentation and transoral incision-less fundoplication.

26. How is GERD diagnosed?
The diagnosis of GERD most often requires taking a multipronged approach and is based on symptom presentation, response to treatment with acid-suppressive therapy, endoscopic evaluation, and reflux monitoring.

Heartburn and regurgitation are the most sensitive and specific symptoms of GERD. A positive response to acid-suppressive therapy is an important marker of underlying GERD.

27. Should barium radiography be used to diagnose GERD?
Barium radiography should not be used to diagnose GERD. Relative to formal pH testing, reflux seen on barium esophagram has poor sensitivity and specificity for GERD. Barium esophagram is appropriate in patients with dysphagia and in those with a higher level of suspicion for an underlying motility disorder.

28. What is the role of high-resolution esophageal manometry (HREM) in diagnosing GERD?
While patients with GERD may have low LES pressure and ineffective esophageal motility, no HREM pattern is specific for GERD. Therefore HREM should not be used to diagnose GERD. HREM should be used for all patients before an antireflux procedure (to rule out achalasia and absent contractility) and in patients with dysphagia in whom there is suspicion of an underlying motility disorder.

29. What is the role of upper endoscopy in patients with GERD?
Invariably, all patients with GERD ultimately undergo upper endoscopy to evaluate the esophageal mucosa. Endoscopy should especially be performed in patients with "alarm symptoms" such as dysphagia, weight loss, bleeding, anemia, and vomiting. Endoscopically, the findings of EE and BE are pathognomonic to GERD. Endoscopy also helps to evaluate alternative diagnoses such as eosinophilic esophagitis (EoE) infection, and pill-induced injury.

30. How is the severity of endoscopic reflux esophagitis classified?
The most widely used scoring system is the LA classification (Fig. 1.2).
- Grade A: One or more mucosal breaks confined to folds, 5 mm or smaller.
- Grade B: One or more mucosal breaks larger than 5 mm confined to folds but not continuous between tops of mucosal folds.
- Grade C: Mucosal breaks continuously between tops of two or more mucosal folds but less than 75% of esophageal circumference is involved.
- Grade D: Mucosal breaks encompass more than 75% of esophageal circumference.

While LA grade A esophagitis is not sufficient enough to make a diagnosis of GERD, LA grade B may be diagnostic, if also found in the presence of typical GERD symptoms and PPI response. LA grades C and D are virtually diagnostic of GERD.

31. Should endoscopy be performed on or off PPI therapy?
The most common finding among patients with GERD undergoing endoscopy is normal esophageal mucosa. PPIs are highly effective in healing EE, and, as a result, underlying esophagitis may be missed by virtue of performing endoscopy while on PPI therapy. In addition, a diagnosis of nonerosive reflux disease can only be diagnosed off

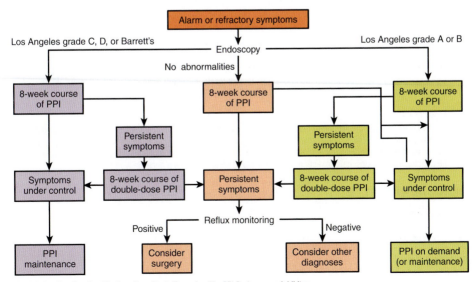

Fig. 1.2 Los Angeles classification of grades A–D esophagitis. *PPI,* Proton pump inhibitor.

of PPI therapy. Ideally, an endoscopy should be performed after PPIs have been held for 2–4 weeks. Furthermore, since PPIs can mask the endoscopic and histologic features of EoE, this cannot be fully excluded if the patient undergoes endoscopy while on PPI therapy.

32. Is histologic analysis important in diagnosing GERD?

Distal esophageal biopsies are not required or recommended to diagnose GERD. Biopsies have low sensitivity and low specificity for this diagnosis. Esophageal biopsies should only be taken when other etiologies of esophagitis are being excluded, such as in patients with suspected EoE or infectious esophagitis.

33. What is the most reasonable initial approach to a patient complaining of GERD and who does not have any alarm symptoms?

In patients with typical symptoms of heartburn or regurgitation, it is reasonable to proceed with an 8-week trial of a once-daily PPI, taken 30–45 minutes prior to their first meal. After 8 weeks, patients should attempt to discontinue their PPI. Endoscopy should then be performed off PPIs for 2–4 weeks in patients who did not respond to that initial PPI therapy and in those whose symptoms return after medication discontinuation.

34. What type of ambulatory esophageal reflux monitoring is available?

The two methods of reflux testing are (1) a wireless telemetry capsule (Bravo; Medtronic, Minneapolis, MN, United States) that is attached to the esophageal mucosa during endoscopy and evaluates for acid reflux over 48–96 hours and (2) a transnasal catheter–based pH and pH-impedance testing, which is generally a 24-hour study. A combination of pH-impedance testing allows the measurement of acid, weak acid, and non–acid reflux episodes.

35. When should ambulatory esophageal reflux monitoring be used?

In patients with a high suspicion for GERD, but in whom the diagnosis is not clear, and endoscopy does not show evidence of esophagitis, reflux testing should be performed off of therapy. Patients who have extraesophageal symptoms without typical heartburn or regurgitation should undergo reflux testing prior to initiating PPI therapy to determine if they truly do have underlying GERD. In patients with documented GERD, but who have persistent symptoms despite twice-daily PPI therapy, pH-impedance testing on therapy can be used to determine if continued symptoms are due to persistent GERD. Reflux testing of acid-suppressive therapy should not be performed to diagnose GERD in patients who have long-segment BE or LA grade C or D esophagitis. In patients who are considering an antireflux surgical intervention, it is critical that the patient has documentation of either abnormal baseline acid reflux or ongoing reflux despite therapy.

PROGNOSIS OF GASTROESOPHAGEAL REFLUX DISEASE

36. What complications can be associated with GERD?

Complications of GERD include EE, peptic stricture, BE, esophageal cancer, and extraintestinal manifestations such as asthma, coughing, and laryngitis.

37. What is BE?

BE occurs when the normal squamous mucosa is replaced by specialized metaplastic columnar epithelial cells. It is estimated that up to 12% of patients with chronic GERD will develop BE. BE is the precursor lesion to esophageal adenocarcinoma (EAC). Single-screening endoscopy should be performed for patients with chronic GERD symptoms and three or more additional risk factors for BE, including male sex, age >50 years, White race, tobacco smoking, obesity, and family history of BE or EAC in a first-degree relative.

38. How is BE managed?

For nondysplastic BE, the American College of Gastroenterology recommends surveillance intervals of 5 years for Barrett segments <3 cm in length and 3 years for segments ≥3 cm in length. Patients with low- or high-grade dysplasia may be candidates for endoscopic eradication therapy, while patients with visible/nodular lesions may be candidates for endoscopic resection. All patients with BE should take a once-daily PPI for life.

CLINICAL VIGNETTE

Available Online.

BIBLIOGRAPHY

Available Online.

CHAPTER 2

ESOPHAGEAL CAUSES OF CHEST PAIN

Anton Jordan De Witte, MD and Dhyanesh A. Patel, MD

 Additional content available online.

1. **What are the epidemiologic factors of noncardiac chest pain (NCCP)?**
   Chest pain is one of the most common chief complaints in outpatient clinics and is known to be the second most common reason for a visit to the emergency department (ED), comprising 5% of ED presentations. Population-based studies have estimated the prevalence of NCCP to be 13%, with an equal sex distribution. There is an inverse relationship between age and prevalence of NCCP.

2. **What should be on the top of the differential for atypical chest pain referred to a gastroenterology clinic? Does a cardiac etiologic factor need to be excluded before starting an evaluation for esophageal chest pain?**
   Cardiac etiology should be the top diagnosis in the differential for any chest pain referral even in gastroenterology clinic as they are potentially life-threatening. In fact, nearly one in three deaths in the United States is due to cardiovascular disease, and only 1%–4% of patients with dysphagia and/or chest pain have a spastic disorder of the esophagus. Patient's history does not reliably distinguish cardiac from esophageal causes, and a thorough cardiac workup should be the first step in any evaluation of chest pain. Patients should be risk stratified based on age and cardiac comorbidities with a referral to a cardiologist as appropriate. Electrocardiogram (ECG) and troponin are not considered to be an adequate cardiac workup and depending on risk factors, provocative testing (such as stress test) should be performed to definitively rule out cardiac etiology before pursuing esophageal workup.

3. **Once a cardiac cause is excluded, what are the causes of NCCP?**
   The source of NCCP can be *gastrointestinal (GI), pulmonary, musculoskeletal, dermatologic, rheumatologic, psychiatric, or referred pain*. A careful history and physical examination can often eliminate many of these potential sources. Pain reproduced by movement or pressing on the chest wall should bring musculoskeletal etiologies higher on the list. Among GI causes of NCCP, gastroesophageal reflux disease (GERD) is the most common cause with a prevalence between 30% and 60%, but pill-induced injury or infectious esophagitis are also in the differential if acute symptoms and have concomitant odynophagia. Only 1%–4% of patients with dysphagia and/or chest pain have a spastic disorder of the esophagus on motility testing.

4. **How is esophageal chest pain transmitted?**
   Both peripheral and central sensitization participate in esophageal hypersensitivity. Although refluxate of noxious agents (acid and/or bile) is the most common cause of esophageal chest pain via stimulation of nociceptive receptors (such as vanilloid receptor 1), acid in the esophagus does not induce symptoms in all individuals, which suggests alternate pain pathways. Mechanoreceptors are sensitive to esophageal distention and abnormal contractions and therefore may be a potential source of pain.

5. **Is a proton pump inhibitor (PPI) test a reasonable first-line approach for diagnosis of GERD?**
   Yes. Because GERD is the most common cause of esophageal chest pain, it is reasonable to give a trial of a PPI for both diagnostic and therapeutic intent if no alarm features are present. Studies show sensitivity and specificity of the "PPI test" for GERD-related NCCP from 69% to 95% and 67% to 86%, respectively. Hence, this is a simple cost-effective approach.

6. **What PPI dosing strategies are used during a PPI test?**
   For patients with classic GERD symptoms with no alarm symptoms, it is generally recommended to initiate an 8-week trial of empiric PPIs once daily before a meal. However, shorter duration, high-dose PPI tests have shown to be as efficacious. One dosing strategy for GERD-associated NCCP is high-dose acid suppression for 1–2 weeks (e.g., omeprazole 40 mg by mouth twice daily or its equivalent) using symptom improvement as a measure of responsiveness. Longer courses (2–3 months) have been more commonly used, but this strategy can be more costly and time-consuming and can delay diagnosis without much increase in sensitivity or specificity. Patients with proven acid reflux on pH studies or those with erosive esophagitis tend to have a greater response and higher diagnostic yield. It is important to ensure a patient does not remain on a high-dose PPI regimen indefinitely. Rather, the PPI should be titrated to the lowest effective dose or discontinued if there is no symptom improvement.

7. **Is there a role for endoscopy in the initial evaluation of esophageal chest pain?**
   Esophagogastroduodenoscopy (EGD) should be reserved for those patients at *high risk* (age >50 years, male sex, Caucasian race, or central obesity) or *with alarm symptoms* (dysphagia, odynophagia, GI bleeding, iron-deficiency anemia, or unintentional weight loss) for the evaluation for erosive esophagitis, Barrett esophagus, or malignancy. Otherwise, nearly 70% of patients with heartburn and no alarm symptoms tend to have normal upper endoscopy and, hence, should not be used as an initial diagnostic tool.

8. **Can esophageal motility disorders induce chest pain?**
   Yes, spastic motility disorders of the esophagus can induce atypical chest pain (distal esophageal spasm, hypercontractile esophagus, or achalasia). Although nonspecific motility abnormalities can be found in up to 30% of non-GERD-related NCCP, spastic motor disorders of the esophagus are only found in 1%–4% of patients undergoing manometry.

9. **How is esophageal motility evaluated?**
   High-resolution manometry (HRM) is the gold standard to evaluate esophageal motility. Fig. 2.1 reviews the classification system for diagnosis of motility disorders based on HRM parameters of integrated relaxation pressure (IRP), distal contractile integral (DCI), and distal latency (DL). IRP assesses the adequacy of swallow-induced lower esophageal sphincter relaxation, DCI is a three-dimensional metric to assess the contractile vigor of the esophageal smooth muscle (taking length, amplitude, and duration of contraction into consideration), and DL can help differentiate between a premature/simultaneous versus peristaltic contraction. Although still in early clinical phases, functional lumen imaging probe (FLIP) is the newest US Food and Drug Administration–approved diagnostic tool to assess esophageal physiology. The FLIP catheter is a distensible balloon encasing multiple pairs of impedance sensors and a single distal pressure sensor that is placed transorally during sedated EGD to detect luminal distensibility. Reduced luminal distensibility is often seen in disorders of esophagogastric junction (EGJ) outflow such as achalasia or EGJ outflow obstruction (EGJOO) and has thus been recommended as a complementary tool to HRM in the setting of inconclusive patterns. EGJ distensibility index of <2 mm^2/mm Hg is considered abnormal.

10. **What is the treatment for esophageal motility disorders?**
    Treatment should be personalized to the type of motility abnormality and the predominant bothersome symptom for the patient. Pneumatic dilation, peroral endoscopic myotomy, and laparoscopic Heller myotomy are primary treatment options for achalasia. If a patient is not a candidate for those options due to significant comorbidities, endoscopic botulinum toxin A injection to the lower esophageal sphincter can be considered. In other motility abnormalities, endoscopic dilation (with or without botulinum toxin A injection for spastic motor disorders), smooth muscle relaxers, or neuromodulators can be considered based on diagnosis and symptoms.

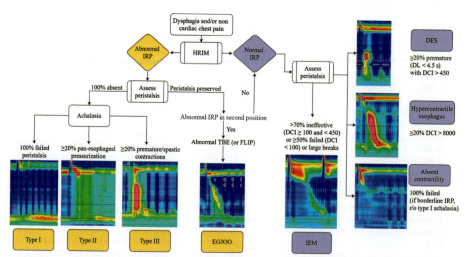

Fig. 2.1 Manometric classification of various esophageal motility disorders based on Chicago Classification v4.0. *DCI,* Distal contractile integral; *DES,* distal esophageal spasm; *DL,* distal latency; *EGJOO,* esophagogastric junction outflow obstruction; *FLIP,* functional luminal imaging probe; *HRIM,* high-resolution impedance manometry; *IEM,* ineffective esophageal motility; *IRP,* integrated relaxation pressure; *TBE,* timed barium esophagogram. (Reproduced with permission from Patel DA, Yadlapati R, Vaezi MF. Esophageal motility disorders: current approach to diagnostics and therapeutics. Gastroenterology. 2022;162(6):1617-1634.)

11. **Is barium esophagogram a useful test in the evaluation of esophageal chest pain?**
Barium esophagogram lacks adequate sensitivity or specificity as an initial test for diagnosing GERD. In fact, it can demonstrate reflux in up to 20% of healthy individuals, and therefore should not be used as a substitute for other higher yield diagnostic modalities for GERD (i.e., PPI test and ambulatory pH study). Barium esophagogram can be helpful in patients when structural evaluation of the esophagus is needed (stricture, malignancy, hiatal hernia, major motility disorder, or diverticulum).

12. **What is the next best test for someone who is partially responsive or unresponsive to PPI?**
Upper endoscopy with ambulatory pH testing OFF PPI therapy. For patients with esophageal chest pain refractory to PPI therapy, it is important to identify any esophageal mucosal abnormalities before proceeding with another form of treatment. Upper endoscopy allows the clinician to evaluate for any mucosal abnormalities (reflux esophagitis, Barrett esophagus, or eosinophilic esophagitis [EoE]). The majority of patients will have normal upper endoscopy, and, in this scenario, ambulatory pH testing should be performed as below to evaluate for GERD.

13. **What is the next step if the upper endoscopy is normal?**
Ambulatory pH monitoring. This testing allows us to determine if there is any abnormal reflux as the etiology of their symptoms by measuring the esophageal acid exposure time (AET) and can give symptom correlation (temporal relationship between chest pain and acid reflux events). Normal pH testing rules out GERD as the underlying etiology and suggests that esophageal hypersensitivity might be playing a major role in symptom generation (if workup for other etiologies was negative).

14. **How is pH monitoring performed?**
Ambulatory pH testing can be performed using transnasal pH catheter-based probes or via wireless pH telemetry capsule monitoring systems. It is recommended to stop PPIs or H2 blockers for at least 7 days prior to initiation of pH monitoring if the diagnosis of GERD is unclear.

15. **What are some of the advantages and disadvantages of the transnasal catheter?**
Advantages:
1. No sedation is needed.
2. Can measure bolus transit, directionality (due to impedance sensors), and all reflux events (acid, nonacid, and gas) when using a multichannel intraluminal (MII-pH) pH-impedance catheter. Can be performed ON or OFF acid-suppressive medications depending on the likelihood of GERD.

Disadvantages:
1. Uncomfortable as it is a transnasal catheter and can lead to altered dietary intake and daily activity, which can affect the accuracy of the test.
2. Limited to only 24 hours of monitoring, which reduces sensitivity for detection of GERD.
3. Cumbersome to read with high variability in interpretation.

16. **What are some of the advantages and disadvantages of the wireless pH monitor?**
Advantages:
1. Endoscopically placed in a sedated patient and allows prolonged monitoring (48–96 hours).
2. Better tolerated from a patient perspective.

Disadvantages:
1. Only measures acid reflux events. Hence, should be done 7–10 days OFF any acid-suppressive medications.
2. Patients can have chest pain with capsule attachment that requires endoscopic removal in up to 2% of patients, and premature detachment can occur in up to 12% of patients.

17. **How do you interpret pH monitoring results?**
As stated above, an ambulatory pH monitoring (off acid-suppressive therapy) measures the degree and duration of esophageal acid exposure with the primary outcome of AET. Fig. 2.2 shows the diagnostic algorithm for NCCP. According to the Lyon Consensus, an AET >6% (time percentage of esophageal pH < 4 over the whole monitoring time) is considered abnormal and diagnostic of nonerosive reflux disease (NERD). An AET <4% is considered normal and should prompt additional testing and/or symptom correlation to determine if the pain is secondary to functional chest pain, reflux hypersensitivity, or esophageal motility disorder. An AET of 4%–6% is inconclusive and requires additional information (reflux burden, symptom association, mucosal integrity testing, or pH-impedance monitoring—postreflux swallow-induced peristaltic wave and mean nocturnal baseline impedance), to differentiate patients with NERD and functional heartburn.

18. **How is functional esophageal chest pain defined?**
According to the ROME IV criteria, functional chest pain of esophageal origin must meet all of the following diagnostic criteria:

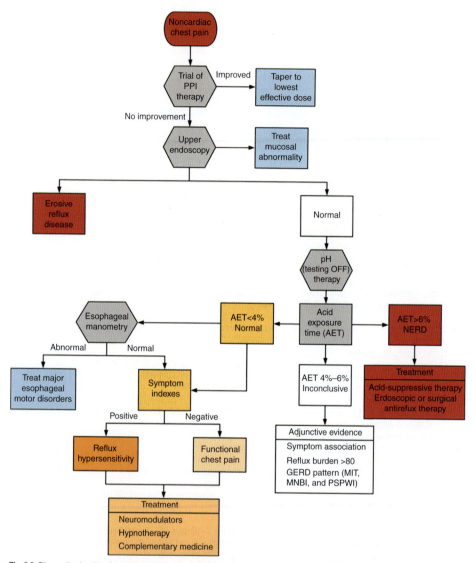

Fig. 2.2 Diagnostic algorithm for patients with noncardiac chest pain. *AET*, Acid exposure time; *GERD*, gastroesophageal reflux disease; *MIT*, mucosal integrity testing; *MNBI*, mean nocturnal baseline impedance; *NERD*, nonerosive reflux disease; *PPI*, proton pump inhibitor; *PSPWI*, postreflux swallow-induced peristaltic wave index. (Reproduced and modified with permission from Patel D, Fass R, Vaezi M. Untangling nonerosive reflux disease from functional heartburn. Clin Gastroenterol Hepatol. 2021;19(7):1314-1326.)

Symptoms must be present for the preceding 3 months, with an onset of more than 6 months with a frequency of at least once a week.
1. Retrosternal chest pain or discomfort; cardiac causes should be ruled out.
2. Absence of associated esophageal symptoms, such as heartburn and dysphagia.
3. Absence of evidence that gastroesophageal reflux or EoE is the cause of the symptom.
4. Absence of major esophageal motor disorders (achalasia/EGJOO, distal esophageal spasm, hypercontractile esophagus, or absent peristalsis).

19. What does a positive symptom correlation mean?
Symptom correlation is the strength of association between symptoms and reflux using statistical probability. There are two indices that are typically used to measure symptom correlation. Symptom index provides data on

Table 2.1 Modalities for Calculating the Association of Symptoms and Reflux Events.

SYMPTOMS SCORING MODALITY	CALCULATION	POSITIVE SCORE (%)
SI	$\dfrac{\text{Symptomatic episodes associated with reflux events}}{\text{Total number of symptomatic episodes}} \times 100$	≥ 50
SAP	Chi-square: Total 24-h pH recording data divided into 2-min segments. Each segment is interpreted for reflux events and reported symptoms. Data are summarized into a 2×2 table and the probability that an association exists is calculated using the Fisher exact test.	≥ 95

SAP, Symptom association probability; *SI*, symptom index; *SSI*, symptom severity index.

the strength of the association between symptoms and reflux events, whereas symptom association probability evaluates the statistical probability that a symptom is due to a reflux event rather than chance alone (Table 2.1). A positive symptom correlation indicates that the patient's subjective symptoms are directly associated with recorded reflux events. Negative symptom correlation, on the other hand, would suggest a discordance between symptoms and reflux events. However, these indices have multiple limitations as they are affected by how often the patient remembers to press the button on the receiver when they truly experience the symptom and how often the symptom occurs during the monitoring period. Of note, none of these methods can reliably predict response to treatment and are therefore viewed as complementary data to support findings on the pH/MII study and clinical suspicions.

20. How do you treat reflux hypersensitivity, functional heartburn, and NCCP?

In patients with normal endoscopy, pH testing, and lack of response to PPI therapy, esophageal hypersensitivity is usually the major driver of underlying symptoms. In patients with normal AET, reflux hypersensitivity is diagnosed with positive symptom correlation, while functional heartburn or functional chest pain syndrome is diagnosed with negative symptom correlation and predominant symptom (heartburn or chest pain). Pain tends to be a perceptive symptom and, hence, neuromodulators are usually the primary treatment option for all three entities. Table 2.2 shows the most commonly used neuromodulators and their level of evidence for NCCP, functional heartburn, and reflux hypersensitivity.

21. Are there any emerging treatments or diagnostic modalities for NCCP?

Mucosal integrity testing. A novel balloon mucosal impedance device has shown promise for differentiating GERD (erosive reflux disease or NERD) and EoE from normal mucosal instantly during endoscopy.

Some novel receptor targets that have gained attention in clinical trials include:

- *N*-Methyl-DD-aspartate receptor antagonist (ketamine) increases sensory threshold without a change in esophageal motility and reduces secondary hyperalgesia. There are considerable adverse drug reactions (central nervous system depression, arrhythmia, or respiratory depression), and it requires intramuscular or intravenous administration.
- Alpha-2-delta ligand (pregabalin) reduces centrally acting pain modulators, glutamate, and substance P.

22. Are any psychiatric diagnoses associated with NCCP?

Yes. Psychiatric comorbidities, most commonly anxiety disorder is frequently present in patients with NCCP. Additional comorbid conditions include major depression, panic disorder, somatization, emotional lability, and poor social support in up to *33% of patients* with NCCP. Treatment of the underlying psychiatric illness remains key to the resolution of symptoms in NCCP, and therapies such as cognitive behavioral therapy, Johrei therapy, and hypnotherapy have been used with significant success.

23. What is the long-term prognosis of NCCP?

Although there is no increase in overall mortality above the general population, several long-term, outcome-based studies have demonstrated a significant impact on the quality of life in patients with NCCP. As many as two-thirds of patients will continue to experience their index symptoms up to 11 years later. Although providing an exact diagnosis may not decrease the frequency or severity of symptoms, patients who understand how hypersensitivity might be driving their pain tend to feel less impaired and use fewer medical resources for ongoing symptoms.

Table 2.2 Randomized Controlled Trials (RCTs) of Neuromodulators for the Treatment of Functional Esophageal Disorders.

CLASS OF DRUG	DOSE	DISORDER	RESPONSE RATE	SIDE EFFECTS
TCAs				
Imipramine	50 mg/d	NCCP	52%	QT prolongation
Imipramine	50 mg/d	NCCP	Significant	Dry mouth and dizziness
Imipramine	50 mg/d	FH and RH	37.2%	Constipation
Amitriptyline	10 and 25 mg/d	NCCP and globus	52% and significant	Excessive sleeping and dizziness
SNRIs				
Venlafaxine	75 mg/d	NCCP	52%	Sleep disturbances
SSRIs				
Sertraline	50–200 mg/d	NCCP	57%	Nausea and restlessness
Sertraline	50–200 mg/d	NCCP	Modest	Dry mouth and diarrhea
Paroxetine	10–50 mg/d	NCCP	Modest	Fatigue and dizziness
Paroxetine	10–50 mg/d	NCCP	21.7%	None
Citalopram	20 mg/d	RH	Significant	None
Fluoxetine	20 mg/d	FH/RH	Significant	Headache and dry mouth
Other				
Melatonin	6 mg/d	FH	75%	Diarrhea
Ranitidine	300 mg/d	FH	Significant	None
Theophylline	200 mg twice/d	NCCP	58%	Nausea, insomnia, and tremor
Gabapentin	300 mg three times/d	Globus	66%	None

FH, Functional heartburn; *NCCP*, noncardiac chest pain; *RH*, reflux hypersensitivity; *SNRI*, serotonin-norepinephrine reuptake inhibitor; *SSRI*, selective serotonin reuptake inhibitor; *TCA*, tricyclic antidepressant.
Reprinted with permission from Gyawali CP, Fass R. Management of gastroesophageal reflux disease. Gastroenterology 2018;154:302-318.

ACKNOWLEDGMENTS

The authors would like to acknowledge the contributions of Dr. Vito V. Cirigliano and Dr. Fouad J. Moawad, MD, FACG, who were the authors of this chapter in the previous edition.

CLINICAL VIGNETTE

Available Online.

BIBLIOGRAPHY

Available Online.

CHAPTER 3

ACHALASIA

Steven Clayton, MD, FAAFP, FACP, FACG

 Additional content available online.

1. What is achalasia?

Achalasia is the quintessential example of an esophageal motility disorder. The term *achalasia* first appeared in the medical literature in an article by Arthur Hertz in 1915. He credits the name designation to his colleague Sir Cooper Perry. The term *achalasia* (Greek a, "not"; χαλάω, "I relax") was used to describe the underlying clinical characteristics of the lower esophageal sphincter (LES) failing to relax, resulting in a functional obstruction at the esophagogastric junction (EGJ). Complicating matters, there is also loss of the esophageal peristaltic function. The combination of a functional obstruction at the LES and aperistalsis results in esophageal bolus stasis, leading to symptoms of dysphagia and voluminous bland regurgitation.

2. How common is achalasia?

Achalasia afflicts humanity as a whole and does not have a preponderance for a particular age, race, and/or sex. Achalasia is a rare disease occurring with an annual incidence of approximately 1 per 100,000 people and a prevalence of 10 per 100,000, owing to the fact that achalasia is a chronic disease with a low mortality rate. Achalasia typically affects people who are in the third to the sixth decade of their life. Achalasia does occur in the pediatric population as well, with an estimated annual incidence of 0.11% in children less than age 16.

3. What is the pathogenesis of achalasia?

Within the esophageal myenteric plexus, there are two types of neurons: excitatory and inhibitory. The primary inhibitory neurotransmitters mediating LES relaxation are nitric oxide (NO) and vasoactive intestinal polypeptide.

Myotomy specimens from patients with achalasia demonstrate prominent inflammation in the esophageal myenteric (Auerbach's) plexus consisting primarily of T lymphocytes resulting in ganglionitis, neuronal apoptosis, and neurofibrosis. This neuronal loss preferentially involves the NO-producing inhibitory neurons. The cholinergic neurons affecting the tonic contraction of the LES are relatively spared. This loss of inhibitory innervation of the LES results in loss of deglutitive reflexive relaxation of the LES, ultimately resulting in EGJ outflow obstruction from a poorly relaxing LES. This functional obstruction at the level of the LES is usually compounded with esophageal body spasm or complete esophageal aperistalsis depending on the achalasia subtype. The exact cause is unknown. There is some evidence to suggest an autoimmune response targeting the neurons, possibly precipitated by an infectious agent.

4. What are common symptoms of achalasia?

The clinical presentation of achalasia is often variable, but typical symptoms are bland, large volume regurgitation, progressive solid and liquid dysphagia, chest pain/fullness, varying degrees of weight loss, and, sometimes, retrosternal burning or heartburn. Respiratory symptoms, including cough, aspiration, and others, have been reported in 40% of patients with achalasia.

As patients with achalasia have bland regurgitation from esophageal stasis, differentiation from gastroesophageal reflux disease (GERD) can be difficult. This leads to many patients with achalasia being inappropriately started on pharmacologic therapies such as proton pump inhibitors and/or sometimes treated with antireflux surgery.

5. How do you evaluate a patient with suspected achalasia?

In patients with clinical symptoms who are suspicious of achalasia, endoscopy, barium esophagram, and esophageal manometry assist with making the diagnosis of achalasia. Endoscopic findings of retained saliva or food in the esophagus, a dilated esophageal lumen, and a rosette (puckered appearance) at the EGJ can suggest achalasia. Endoscopy is of paramount importance to exclude pseudoachalasia caused by malignancy or other mechanical obstructions at the EGJ that may result in symptoms similar to achalasia.

Barium esophagram demonstrating a dilated and sometimes tortuous esophagus with a narrowing at the EGJ and liquid barium stasis in the upright position strongly suggests the diagnosis (Fig. 3.1).

High-resolution manometry (HRM) is the accepted gold standard for assessing for disorders of esophageal motility, including achalasia. The HRM catheters consist of solid-state pressure sensors spaced 1 cm apart. The catheter is positioned to span the length of the esophagus extending from the hypopharynx to the stomach. Computer software generates esophageal pressure topography plots that represent esophageal

19

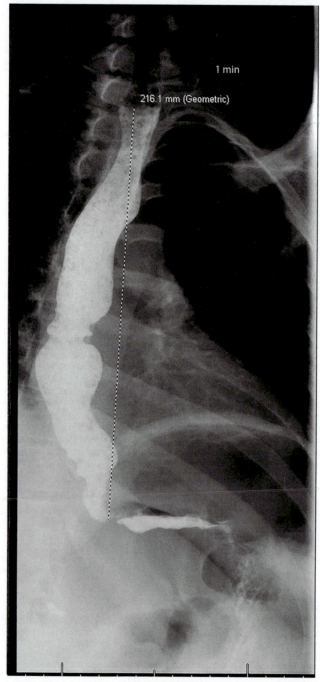

Fig. 3.1 Image of a barium esophagram demonstrating a dilated and tortuous esophagus with a narrowing at the esophagogastric junction and liquid barium stasis in the upright position consistent with achalasia.

motility and sphincter function on color-coded, pressure-space-time plots called a Clause plot. Achalasia is the best known esophageal disorder and has been defined as having an elevated IRP (>15 mm Hg) without identifiable esophageal smooth muscle peristalsis.

6. What is the role of endoscopy in the evaluation of suspected achalasia?

Endoscopic evaluation is of paramount importance to evaluate for an obstructing esophageal lesion at the level of the EGJ that could create an achalasia-like picture. Other endoscopic findings can suggest achalasia, such as the appearance of foam and/or retained saliva in the esophagus. Puckering of EGJ that requires more than usual pressure to traverse endoscopically is frequently observed. In the later stages of achalasia, a dilated or sigmoid esophagus may be present. If these endoscopic features are present, achalasia should be confirmed with HRM.

7. What are the manometric subtypes of achalasia, and why is subtyping important?

HRM allows achalasia to be differentiated into three subtypes based on manometric patterns: type I achalasia (classic) has absent smooth muscle contractility in the esophageal body with an elevated integrated relaxation pressure (IRP), type II achalasia has ≥20% of swallows with panesophageal pressurization and an elevated IRP, and type III achalasia (spastic/vigorous) has shortened distal latency (<4.5 seconds), distal contractile integral (DCI) > 450 mm Hg cm/s, and an elevated IRP. Fig. 3.2 shows representative swallow examples of the three subtypes of achalasia. When evaluating for achalasia, normal esophageal peristalsis should not be present. Differentiating achalasia is of clinical importance as the three subtypes present similarly but their treatment response varies

8. How does manometric subtyping of achalasia predict response to therapy?

Historically, achalasia was treated with laparoscopic Heller myotomy (LHM) and pneumatic dilation (PD). As a result, there is a robust literature examining the outcomes between these treatment modalities. Overall, patients with type II achalasia have the most clinical improvement, while patients with type III achalasia have the least improvement with traditional therapies. In 2009 a new endoscopic approach to performing myotomy of the LES was introduced, the peroral endoscopic myotomy (POEM). Since the introduction and widespread usage of POEM, the literature supports POEM as a safe, effective, and minimally invasive treatment option for achalasia. The advantage of POEM compared with traditional therapies is the ability to perform a tailored esophageal smooth muscle myotomy. POEM has become the preferred treatment option in type III achalasia when a longer myotomy is needed to treat both the functional obstruction at the LES and the esophageal body smooth muscle spasm.

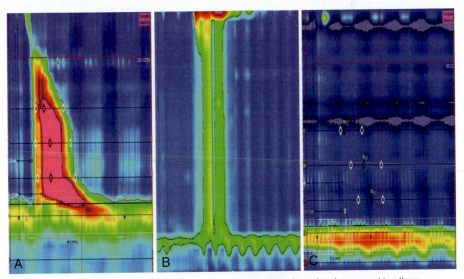

Fig. 3.2 High-resolution manometry allows achalasia to be differentiated into three subtypes based on manometric patterns: (A) type III achalasia (spastic/vigorous) has shortened distal latency (450 mm Hg cm/s) and an elevated median IRP >15 mm Hg; (B) type II achalasia has ≥20% of swallows of panesophageal pressurization and an elevated median integrated relaxation pressure (IRP) >15 mm Hg; and (C) type I achalasia (classic) has absent smooth muscle contractility in the esophageal body with an elevated median IRP >15 mm Hg.

9. **What is functional lumen imaging probe (FLIP), and how is it used in the diagnosis of achalasia?**

   The FLIP is a catheter placed in the esophagus straddling the LES (Fig. 3.3) at the time of endoscopy that can be used to measure pressure, diameter, compliance, cross-sectional area, and distensibility of the LES. FLIP is a complementary diagnostic tool to HRM in the evaluation and diagnosis of achalasia. FLIP evaluates esophageal function in nonobstructive dysphagia by detecting an abnormal response to volumetric balloon–mediated esophageal distension. Furthermore, FLIP can characterize achalasia subtypes by detecting esophageal body contraction patterns. FLIP can also help in clarifying the diagnosis of achalasia in patients with the inconclusive diagnosis of achalasia on HRM. Fig. 3.4 demonstrates the timed barium esophagram (TBE) (A), the HRM (B), and the FLIP (C) in a type I achalasia patient with poor esophageal emptying. The FLIP (C) demonstrates reduced distensibility in red (1) with the absence of peristalsis proximally (2).

10. **What are the diseases or conditions that mimic achalasia?**

    Chagas disease is an infectious disease caused by the protozoan *Trypanosoma cruzi* in Central and South America. Chagas disease is spread by bites from the reduviid (kissing) bugs. Ganglionitis occurs throughout the body causing esophageal, duodenal, colonic, and rectal damage. The esophageal disease is similar to achalasia (functional obstruction at the level of the LES and a dilated esophagus). Many patients have concomitant cardiac disease, which is the leading cause of death in patients with Chagas.

    "Pseudoachalasia" is a term used to describe an anatomic obstruction at the EGJ that creates esophagogastric outflow obstruction resulting in an achalasia-like syndrome with similar symptoms, radiographic features, and manometric to primary achalasia. The prevalence of pseudoachalasia is about 5% of patients presenting with an achalasia-like syndrome.

    Malignancy is the most common etiology and should be suspected in older adult patients with rapidly progressing dysphagia and weight loss. The most common types of cancer resulting in pseudoachalasia are adenocarcinoma of the esophagus and stomach. Upper endoscopy is the preferred diagnostic modality for diagnosing esophageal and gastric malignancy. In addition, pseudoachalasia has been associated with surgical procedures such as a tight fundoplication or a migrated laparoscopic gastric band.

11. **What are the goals for the treatment, and what treatment options are available for achalasia?**

    Achalasia is a chronic condition without a cure at this time. No treatment can restore normal smooth muscle function or sphincter activity to the esophagus. Treatment is directed at alleviating symptoms, improving esophageal emptying, and preventing disease progression and dilation of the esophagus. The currently available treatment options for achalasia include pharmacologic, endoscopic, and surgical therapies.

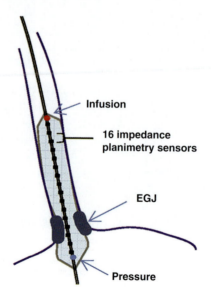

Fig. 3.3 Image demonstrating the correct placement of the functional lumen imaging probe catheter. (With permission from Hirano I, Pandolfino JE, Boeckxstaens GE. Functional lumen imaging probe for the management of esophageal disorders: expert review from the Clinical Practice Updates Committee of the AGA Institute. Clin Gastroenterol Hepatol. 2017;15(3):325-334.)

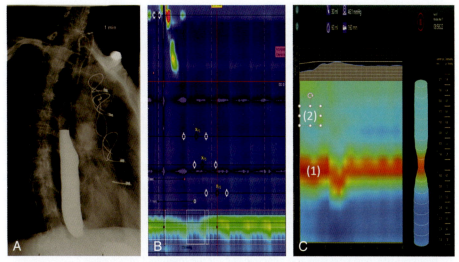

Fig. 3.4 TBE, HRM, and FLIP from a patient with type I achalasia. (A) The TBE shows a 20 cm column of retained liquid barium at 1 min representing significant esophageal stasis. (B) The HRM reveals the complete absent smooth muscle contractility in the esophageal body with an elevated median IRP > 15 mm Hg (type I achalasia). (C) The FLIP reveals reduced distensibility at the lower esophageal sphincter displayed as a red band (1) with complete aperistalsis in the esophageal body (2). *FLIP*, Functional lumen imaging probe; *HRM*, high-resolution manometry; *TBE*, timed barium esophagram.

12. How effective is pharmacologic therapy to treat achalasia, and what agents are available?

Nitrates and calcium channel blockers are the most common medications used to treat achalasia. Nitrates increase NO concentration in smooth muscle cells resulting in smooth muscle relaxation. Calcium channel blockers diminish cellular calcium uptake and have been shown to lower LES pressure by nearly 50%. Isosorbide dinitrate (5 mg) and nifedipine (10–30 mg) both are used to treat achalasia. Typically, they are administered 30 minutes before meals and at bedtime. A major disadvantage of medical therapy is side effects, with many patients experiencing hypotension, headaches, and dizziness.

Overall, pharmacologic therapy is the least effective treatment available for achalasia. Endoscopic and surgical therapies have better and more durable efficacy compared to medications. Medical therapy should be reserved only for patients with achalasia who are poor candidates for surgical or endoscopic therapy.

13. How is botulinum toxin used to treat achalasia?

Botulinum toxin A is injected intramuscularly into the LES and is the most common endoscopically administered drug used to treat achalasia. Botulinum toxin is a neurotoxin that blocks exocytosis of acetylcholine from the nerve synapsis resulting in a short-term paralysis of the LES, diminishing the functional obstruction at the EGJ. The effect is temporary but durable for 3–12 months. In the treatment of achalasia, 100 units of botulinum toxin is typically delivered 1–2 cm proximal to the squamocolumnar junction using a sclerotherapy needle in 0.5–1 mL aliquots and is distributed circumferentially around the LES. Botulinum toxin should not be given to patients with an egg allergy. Otherwise, the drug is safe and simple to administer. Around 80% of patients experienced clinical improvement within 1 month by using 100 units of botulinum toxin, but less than 40% are in remission at 1 year. Of those responding to the first injection, 75% respond to a second botulinum toxin injection.

14. Which patients with achalasia should be treated with botulinum toxin?

Botulinum toxin is an effective initial treatment for achalasia; however, the effectiveness of botulinum toxin treatment dwindles over time. Therefore botulinum toxin is a suboptimal intervention for patients with a reasonable life expectancy and those who are well enough for more efficacious and long-lasting therapies for achalasia. Ideally, botulinum toxin injections should be reserved for patients with severe comorbid conditions such that the patient is not a candidate for myotomy or PD.

15. What is PD of the LES, and how is it performed?

PD disrupts the LES by stretching the sphincter muscle fibers using a noncompliant polyethylene balloon. These balloons come in three diameters (30, 35, and 40 mm) mounted on a flexible catheter and placed over a guidewire during endoscopy. The PD balloon is positioned across the LES using either fluoroscopic or endoscopic positioning.

The PD balloon is inflated slightly until a *waist* (a narrowing in the balloon under fluoroscopy representing the nonrelaxing LES) is identified. The pressure required to obliterate the fluoroscopic *waist* is usually 10–15 psi of air held for 15–60 s. PDs are usually started with the smallest balloon (30 mm) and then repeated at 2- to 4-week intervals, with sequentially larger diameter balloons until the patient experiences symptom relief and improved esophageal emptying on the TBE.

16. What are the results of PD?

PD is a safe and effective treatment for achalasia and should be part of any tertiary referral centers' achalasia treatment armamentarium. PD has proven clinical efficacy, resulting in good to excellent symptoms relief with 30, 35, and 40 mm in 74%, 86%, and 90% of patients, respectively, with an average follow-up of 1.6 years. Over 5 years, nearly one-third of patients have symptom relapses. Therefore serial PD usually is needed and has a similar efficacy to LHM at 2 (85% vs 90%, respectively) and 5 years (82% vs 84%, respectively), based on a large randomized control trial from Europe.

17. Are there subsets of patients who respond better with PD?

Patients that have the most optimal treatment response after treatment with PD include the following: older age (>45 years), female, narrow (nondilated) esophagus, and LES pressure after PD of <10 mm Hg. Achalasia subtyping with HRM is important as patients with types I and II achalasia have better therapeutic benefit with PD in comparison with type III achalasia. PD is highly cost-effective compared with both LHM and POEM and has the least risk of post-LES intervention GERD.

18. What is LHM, and how safe and effective is it for the treatment of achalasia?

The classic surgical treatment of achalasia is a Heller myotomy with a partial fundoplication. During this operation, a 6 cm esophageal myotomy is created that extends 2–3 cm onto the upper stomach and is usually performed in conjunction with an antireflux fundoplication (Dor or Toupet) to reduce subsequent GERD. Implemented in 1992, LHM allows improved visualization of the distal esophageal muscle layers and gastric sling fibers of the upper stomach, resulting in a shorter surgical duration and recovery time.

Campos et al. performed a large systematic review with a mean follow-up of 4 years affirming that LHM is safe and effective. They found that the mean symptom relief was 90% (range 76%–100%). In 2019 a European randomized trial assigned 109 patients to undergo LHM with Dor fundoplication and 112 patients to undergo POEM. At 2 years, the improvement of dysphagia symptoms and LES residual pressure were similar in both groups: 81.7% for LHM and 83% for POEM. However, in the POEM group, GERD and esophagitis were twice as high (44%) compared to the LHM group (29%). Serious complications occurred in both groups but more complications in the LHM group versus POEM ($n = 9$ [7.3%] vs $n = 3$ [2.7%]; absolute between-group difference, 4.6 percentage points; 95% CI −1.1 to 10.4).

Predictors of success for LHM include young age (< 40 years), lower esophagus sphincter pressure greater than 30 mm Hg, a straight and nontortuous esophagus, and patients with types I and II achalasia.

19. What is POEM, and how safe and effective is it for the treatment of achalasia?

POEM is the endoscopic creation of a long submucosal tunnel proximal to the LES followed by endoscopic myotomy of the circular muscle bundles within the LES and cardia. The length of myotomy within the esophagus can be tailored depending on the subtype of achalasia being treated. As POEM is performed through an endoscopically created submucosal tunnel, this technique avoids some of the difficulties and complications of performing a myotomy from either a thoracic or laparoscopic approach, including the need for a mediastinal dissection, decreased risk of vagal nerve injury, and diminished risk of development of intra-abdominal adhesions.

In 2019 a randomized multicenter trial compared the efficacy of POEM ($n=67$) and PD. In this study, PD was only performed with the 30- and 35-mm balloons ($n=66$). The rates of treatment success (Eckardt score ≤ 3 and the absence of severe complications or re-treatment) at the 2-year follow-up were significantly greater in the POEM group when compared with PD group (92% vs 54%, $P<.001$). A major limitation of this trial was that patients treated with PD were not treated with a third dilation using a 40-mm balloon prior to being declared treatment failures. Some patients in the study did undergo a 40-mm balloon dilation and success improved from 54% to 76% on the post hoc analysis, but the treatment success rate of POEM was still significantly higher than PD (92%, $P=.008$). The authors of this study stated that the major disadvantage of POEM is the high incidence of reflux esophagitis. In their study, 49% of the patients had reflux esophagitis at the 1-year follow-up, and 8% had a severe grade compared to PD.

A 2019 metaanalysis of 20 studies (1575 patients) compared the therapeutic success of POEM versus LHM. The authors concluded that POEM was associated with greater therapeutic success rates than LHM for achalasia type I (OR 2.97, 95% CI 1.09–8.03; $P=.032$) and type III (OR 3.50, 95% CI 1.39–8.77; $P=.007$) achalasia. POEM and LHM were associated with similar rates of therapeutic success for type II achalasia (OR 1.31, 95% CI 0.48–3.55; $P=.591$). The study demonstrated the treatment efficacy of POEM in all subtypes of achalasia, but POEM is especially beneficial in treating type III achalasia given the ability to perform a longer myotomy.

20. **What are the major problems with POEM, and which patients with achalasia should avoid POEM?**

As stated earlier, POEM is effective for most patients with achalasia but especially patients with type III achalasia. The major downside of POEM is the risk of post-POEM GERD. The American Gastroenterological Association has advised that patients with achalasia treated with POEM are considered at high risk of developing reflux esophagitis. Prior to POEM, patients should be counseled about potential post-POEM GERD and the possible need for indefinite use of antisecretory therapy and/or surveillance endoscopy. POEM should be avoided in patients with a known hiatal hernia and morbid obesity (body mass index [BMI] > 40) secondary to the risk of post-POEM GERD. Other contraindications include the following: liver cirrhosis with portal hypertension, history of radiation therapy involving the distal esophagus, previous endoscopic mucosal resection of the distal esophagus, or radiofrequency ablation of the distal esophagus.

21. **How should we follow a patient with treated achalasia?**

Patients with achalasia, regardless of the type of treatment or symptoms, need physiologic follow-up as all therapies are palliative and focus on alleviating the functional obstruction at LES. There are no guidelines available about the appropriate follow-up interval posttherapy for achalasia, but most experts would recommend yearly to biannual follow-up to assess for symptom recurrence in conjunction with a TBE. The TBE protocol begins with the administration of 240 mL (8 oz) of low-density barium in the standing position; two-on-one spot films are obtained at 1 and 5 minutes to assess liquid emptying and for esophageal stasis. After the assessment of liquid barium emptying, a 13-mm barium tablet is administered. Tablet retention at EGJ for $\geq$ 5 minutes is abnormal. Studies have demonstrated that near complete esophageal emptying (<1 cm retained barium at 1 minute) on TBE is associated with long-term symptom relief. Conversely, postintervention retention of a liquid barium column greater than 50% of the baseline TBE is predictive of symptom persistence and treatment failure. Therefore patients with persistent symptoms or poor esophageal emptying warrant further treatment.

22. **Is achalasia a premalignant condition?**

Longstanding achalasia is associated with the risk of developing squamous cell carcinoma (SCC) of the esophagus. Currently, there are no screening/surveillance guidelines in practice. The presence of a megaesophagus and poor esophageal emptying are important risk factors in developing SCC. Therefore it is reasonable to recommend initiating screening upper endoscopy in patients with achalasia longer than 15 years with concomitant esophageal dilation or tortuosity.

23. **What is the best therapy for a patient with achalasia?**

With the advent and widespread adoption of HRM, the diagnosis of achalasia has increased in both academic medical centers and the community. There are specific examples where the treatment is relatively straightforward. For example, botulinum toxin injection is best utilized in a patient with significant comorbid diseases or a short life expectancy that precludes definitive therapy. POEM is a better therapeutic option in most patients with type III achalasia but should be avoided in patients with a known hiatal hernia and/or morbid obesity (BMI > 40)

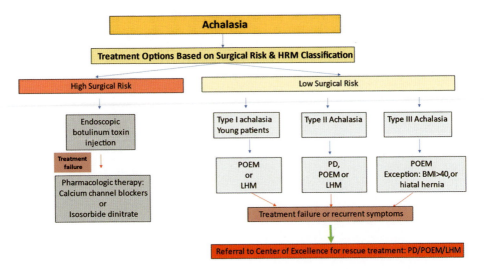

Fig. 3.5 A generalized algorithmic treatment approach to assist with optimal treatment selection in patients with achalasia. *BMI,* Body mass index; *HRM,* high-resolution manometry; *LHM,* laparoscopic Heller myotomy; *PD,* pneumatic dilation; *POEM,* peroral endoscopic myotomy.

secondary to the risk of post-POEM GERD. Younger patients do better with myotomy or POEM. Fig. 3.5 is a suggested treatment approach for patients with achalasia. If available, most experts would advocate a multidisciplinary approach to treat patients with achalasia. The multidisciplinary approach gives our patients the best opportunity for long-term therapeutic success and helps avoid long-term complications.

CLINICAL VIGNETTE

Available Online.

BIBLIOGRAPHY

Available Online.

CHAPTER 4

SWALLOWING DISORDERS AND DYSPHAGIA

Peter R. McNally, DO, MSRF, MACG

 Additional content available online.

1. **What are the five phases of swallowing?**
   - *Anticipatory phase (involuntary)*: Sensing food through sight, smell, and taste stimulates saliva production in anticipation of intake. Saliva lubricates the bolus and makes chewing and swallowing easier.
   - *Oral preparatory phase (voluntary)*: Controlled by the cortex and brainstem, the tongue, teeth, and palate transform food into a bolus that is determined by learned memory to be sufficiently prepared to transport into the pharynx.
   - *Oral transport phase*: Food bolus is propelled into the hypopharynx by the tongue. Once the bolus reaches the tonsillar pillars, it triggers the swallow reflex.
   - *Pharyngeal phase (involuntary)*: Multiple coordinated, but involuntary, muscular contractions and relaxations are triggered by the swallow reflex. They include four subphases: velopharyngeal closure (prevents bolus regurgitation into the nasopharynx), peristaltic contraction of pharyngeal constrictors (propels the food bolus through the pharynx), laryngeal elevation and closure (provides airway protection and prevents aspiration), and upper esophageal sphincter (UES) opening (allowing the bolus to pass from the larynx to esophagus).
   - *Esophageal phase*: The food bolus passes through the UES via involuntary peristaltic contractions. This peristaltic wave clears residue from the pharynx and the esophagus. At the instant that food enters the esophagus, the lower esophageal sphincter (LES) relaxes and remains relaxed until the bolus passes into the stomach via peristalsis.

2. **What is the definition of** *dysphagia?*
   Dysphagia derives from the Greek words *dys* (which means "difficult") and *phagia* (which means "eating") and refers to a subjective difficulty or abnormality in swallowing or passage of food or liquid from the mouth to the stomach. Dysphagia is common, and approximately 1 million new cases are diagnosed annually in the United States. Given the natural atrophy of swallowing muscles (sarcopenia) and changes in mental alertness that often accompany aging, symptoms of dysphagia are especially prevalent in the elderly. Up to 60% of nursing home residents experience dysphagia, and up to half of Americans by the age of 60 experience some swallowing disorder. Aspiration pneumonia is one of the most concerning complications among the elderly.

3. **How is dysphagia clinically classified?**
   Dysphagia can be clinically classified based on either location or etiologic factors. If classified by location, dysphagia can generally be separated into either oropharyngeal dysphagia (also referred to as transfer dysphagia) or esophageal dysphagia (Fig. 4.1). If classified by etiologic factors, dysphagia can be separated into a mechanical disorder (often characterized by dysphagia to solid foods only) or a motility disorder (generally characterized by dysphagia to both solids and liquids).

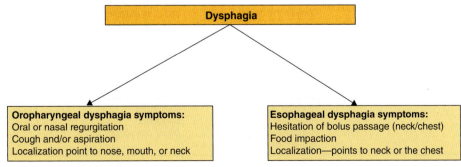

Fig. 4.1 Key clinical features to distinguish between oropharyngeal and esophageal dysphagia.

Oropharyngeal dysphagia is further separated into two categories: oral phase and pharyngeal phase. *Oral-phase* dysphagia is associated with poor formation of and control of the food bolus, which typically results in prolonged retention of the bolus in the oral cavity. It can be accompanied by drooling, food leakage from the mouth, and difficulty initiating swallowing. The *oral phase* of the swallowing mechanism is under voluntary control and can be impaired by decreased lip closure, decreased strength in the muscles of mastication, and limited tongue coordination or movement. *Pharyngeal-phase* dysphagia typically results either from poor propulsion of the bolus by the tongue or obstruction at the UES. The *pharyngeal phase* is under involuntary control, and impairments here may be present as delayed swallow reflex, decreased velopharyngeal closure, resulting in nasal regurgitation, decreased epiglottic movement and decreased laryngeal elevation on swallowing, or disorders or injury to the UES. Depending on the cause of oropharyngeal type, patients may feel a globus sensation in the neck or experience nasal regurgitation, aspiration, and symptoms of reflux.

4. What are the clinical features of oropharyngeal dysphagia?

Oropharyngeal dysphagia results in difficulty transferring food from the mouth to the posterior pharynx. This can lead to symptoms of subjective obstruction in the neck, coughing, choking, regurgitation with either solids or liquids (including nasal regurgitation), drooling, dysphonia, and aspiration pneumonia. Specific physical maneuvers may aid oropharyngeal function and may be used to compensate for deficits.

5. What is the differential diagnosis for oropharyngeal dysphagia?

Oropharyngeal dysphagia can result from discoordination, weak propulsion, or structural abnormalities. Although the differential diagnosis is broad, neurologic or muscular etiologic factors are most commonly seen in practice and account for approximately 80% of cases in older adults. Of that group, cerebrovascular accidents account for the vast majority. See Table 4.1 for a more extensive differential and Fig. 4.2 for a helpful screening and diagnostic clinical algorithm for oropharyngeal dysphagia.

Table 4.1 Differential Diagnosis for Oropharyngeal Dysphagia.

IATROGENIC	METABOLIC	MYOPATHIC
Corrosive (pill injury or ingestion)	Amyloidosis	Connective tissue disease
Functional dysphagia	Cushing syndrome	(scleroderma, Sjögren syndrome, systemic
Medication side effects (chemotherapy, neuroleptics, anticholinergics, antihistamines, antihypertensives, steroids, and others less common)	Hypothyroidism with myxedema	lupus erythematosus)
Postsurgical	Thyrotoxicosis	Dermatomyositis
Radiation	Wilson disease	Myotonic dystrophy
		Myasthenia gravis
		Metabolic myopathy
		Oculopharyngeal dystrophy
		Polymyositis
		Paraneoplastic syndromes
		Sarcoidosis

INFECTIOUS	NEUROLOGIC	STRUCTURAL
AIDS (CNS involvement)	Amyotrophic lateral sclerosis	Cervical webs
Botulism	Brainstem tumors	Congenital disorders (cleft
Diphtheria	Cranial nerve palsies	palate, for example)
Lyme disease	Cerebrovascular accident	Cricopharyngeal bar
Mucosal inflammation	Dementia	Dental anomalies
(abscess,	Guillain-Barré syndrome	Extrinsic compression (goiter,
Candida, CMV, HSV, pharyngitis,	Head trauma	lymphadenopathy, neoplasm)
tuberculosis)	Huntington disease	Oropharyngeal neoplasm
Rabies	Metabolic encephalopathies	Prosthetics
Syphilis	Multiple sclerosis	Skeletal abnormalities and
	Parkinson disease	osteophytes
	Poliomyelitis (bulbar)	Xerostomia
	Post-polio syndrome	Zenker diverticulum
	Tardive dyskinesia	

AIDS, Acquired immune deficiency syndrome; *CMV*, cytomegalovirus; *CNS*, central nervous system; *HSV*, herpes simplex virus.

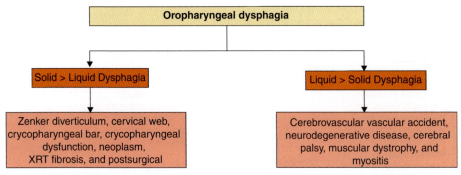

Fig. 4.2 Categories of oropharyngeal dysphagia distinguished by the severity of solid versus liquid dysphagia. *XRT*, Radiation.

6. What is the best test to evaluate oropharyngeal dysphagia?

A careful history and detailed physical examination are essential first steps, and most patients with oropharyngeal dysphagia will require radiographic imaging. Because of the rapid sequence of events that comprise a swallow, static barium studies are often not adequate to evaluate the oropharynx. The preferred initial study is video fluoroscopy or modified barium swallow. Some centers may also perform a fiberoptic endoscopic evaluation of swallowing, which allows direct imaging for structural abnormalities and the acquisition of biopsies if required. Routine esophagogastroduodenoscopy and esophageal manometry have a limited and complementary role in this population.

7. What is the definition of *odynophagia?*

Odynophagia derives from the Greek roots *odyno* (which means "pain") and *phagia* (which means "eating") and refers to pain with swallowing. Odynophagia can accompany dysphagia or exist independently.

8. What is the definition of globus sensation?

Globus sensation is defined as an intermittent or persistent sensation of a foreign body or lump in the throat between meals and in the absence of dysphagia or odynophagia. This was previously referred to as *globus hystericus* because of erroneous suspicion by prior generations of physicians that the cause may stem from factors produced by the uterus.

9. Is dysphagia an alarming symptom?

Yes. The presence of dysphagia suggests an organic abnormality and mandates additional evaluation. Although dysphagia may occur because of benign processes, it is neither a natural phenomenon nor a normal result of aging and always requires additional evaluation.

10. When is it appropriate to evaluate dysphagia related to a cerebrovascular accident?

Dysphagia is common after a stroke (at least 25% of patients) and is a risk factor for pneumonia and aspiration. Although early evaluation is reasonable to minimize these complications, most patients with dysphagia after a cerebrovascular accident will note improvement within the first 2 weeks. Because of this, invasive procedures such as percutaneous gastrostomy should be avoided for at least the first 2 weeks after a cerebrovascular accident, with the hope that there will be an improvement in the interim.

11. Do patients accurately localize the site of dysphagia?

Patients with oropharyngeal dysphagia generally recognize that their dysfunction is in the oropharynx and often point to the cervical region when asked to localize the source of their symptoms. For patients with esophageal dysphagia, however, symptoms may not be a reliable predictor of location. Localization of dysphagia to the distal esophagus (near the xiphoid process) is generally viewed as specific for a distal esophageal process; however, suprasternal (or upper chest) localization can be referred from a distal process in approximately one-third of cases and is viewed as less specific.

12. What is the differential diagnosis of esophageal dysphagia?

Esophageal dysphagia is generally related to either a motility disorder (such as achalasia, spasm, nutcracker esophagus, scleroderma) or a mechanical disorder (stricture, rings, web, diverticulum, cancer). *A motility disorder is suggested by dysphagia to solids and liquids, whereas a mechanical disorder is suggested by dysphagia to solids only.* See Table 4.2 for a more extensive differential diagnosis.

Table 4.2 Differential Diagnosis for Esophageal Dysphagia.

MECHANICAL	MOTOR
Caustic of NG tube stricture	Achalasia
Cardiovascular compromise (dysphagia lusoria)	Diffuse esophageal spasm
Diverticulum	Esophagogastric junction outflow obstruction
Eosinophilic esophagitis	Functional dysphagia
Esophageal rings or webs	Ineffective esophageal motility
Infectious esophagitis	Jackhammer esophagus
Medication-induced injury	Nutcracker esophagus
Peptic stricture	Scleroderma
Radiation injury	
Tumor (benign or malignant)	

NG, Nasogastric.

13. **What are the key questions to ask of a patient with suspected esophageal dysphagia?**

A careful history can often clarify the etiologic factors of esophageal dysphagia. The key points to clarify on the initial evaluation are as follows:
- *Chronology:* How long have symptoms been present? How often do they occur? Are they progressing with time?
- *Dysphagia:* What type of foods cause problems (solids, liquids, or both)? Where does the food become stuck? How long does it stick for?
- *Regurgitation:* Does food or liquid come back up to the throat or mouth? Does this occur when eating, soon after the meal is over, or at a much later time? Can this occur hours after the meal is complete? Is it more likely to occur when lying down or sitting up? Does it taste sour or bitter?
- *Cough:* Is there coughing or choking during or after eating? Does this occur with swallows, soon after swallowing, or after the meal is over?
- *Pain:* Is there throat or chest pain either while eating or afterward? Where is the pain located? Does it radiate anywhere else?

14. **At what luminal diameter will most patients experience symptoms of dysphagia?**

This exact issue was evaluated by radiologist Richard Schatzki in the 1950s and 1960s. He reported that for patients with a distal esophageal ring (now named the *Schatzki ring*), *dysphagia was almost universal if the diameter of the lumen was less than 13 mm. If the diameter was greater than 20 mm, no one was symptomatic.* Intermittent symptoms could be seen in some people at ranges in between. It is because of these seminal studies that most barium tablets used in a traditional radiographic dysphagia evaluation are 13 mm in diameter.

15. **What diagnostic studies are available to evaluate a patient with esophageal dysphagia?**

Much can be deciphered by a careful history; however, diagnostic studies are usually necessary to arrive at a diagnosis and optimize therapy. To evaluate dysphagia, three main diagnostic modalities are currently employed, plus other emerging studies. The key studies appear in the following list. Figs. 4.3, 4.4, and 4.5 show a representative example of achalasia using fluoroscopy, endoscopy, and manometry, respectively.
- *Fluoroscopy:* The classic fluoroscopic study employed is a barium esophagram, in which contrast is ingested while serial x-rays are obtained. This allows visualization of structural lesions such as rings, webs, bars, strictures, masses, diverticula, and fistulas. It also may detect any gross motility abnormalities such as spasms and achalasia.
- *Timed barium esophagogram:* While standing, the patient swallows 100–250 mL of barium sulfate (45% weight/volume) over 15–20 seconds, then plain radiographs of the esophagus are taken at 1, 2, and 5 minutes in the left posterior oblique position. The height at each time interval is measured from the horizontal line at the bottom and the top of the barium column. The diameter of the esophagus is measured at the widest part of the barium column perpendicular to the long axis of the esophagus.
- *Endoscopy:* A flexible fiberoptic tube is passed from the mouth to the small bowel and allows direct visualization, biopsy acquisition, and potential therapeutic options (such as dilation). This can also be combined with endoscopic ultrasound if available to evaluate for possible extrinsic compression or submucosal processes.
- *Manometry:* A catheter with numerous pressure sensors is placed, allowing measurement of the UES, esophageal body, and LES. This study evaluates intraluminal pressure and coordination of pressure activity. This is the most sensitive study for the detection of an esophageal motility disorder but is usually reserved for those cases in which the diagnosis is not readily apparent with the tests detailed previously.

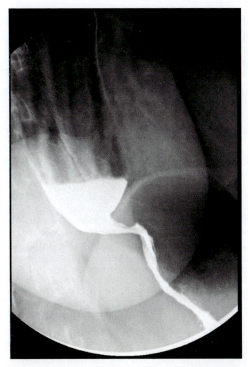

Fig. 4.3 A representative fluoroscopic image of a patient with established achalasia. Note the dilated esophagus and classic bird's beak appearance (representing the tonically contracted lower esophageal sphincter).

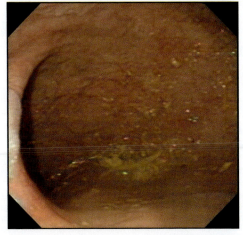

Fig. 4.4 An extreme endoscopic image of a patient with advanced achalasia. Note the dilated esophagus, atonic mucosa, and scant-retained food particles.

- *Impedance*: Impedance allows direct measurement of bolus flow and can be a useful adjunct to manometry. It is mainly used for the detection of nonacid reflux but can be employed if needed in the work-up of dysphagia.
- *Impedance planimetry (EndoFLIP)*: It can be used to evaluate esophageal compliance and has been shown to have benefits in predicting prognosis for patients with achalasia, eosinophilic esophagitis (EoE) and the evaluation of patients with esophageal unresponsive to proton pump inhibitor (PPI) therapy (Fig. 4.6).

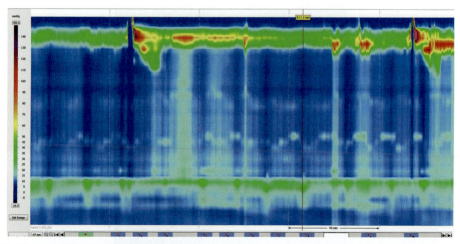

Fig. 4.5 A representative high-resolution esophageal manometry showing a patient with achalasia (type II pattern). Note the absence of any esophageal peristaltic waves in this patient with achalasia, as compared with normal peristalsis shown in eFig. 4.1. Manometry is the most sensitive test for the detection of achalasia and may detect abnormalities before either radiographic or endoscopic changes are noted. *2–6-FEDAETEGJ-DIEGJOOEoEFLIPLA BPPI* . (Adapted from Triggs J, Pandolfino J. Recent advances in dysphagia management [version 1; peer review: 3 approved]. F1000Res 2019;8(F1000 Faculty Rev):1527. https://f1000research.com/articles/8-1527.)

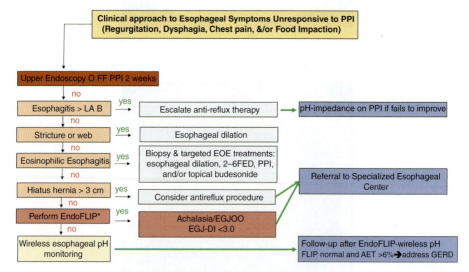

Fig. 4.6 Clinical approach for patients presenting with esophageal symptoms unresponsive to PPI. *2–6FED*, Two to six food elimination diets; *AET*, acid exposure time; *EGJ-DI*, esophagogastric junction-distensibility index; *EGJOO*, esophagogastric junction outflow obstruction; *EoE*, eosinophilic esophagitis; *FLIP*, functional luminal imaging probe; *LA B*, Los Angeles classification B; *PPI*, proton pump inhibitor. (Adapted from Triggs J, Pandolfino J. Recent advances in dysphagia management [version 1; peer review: 3 approved]. F1000Res 2019;8(F1000 Faculty Rev):1527. https://f1000research.com/articles/8-1527.)

16. What is the best initial test for a patient with esophageal dysphagia?

This is a controversial area and there is a debate as to whether a barium esophagram or endoscopy should be the initial test of choice. Endoscopy offers diagnostic value as well as the ability to obtain biopsies to clarify etiologic factors and the ability to perform a therapeutic intervention, such as dilation. Barium studies may provide more information on patients with proximal lesions or motility disorders. There are no official guidelines recommending one approach versus the other, and the initial test of choice is often based on local practice patterns and regional expertise.

17. What is the most common cause of dysphagia in young patients today?
EoE is the most common cause of dysphagia in young patients today and is increasing in both incidence and recognition. The etiologic impetus of EoE is believed to be an allergic diathesis in which eosinophilic deposition leads to remodeling of the esophagus and decreased distensibility, characterized by the development of rings and strictures. The diagnosis is made by esophageal biopsy demonstrating more than 15 eosinophils per high-powered field. Typical endoscopic findings include circumferential rings, longitudinal furrows, and white plaques (representing eosinophilic microabscesses), although up to 20% of endoscopies may appear normal on gross appearance. For this reason, biopsies of the esophagus should be taken during endoscopy for all patients with dysphagia.

18. What is the preferred treatment for patients with documented esophageal eosinophilia?
Approximately 25% of patients with esophageal eosinophilia will have marked improvement or resolution of their symptoms with PPIs. For this reason, the term *eosinophilic esophagitiseosinophilic esophagitis* is reserved for those patients with continued eosinophilic tissue deposition despite acid suppressive therapy. For these patients, there is data to support the use of steroids (both topical and systemic), dietary modification, and intermittent endoscopic dilation. There is no clear consensus as to what the optimal initial therapy should be and no good head-to-head trials at present. Most authorities initiate treatment with topical steroids, usually either swallowed fluticasone (220–440 mcg twice daily) or viscous budesonide (1 mg twice daily).

19. Is it safe to perform endoscopic dilation for patients with EoE?
Early reports of dilation for patients with EoE suggested deep mucosal tears and an increased risk of perforation, prompting the medical establishment to recommend against dilation unless medical therapy had failed and a clear stricture was present. However, more recent studies have suggested that the rate of perforation in expert hands is much lower than previously reported (approximately 0.3% in the largest series to date) and may be a safe treatment option if performed with care. Of note, although dilation is effective for relieving dysphagia, it has no effect on the underlying inflammation and therapeutic relief will likely be transient.

20. What is a Schatzki ring?
A Schatzki ring is a thin membrane found at the squamocolumnar junction (separating the esophagus and stomach) composed of mucosa and submucosa. There is debate as to whether it is a vestigial structure or a result of reflux and inflammation. It is seen in approximately 15% of adults older than the age of 50 and is a benign process. It can cause intermittent dysphagia to solids and is treated with dilation. There are data to suggest that acid suppressive therapy may decrease the recurrence of the ring after dilation. The classic clinical scenario is the "steakhouse syndrome" wherein a businessperson is eating dinner at a steakhouse, socializing and taking larger bites than normal, and subsequently develops food impaction from a piece of meat lodging at the ring.

21. What is Plummer-Vinson syndrome?
Plummer-Vinson syndrome is a rare condition characterized by the presence of an esophageal web, dysphagia, and iron-deficiency anemia. An esophageal web is a thin, horizontal membrane of stratified squamous epithelium, which typically is eccentric and does not circle the entire lumen. Treatment consists of iron repletion and dilation and rupture of the esophageal web. Patients with Plummer-Vinson syndrome have a higher risk of developing esophageal squamous carcinoma.

22. What is a Zenker diverticulum?
A Zenker diverticulum is a mucosal outpouching (or diverticulum) in the hypopharynx. This is immediately proximal to the cricopharyngeus and often is a result of a relative obstruction in this region. Symptoms consist of dysphagia and regurgitation, often delayed. The best study to identify a Zenker diverticulum is a barium swallow. Treatment consists of surgical diverticulectomy with or without myotomy, rigid endoscopic myotomy, and flexible endoscopic cricopharyngeal myotomy.

23. What is the Chicago classification of esophageal motility?
Because of the increased data presented with high-resolution esophageal manometry, new classification schemes have been proposed to guide the use of results. The Chicago classification is currently the main system in use for the classification of esophageal motility disorders via high-resolution esophageal manometry. The main steps of the Chicago classification are the following: (1) assessment of the gastroesophageal junction and (2) assessment of esophageal contractility. Based on these two parameters, studies can be divided into disorders that are clearly abnormal and not seen in normal individuals, as compared with borderline abnormalities of uncertain clinical significance. The main classification categories of the Chicago classification are listed in Box 4.1.

Box 4.1 Chicago Classification of Esophageal Motility: High-Resolution Manometry

Achalasia
EGJ outflow obstruction
Abnormal motor function
Esophageal spasm
Hypercontractile (jackhammer) esophagus
Absent peristalsis
Borderline motor function
Frequent failed peristalsis
Weak peristalsis
Rapid contraction
Hypertensive (nutcracker) esophagus
Normal

EGJ, Esophagogastric junction.

---

24. What is nutcracker esophagus?

The phrase *nutcracker esophagus* was coined by Dr. Donald Castell, who is perhaps the world's foremost author-ity on esophageal motility. The term was used to describe a condition in which the esophageal pressures are so high that they could perhaps crack a nut (hence the name). The normal amplitude of esophageal contractions is between 30 and 180 mm Hg, and nutcracker esophagus was defined as an average esophageal amplitude of more than 180 mm Hg. Symptoms of chest pain and dysphagia have both been reported with this condition, although it remains unclear whether the high amplitude is a direct cause of symptoms or a result of some other process. Treatment consists of reflux therapy (if appropriate) and smooth muscle relaxants (such as calcium channel block-ers or nitrates).

25. How common is esophageal spasm?

Esophageal spasm has been defined as an uncoordinated or rapid contraction in association with symptoms such as chest pain and dysphagia. Although this is commonly cited as the source of unexplained chest pain and dysphagia, several large studies suggest that this is actually uncommon, with one large study suggesting spasm is present in only 3% of patients with unexplained chest pain or dysphagia. The gold standard for diagnosis is esophageal manometry, although barium radiography can also be highly suggestive. Treatment consists of reflux therapy (if appropriate) and smooth muscle relaxants (such as calcium channel blockers or nitrates).

26. What is a scleroderma esophagus?

Scleroderma is associated with esophageal motility disorders in greater than 90% of patients. The characteristic pattern is a hypotensive LES and either aperistalsis or weak peristalsis; however, multiple variations can be seen and not all patients with scleroderma have this pattern. Colloquially, a manometry pattern of aperistalsis with a hypotensive LES has been referred to as a *scleroderma pattern* or as *scleroderma esophagus.* However, it should be noted that this pattern is not pathognomonic for scleroderma and can be seen in other conditions.

27. Can cardiovascular abnormalities cause dysphagia?

Occasionally, vascular anomalies can cause dysphagia by compressing the esophagus. This is referred to as *dys-phagia lusoria* but is relatively rare. The diagnosis can be suggested by barium esophagram and can be confirmed by endoscopic ultrasound or computed tomography. In our experience, treatment is usually conservative. In older adults, a large aneurysm of the thoracic aorta or severe atherosclerosis can result in impingement of the esopha-gus and is referred to as *dysphagia aortica.*

28. What is functional dysphagia?

Functional dysphagia is defined by the Rome III criteria as a sense of solid or liquid food lodging or passing abnor-mally through the esophagus in the absence of gastroesophageal reflux, a structural disorder, or a defined motil-ity disorder. Although the cause is not known, this is believed to be a manifestation of visceral hypersensitivity. Patients should be reassured and instructed to avoid any known precipitants. Treatment is largely supportive.

29. How should I approach a patient with esophageal dysphagia?

The evaluation of dysphagia is not standardized, and variation can exist based on local practice patterns. Societal guidelines have not been updated in more than a decade, and it remains controversial whether an upper endos-copy or barium esophagram should be the initial study. A suggested algorithm is detailed in Fig. 4.7.

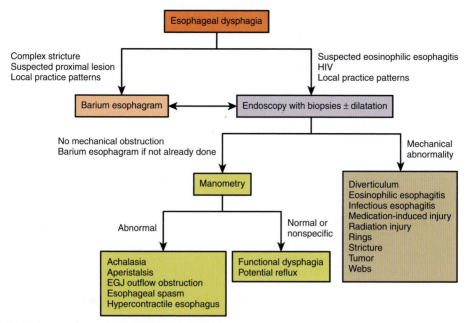

Fig. 4.7 A suggested approach to esophageal dysphagia. *EGJ*, Esophagogastric junction; *HIV*, human immunodeficiency virus.

ACKNOWLEDGMENTS

The author acknowledges the previous contributions to this chapter by Francis C. Okeke, MD, MPH, and John O. Clarke, MD.

CLINICAL VIGNETTE

Available Online.

BIBLIOGRAPHY

Available Online.

WEBSITES

Available Online.

CHAPTER 5

ESOPHAGEAL CANCER

Nimish Vakil, MD, FACP, FACG, AGAF, FASGE

 Additional content available online.

1. How common is esophageal cancer?

Cancer of the esophagus accounts for 1% of all newly diagnosed cancers in the United States. The American Cancer Society's estimates for esophageal cancer in the United States for 2022 are about 20,640 new esophageal cancer cases diagnosed (16,510 in men and 4,130 in women) and about 16,410 deaths from esophageal cancer (13,250 in men and 3,160 in women). The lifetime risk of esophageal cancer in the United States is approximately 1 in 125 men and 1 in 435 women.

2. Is the incidence of esophageal cancer increasing?

No, the incidence of esophageal carcinoma in the United States has plateaued for the last decade. However, significant changes have been observed in the cell types of esophageal cancer seen. Forty years ago, squamous cell carcinoma (SCCA) was the most common form of esophageal cancer in the United States; now, adenocarcinoma (AdenoCA) is the most common form of esophageal carcinoma (Fig. 5.1).

Esophageal cancer was once much more common in Black patients than in Whites, but it is now about equally as common, as rates have fallen in Blacks and increased slightly in Whites during the past few decades. SCCA is the most common type of cancer of the esophagus among Blacks, whereas AdenoCA is more common in Whites.

3. Are there geographical variations in the incidence of esophageal cancer?

Yes. The incidence of esophageal cancer varies internationally by nearly 16-fold. For example, esophageal cancer rates in the "esophageal cancer belt" (Iran, Northern China, India, and parts of Africa) are 10–100 times higher than in the United States. Exposure to tobacco, low levels of soil selenium, high ingestion of nitrosamines and hot liquids, and low intake of fruits and vegetables are thought to be causative factors. Some countries in Asia (such as Singapore) are reporting an increase in the rate of esophageal AdenoCA suggesting a change may be taking place in the epidemiology of cancer in Asia.

4. What are the most common types of esophageal cancer?

Worldwide, the most common type of esophageal cancer is SCCA (90%–95% of all esophageal cancers), whereas in the United States, the incidence of SCCA has dwindled during the last 40 years. Prior to 1970, SCCA was the most common cell type in the United States, but in recent years, AdenoCA has become the most common type of

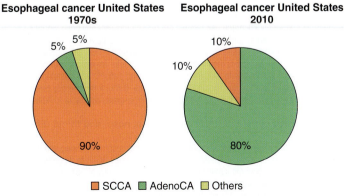

Trends in esophageal cancer cell type
1970s versus 2010

Esophageal cancer United States 1970s

Esophageal cancer United States 2010

■ SCCA ■ AdenoCA ■ Others

Fig. 5.1 Comparison of esophageal cancer cell types: 1970s versus 2010 demonstrating a shift from squamous cell carcinoma (SCCA) as the predominant esophageal cancer cell type in the 1970s to adenocarcinoma (AdenoCA) cell type in 2010.

esophageal cancer (Fig. 5.1). A decline in tobacco use and smoking is thought to be responsible for the decline in SCCA, whereas the epidemic of obesity and gastroesophageal reflux disease (GERD) are responsible for the increase in AdenoCA. Recent studies suggest that while esophageal AdenoCA increased at a rapid rate in the United States from 2004 to 2014, the rate of increase may be slowing.

5. What is the association between bisphosphonates and esophageal cancer?

The use of bisphosphonates has been linked to esophageal AdenoCA and SCCA in postmarketing surveillance. Recommendations were made in the past to avoid bisphosphonates in the Barrett esophagus (BE). Recent studies have cast doubt on this association and there is no clear consensus on avoiding bisphosphonates in BE.

6. What are the current recommendations for screening of esophageal cancer in the United States?

Currently, there is no cost-effective method of screening for esophageal cancer in the United States. Several patient subgroups are at increased risk for esophageal cancer and should be independently considered for endoscopic screening. These are patients with:
- Achalasia
- Lye ingestion
- Plummer-Vinson syndrome
- Tylosis

There are no strict guidelines for endoscopic cancer screening for patients with achalasia or previous lye ingestion, but some experts suggest endoscopic examination and biopsy at the 15-year mark and the need for a low threshold to investigate dyspeptic and dysphagia symptoms. Dysphagia symptoms associated with Plummer-Vinson syndrome should be investigated with endoscopy and biopsy and iron deficiency corrected. Patients with tylosis should begin endoscopic surveillance at the age of 30 years. Most cases of esophageal cancer in these patients have been noted in the distal esophagus, so attention should be focused on this area during the examination. BE is associated with increased risk for AdenoCA of the esophagus. However, optimal cost-effective screening for the identification of BE is debated. New guidelines from the American College of Gastroenterology recommend a single-screening endoscopy in patients with GERD with three or more risk factors. The risk factors to be considered are male sex, age >50 years, White race, tobacco smoking, obesity, and a family history of BE or esophageal cancer in a first-degree relative. Once BE is identified, periodic esophagogastroduodenoscopy (EGD) and biopsy are recommended. The reader is referred to Chapters 7 and 62 for additional information.

7. What gastrointestinal disorders are associated with increased risk for esophageal cancer?
- Achalasia: SCCA
- Plummer-Vinson syndrome: SCCA
- BE: AdenoCA
- Celiac disease: SCCA
- Prior gastrectomy: SCCA

8. What are the typical clinical features of esophageal cancer?

Although SCCA typically occurs in the upper and middle esophagus and AdenoCA typically occurs in the distal esophagus, both have similar clinical presentations. The most common age of onset for esophageal cancer is 65–74 years. Typical clinical features of esophageal cancer are shown in Table 5.1.

9. What are the risk factors for esophageal cancer?

Risk factors for esophageal cancer vary according to cell type and are outlined in Table 5.2. Tobacco and alcohol are the most commonly identified risk factors, but obesity has recently been identified as an important independent risk factor. BE is an acquired condition associated with metaplastic replacement of normal squamous epithelium with a columnar lining caused by chronic gastroesophageal reflux. The incidence of AdenoCA increases nearly 40-fold in patients with BE and is the most significant risk factor for esophageal cancer. It is estimated that 5% of patients with BE will eventually develop invasive cancer, and patients with histologically proven BE require lifelong surveillance because of this risk. The annual risk is 0.4%–0.5%. It is generally believed that the disease progresses from Barrett metaplasia to low-grade dysplasia to high-grade dysplasia to AdenoCA.

10. Is there a link between current or past history of ear, nose, and throat (ENT) conditions and esophageal cancer?

Yes. This probably reflects exposure to common SCCA risk factors, such as smoking and alcohol. Although some studies have suggested the incidence of synchronous or metachronous SCCA to be between 3% and 14%, there are no accepted guidelines for periodic surveillance. The American Society of Gastrointestinal Endoscopy does recommend a single EGD to evaluate for synchronous esophageal cancer in patients with ENT malignancy. It is prudent for caregivers to have a low threshold for the investigation of aerodigestive symptoms among these patients and to engage in a regular, directed inquiry about symptoms of dysphagia.

Table 5.1 Clinical Features of Esophageal Cancer.

CLINICAL FEATURES	FREQUENCY (%)	SIGNIFICANCE
Peak age at onset	65–75	Comorbidities often preclude operability
Sex (male:female)	4:1	Much more common in men
Race (Black:White)	50:50	SCCA > Black men AdenoCA > White men
Dysphagia	90	Often advanced disease
Anorexia and weight loss	75	
Odynophagia	50	Suggests tumor ulceration
Chest pain, often radiates to back	Less frequent	Implies invasion of neuromediastinal structures
Vocal cord paralysis	Less frequent	Suggests invasion more typical of SCCA
Cough and pneumonia	Less frequent	Esophageal obstruction, aspiration, fistula
Hoarseness	Less frequent	High GERD, coincident ENT malignancy, SCCA invasion
Hiccups	Less frequent	Diaphragmatic involvement

AdenoCA, Adenocarcinoma; *ENT,* ear, nose, and throat; *GERD,* gastroesophageal reflux disease; *SCCA,* squamous cell carcinoma.

Table 5.2 Risk Factors for Esophageal Cancer.

RISK FACTORS	SQUAMOUS CELL CARCINOMA	ADENOCARCINOMA
Tobacco use	+	+
Alcohol use	+	−
Barrett esophagus	−	+
Frequent gastroesophageal reflux	−	+
Body mass index >30 kg/m²	−	+
Low socioeconomic status	+	−
Prior caustic lye ingestion	+	−
Diet: high *N*-nitroso compounds, pickled vegetables, toxic fungi, areca nuts or betel quid, hot beverages, low selenium, and zinc	+	−
Human papillomavirus	+	?

11. What genetic condition is highly associated with SCCA of the esophagus?

Nonepidermolytic palmoplantar keratoderma (tylosis) is a rare autosomal-dominant disorder defined by a genetic abnormality at chromosome 17q25 and is the only recognized familial syndrome that predisposes patients to SCCA of the esophagus. It is characterized by hyperkeratosis of the palms and soles, as well as by thickening of the oral mucosa, and in affected families, it confers up to a 40%–92% risk of SCCA of the esophagus by the age of 70 years.

12. What types of cancer have been reported to metastasize to the esophagus?

Metastatic carcinoma of the esophagus is unusual, but melanoma and breast cancer are the most common.

13. **What is the prognosis for esophageal cancer presenting with dysphagia?**

The prognosis is poor; 50%–60% of patients presenting with dysphagia have incurable locally advanced disease or metastasis. Two factors seem to be responsible for this: tumors are usually far advanced before sufficient luminal narrowing occurs to cause obstructive symptoms, and the lack of an outer esophageal serosa reduces the resistance to local spread. Recent studies show that the overall 5-year survival rates of esophageal cancer are improving. This may be due to improvements in surgical techniques and adjuvant therapy. Endoscopic surveillance programs in BE may also play a role in identifying early esophageal cancer.

14. **Is infection with *Helicobacter pylori* associated with increased risk for esophageal cancer?**

No. There is actually an inverse relationship between *H. pylori* infection and the risk for the development of AdenoCA in the esophagus. The prevalence of the more virulent cagA+ strain of *H. pylori* is lower in patients with more severe complications of GERD. Also, the odds of having BE complicated by dysplasia or cancer are reduced more than twofold in patients infected with cagA+ strains.

15. **What are the American Joint Committee on Cancer (AJCC) tumor, node, metastasis (TNM) staging criteria for esophageal cancer?**

(**T**) the extent of the **t**umor growth, (**N**) lymph **n**ode involvement, and (**M**) **m**etastatic spread of the tumor, see https://www.cancer.org/cancer/types/esophagus-cancer/detection-diagnosis-staging/staging.html.

16. **What are the general principles that guide the management of esophageal cancer?**

Interdisciplinary planning is essential in the management of patients with esophageal cancer. Interventions are based on operability ("fitness" to tolerate surgery), stage of disease, and cell type.

17. **What AJCC stage of esophageal cancer is considered amenable to endoscopic treatment?**

Consideration of endoscopic resection (ER) for early esophageal cancer requires precise staging and the use of high-frequency endoscopic ultrasound (EUS) (Fig. 5.2). A comprehensive subclassification scheme has been proposed for early esophageal cancers and is useful in deciding on ER. According to this classification, mucosal tumors are divided into types based on the depth of invasion:

Tis: Malignant cells confined to the epithelium by the basement membrane.

T1: Tumor invades the lamina propria, muscularis mucosa, or submucosa.

T1a: Tumor invades the lamina propria or muscularis mucosa.

T1b: Tumor invades the submucosa.

Endoscopic therapies are now the preferred treatment for Tis and T1a lesions while esophagectomy is an alternative.

ER techniques include endoscopic mucosal resection (EMR) and endoscopic submucosal dissection. Both techniques require specialized skill and equipment and carry potential procedural risks (postresection bleeding [10%], perforation [2%–5%], and stricture [5%–17%]) that need to be thoroughly discussed with the patient. Description of these ER techniques and other evolving ablative therapies is beyond the scope of this chapter (see the referenced website for video demonstration and further description).

18. **What is the standard of care for "fit" patients with localized tumors?**

Endoscopic therapies are now the preferred treatment for Tis and T1a lesions (Figs. 5.3 and 5.4). Surgical resection is still the standard of care for T1b disease. In expert surgical hands, patients with stage I disease have a 5-year survival of 40%–50%. The reader is referred to Chapter 73 for details about surgical options. Radiation therapy alone can cure a minority of patients with SCCA and has been supplanted by combination therapy. Preoperative chemotherapy is of benefit in patients with AdenoCA. Preoperative chemoradiation has been shown to confer a survival benefit, and a meta-analysis supports the use of chemoradiation preoperatively. However, postoperative mortality may be increased and the exact population that benefits is not clear. Chemotherapy alone is now increasingly used as an induction therapy prior to surgery. Stage-directed therapy is evolving as new endoscopic and minimally invasive surgical modalities become available.

19. **What are the treatment options for limited disease (stage I)?**

Figs 5.3 and 5.4 show the stage-based approach to treatment of esophageal cancer. Surgery is the treatment of choice for localized SCCA and AdenoCA, if the submucosa or muscularis are involved. Chemotherapy and radiation are not used as adjuvants for early mucosal cancers. Surgical therapy consists of resection of the tumor with anastomosis of the stomach with the cervical esophagus (gastric pull-up) or interposition of the colon to reestablish gastrointestinal continuity (Chapter 73). Results are better in hospitals that perform this surgery frequently and poorer in small hospitals that perform the surgery infrequently.

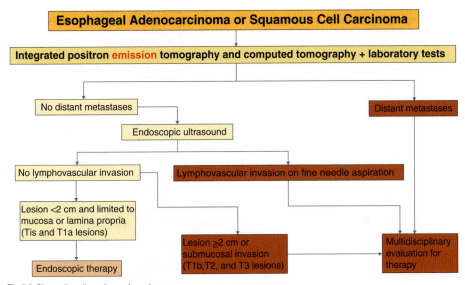

Fig. 5.2 Diagnostic pathway in esophageal cancer.

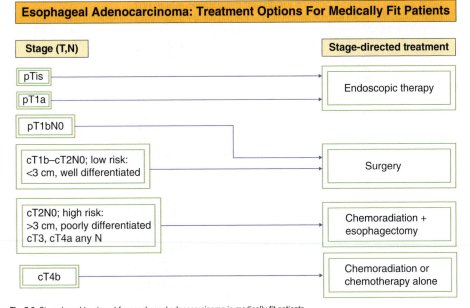

Fig. 5.3 Stage-based treatment for esophageal adenocarcinoma in medically fit patients.

20. **What are the treatment options for locally advanced disease (stages II and III)?**

Figs 5.3 and 5.4 show the approach to patients with stage II and III disease. A recent meta-analysis has shown that a multimodality approach consisting of chemotherapy and radiation followed by surgery (triple therapy) offers the best likelihood of cure. Triple therapy is aggressive and expensive and has a high side-effect rate. Patients who are in poor general condition may elect to have palliative therapy after balancing the low probability of cure against the morbidity of treatment. Combined modality therapy using chemoradiation followed by surgery or definitive chemoradiation in patients who cannot or will not undergo surgery are the currently recommended treatments.

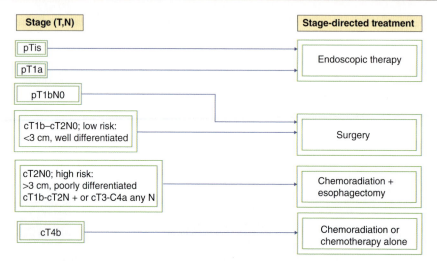

Esophageal Squamous Cell Carcinoma: Treatment Options For Medically Fit Patients

Stage (T,N)

Stage-directed treatment

| pTis | | |
| pT1a | → | Endoscopic therapy |

| pT1bN0 | | |
| cT1b–cT2N0; low risk: <3 cm, well differentiated | → | Surgery |

| cT2N0; high risk: >3 cm, poorly differentiated cT1b-cT2N + or cT3-C4a any N | → | Chemoradiation + esophagectomy |

| cT4b | → | Chemoradiation or chemotherapy alone |

Fig. 5.4 Stage-based treatment for squamous cell carcinoma in medically fit patients.

21. **What are the treatment options for distant metastases (stage IV)?**

Distant metastases make esophageal cancer incurable and therapy is palliative. External beam irradiation, radiation therapy, and chemotherapy are frequently used and may offer small increases in survival rates with the trade-off of systemic side effects. In patients with dysphagia, a number of palliative measures are possible but do not prolong survival.

   Endoscopic options for palliation of malignant dysphagia include the following:
   - Esophageal dilation—transient relief
   - Endoscopic laser (ND:YAG)
   - Endoscopic injection (absolute alcohol)
   - Argon plasma coagulation
   - EMR
   - Photodynamic therapy
   - Placement of prosthetic self-expanding plastic stent or self-expanding metal stent

22. **What does the future hold for patients at risk for the development of esophageal cancer?**

Prevention of esophageal cancer by lifestyle modification is a goal, but the US epidemic of obesity and resurgence in the popularity of tobacco and alcohol among young adults is cause for pessimism that we will achieve this goal. Early detection (selective screening of at-risk groups) and refinement of endoscopic and minimally invasive surgical techniques complemented with targeted radio- and chemotherapy offer great optimism for improved survival and decreased morbidity caused by this devastating disease. Advances in the chemoprevention of esophageal cancer hold great promise. Although definitive proof is lacking, there is a significant amount of suggestive evidence that aspirin, nonsteroidal anti-inflammatory drugs, cyclooxygenase-2 inhibitors, proton pump inhibitors (PPIs), and even statins may have a beneficial role in chemoprevention for selected patients. A recent study in BE showed that high-dose PPI therapy with aspirin reduced the rate of dysplasia and cancer in BE. Immunotherapy may offer survival benefits for patients with advanced disease in the future.

CLINICAL VIGNETTE

Available Online

BIBLIOGRAPHY

Available Online

WEBSITES

Available Online

CHAPTER 6

ESOPHAGEAL ANOMALIES, INFECTIONS, AND NONACID INJURIES

Meghana Golla, MD and Dhyanesh A. Patel, MD

 Additional content available online.

1. **What is the difference between a ring and a web?**
   Web: Thin (<2 mm), eccentric membrane that protrudes into the esophageal lumen and most commonly occurs in the *proximal* esophagus (Fig. 6.1A).
   Ring: Thin (2–5 mm), concentric extension of tissue in the *distal* esophagus containing squamous and columnar epithelium (Fig. 6.1B). They are often associated with a hiatal hernia.

2. **What are the three different types of esophageal rings?**
   Different types of esophageal rings are depicted in Table 6.1.

3. **What are the clinical symptoms associated with esophageal webs and rings?**
   Symptomatic patients typically present with intermittent dysphagia, particularly to solids such as meat or bread. Patients with an esophageal lumen narrowing of less than 13 mm (39 French) will usually experience solid-food dysphagia. Hence, clinical history of dysphagia to primarily solids should bring mechanical stricture (creating luminal narrowing) higher on the differential.

4. **How do you diagnose rings and webs?**
   In patients with primarily solid-food dysphagia, endoscopy is typically the first step as it serves as both diagnostic and therapeutic options. Barium esophagram with a 13-mm barium tablet can also be used as a noninvasive test. This might show a transient delay in the passage of the 13 mm tablet at the site of a Schatzki ring. Given that

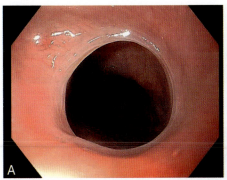 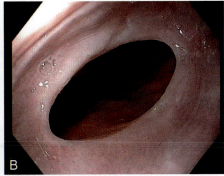

Fig. 6.1 Endoscopic view of a cervical esophageal web (A) and Schatzki ring (B).

Table 6.1 Types of Esophageal Rings.		
TYPE	**LOCATION**	**SYMPTOMATIC**
A	1.5 cm proximal to squamocolumnar junction	Rare
B (Schatzki ring)	At the squamocolumnar junction or proximal border of a hiatal hernia	Often
C	Indentation caused by the diaphragmatic crura	Never

esophageal webs are usually located in the proximal esophagus, video fluoroscopy has higher sensitivity compared to endoscopy.

5. **What are the treatment options for esophageal webs and rings?**
Upper endoscopy with esophageal dilation is the primary therapeutic option with the goal of disrupting the mucosal ring or web. This can be achieved with either bougie dilators or scope balloon dilators. Given that subtle webs and rings can often be missed during endoscopy, in patients with primarily solid dysphagia, empiric esophageal dilation can also be considered. Schatzki rings are often associated with gastroesophageal reflux disease (GERD); hence, in patients with concomitant heartburn or regurgitation, acid-suppressive therapy should also be considered.

6. **What triad is classically associated with Plummer-Vinson syndrome?**
Triad: Iron-deficiency anemia, upper esophageal web, and dysphagia.
    Other symptoms: Glossitis, koilonychia, and cheilitis. This syndrome has been identified as a risk factor for developing esophageal cancer.

7. **What other conditions are associated with esophageal webs?**
Zenker diverticulum, bullous pemphigoid, pemphigus vulgaris, and chronic graft-versus-host disease have been associated with webs.

8. **What condition can cause diffuse concentric esophageal rings?**
Diffuse mucosal rings (rather than localized) should bring eosinophilic esophagitis higher on the differential (Fig. 6.2). During endoscopy, one can see "trachealization" of the esophagus, longitudinal furrows, mucosal edema, and white patches (suggestive of eosinophilic microabscesses). In this setting, esophageal biopsies should be obtained for evaluation; ≥15 eosinophils per high-power field on pathology is considered diagnostic for eosinophilic esophagitis. This condition is more common in younger patients with solid-food dysphagia, history of food impaction, or atopic diseases (eczema, asthma, or seasonal allergies).

9. **What are the types of esophageal diverticula? What is the pathogenesis of each?**
Information on the types of esophageal diverticula is given in Table 6.2.

10. **How do patients with Zenker diverticulum present?**
Most of the small Zenker diverticula tend to be asymptomatic. However, early on, some patients can present with oropharyngeal dysphagia (coughing immediately with swallows of solids or liquids). As the diverticulum becomes large enough to retain food contents, patients may have halitosis, regurgitation, and gurgling. Patients often experience weight loss.

11. **How do you manage Zenker diverticulum?**
Symptomatic patients with diverticula >1 cm can be treated surgically with a cricopharyngeal myotomy and diverticulectomy. There are also data supporting a newer technique using a transoral endoscopic approach to cricopharyngeal myotomy using Zenker peroral endoscopic myotomy. Both are reasonable options depending on available expertise.

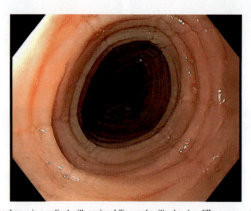

Fig. 6.2 Endoscopic view of esophagus in a patient with eosinophilic esophagitis showing diffuse mucosal rings (trachealization), longitudinal furrows, and mucosal edema.

Table 6.2 Types, Anatomical Location, and Pathogenesis of Various Esophageal Diverticula.

NAME	ANATOMICAL LOCATION	PATHOGENESIS
Zenker diverticula (Fig. 6.3A)	Cervical (posterior)	Pressure during swallowing causes an outpouching in a natural area of weakness in the posterior wall of the pharyngoesophageal segment just *above the cricopharyngeus*
Killian-Jamieson diverticula	Cervical (anterolateral location)	Originates in the gap *below the cricopharyngeus* and lateral to the longitudinal tendon of the esophagus (i.e., the Killian-Jamieson space)
Traction diverticula (Fig. 6.3B and D)	Middle third (mid-esophagus), near bifurcation of the trachea	Mediastinal inflammation (tuberculosis, histoplasmosis), or mediastinal lymphadenopathy (malignancy) causing contracture in proximity to esophageal wall
Epiphrenic diverticula (Fig. 6.3C)	Distal esophagus (immediately above the lower esophageal sphincter)	Associated with motility disorders, particularly achalasia

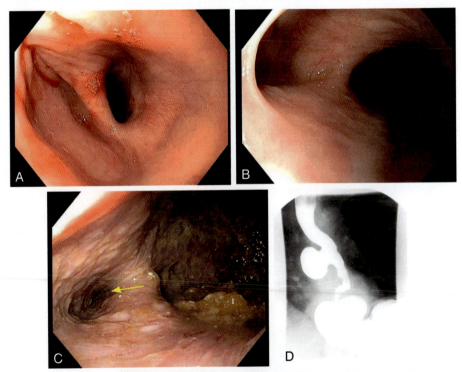

Fig. 6.3 Endoscopic views of Zenker diverticulum in the cervical esophagus (A), traction diverticulum in the mid-esophagus (B), and large epiphrenic diverticulum in the distal esophagus (C) with an *arrow* showing the lower esophageal sphincter. (D) A mid-esophageal diverticulum on a barium esophagram.

12. What are the treatment options for epiphrenic diverticulum?

Nearly 80% of epiphrenic diverticula are associated with an esophageal motility disorder. Hence, preoperative endoscopy and esophageal manometry should be performed. Treatment usually involves surgery with resection of the diverticula and myotomy (due to the high likelihood of associated motility disorder).

13. **What is an inlet patch?**
An inlet patch is ectopic gastric mucosa: a discrete area resembling gastric mucosa found in the proximal esophagus (often the first 3 cm). It is a benign lesion, with an approximated prevalence of 2%–10% of the population. The majority of these lesions are found incidentally on endoscopy with no associated symptoms. However, some do report globus sensation or hoarseness.

14. **How do patients with a tracheoesophageal fistula present?**
Patients present with coughing following solid and liquid intake (Ono sign), recurrent pneumonia and bronchitis, and malnutrition. They can be diagnosed using multiple modalities: endoscopy, cross-sectional body imaging, or barium esophagram.

15. **What are the most common etiologies of tracheoesophageal fistulas?**
More than 50% of tracheoesophageal fistulas are secondary to malignancy (particularly esophageal or lung cancer). They can also be caused by prolonged endotracheal intubation, surgical/endoscopic intervention history, radiation, or mediastinal granulomas.

INFECTIONS

16. **What are the presenting symptoms for patients with infectious esophagitis?**
Patients typically present with dysphagia, odynophagia (pain with swallowing), or retrosternal chest pain. Immunocompromised (i.e., organ transplant, chemotherapy, chronic steroid use, and human immunodeficiency virus [HIV]/acquired immunodeficiency syndrome) patients are predisposed to infectious etiologies of esophagitis.

17. **What is the most common pathogen for infectious esophagitis?**
Candida albicans is the most common pathogen. *Candida* should be suspected in any immunocompromised patient using inhaled corticosteroids and presenting with odynophagia. Oral thrush may be absent.

18. **How do you diagnose *Candida* esophagitis?**
Direct visualization with endoscopy is the primary diagnostic modality with characteristic white or yellow mucosal plaques that cannot be washed off (Fig. 6.4). Confirmation is made by brushing the lesion followed by a cytologic examination or biopsy, which can show yeast and pseudohyphae with inflammation.

19. **How do you treat *Candida* esophagitis?**
Patients should be treated with systemic antifungals, specifically fluconazole 400 mg (oral) on the first day followed by 200–400 mg daily for 14–21 days.

20. **What are the viral esophagitis pathogens and populations?**
The viral esophagitis pathogens and populations are given in Table 6.3.

21. **How do you treat herpes simplex virus (HSV) esophagitis in immunosuppressed patients?**
In immunocompetent patients, their symptoms typically self-resolve in 1–2 weeks; however, they can be treated with acyclovir 400 mg by mouth three times a day for 7–10 days to expedite recovery. Immunosuppressed patients should be treated with valacyclovir 1 g three times a day or oral acyclovir therapy 400 mg five times a day for 2–3 weeks.

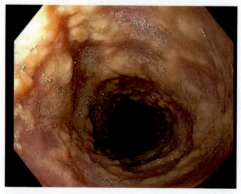

Fig. 6.4 Endoscopic view of *Candida* esophagitis with characteristic white/yellow plaques coating the entire esophagus.

Table 6.3 Clinical, Endoscopic, and Histologic Features Along With Treatment Options of Herpes Simplex Virus (HSV) and Cytomegalovirus (CMV).

	HSV	CMV
Patient population	Immunosuppressed and immunocompetent patients	Immunosuppressed patients
Endoscopic features	Multiple shallow ulcers with vesicles	Deep, punched out, and longitudinal ulcers
Location	Distal esophagus	Middle to distal esophagus
Biopsy	Edge	Center (C for CMV)
Histologic findings	Multinucleated giant cells, ground-glass nuclei, and eosinophilic Cowdry type A inclusion bodies	Intranuclear inclusions, perinuclear halo, and cytoplasmic inclusions
Treatment	Oral acyclovir 400 mg three times daily for 7–10 days Oral valacyclovir 10 mg three times daily for 7–10 days	Intravenous ganciclovir 5 mg/kg for 14 days Oral valacyclovir

22. What esophageal findings can you see with HIV?

Patients with HIV are predisposed to the above infectious etiologies; however, patients with CD4 counts <200 can additionally form benign HIV-associated idiopathic giant esophageal ulcers. Pathology testing will be negative for infectious etiologies such as cytomegalovirus, HSV, or fungal infection. In this setting, treatment is typically focused on antiretroviral therapy in combination with corticosteroids.

23. What infection should you suspect in patients with dysphagia from Latin/South America?

You should suspect Chagas disease, an infection caused by the vector-borne parasite *Trypanosoma cruzi*. Patients typically present in the chronic phase, more than 10 years after infection, with symptoms of progressive dysphagia, regurgitation, retrosternal pain, and progressive constipation.

24. How do you diagnose Chagas disease?

Chagas disease is diagnosed with positive serologic testing for *T. cruzi*. When available, barium esophagram and manometry will appear like achalasia. An upper endoscopy should be performed to exclude malignancy at the esophagogastric junction.

25. How do you treat Chagas megaesophagus?

Treatment options are similar to patients with idiopathic achalasia, given antiparasitic treatment has not shown significant benefit. Pharmacologic therapy includes nitrates and nifedipine aimed at decreasing the lower esophageal sphincter pressure, but patients often develop tachyphylaxis and side effects. Procedural interventions, including laparoscopic heller myotomy, peroral endoscopic myotomy, and pneumatic dilation, are primary first-line treatment options. For refractory disease, patients may require esophagectomy.

PILL AND NONACID INJURY

26. When should you suspect pill-induced esophageal injury?

Patients will present with sudden-onset retrosternal pain and odynophagia after ingestion. Specifically, this pain will be exacerbated by swallowing.

27. What are the risk factors that predispose patients to pill-induced esophageal injury?

Overall, slowed esophageal transit predisposes patients to pill-induced injury. Risk factors include the following:
1. disorders of esophageal motility
2. abnormal anatomy (esophageal diverticula, aortic aneurysms, enlarged left atrium, and strictures)
3. decreased salivary flow (sicca syndrome and anticholinergic medications)
4. bedridden, older adult patients.

28. What medications are associated with pill-induced esophagitis?

Numerous medications have been identified but most commonly include antibiotics (tetracyclines and clindamycin), bisphosphonates, nonsteroidal anti-inflammatory drugs, potassium chloride, and ferrous sulfate. Table 6.4 lists the more common offending agents.

Table 6.4 Common Medications Associated With Pill Esophagitis.

- Antibiotics: amoxicillin, azithromycin, bactrim, clindamycin, doxycycline, and tetracycline
- Antihypertensives: alprenolol, captopril, and nifedipine
- Bisphosphonates: alendronate
- Nonsteroidal anti-inflammatory drugs: aspirin, ibuprofen, and naproxen
- Supplements: ascorbic acid, ferrous sulfate, and potassium chloride
- Miscellaneous: glucocorticoids and quinidine

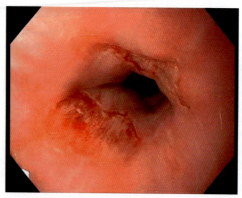

Fig. 6.5 Classic endoscopic appearance of "kissing ulcers," which might suggest pill-induced esophageal injury.

29. **When should patients with suspected pill-induced esophagitis undergo upper endoscopy?**

    Clinical diagnosis can be made with the appropriate history of sudden-onset dysphagia or pain after medication ingestion. Endoscopy should be considered when symptoms are severe (i.e., hematemesis and dysphagia) or if symptoms persist for 1 week after discontinuation of the medication. The typical endoscopic appearance of pill-induced esophageal injury is a discrete ulcer with normal surrounding mucosa or classic "kissing ulcers" with ulcers facing each other as shown in Fig. 6.5.

30. **Where are the most common sites of injury?**

    The proximal esophagus (near the compression from the aortic arch) is most commonly affected. Patients with left atrial enlargement often have injury of the distal esophagus.

31. **How should patients with pill esophagitis be treated?**

    The culprit medication should be discontinued or transitioned to a liquid formulation until patients' symptoms resolve. Most cases of medication-induced esophageal injury heal within a few days. After symptoms resolve, the medication can be resumed unless patients have a predisposing risk factor as above. If the patient has an esophageal stricture, dilation may help long term.

32. **How do you prevent pill-induced esophagitis?**

    Patients with risk factors as above should avoid medications associated with pill esophagitis. Patients should be advised to take medication with at least 8 oz of water, to sit upright for at least 30 minutes, and to eat a meal afterward.

33. **What are peptic strictures?**

    Peptic strictures are the most common type (90%) of benign esophageal strictures. They are associated with reflux and have been decreasing in incidence since the 1990s with the increased prevalence of proton pump inhibitors (PPIs).

34. **How do peptic strictures appear on endoscopy?**

    These strictures are typically short in length (1–4 cm) and located at the squamocolumnar junction. Endoscopy may also reveal adjacent reflux esophagitis as shown in Fig. 6.6.

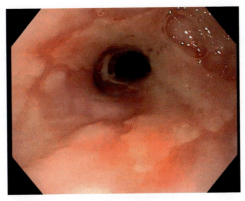

Fig. 6.6 Peptic stricture in the distal esophagus with associated esophagitis.

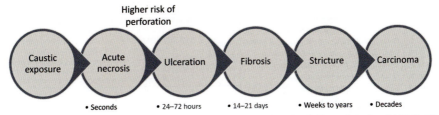

Fig. 6.7 Timing of tissue damage and repair after caustic injury of the esophagus. (Reproduced with permission from Patel D. Caustic injuries of the esophagus. In Richter, JE, Castell, DO, Katzka, DA, Katz, PO, Smout, A, Spechler, S, et al, eds. The Esophagus. 6th ed. John Wiley and Sons; 2022:757-768.)

35. How do you manage peptic strictures?

During endoscopy, esophageal dilation can be performed to improve dysphagia. Patients should also be started on PPIs to prevent stricture recurrence once they have been dilated.

36. What type of caustic ingestion is most common?

Alkali ingestion (drain cleaner, detergent, and bleach) is most common. Concentrated acids such as toilet bowl or pool cleaners are less commonly ingested. Overall, caustic ingestions in adults are typically purposeful. The degree of injury depends on the concentration of the solution, time of contact, and volume ingested.

37. Describe the pathogenesis of alkali- versus acid-induced injury.

Acid injury occurs via coagulation necrosis. Alkali injury occurs via liquefactive necrosis, which can rapidly disintegrate through the mucosa, potentially causing perforation. It can lead to ulceration over the following days, then fibrose into strictures. Long term, these patients are predisposed to esophageal cancer. Fig. 6.7 shows the timing of tissue damage and repair after caustic injury of the esophagus.

38. What should the initial evaluation of these patients be?

The primary focus of the initial evaluation is to distinguish patients with severe life-threatening injuries who require emergency surgery from patients with mild injuries who can be monitored with supportive measures. Patients with oropharyngeal symptoms concerning for airway compromise should be intubated. Patients with signs of perforation should undergo emergency surgery. If patients have no signs of perforation, they should undergo endoscopic or imaging evaluation for staging. Fig. 6.8 shows an algorithm for evaluation, classification for grading the severity of injury, and management of patients with caustic ingestion.

39. What is the recommended timing for upper endoscopy in caustic ingestion?

When there is no evidence of perforation, endoscopic evaluation is recommended within the first 48 hours to evaluate damage and guide management. Endoscopic and CT grading can help determine prognosis in terms of stricturing, mortality, and potential need for esophageal resection as shown in Fig. 6.8. CT grading has been shown to be superior at predicting the risk of late complications compared to endoscopy in recent studies.

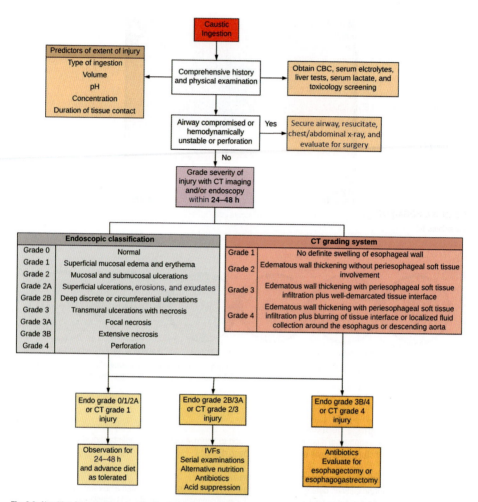

Fig. 6.8 Algorithm for evaluation, classification for grading the severity of injury, and management of patients with caustic ingestion. *CBC,* Complete blood count; *CT,* computed tomography; *IVF,* in vitro fertilization. (Reproduced with permission from Patel D. Caustic injuries of the esophagus. In Richter, JE, Castell, DO, Katzka, DA, Katz, PO, Smout, A, Spechler, S, et al, eds. The Esophagus. 6th ed. John Wiley and Sons; 2022:757-768.)

40. What are the late complications of caustic ingestion?

Strictures are the most common esophageal complication of caustic ingestion. Three to six weeks after the initial injury, patients are reevaluated endoscopically and may undergo dilation. Caustic ingestion can increase the risk of squamous cell carcinoma; thus surveillance endoscopies starting a decade after ingestion are recommended every 2–3 years.

41. What is a Mallory-Weiss tear?

It is an *intraintra*mural dissection of the distal esophagus. Mallory-Weiss tears account for 8%–15% of upper gastrointestinal bleeds. They are induced by a sudden increase in intrabdominal pressure such as during vomiting.

42. How do you diagnose Mallory-Weiss tears?

Mallory-Weiss tears should be suspected in patients with acute-onset hematemesis after an antecedent vomiting history. Definitive diagnosis is made with endoscopy to rule out other etiologies. A majority of these tears will heal within 24–48 hours, so may be missed if the endoscopy is delayed.

43. **What is Boerhaave syndrome?**

It is a *trans*mural dissection or rupture of the esophagus. This condition has high morbidity and mortality. Patients present with chest pain and crepitus due to subcutaneous emphysema, and may be clinically unstable. On imaging, they may have subcutaneous or peritoneal free air.

44. **What are the risk factors for radiation-induced esophageal injury?**

Higher radiation doses, use of concurrent chemotherapy, radiation technique, and presence of underlying esophageal disease (i.e., GERD) all increase the likelihood of radiation-induced esophagitis.

45. **What are the early and late manifestations of radiation esophagitis?**

Early symptoms due to mucosal inflammation include dysphagia, odynophagia, and retrosternal discomfort. These symptoms occur within weeks of radiation initiation and may self-resolve with mucosal healing. Late manifestations, months after radiation, include esophageal strictures, altered motility due to fibrosis or nerve injury, and chronic ulceration. Rarely, patients may develop tracheoesophageal fistulas.

ACKNOWLEDGMENT

The authors acknowledge the contributions of Dr. Atia and Dr. Ramirez, who were the authors of this chapter in the previous edition.

CLINICAL VIGNETTE

Available Online.

BIBLIOGRAPHY

Available Online.

CHAPTER 7

BARRETT ESOPHAGUS

Nimish Vakil, MD, FACP, FACG, AGAF, FASGE and Heather Korus, MSN, APNP, FNP-BC

 Additional content available online.

1. **How is Barrett esophagus (BE) defined?**

   BE may be simply defined as the presence of columnar metaplasia of the anatomic esophagus. It is a complication of chronic gastroesophageal reflux disease (GERD). The current American Society of Gastroenterology (ASGE) guidelines define BE as a premalignant condition for esophageal adenocarcinoma (EAC) and is characterized by the replacement of the normal squamous epithelium of the distal esophagus with metaplastic intestinal-type columnar epithelium.

2. **Why is BE important?**

   BE is a precancerous lesion diagnosed in about 7%–10% of individuals with chronic GERD. Every year, about 0.3% of patients with BE will go on to develop EAC. Without proper surveillance, most patients with EAC are diagnosed with late-stage disease and as such have a less than 20% survival rate. The incidence of EAC is one of the fastest growing in the Western world, and given the high mortality rate, surveillance using endoscopy is important to identify patients with early disease.

3. **What are the risk factors for BE?**
   - Age $\geq$50 years
   - GERD symptoms $\geq$5 years
   - White race
   - Male sex
   - Obesity
   - First-degree relative with BE or EAC
   - Hiatal hernia
   - Truncal obesity
   - Smoking

4. **What are the endoscopic appearance and characterization of BE?**

   BE has a typical endoscopic appearance. It is generally described as a salmon-pink area of mucosa within the tubular esophagus, in contrast to the light gray appearance of the esophageal squamous mucosa (Fig. 7.1). It should be emphasized that histologic examination of esophageal biopsy samples is required to confirm the diagnosis of BE. The Prague classification is a standardized method of reporting the extent of BE and is recommended for routine endoscopy. The vertical extent of Barrett epithelium that is circumferential is measured from the top of the gastric folds and designated as the C length. Longitudinal columns of Barrett epithelium are designated by the letter M, followed by the vertical length. For example, a patient with a circumferential change of 2 and 1 cm tongues of Barrett epithelium extending upward from the circumferential segment is designated as C2M1 based on the Prague classification (Fig. 7.2). Short-segment BE is defined by the presence of intestinal metaplasia identified in biopsies obtained from the esophagus with an endoscopic appearance suggestive of BE that extends $\leq$3 cm into the esophagus. Long-segment BE is defined by segments of abnormal epithelium $\geq$3 cm.

5. **What is the risk of cancer in BE?**

   Projections of the annual incidence of cancer in patients with BE have ranged from 0.1% to almost 3.0%, with most studies suggesting a rate of 0.1%–0.4% per year. Though the risk of developing esophageal cancer is increased by 30-fold in patients with BE, the absolute risk of developing cancer for an individual patient with nondysplastic BE is low.

6. **What are the risk factors for the development of dysplasia and cancer in BE?**

   It is uncertain if the risk increases or decreases with the passage of time, but dysplasia and cancer are typically found after the age of 50 years. There is good evidence to suggest a higher risk for patients with long-segment BE and a greater risk in males compared with females. Obesity is a major risk factor that is amenable to intervention. Smoking has been shown to increase risk in some studies but not in others.

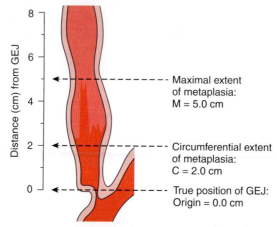

Fig. 7.1 Diagrammatic representation of endoscopic Barrett esophagus showing an area classified as C2M5. *C*, Extent of circumferential metaplasia; *GEJ*, gastroesophageal junction; *M*, maximum extent of metaplasia (C plus a distal "tongue" of 3 cm). (From Sharma P, Dent J, Armstrong D, Bergman JJGHM, Gossner L, Hoshihara Y, et al. The development and validation of an endoscopic grading system for Barrett's esophagus: the Prague C & M criteria. Gastroenterology. 2006;131(5):1392-1399.)

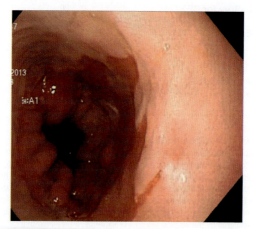

Fig. 7.2 Barrett esophagus seen at conventional white light endoscopy. Note the salmon-colored epithelium that contrasts with the normal gray epithelial lining of the esophagus.

7. What is the risk of progression to cancer once dysplasia develops?

Once dysplastic BE is present, the progression to EAC is at a rate of 0.2%–14% per year based on the degree of dysplasia. Low-grade dysplasia (LGD) evolves into cancer at a rate of about 0.54% per year, whereas high-grade dysplasia (HGD) evolves into cancer at a rate of 4%–8% per year. Indefinite for dysplasia appears to progress to EAC at a rate of 0.2%–1.2% per year.

8. Does medical therapy prevent the risk of dysplasia or cancer?

There is no high-level evidence to tell with certainty. Treatment with proton pump inhibitors (PPIs) has been shown to reduce the risk of dysplasia and cancer in observational studies. The combined use of a statin and aspirin has been shown to significantly reduce the risk of developing adenocarcinoma or HGD. Similarly, there is evidence to suggest that a high-dose PPI combined with a full-dose aspirin may prevent progression to EAC, HGD, and all-cause mortality, but the difference between the aspirin group and nonaspirin group was modest and not statistically significant, so this is not routinely implemented as a prevention strategy. Fundoplication has not been convincingly shown to prevent cancer.

9. Is there a role for screening upper endoscopy to identify BE?

Routine screening for BE is not recommended. A strategy based on screening high-risk individuals is recommended by several societies. Criteria that identify patients at high risk include male sex, White race, reflux disease for longer than 5 years, a history of esophageal cancer, or BE in a first-degree relative.

10. What is the goal of medical treatment in BE?

- Treat the symptoms of GERD commonly associated with BE.
- Prevent complications by decreasing mucosal inflammation in the esophagus.
- Monitor for the development of dysplasia or cancer of the esophagus so that early intervention may be offered to the patient.

11. What is the recommendation for endoscopic surveillance in BE?

- Surveillance intervals should vary based on BE length:
- <1 cm (an irregular Z-line): no routine biopsies or surveillance.
- 1–3 cm: surveillance should be repeated every 5 years.
- ≥3–10 cm: surveillance should be every 3 years.
- ≥10 cm should be referred to a BE expert center for surveillance endoscopies.
- Patients with ≥75 years and/or limited life expectancy should no longer undergo endoscopic surveillance.

12. What is the recommended biopsy protocol for BE?

In patients undergoing BE surveillance, we recommend using chromoendoscopy, including virtual chromoendoscopy and biopsy sampling, compared with white light endoscopy with biopsy sampling. Virtual chromoendoscopy, also known as narrow-band imaging (NBI), is now widely available and uses a narrow spectrum of light to illuminate the Barrett epithelium. NBI does not impose any additional costs and can be advantageous during the workup of patients with early neoplasia. Chromoendoscopy is another technique using dye (methylene blue or indigo carmine) sprayed over Barrett epithelium to identify surface abnormalities.

The American College of Gastroenterology (ACG) recommends using four-quadrant biopsy sampling at 2-cm intervals in patients without dysplasia and at 1-cm intervals in patients with prior dysplasia, along with targeted biopsy sampling from any mucosal abnormality (Fig. 7.3).

13. What is the management strategy for indefinite for dysplasia?

For patients whose biopsies show indefinite for dysplasia, a repeat endoscopy after optimization of acid-inhibitory medications for 3–6 months is recommended. If a subsequent endoscopy again shows indefinite for dysplasia, the patient should undergo surveillance every 12 months.

14. How reliable is the pathologic diagnosis of HGD?

Interobserver variability between pathologists in identifying HGD and early cancer is common. The ASGE and ACG recommend that the diagnosis of any degree of dysplasia (including "indefinite for dysplasia") requires confirmation by an expert gastrointestinal pathologist.

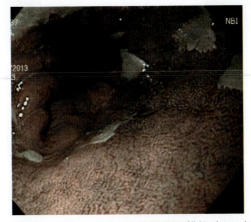

Fig. 7.3 Narrow-band imaging (NBI) of Barrett esophagus. Using a narrow spectrum of light enhances detail and allows clearer visualization of the surface characteristics. It allows sharp demarcation from the normal squamous epithelium.

15. How reliable is pathologic diagnosis of LGD in BE?

The criteria for the definition of LGD are not well defined and vary in different regions of the world. In 30% of patients with a single endoscopy diagnosis of LGD, the diagnosis will not be reproduced on subsequent endoscopies. There is a tendency to overdiagnose LGD as a result of misinterpretation of regenerative changes. A single diagnosis of confirmed LGD does not justify ablation therapy and a second expert GI pathologist should confirm the diagnosis (per ASGE). In patients with confirmed LGD, endoscopic ablation therapy is recommended.

16. What is the risk of progression in LGD?

The current consensus is that patients with LGD progress to cancer at a rate of 0.54% per year, although it is difficult to predict precisely.

17. How should LGD be managed?

LGD is a risk factor for malignancy. The risk for progression may have been underestimated in the past, and currently, the risk is poorly defined with a major factor being the differences in how study pathologists diagnose LGD. The diagnosis of LGD should first be confirmed by a second pathologist. In patients who have not previously been treated for reflux disease, treatment with PPIs followed by repeated biopsy is recommended. Patients with persistent LGD should be offered the option of surveillance or radiofrequency ablation (RFA), which may be preferable to patients who are willing to accept the procedural risks. Patients who undergo RFA are less likely to progress to HGD or cancer compared with those who do not, although uncertainty remains around the durability of the ablation procedure.

18. What is the management of HGD in BE?

Endoscopic treatment is preferred over endoscopic surveillance for the management of most patients with BE who have HGD or intramucosal cancer of the esophagus (Fig. 7.4). Endoscopic therapy is also preferred to surgical intervention in this setting. The commonly used options for endoscopic therapy are RFA and photodynamic therapy. Both have shown a high degree of success in ablating the dysplastic epithelium and preventing recurrence.

19. What is the management of early esophageal cancer in BE?

Endoscopic therapy for BE is recommended for intramucosal cancer (T1a). Endoscopic therapy is an alternative to surgery in T1b lesions with submucosal involvement if *all* of the following are present:
1. Submucosal invasion limited to <500 µm.
2. Tumor differentiation grade: well or moderate.
3. Absence of tumor invasion in lymphatic or blood vessels.
4. Absence of tumor infiltration in the deep resection margin.

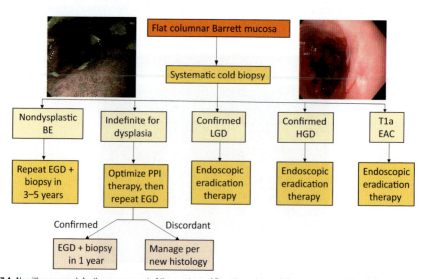

Fig. 7.4 Algorithm approach for the management of the spectrum of Barrett esophagus (BE) based on histologic criteria. *EAC,* Esophageal adenocarcinoma; *EGD,* esophagogastroduodenoscopy; *HGD,* high-grade dysplasia; *LGD,* low-grade dysplasia; *PPI,* proton pump inhibitor.

Endoscopic submucosal dissection (ESD) and endoscopic mucosal resection (EMR) are both highly effective. EMR is preferred due to the higher risk of complications and difficulty with ESD, although ESD can be considered for bulky lesions and for lesions where submucosal invasion is suspected.

BIBLIOGRAPHY

Available Online.

CHAPTER 8

ESOPHAGEAL AND STOMACH PATHOLOGY

Shalini Tayal, MD

 Additional content available online.

ESOPHAGUS

1. Describe a normal esophagus lining.
   - Esophagus consists of mucosa, lamina propria, muscularis mucosae, submucosa, muscularis propria, and adventitia (lacks serosa) (Fig. 8.1A).
   - Sebaceous glands can be seen normally in the submucosa.
   - Normal gastroesophageal (GE) junction (Fig. 8.1B) shows squamous and columnar epithelium.

2. What are the histologic features of GE reflux disease (GERD) and eosinophilic esophagitis (EE)?
   Histologic features of GERD include the following (Fig. 8.2A):
   - Distal esophagus is more severe than proximal esophagus.
   - Basilar hyperplasia is present.
   - Elongation of vascular papillae occurs.
   - Intraepithelial neutrophils and eosinophils increase (~8 eosinophils per high power field [HPF]).
   - Balloon cells (enlarged squamous cells with abundant accumulation of plasma proteins) indicate chemical injury.
   Histologic features of EE are the following (Fig. 8.2B):
   - Proximal esophagus is more commonly affected than distal esophagus.
   - Distribution can be patchy.
   - Obtain biopsy samples from upper, mid, and distal esophagus.
   - Intraepithelial eosinophils in the upper layers of epithelium are increased (>15–20 eosinophils/HPF).
   - Eosinophilic microabscesses appear in the superficial layers of epithelium.
   - Extensive degranulation of eosinophils is more common.
   - *GERD can coexist in 30% of cases and is difficult to distinguish histologically.*

3. Discuss the infectious causes of esophagitis.
   The infectious causes of *fungal esophagitis* are the following:
   - *Candida esophagitis* (Fig. 8.3A and B): *C. albicans* is the most common of the *Candida* species. Others include *C. glabrata, C. tropicalis, C. parapsilosis*, and *C. krusei*. Endoscopy shows whitish, raised plaques with erosions

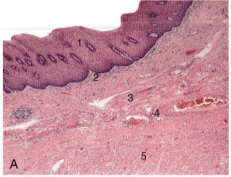
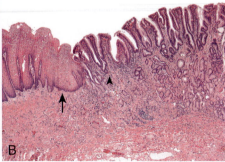

Fig. 8.1 Photomicrographs of (A) normal esophagus lining: (1) mucosa, (2) lamina propria, (3) muscularis mucosae, (4) submucosa, and (5) muscularis propria (adventitia is not shown) (hematoxylin and eosin [H&E] stain). (B) Normal gastroesophageal junction showing squamous mucosa (*arrow*) and columnar mucosa (*arrowhead*) (H&E stain).

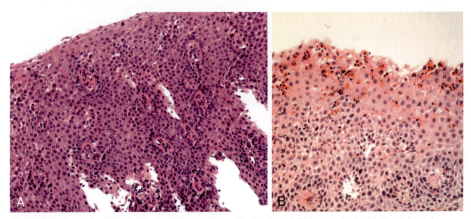

Fig. 8.2 Photomicrographs of (A) reflux esophagitis (gastroesophageal reflux disease). Basilar hyperplasia and elongated vascular papillae (hematoxylin and eosin [H&E] stain). (B) Eosinophilic esophagitis. Note the increased intraepithelial eosinophils in this biopsy sample from the midesophagus (H&E stain).

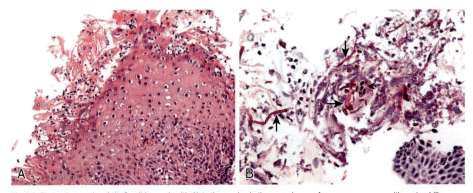

Fig. 8.3 Photomicrographs of (A) *Candida esophagitis*. Note the erosion in the upper layers of squamous mucosa with neutrophilic infiltrate forming microabscesses (hematoxylin and eosin stain). (B) Yeast (*arrowhead*) and pseudohyphae (*arrows*) are highlighted by periodic acid–Schiff stain.

or ulcerations. Histologic examination reveals erosion of superficial layers of squamous epithelium or ulceration with yeast and pseudohyphal forms (highlighted by special stains such as Grocott methenamine silver or periodic acid–Schiff stain [PAS]). The key to diagnosis is the presence of pseudohyphal forms, which indicates infection. The presence of yeast forms alone suggests oral contamination.

- *Histoplasma:* In the United States, *Histoplasma* is endemic around the Mississippi and Ohio River valleys. It is also endemic to Central and South America and the Caribbean islands. Endoscopy may appear normal. Histologic examination reveals subepithelial necrotizing granulomas with giant cells that contain organisms of 2–4 μm in diameter.
- *Aspergillus:* The most common species are *A. fumigatus* and *A. flavus*. Seen as branching (at 45 degrees) septate hyphae 4 μm in diameter.
- *Mucormycosis:* Mucormycosis can be seen in immunocompromised hosts as nonseptate parallel hyphae (10–15 μm in diameter) that branch at right angles.

The infectious causes of *viral esophagitis* are the following:

- *Herpes esophagitis* (Fig. 8.4): Herpes esophagitis is seen in immunocompromised patients.
  - Endoscopy: May reveal vesicles or coalesced shallow ulcers.
- Histology: Infected epithelial cells show multinucleation with molding and smudged intranuclear inclusions.
- *Cytomegalovirus:* Seen in immunocompromised patients. The viral cytopathic effect includes intracytoplasmic and intranuclear inclusions seen in endothelial cells, epithelial cells, histiocytes, or fibroblasts.

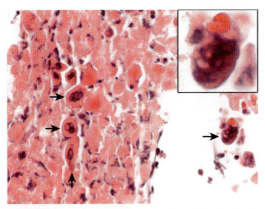

Fig. 8.4 Photomicrograph of herpes esophagitis. Note the multinucleated cells with molding (*arrows*) and smudged eosinophilic viral inclusions (*inset*) (hematoxylin and eosin stain).

4. **What is the most important differential to be considered in biopsy samples to evaluate graft-versus-host disease (GVHD)?**
   Infectious etiologic factors must be ruled out with the use of special stains (fungal and viral) and with serologic and tissue culture examinations. In general, the upper esophagus is usually affected.
   - Histology: GVHD is graded as mild, moderate, or severe based on the degree of damage seen. Apoptotic bodies are seen in the squamous epithelium; there are intraepithelial lymphocytes and basal vacuolization and, in severe cases, ulceration and necrosis.

5. **What is the histologic prevalence of esophageal Crohn's disease in endoscopically normal studies?**
   Histologic prevalence varies from 5% to 42% and does not correlate with endoscopic findings. Crohn's esophagitis may be seen with severe cases of ileocolic disease.
   - Histology: Varies from mild inflammation with epithelioid nonnecrotizing granulomas in the lamina propria to ulcerations and transmural involvement with fistula formation.

6. **What are other miscellaneous esophageal conditions?**
   - Glycogen acanthosis:
     - Endoscopy: Small, white-gray plaques in the midesophagus. There is an association with Cowden syndrome.
     - Histology: Squamous cells distended with increased intracellular glycogen.
   - Gastric inlet patch:
     - Endoscopy: Reveals a patch (2 mm–3 cm) of gastric-appearing mucosa located just below the cricopharyngeus muscle.
     - Histology: Oxyntic (parietal)-type mucosa. Intestinal metaplasia may be found.
   - Pancreatic heterotopia:
     - Endoscopy: Often not apparent to the eye. This tissue is often seen in biopsy samples at the GE junction or distal esophagus. It may represent metaplasia or ectopic foci of pancreatic tissue.
     - Histology: Acinar cells with dense, coarse eosinophilic granules are seen.
   - Melanosis:
     - Endoscopy: Tiny 1- to 2-mm brown-black spots. Melanocytes may be seen in the basal layer of squamous epithelium. The differential diagnosis is malignant melanoma. The melanocytes in melanosis are benign appearing and mature. Pigment can be seen in the upper layers of mucosa and in the adjacent lamina propria.

7. **List the dermatologic conditions that can affect the esophagus.**
   Dermatologic conditions that affect the esophagus are pemphigus vulgaris, bullous pemphigoid, erythema multiforme, Behçet syndrome, lichen planus, dermatitis herpetiformis, scleroderma, and toxic epidermolysis necrosis.

8. **Discuss the histologic characteristics of Barrett esophagus and the grading of dysplasia.**
   Barrett esophagus is an endoscopic change in esophageal epithelium of any length, confirmed to have intestinal metaplasia at biopsy. Histologic findings include squamocolumnar junctional mucosa with intestinal metaplasia recognized by the presence of goblet cells (Fig. 8.5A), which stain blue with Alcian blue stain at pH 2.5 (Fig. 8.5B). Dysplasia in Barrett esophagus is graded as follows:

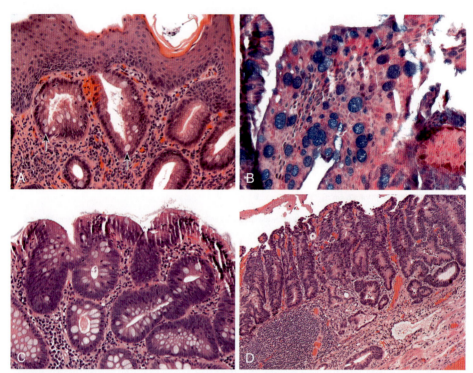

Fig. 8.5 Photomicrographs of Barrett esophagus. (A) Intestinal metaplasia is recognized by the presence of goblet cells (*arrows*) in the glandular epithelium (hematoxylin and eosin [H&E] stain). (B) Alcian blue stain at pH 2.5 stains the acidic mucin of goblet cells *blue*. (C) Barrett esophagus with low-grade dysplasia. There is a lack of surface maturation, and the glandular epithelium shows nuclear stratification with hyperchromasia (H&E stain). (D) Barrett esophagus with high-grade dysplasia and invasion into the lamina propria (intramucosal carcinoma) seen next to the lymphoid aggregate (H&E stain).

None: There is no evidence of dysplasia.

Indefinite for dysplasia: This grading is assigned when a distinction cannot be made between low-grade dysplasia and inflammation-associated changes. The surface epithelium shows maturation, but the deeper glands show architectural crowding, nuclear hyperchromasia, and, occasionally, increased mitotic activity.

Low-grade dysplasia (Fig. 8.5C): Lack of surface maturation and glandular epithelium shows amphophilic cytoplasm with mucin depletion and nuclear hyperchromasia. Architectural crowding is similar to that seen in colonic tubular adenomas.

High-grade dysplasia: Lack of surface maturation usually, with dysplastic cells showing marked cytologic atypia characterized by loss of polarity, high nuclear-to-cytoplasm ratio, irregular nuclear contours, and prominent large nucleoli. The architecture becomes complex with focal areas of cribriforming. Cytologic abnormalities supersede architectural complexity in diagnosing high-grade dysplasia.

High-grade dysplasia with invasion or intramucosal carcinoma—T1 (Fig. 8.5D): Invasion into the lamina propria or muscularis mucosae has prognostic implications in the esophagus, unlike in the colon, because of the presence of lymphatics in the former. Lymph node metastasis has been reported in 13% of T1 tumors. Duplication of muscularis mucosae can at times be present and should not be mistaken for invasion into the submucosa.

9. **What histologic patterns can be seen in the biopsy samples from the GE junction that do not show typical endoscopic findings of Barrett esophagus?**
   - Gastric-type mucosa without goblet cells—gastric-cardiac mucosa, mostly associated with inflammation (gastric carditis).
   - Prominent Z-line showing gastric-cardiac mucosa with goblet cells.
   - In endoscopically uncertain cases, the presence of goblet cells may suggest either early Barrett mucosa or gastric cardia with goblet cells.

STOMACH

10. **What are the histologic features of the mucosal lining in different parts of the stomach?**
    The five layers of the stomach are the following:
    - Mucosa
    - Muscularis mucosae
    - Submucosa
    - Muscularis propria (innermost oblique, inner circular, and outermost longitudinal layers)
    - Serosa
      The mucosa has three zones that vary by function in different locations of the stomach.
      Superficial layer of neutral mucin secretes foveolar epithelium and lines the entire luminal surface of the stomach, followed by the isthmus (neck) and deep glandular layer.
      Fundus and *body mucosa* have similar features and contain pyramid-shaped parietal or oxyntic (acid-secreting and intrinsic factor–producing) cells and the chief cells (enzyme-producing) in the isthmus and base with scattered endocrine cells. The lining of the foveolar layer is short. The isthmus also contains mucus-secreting cells.
      Cardia and *antrum* have similar features and have a broad, superficial zone of foveolar epithelial cells. The gastric antrum also contains gastrin-secreting G cells. The other enteroendocrine cells have been shown to secrete serotonin, somatostatin (D cells), and vasointestinal polypeptide–like substance.

11. **What are the histologic patterns of gastritis?**
    The two major histologic patterns of gastritis are the following:
    - *Acute gastritis:* Onset is acute. Neutrophilic inflammation, edema, and hemorrhage may all be seen. Acute gastritis is associated with hemorrhage or erosions and ulcerations.
    - *Chronic gastritis with or without activity:* Mixed inflammation with predominant mononuclear cell infiltration and foveolar hyperplasia occurs, with or without intestinal metaplasia and atrophy. Activity can be graded based on the extent of acute inflammation present (mild, moderate, or severe).

12. **What is *Helicobacter heilmannii*–associated gastritis?**
    H. heilmannii (Gastrospirillum hominis) is a rare, long, tightly coiled Gram-negative, urease-producing bacteria that causes gastritis of mild severity.

13. **What are the salient histologic features of chemical and reactive gastropathy?**
    - Histology: Foveolar hyperplasia with glandular tortuosity, edema in the lamina propria, dilated superficial vessels, vertical muscle fibers in the lamina propria, and minimal inflammation (Fig. 8.6).
    - Etiology: Nonsteroidal anti-inflammatory drugs, alcohol, and alkaline reflux (bile).

14. **What is lymphocytic gastritis, and with which disease processes is it associated?**
    - Lymphocytic gastritis occurs in the fundus and body of stomach, but the antrum is affected in celiac disease.
    - Histology: Demonstrates chronic gastritis pattern with increased intraepithelial lymphocytes.

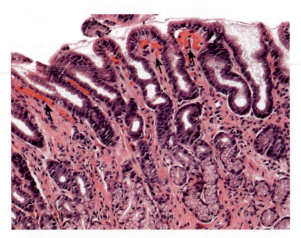

Fig. 8.6 Photomicrograph of chemical-reactive gastropathy. Note the foveolar hyperplasia, glandular tortuosity, ectatic vessels in the lamina propria (*arrow*), and minimal inflammation (hematoxylin and eosin stain).

- Etiology: Most commonly celiac disease and *H. pylori* infection. Less common etiologic factors include varioliform gastritis, lymphocytic gastroenterocolitis, human immunodeficiency virus infection, and lymphoma.

15. What is the differential diagnosis of granulomatous gastritis?
- Histology: Granulomas that may be necrotizing or nonnecrotizing.
- Etiology: Infectious (tuberculous and fungal), Crohn's disease, sarcoid, drug reaction, vasculitis, or idiopathic (isolated granulomatous gastritis) causes.

16. Histologically, how are gastric antral vascular ectasia (GAVE), portal hypertensive gastropathy, Dieulafoy lesion, and radiation injury differentiated?
GAVE on endoscopic evaluation demonstrates red longitudinal stripes usually located in the antrum of the stomach; this is often referred to as "watermelon stomach." Histologic examination reveals dilated, congested vessels; fibrin thrombi and reactive changes such as foveolar hyperplasia; and strands of muscle fibers in the lamina propria.
- *Portal hypertensive gastropathy* on endoscopic evaluation demonstrates the "tiger skin" pattern of dilated mucosal vessels in the body and fundus of the stomach. Histologic biopsy is not recommended. Histologic features include dilated ectatic vessels, foveolar hyperplasia, and fibrosis in the lamina propria with minimal inflammation. The lack of fibrin thrombi can distinguish this from GAVE.
- *Dieulafoy lesion* on endoscopic evaluation usually reveals a *pigmented protuberant vessel* in the proximal stomach without mucosal ulceration. Histologic examination finds an abnormal large artery in the superficial submucosa, which may erode and cause massive hemorrhage. The histologic features include erosion with fibrin and hemorrhage and a large vessel in the submucosa.
- *Radiation injury* on endoscopic evaluation demonstrates numerous mucosal red vascular ectasias located in the radiation port. Histologic examination demonstrates dilated vessels with hyalinized walls. The epithelial and stromal cells show marked atypia, raising the suspicion of dysplasia. Clinical history is important to rule out other causes of angiectasias such as GAVE and portal hypertensive gastropathy.

17. What are the histologic features of giant mucosal folds seen in Ménétrier disease and Zollinger-Ellison syndrome?
- Endoscopic examination finds enlarged gastric folds greater than 8 mm.
- Histologic examination demonstrates that the giant folds are due to hyperplasia of foveolar epithelium or oxyntic epithelium. Ménétrier disease resembles hyperplastic polyp and shows elongated hyperplastic foveolar epithelium with loss of oxyntic glands in the gastric mucosa. Expansion of oxyntic glandular zone resulting in hypertrophic gastropathy is seen in Zollinger-Ellison syndrome. Large folds can also be seen in *H. pylori*–associated gastritis.

18. Compare gastric dysplasia and adenoma.
Gastric dysplasia refers to a flat lesion showing dysplasia (*flat adenoma*). A similar lesion with a polypoid appearance is referred to as an *adenoma*, which consists of tubular, or tubulovillous, architecture. Fig. 8.7 depicts a gastric adenoma showing strong immunoreactivity with p53 antibody. The flat lesion is more likely to be multifocal and associated with high-grade dysplasia. Mapping biopsies are required to rule out invasive carcinoma in both. The adenomas can have morphologic characteristics of the intestinal type (goblet or Paneth cells) or gastric type. Adenocarcinoma is more commonly associated with intestinal-type morphologic characteristics.

19. What are the histologic types of gastric adenocarcinoma?
The WHO classification describes multiple histologic patterns of adenocarcinoma:
- Tubular adenocarcinoma
- Parietal cell carcinoma
- Adenocarcinoma with mixed subtype
- Papillary adenocarcinoma
- Micropapillary carcinoma
- Mucoepidermoid carcinoma
- Mucinous adenocarcinoma
- Signet ring cell carcinoma (Fig. 8.8)
- Poorly cohesive carcinoma
- Medullary carcinoma with lymphoid stroma
- Hepatoid adenocarcinoma
- Paneth cell carcinoma

Other rare variants include adenosquamous carcinoma, squamous cell carcinoma, and undifferentiated carcinoma.

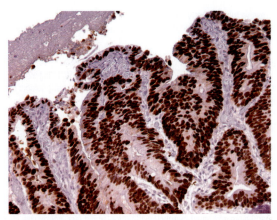

Fig. 8.7 Photomicrograph of gastric adenoma showing strong nuclear immunoreactivity with p53 antibody (immunohistochemical stain).

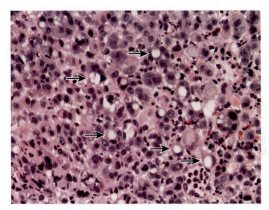

Fig. 8.8 Photomicrograph of gastric adenocarcinoma with signet ring cell morphology (*arrows*) (hematoxylin and eosin stain).

20. What is the histologic classification of neuroendocrine tumors of the stomach?
   - Well-differentiated neuroendocrine tumor (grade 1, grade 2, and grade 3).
   - The recommended grading system for well-differentiated gastric neuroendocrine tumors includes evaluating mitotic activity and Ki-67 labeling index (Ki-67 index is assessed using immunohistochemical stain) (Table 8.1).

Table 8.1 Recommended Grading System for Well-Differentiated Gastroenteropancreatic Neuroendocrine Tumors.

GRADE	MITOTIC RATE (PER 2 MM²)	KI-67 INDEX (%)
Well-differentiated neuroendocrine tumor, G1	<2	<3
Well-differentiated neuroendocrine tumor, G2	2–20	3–20
Well-differentiated neuroendocrine tumor, G3	>2	>2

From College of American Pathologists. Protocol for the examination of specimens from patients with well-differentiated neuroendocrine tumors (carcinoid tumors) of the stomach. Version: 4.1.0.0. Published June 2021.

The neuroendocrine carcinoma is a separate category and includes the following:
   - Small cell neuroendocrine carcinoma
   - Large cell neuroendocrine carcinoma

These are highly aggressive tumors rarely originating in the stomach.

Mixed neuroendocrine and non-neuroendocrine neoplasm show both neuroendocrine and adenocarcinoma components.

21. **What is the differential diagnosis of gastric stromal tumors?**

Gastric stromal tumors are seen as submucosal masses, and the differential diagnosis includes *schwannoma, leiomyoma, GI stromal tumor (GIST),* and *inflammatory fibroid polyps.* The morphologic characteristics are similar to those seen in other sites.

GASTROINTESTINAL STROMAL TUMORS

GISTs are most commonly seen in the stomach (50%), followed by the small bowel (25%), the colon and rectum (10%), and the esophagus (5%). Histologically, these can be spindled or epithelioid and show strong reactivity with CD117 (95%) and positive staining with CD34 (60%–70%). These also stain positive with DOG 1 (*Di*scovered *On GIST*) antibody (including some of *kit* negative tumors). Approximately one-third can also show reactivity with smooth muscle markers (e.g., smooth muscle actin [SMA]). These arise from interstitial cells of Cajal, and *kit* mutations are seen in 85%–90% of GISTs. Approximately 5% show mutation within the *PDGFRA* gene; these are seen in gastric GISTs and have epithelioid morphologic features and a less-aggressive clinical course. All the GISTs are potentially aggressive. The clinical behavior can be predicted on the basis of size, mitotic figures, and site. Gastric GISTs have a better prognosis than small bowel GISTs. The GISTs with exon 11 mutation have a low risk for progressive disease (as opposed to exon 9 mutation).

INFLAMMATORY FIBROID POLYPS

Inflammatory fibroid polyps are bland spindle cells accentuated around vessels and accompanied by a mixed inflammatory infiltrate in the stroma. These are negative for CD117 and may show immunoreactivity with CD34.

22. **What are the different types of gastric lymphomas?**

Mucosa-associated lymphoid tissue (MALT) lymphomas (also known as *extramarginal zone B cell lymphoma*) are low grade and show lymphoepithelial lesions (lymphoma cells infiltrating the gland epithelium). They extend deep into the muscularis mucosae, unlike reactive lymphoid hyperplasia, which is generally more superficial and a major differential diagnosis in these cases. These cells are CD20 (B cell marker) positive; may coexpress CD43; and are CD5 negative, CD10 negative, and positive for bcl-2 protein. *Helicobacter* organisms may be seen. Distinction between reactive infiltrate versus neoplastic can be difficult in small biopsy specimens. Flow cytometry and cytogenetics are useful studies in these cases requiring submission of biopsies in appropriate media (not formalin). Gene rearrangement studies generally help determine the clonality in atypical lymphoid aggregates.

The other lymphomas that can involve the GI tract include mantle cell lymphoma, large B cell lymphoma, enteropathy-like T cell lymphoma, and Burkitt lymphoma.

ACKNOWLEDGMENT

Special thanks are given to Lisa Litzenberger for her superb photographic technical assistance.

BIBLIOGRAPHY

Available Online.

WEBSITES

Available Online.

GASTRITIS, PEPTIC ULCER DISEASE, NONSTEROIDAL ANTI-INFLAMMATORY DRUGS, AND *HELICOBACTER PYLORI* INFECTION

CHAPTER 9

David T. Dulaney, MD and Anish Patel, DO

 Additional content is available online.

1. What is gastritis?

Patients typically refer to the symptom of dyspepsia as *gastritis*. Gastroenterologists use the term *gastritis* to describe endoscopic observations. Pathologists refer to a histologic finding. Most would agree that gastritis requires a mucosal biopsy as it is a histopathologic diagnosis. Inflammation of the gastric mucosa can be classified into two types: *gastritis* or *gastropathy*. The gastric mucosa can have an injury to its epithelium and regeneration without having significant inflammation. When this happens, it is referred to as *gastropathy*. *Gastritis*, however, refers to inflammation of the gastric mucosa with an associated inflammatory infiltrate. Although gastritis c an be either acute or chronic, most cases are truly chronic, as acute gastritis is infrequently diagnosed soon after initiation of the inflammatory process.

2. What are the endoscopic findings associated with gastritis?

There is not one endoscopic entity that defines gastritis. Both gastroenterologists and pathologists have realized that endoscopic appearance frequently does not predict changes in histology (i.e., the presence of inflammation). Endoscopists use the word *gastritis* to describe various findings, including erythema, edema, enlarged gastric folds, polyps, the presence of erosions or ulcers, mucosal bleeding, or atrophy. A normal endoscopic appearance is the most common endoscopic finding associated with histologically diagnosed gastritis.

3. What is the Sydney system for the diagnosis of gastritis?

The Sydney system is a gastric biopsy protocol indicating where gastric mucosal biopsies should be obtained to optimize a diagnosis of gastritis implicated by *Helicobacter pylori*. Five biopsy specimens are taken: two from the antrum within 2–3 cm of the pylorus (one from the distal lesser curvature and one from the distal greater curvature), two from the corpus approximately 8 cm from the cardia (one from the lesser and the other from the greater curvature), and one from the incisura angularis. Samples from the antrum, corpus, and incisura angularis should be separately identified. Duodenal biopsies may be helpful in certain settings (e.g., suspected celiac disease and lymphocytic gastritis, or duodenal Crohn's disease and granulomatous gastritis).

4. What are the common causes of chronic gastritis?

The most common cause of chronic gastritis is *H. pylori* infection. Autoimmune gastritis (atrophic gastritis) accounts for the most common cause of *H. pylori*–negative chronic gastritis (roughly 5%); less common causes include infections, eosinophilic gastritis, lymphocytic gastritis, granulomatous gastritis, graft-versus-host disease, and inflammatory bowel disease (Table 9.1). As mentioned previously, most cases of gastritis are "chronic" because patients with acute gastritis are rarely diagnosed.

5. What are the common etiologic factors of reactive gastropathy?

Medications (particularly nonsteroidal anti-inflammatory drugs [NSAIDs]), toxins, tobacco, alcohol, portal hypertensive gastropathy, cocaine, stress, radiation, bile reflux, ischemia, mechanical injury from gastric cardia prolapsing to the esophageal lumen during retching or vomiting, aging, and certain infections are commonly associated with reactive gastropathy.

6. What medications are frequently associated with gastropathy?

- Acetylsalicylic acid (even low dose) and NSAIDs
- Oral iron
- Potassium chloride
- Bisphosphonate

Table 9.1 Types of Gastritis.

PATHOLOGIC DIAGNOSIS	HISTOLOGIC FINDINGS	ETIOLOGIC FACTORS	ENDOSCOPIC FINDINGS	CLINICAL ASSOCIATIONS
Acute suppurative gastritis	Neutrophilic inflammation	Acute *Helicobacter pylori* and *Streptococcal* gastritis or other bacteria	May be normal or have mucosal fold swelling; dark red, distended stomach; pus	Acute gastroenteritis–like illness, perforation, and gangrene
Chronic and chronic active gastritis	Mixed inflammatory infiltrates (neutrophils, plasma cells, and eosinophils) with or without foveolar hyperplasia, lymphoid aggregates, erosions, ulcers, intestinal metaplasia, and atrophy (late stages)	Chronic *H. pylori* gastritis	Typically normal; may present with erythema, friability, nodularity, or in some cases erosions or ulcerations	Varies; most may be asymptomatic; can present with duodenal ulcer, gastric ulcer, and gastric adenocarcinoma; some association with functional dyspepsia
Lymphocytic gastritis	Chronic active inflammation with increased intraepithelial lymphocytes with or without foveolar hyperplasia, erosions, and ulcers	Hypersensitivity to gliadin, hypersensitivity to unknown agents, and autoimmune	Varioliform or chronic erosive gastritis (nodules with central ulceration); picture of Ménétrier disease	Celiac sprue; Ménétrier disease
Granulomatous gastritis	Multifocal (frequently necrotizing) active chronic inflammation with epithelioid granulomas	Idiopathic isolated granulomatous gastritis; Crohn's disease; fungal, mycobacterial, and spirochetal infections; sarcoidosis; vasculitis; and drug reactions	Variable, including thickened folds and ulcerations	Depends on underlying disease
Eosinophilic gastritis	Sheets of eosinophils	Idiopathic food allergy, drug allergy, and parasitic disease	Prominent folds, hyperemia, nodularity, ulcer, or may be normal	Pain, nausea, and vomiting; early satiety; weight loss and anemia
Hypertrophic lymphocytic gastritis	Lymphocytic gastritis with extreme foveolar hyperplasia	Clinical syndrome identical to Ménétrier gastropathy; etiologic factors presumed different	Same as hypertrophic gastropathy	Same as hypertrophic gastropathy

Adapted from Carpenter HA, Talley NJ. Gastroscopy is incomplete without biopsy: clinical relevance of distinguishing gastropathy from gastritis. Gastroenterology. 1995;108(3):917-924.

Box 9.1 Gastric Epithelial Defense Mechanisms

Pre-epithelial

The mucus barrier forms a continuous gel into which bicarbonate-rich fluid is secreted, forming a protective pH gradient by maintaining a neutral pH.

Epithelial

Surface epithelial cells can withstand acidic environments as low as pH 2.5 and are designed to rapidly repair themselves through a process known as *mucosal restitution*.

Post-epithelial

Rich vascular anatomy within the gastric mucosa ensures delivery of the newly released bicarbonate by parietal cells to the gastric epithelium to neutralize neutrons.

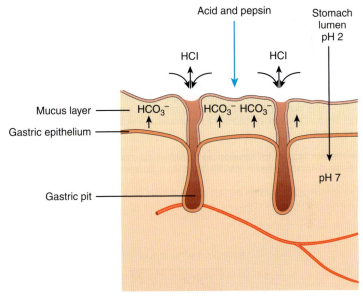

Fig. 9.1 Gastric mucosa protective mechanisms include mucus layer thickness, pH gradient, cell membrane hydrophobicity, bicarbonate (HCO_3^-) secretion, and mucosal blood flow. These mechanisms are mostly mediated by prostaglandins. *HCl*, Hydrochloric acid.

- Fluoride
- Systemic chemotherapy
- Hepatic arterial infusion of chemotherapy
- Toxic ingestion of heavy metals

7. **How does the gastric mucosa normally protect itself from injury given its acidic environment?**

   The stomach has epithelial defense mechanisms that serve to maintain its mucosal integrity. These protective mechanisms are often characterized by three components: pre-epithelial, epithelial, and post-epithelial, all of which are prostaglandin dependent. See Box 9.1 and Fig. 9.1.

8. **What are the common causes of gastric or duodenal ulcers?**

   Very common (>95%):
   - *H. pylori* infection
   - NSAIDs

   Less common (≈5%):
   - Gastric malignancy (adenocarcinoma or lymphoma)
   - Stress ulceration (central nervous system trauma and burn patients)
   - Viral infection (herpes simplex virus type 1 or cytomegalovirus)

Uncommon or rare (<1%):
- Zollinger-Ellison syndrome
- Cocaine use
- Crohn's disease
- Systemic mastocytosis
- Myeloproliferative disorders with basophilia
- Idiopathic (non-*H. pylori*) hypersecretory duodenal ulcer
- Abdominal radiotherapy
- Hepatic artery infusion of 5-fluorouracil

9. What is the role of NSAIDs in the pathogenesis of gastroduodenal ulcers?

There are *two* principal pathogenic mechanisms by which NSAIDs cause ulceration (Fig. 9.2):
- Reduction of gastrointestinal mucosal prostaglandins
- Local, topical injury to surface epithelial cells
  - Prostaglandins protect against injury in the gastrointestinal tract. NSAIDs inhibit cyclooxygenase (COX), the rate-limiting enzyme in prostaglandin synthesis, leading to a reduction in prostaglandin concentrations and loss of a primary mechanism of protection and predisposition to injury. There are two COX isoforms: COX-1 and COX-2. COX-1 is the predominant isoform present in the gastrointestinal tract. COX-2 is primarily present at sites of inflammation; NSAIDs that inhibit COX-2 primarily cause less reduction in gastrointestinal prostaglandins and thus lower rates of NSAID-induced ulcers.

10. What are NSAID-related gastrointestinal complications?

The most common gastrointestinal *finding* associated with NSAID use is symptomatic ulcers. However, most of these ulcers have a benign course, and most do not progress to complications. Among the possible complications of NSAID-related ulcers, gastrointestinal bleeding, perforation, and gastrointestinal obstruction are frequent occurrences. The most common gastrointestinal *complication* of NSAID use is bleeding from peptic ulcer disease, mainly in the stomach.

11. What are the risk factors for developing NSAID-related complications?

H. pylori infection also increases the risk of NSAID-related ulcers. Treatment of *H. pylori* reduces the risk of rebleeding.

Selective serotonin reuptake inhibitors increase the risk of upper gastrointestinal bleeding threefold. Concurrent use of NSAIDs potentiates this effect.

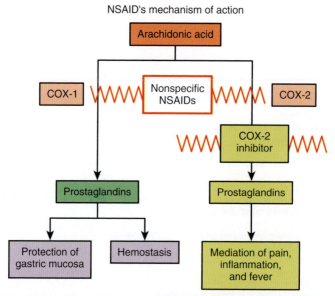

Fig. 9.2 Nonsteroidal anti-inflammatory drugs' (NSAIDs) main mechanism of mucosal injury is via local irritation of gastric mucosa and by inhibition of cyclooxygenase (COX), which subsequently leads to a reduction in prostaglandins.

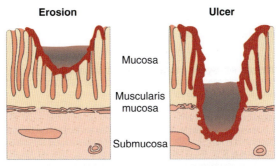

Fig. 9.3 Difference between an erosion and an ulcer mainly involves the depth of mucosal injury.

Box 9.2 Difference Between Erosion and Ulcer

Erosion	Well-defined hemorrhagic lesions 1–2 mm in size; superficial lamina necrosis—endoscopically defined as <3 mm in diameter
Ulcer	Extends to the muscularis mucosa

Concurrent clopidogrel (Plavix) with aspirin increases the risk of upper gastrointestinal bleeding. The need for anti-platelet agents should be reviewed. In patients with established cardiovascular disease who require antiplatelet therapy, proton pump inhibitor (PPI) co-therapy should be provided long term.
- Older age
- Previous gastrointestinal event (e.g., previous ulcer or gastrointestinal bleeding)
- Concomitant use of anticoagulants
- Corticosteroids
- Other NSAIDs, including low-dose aspirin and high-dose NSAID therapy
- Chronic debilitating disorders such as cardiovascular disease

12. How is an erosion different from an ulcer?
An erosion is differentiated from an ulcer according to the depth of the mucosal injury. Erosions do not extend into or below the muscularis mucosae, whereas ulcers do (Fig. 9.3 and Box 9.2).

Unlike erosions, ulcers extend to the muscularis mucosa and submucosa; therefore, healing an ulcer requires tissue regeneration, whereas superficial erosion heals with the adjacent mucosa.

13. What is the typical presentation of uncomplicated ulcer disease?
- Burning, sharp, deep epigastric pain that usually arises 1–3 hours after eating
- Vague abdominal discomfort or nausea rather than pain
- Relief of symptoms by eating or taking antacids
- Occurrence of symptoms when the stomach is empty or at night (nocturnal acid production)
- History of self-treatment with antacids, frequent and long-standing use of H_2-receptor antagonists, or cigarette smoking
- Symptoms recurring over months or years
- Epigastric tenderness on palpation (with active symptomatic ulcers)

14. How is the endoscopic diagnosis of an ulcer made?
It is important to differentiate between an erosion and an ulcer. Whereas an erosion involves only the superficial mucosa, an ulcer generally extends to the submucosa where vessels reside. According to the most current guidelines from the American College of Gastroenterology (ACG), although the diagnosis of an ulcer requires histologic depth, we rely on the endoscopist to interpret the depth of the ulcer and to provide clues about the endoscopic appearance of the ulcer to help guide its management.

15. What is *H. pylori* infection?
H. pylori is a major pathogen in humans. *H. pylori* is a small, curved, microaerophilic, Gram-negative, rod-shaped bacterium that can infect the human gastric mucosa and become persistent. Although many people infected with *H. pylori* may be asymptomatic, infection may lead to complications such as gastric and duodenal ulcers, multifocal atrophic gastritis, mucosa-associated lymphoid tissue (MALT) lymphoma, and gastric cancer.

16. **How is *H. pylori* transmitted?**
    Transmission of *H. pylori* appears to occur by direct, person-to-person contact, especially gastro-oral. Fecal-oral, oral-oral, and salivary routes of transmission have been reported.

17. **What is cagA⁺+ *H. pylori*?**
    H. pylori strains that possess the *cagA* gene are associated with severe forms of gastroduodenal disease. *CagA* is a gene that codes for an immunodominant antigen. The genetic locus that contains *cagA* (*cag*) is part of a 40-kb DNA insertion that likely is acquired horizontally.

18. **What is the prevalence of *H. pylori*?**
    The prevalence of *H. pylori* varies worldwide. According to the Centers for Disease Control and Prevention, close to 50% of the world's population is infected with *H. pylori*. A recent meta-analysis showed that the overall prevalence of *H. pylori* in the United States is 35.6% (95% confidence interval [CI]: 30.0%–41.1%). However, the incidence is much higher in indigenous populations, such as the Alaskan indigenous population (74.8%; 95% CI: 72.9%–76.7%). Worldwide, the regions with the highest prevalence of *H. pylori* are Africa (70.1%; 95% CI: 62.6%–77.6%), South America (69.4%; 95% CI: 63.9%–74.9%), and Western Asia (66.6%; 95% CI: 56.1%–77.0%).

19. **What are the typical pathologic findings associated with *H. pylori* infection?**
    H. pylori is usually found in the antrum, although it may be found in the corpus. An inflammatory infiltrate consisting of neutrophils within the lamina propria can be seen crossing the basement membrane. Intraepithelial neutrophils and subepithelial plasma cells are pathognomonic for *H. pylori* infection. Lymphoid aggregates are frequently present.

20. **How does *H. pylori* infection lead to peptic ulcer disease?**
    An antral-predominant pattern of *H. pylori* infection generally spares the body and fundus. This infection preferentially alters the total mass of antral D cells, which secrete somatostatin. Lowered somatostatin levels prevent the usual downregulation of gastrin-secreting G cells. Thus antral-predominant infection leads to unopposed gastrin secretion. This leads to increased parietal cell mass, hyperchlorhydria, and lower intraluminal pH, which causes mucosal injury and ulceration.

21. **How does *H. pylori* infection lead to gastric atrophy or atrophic gastritis?**
    Long-standing corpus-predominant *H. pylori* infection can lead to depletion of parietal cell mass in the fundus and body of the stomach. This is often referred to as *multifocal atrophic gastritis*. It tends to be characterized by antrum-predominant gastritis or pan-gastritis, where the normal mucosa is subsequently replaced by the mucosa that is not normally there (metaplasia). In the setting of *H. pylori* infection, atrophy and intestinal metaplasia invariably involve the antrum and could involve the corpus as well.

22. **How does *H. pylori* infection lead to gastric cancer?**
    See Fig. 9.4.
    Presently, *H. pylori* is considered a Group I carcinogen by the International Agency for Research on Cancer, and it is considered a necessary but insufficient cause of gastric adenocarcinoma. Eradication of *H. pylori* is associated with a reduction in gastric cancer incidence.

23. **What diagnostic tests are available for testing for *H. pylori* and what are their sensitivity and specificity?**
    See Table 9.2.

24. **Who should be tested and treated for *H. pylori* infection?**
    - A test-and-treat strategy for *H. pylori* is encouraged. According to the 2017 ACG guidelines, those with active peptic ulcer disease (gastric or duodenal ulcer), those with a confirmed history of peptic ulcer disease (without a documented test of cure for *H. pylori*), those with low-grade gastric MALT lymphoma, those who have had endoscopic resections of early gastric cancer, and those with un-investigated dyspepsia who are under 60 years of age and without alarm features who live in areas of high *H. pylori* prevalence should be tested for *H. pylori* and treated.
    - It is recommended that those taking long-term, low-dose aspirin should be considered for *H. pylori* testing to reduce the risk of ulcer bleeding. Similarly, those taking chronic NSAID therapy should be tested and offered eradication therapy if found to be positive.
    - Patients with idiopathic thrombocytopenic purpura should be tested and offered eradication therapy if testing is positive.
    - Patients with unexplained iron-deficiency anemia, despite an appropriate evaluation, should be tested for *H. pylori* and offered eradication treatment if positive.

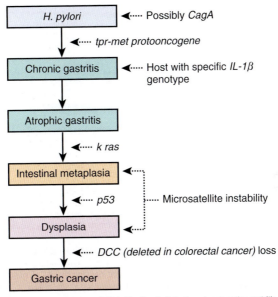

H. Pylori infection and gastric cancer:
the correa cascade

Fig. 9.4 Well-defined precancerous sequential stages initiated by *H. pylori* infection: chronic active gastritis → chronic atrophic gastritis → intestinal metaplasia → dysplasia (also called *intraepithelial neoplasia*) and carcinoma. *IL-1β*, Interleukin-1β.

Table 9.2 Comparison of Diagnostic Tests for *Helicobacter pylori*.		
DIAGNOSTIC TESTS	**SENSITIVITY (%)**	**SPECIFICITY (%)**
Invasive (Endoscopy)		
Gastric biopsies, histologic examination	93–99	95–99
Clo-test (rapid urease assay)	89–98	93–98
Culture	58	100
Noninvasive (Nonendoscopic)		
Serologic evaluation	88–99	93–98
Urea breath test	90–97	90–100
Stool antigen	90–96	97–98

Adapted from McNally PR. GI/Liver Secrets Plus. 4th ed. Philadelphia, PA: Mosby; 2010; Kanna S, Maradey-Romero C, Fass R. Diagnostic tests for *Helicobacter pylori*. In Gastroenterology & Endoscopy News. McMahon Publishing; 2013.

25. What is the recommended initial treatment for *H. pylori* infection?

Recent guidelines from the ACG suggest that the choice of first-line treatment option should be based on that which has the greatest likelihood of eradication when considering local resistance patterns of *H. pylori* and patient factors (e.g., penicillin [PCN] allergy or macrolide exposure for any reason in areas with >15% clarithromycin resistance). See Fig. 9.5.

Presently, the recommended first-line treatment regimens are clarithromycin triple therapy, bismuth quadruple therapy, and concomitant therapy. Suggested first-line treatment regimens include sequential therapy, hybrid therapy, levofloxacin triple therapy, and fluoroquinolone therapy.

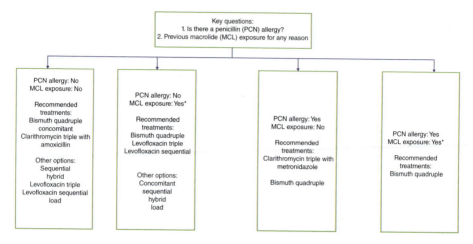

*In regions with clarithromycin resistance >15%.

Fig. 9.5 Algorithm of selection of first-line therapies for *Helicobacter pylori* per recent American College of Gastroenterology guidelines. (From Chey WD, Leontiadis GI, Howden CW, Moss SF. ACG clinical guideline: treatment of *Helicobacter pylori* infection. Am J Gastroenterol. 2017;112:212-239.)

26. What are the treatment regimens for *H. pylori* eradication per the ACG guidelines?
See Table 9.3. Longer treatment durations provide higher success rates of eradication.

27. How is eradication of *H. pylori* confirmed?
Per the current ACG guidelines, testing for proof of eradication should be performed using urea breath test, fecal antigen testing, or biopsy-based testing. This should be performed at least 4 weeks after the completion of antibiotic therapy and after PPI therapy has been withheld for 1–2 weeks.

28. What are the causes of the failure of eradication of *H. pylori*?
Failure of eradication of *H. pylori* is impacted by host, system, and microbial factors. Host factors are generally dictated by nonadherence to treatment or factors that affect the intragastric pH. Patients with metabolism-enhancing polymorphisms of *CYP2C19*, a gene of cytochrome P450 that is responsible for the metabolism of earlier-generation PPIs, have higher rates of eradication failure, particularly when using PPIs metabolized through this pathway (e.g., omeprazole and lansoprazole). Microbial factors such as antibiotic resistance can lead to eradication failure. Furthermore, systemic factors such as lack of local and national surveillance registries and local resistance patterning can lead to incorrect antibiotic choices and eradication failure.

29. What are the salvage therapies for first-line failure of *H. pylori* treatment?
Failure of eradication from first-line therapies requires the use of salvage therapies for treatment. As a general principle, the use of the same antibiotic should be avoided. The salvage therapies are shown in Table 9.4. The algorithm for the selection of salvage therapies is included in Fig. 9.6.

If bismuth quadruple therapy failed as a first-line treatment, the recommended second-line options should include levofloxacin or rifabutin-based triple-therapy regimens with high-dose PPI, and amoxicillin or alternative bismuth-containing quadruple therapy. Also, when considering treatment failure, inadequate acid suppression must be addressed with the use of high doses of more potent PPIs, PPIs not metabolized via *CYP2C19*, or potassium-competitive acid blockers, where available.

For patients in whom PCN-based therapies were avoided due to reported history of PCN allergy, a referral to an allergist and allergy testing should be performed after failure of first-line therapy.

After two failed therapy courses, *H. pylori* susceptibility testing should be considered to guide the selection of future treatment regimens.

30. What is autoimmune atrophic gastritis?
Autoimmune gastritis refers to an autoimmune process that progressively destroys the normal parietal cells in the stomach, also referred to as *oxyntic cells*, and leads to gastric atrophy.

Table 9.3 Recommended First-Line Treatment Regimens for *Helicobacter pylori* Infection.

REGIMEN	DRUGS (DOSES) AND FREQUENCY	DURATION	COMMENTS
Clarithromycin triple	PPI* (high dose) twice daily, clarithromycin (500 mg) twice daily, amoxicillin (1000 mg) twice daily, or metronidazole (500 mg) three times daily	14 days	Remains a first-line option for treatment in regions where clarithromycin resistance is below 15% Avoid if local resistance to clarithromycin is high (>15%) Avoid if previous exposure to macrolides for any reason
Bismuth quadruple	PPI* (standard dose) twice daily, bismuth subcitrate (120–300 mg) or subsalicylate (300 mg) four times daily, tetracycline (500 mg) four times daily, and metronidazole (250 mg) four times daily or (500 mg) three to four times daily	10–14 days	Initial treatment regimen of choice for patients in regions with high clarithromycin resistance or in patients previously treated with macrolides for any reason
Concomitant	PPI* (standard dose) twice daily, clarithromycin (500 mg) twice daily, amoxicillin (1000 mg) twice daily, and nitroimidazole (500 mg) twice daily	10–14 days	Similar tolerance and compliance with clarithromycin triple therapy At least as effective as clarithromycin triple therapy Considered a recommended first-line treatment option in North America
Sequential	PPI* (standard dose) and amoxicillin (1000 mg) twice daily twice daily PPI* (standard dose) twice daily, clarithromycin (500 mg) twice daily, nitroimidazole (500 mg) twice daily	5–7 days for PPI and amoxicillin followed by 5–7 days for PPI, clarithromycin, and nitroimidazole	Complexity of therapy detracts from relevance as first-line therapy 10 days of therapy is viable alternative to 14-day clarithromycin triple therapy, but not superior to it
Hybrid	PPI* (standard dose) twice daily and amoxicillin (1000 mg) twice daily PPI* (standard dose) twice daily, amoxicillin (1000 mg) twice daily, clarithromycin (500 mg) twice daily, and nitroimidazole (500 mg) twice daily	7 days for PPI and amoxicillin followed by 7 days for PPI, amoxicillin, clarithromycin, and nitroimidazole	Similar tolerability to clarithromycin triple therapy At least as effective as clarithromycin triple therapy
Levofloxacin triple	PPI* (standard dose) twice daily, levofloxacin (500 mg) once daily, and amoxicillin (1000 mg) twice daily	10–14 days	Little data exist addressing the efficacy of first-line levofloxacin regimens Little data is present to address fluoroquinolone resistance rates or their impact on efficacy
Levofloxacin sequential	PPI* (standard or high dose) twice daily, amoxicillin (1000 mg) twice daily PPI* (standard or double dose) twice daily, amoxicillin (1000 mg) twice daily, levofloxacin (500 mg) once daily, and nitroimidazole (500 mg) twice daily	5–7 days for PPI and amoxicillin followed by 5–7 days for PPI, amoxicillin, levofloxacin, and nitroimidazole	
LOAD	Levofloxacin (500 mg) daily, PPI* (high dose) daily, nitazoxanide (500 mg) twice daily, and doxycycline (100 mg) daily	7–10 days	

PPI, Proton pump inhibitor.
From Chey WD, Leontiadis GI, Howden CW, Moss SF. ACG clinical guideline: treatment of *Helicobacter pylori* infection. Am J Gastroenterol. 2017;112:212–239.

Table 9.4 Salvage Therapies for *Helicobacter pylori* After First-Line Therapy Failure.

REGIMEN	DRUGS (DOSES)	DURATION	COMMENTS
Bismuth quadruple	PPI[a] (standard dose) twice daily, bismuth subcitrate (120–300 mg) or subsalicylate (300 mg) four times daily, tetracycline (500 mg) four times daily, and metronidazole (250 mg) four times daily or (500 mg) three to four times daily	14 days	Preferred treatment options if the patient received first-line treatment with clarithromycin
Levofloxacin triple	PPI[a] (standard dose) twice daily, levofloxacin (500 mg) once daily, and amoxicillin (1000 mg) twice daily	14 days	Preferred if first-line therapy contained clarithromycin or for first-line bismuth quadruple therapy
Concomitant	PPI[a] (standard dose) twice daily, clarithromycin (500 mg) twice daily, amoxicillin (1000 mg) twice daily, and nitroimidazole (500 mg) twice daily or three times daily	10–14 days	
Rifabutin triple	PPI[a] (standard dose) twice daily, rifabutin 300 mg daily, and amoxicillin (1000 mg) twice daily	10 days	
High-dose dual	PPI[a] (standard to high dose) three to four times daily and amoxicillin (1000 mg) three times daily or (750 mg) four times daily	14	

PPI, Proton pump inhibitor.
[a]Standard dose varies by PPI.
From Shah SC, Iyer PG, Moss SF. AGA clinical practice update on the management of refractory *Helicobacter pylori* infection: expert review. Gastroenterology. 2021;160:1831-1841.

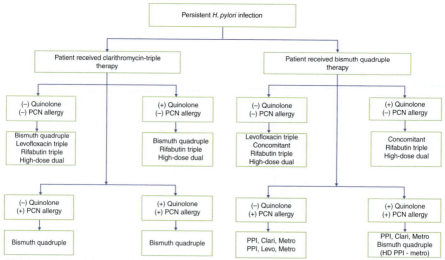

(-) Quinolone = no previous quinolone exposure; (+) Quinolone = previous quinolone exposure; (-) PCN allergy= no penicillin allergy; (+) PCN allergy penicillin allergy
PPI=proton pump inhibitor, Clari = clarithromycin, Levo = levofloxacin; Metro = metronidazole; HD = high dose

Fig. 9.6 Algorithm for the selection of salvage treatment regimen for persistent *Helicobacter pylori* infection following the failure of first-line therapy per recent American College of Gastroenterology guidelines. (From Chey WD, Leontiadis GI, Howden CW, Moss SF. ACG clinical guideline: treatment of *Helicobacter pylori* infection. Am J Gastroenterol. 2017;112:212-239.)

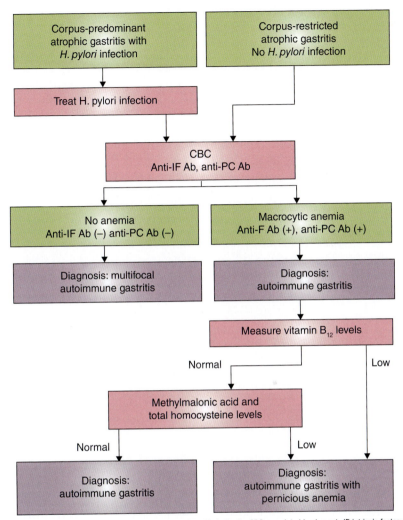

Fig. 9.7 Proposed algorithm for diagnosis of autoimmune gastritis. *Ab*, Antibody; *CBC*, complete blood count; *IF*, intrinsic factor; *PC*, parietal cell. (From Neumann WL, Coss E, Rugge M, Genta RM. Autoimmune atrophic gastritis-pathogenesis, pathology and management. Nat Rev Gastroenterol Hepatol. 2013;10(9):529-541.)

31. How is autoimmune atrophic gastritis different from multifocal atrophic gastritis?

Autoimmune atrophic gastritis tends to be restricted to the corpus, whereas *H. pylori* multifocal atrophic gastritis involves the antrum. Autoimmune atrophic gastritis can be associated in its severe form with vitamin B_{12}–deficiency anemia, also known as *pernicious anemia*.

32. How is autoimmune atrophic gastritis diagnosed?

Patients with autoimmune atrophic gastritis often present with vague clinical symptoms, including fatigue, or symptoms related to iron-deficiency anemia, which is what prompts an endoscopic evaluation, usually with endoscopy and colonoscopy. The diagnosis of autoimmune atrophic gastritis relies on biopsies but can be substantiated by demonstrating autoantibodies against intrinsic factors and parietal cells. Fig. 9.7 is a diagram with a proposed algorithm for a treatment approach for a patient with suspected autoimmune atrophic gastritis.

BIBLIOGRAPHY

Available Online.

CHAPTER 10

GASTRIC CANCER

Prashant Vasanth Krishnan, MD

 Additional content available online.

EPIDEMIOLOGY

1. **What are the incidence and ethnic and geographic distributions of gastric adenocarcinoma?**

   Every year, approximately 1 million people are diagnosed with gastric cancer worldwide. Incidence rates are the highest in East Asia, Central Asia, Eastern Europe, and South America, whereas the lowest rates are in North America, North Africa, and East Africa. Although the incidence and mortality of gastric cancer have decreased over recent decades, it remains the fifth most commonly diagnosed cancer and the third leading cause of cancer mortality (Fig. 10.1).

2. **How common is gastric cancer in the United States?**

   The American Cancer Society estimates that there were 26,380 new cases of stomach cancer (with 11,090 deaths) in the United States in 2022.

3. **How is the incidence of gastric adenocarcinoma changing?**

   Gastric adenocarcinoma has two major sites of presentation: carcinoma gastric cardia (CGC, within 5 cm of the gastroesophageal [GE] junction) or distally, referred to as non-CGC (NCGC). Worldwide, NCGC is the most common, with chronic *Helicobacter pylori* infection responsible for roughly 90% of cases. Rates of NCGC in the United States continue to decrease among adults 50 years or older; however, the incidence of NCGC among persons less than 50 years is increasing, particularly among Hispanics, non-Hispanic Blacks, and Asian and Pacific Islanders. Conversely, worldwide, CGC has been increasing rapidly, probably related to obesity and reflux of gastric contents.

4. **What is the role of diet in the development of gastric cancer?**

   Dietary factors appear to be important in the development of gastric cancer. In general, the incidence of gastric cancer is higher when a greater proportion of the diet is obtained from salted or smoked meats or fish; fruits and vegetables appear to be protective. Dietary factors are thought to explain a large part of the variation in gastric

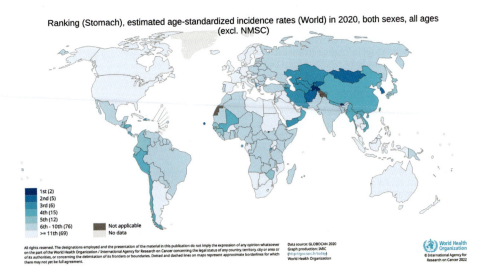

Ranking (Stomach), estimated age-standardized incidence rates (World) in 2020, both sexes, all ages (excl. NMSC)

1st (2)
2nd (5)
3rd (6)
4th (15)
5th (12)
6th - 10th (76)
>= 11th (69)
Not applicable
No data

Data source: GLOBOCAN 2020
Graph production: IARC
(http://gco.iarc.fr/today)
World Health Organization

World Health Organization
© International Agency for Research on Cancer 2022

Fig. 10.1 Global estimated age-standardized incidence rates for stomach cancer in 2020.

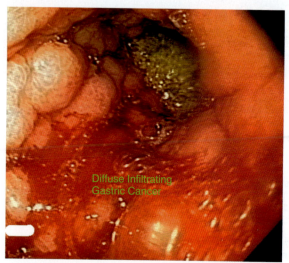

Diffuse Infiltrating
Gastric Cancer

Fig. 10.2 Endoscopic view of infiltrating gastric adenocarcinoma.

cancer occurrence from country to country and may be responsible for the decrease in gastric cancer incidence seen when subjects migrate from high- to low-incidence areas.

ETIOLOGY/PATHOGENESIS

5. **What inherited genetic syndromes are associated with gastric adenocarcinoma?**
   Approximately 10% of gastric cancer appears to be familial, independent of *H. pylori* status. Familial adenomatous polyposis patients have a 10-fold increase in gastric cancer over the general population. Approximately 10% of patients with Lynch syndrome develop gastric cancer. Families with specific mutations in the E-cadherin gene (*CDH1*) have been reported to have a 100% chance of developing diffuse gastric cancer (Fig. 10.2). *Gastric adenocarcinoma and proximal polyposis of the stomach*, an autosomal dominant syndrome, is characterized by fundic gland polyposis (a condition previously believed to be benign) and intestinal-type proximal gastric cancer.

6. **What is the role of *H. pylori* in gastric adenocarcinoma?**
   H. pylori infection appears to increase the lifetime risk of gastric cancer. Infected persons have approximately a twofold increase in the risk of acquiring gastric adenocarcinoma; however, the overall risk is still very low. *H. pylori* infection results in a rather marked inflammatory state in the stomach, which can eventually lead to atrophic gastritis and achlorhydria. Some reports suggest that host factors, including a proinflammatory host genotype, lead to both achlorhydria and gastric cancer development.

7. **What is the role of achlorhydria in gastric cancer?**
   Achlorhydria is caused by destruction of the parietal cells, either from autoimmune conditions or from *H. pylori* infection, often presenting with cobalamin (B_{12}) deficiency. People with achlorhydria, independent of *H. pylori*, have a significant increase in the incidence of gastric cancers, possibly related to the associated elevation in gastrin levels, as well as the inflammation leading to parietal cell destruction.

8. **Should *H. pylori* infection be eradicated to prevent gastric cancer from occurring?**
   A systematic review and meta-analysis showed that *H. pylori* eradication decreases gastric cancer incidence, applicable to all levels of baseline risk, such as genetics, diet, and tobacco use.

9. **What is gastric stump cancer?**
   After partial gastric resection, the incidence of gastric cancers at the gastrointestinal anastomosis (Fig. 10.3) appears to be increased twofold. The median interval time from initial surgery to cancer is 16.5 years. In the initial 5 years after partial gastrectomy, there may be an actual decrease in cancer risk. Resection may impart a pro-cancer effect, and over time, cancers start to form. Although there are no firm recommendations, if surveillance is considered, it should be instituted 15–20 years after the original gastric surgery.

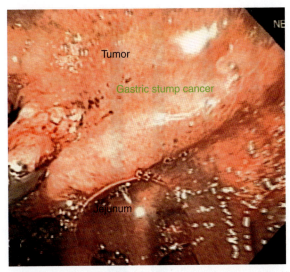

Fig. 10.3 Endoscopic view of gastric stump cancer at the gastrojejunostomy anastomosis using narrow band imaging.

HISTOLOGIC CLASSIFICATION

10. **What are the histologic types of gastric cancer?**
    More than 80% of gastric cancers are adenocarcinomas. Less common types include lymphomas (low grade and high grade), endocrine tumors such as carcinoid or small cell cancers, mesenchymal tumors, and metastatic tumors (e.g., melanoma and breast cancer).

11. **What are mesenchymal tumors of the stomach?**
    The mesenchyme is the loosely packed, unspecialized cells from which connective tissue, bone, cartilage, and the circulatory and lymphatic systems develop. These tissues can undergo transformation. In the stomach, these tumors appear to be subepithelial. The histologic findings can be varied, and the final identification often relies on immunohistochemistry. The most common mesenchymal tumor of the stomach is the gastrointestinal stromal tumor (GIST), which stains for c-KIT/CD117 and CD34.

12. **What is a signet ring cell carcinoma?**
    Signet ring carcinomas are adenocarcinomas in which more than 50% of the malignant cells have intracytoplasmic mucin, pushing the nucleus off to the side. Signet ring cell carcinoma, an aggressive subtype, produces a desmoplastic (fibrous stromal) reaction.

13. **What is linitis plastica?**
    Linitis plastica is a form of gastric adenocarcinoma that infiltrates the stomach wall, causing an associated desmoplastic reaction. The stomach becomes poorly distensible and resembles a "leather bottle." This presentation generally has a poor prognosis.

STAGING/PROGNOSIS

14. **What is early gastric cancer?**
    Early gastric cancer is a gastric adenocarcinoma in which the primary tumor is confined to the mucosa or submucosa, independent of nodal status.

15. **What is the staging scheme for gastric adenocarcinoma?**
    Tumor-node-metastasis (TNM) staging is generally used. T stage is primarily determined by the relation of the tumor to the muscularis propria (above = T1, into = T2, or through = T3). T4a is through serosa and T4b is into adjacent structures (Fig. 10.4). N stage is determined by the number and location of the affected nodes (local versus distant). M stage is determined by whether distant metastases are present.

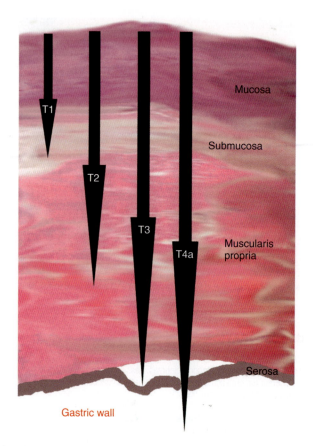

Fig. 10.4 T staging scheme for gastric adenocarcinoma.

16. **How does staging help in treating gastric cancer?**
    Survival after gastrectomy for gastric cancer is directly correlated with the stage as reported in the Surveillance, Epidemiology, and End Results data. For instance, stage-stratified 5-year relative survival rates in a study of more than 50,000 cases of gastric cancer in the United States were as follows: stage IA 78%, stage IB 58%, stage II 34%, stage IIIA 20%, stage IIIB 8%, and stage IV 7%. Therapy, prognosis, and follow-up can be tailored based on initial staging.

17. **What is the role of endoscopic ultrasonography (EUS) in staging gastric cancer?**
    EUS is the most accurate method of T and N staging of gastrointestinal tumors and has the advantage of biopsy capability. EUS can detect small amounts of ascites in staging gastric cancer, suggesting unresectability. Lymph node staging is approximately 80% accurate. EUS imaging can provide a roadmap, but surgical and pathologic staging is more definitive than image-based staging. See Chapter 71.

TREATMENT

18. **What is the role of endoscopy in the treatment of early gastric cancer?**
    Early gastric cancer with a surface diameter of less than 2 cm is amenable to endoscopic removal. The cure rate with endoscopic resection is higher than 95% if the tumor shows no evidence of lymphovascular invasion, is confined to the mucosa, and has intestinal histologic characteristics. EUS is a valuable adjunct to endoscopic resection because detection of nodal involvement precludes definitive endoscopic management of the tumor.

19. **What are gastric endoscopic mucosal resection (EMR) and gastric endoscopic submucosal dissection (ESD)?**
    Both methods generally employ the injection of a fluid between the mucosa and the gastric wall to separate the lesion from deeper structures. EMR often uses suction devices and a snare to remove the tumor, whereas ESD

employs an endoscopic cautery knife to dissect the lesion free from the underlying tissue. EMR is easier to perform and has a lower complication rate, but ESD can be used for en bloc resection of larger lesions.

20. **What is the extent of surgery when trying to remove locally advanced gastric adenocarcinoma?**
    Surgery is a potentially curative therapy for localized gastric adenocarcinoma. The prognosis is based on TNM staging. The extent of resection is somewhat controversial. Japanese literature suggests that an extended lymphadenectomy plus omentectomy (D2 operation) is superior to a limited lymphadenectomy with omentectomy (D1 procedure) or limited lymphadenectomy (D0 procedure). In a randomized European study, patients undergoing D2 resection had twice the operative mortality as those undergoing D1 resection, and there was no survival benefit.

21. **What is the role of neoadjuvant therapy in gastric adenocarcinoma?**
    Neoadjuvant therapy is a treatment given before an attempt at curative surgical resection. The hypothesis is that this therapy shrinks the primary tumor and possibly treats small foci of disease outside the operative field. Some studies suggest neoadjuvant chemotherapy is beneficial for proximal gastric cancer with a more advanced local stage.

22. **What is the role of adjuvant therapy in gastric adenocarcinoma?**
    Adjuvant therapy is an additional treatment given to patients after attempted curative surgery. Adjuvant treatment is given if there is no evidence of remaining disease. Adjuvant radiation and chemotherapy improve the outcome in treating gastric cancer. A meta-analysis also suggests that adjuvant chemotherapy without radiation therapy provides benefit after curative-intent surgery.

SCREENING

23. **Who should be screened for gastric cancer?**
    In Japan, where gastric cancer is the leading cause of cancer death, annual screening is recommended after the age of 40 years. There are no screening recommendations for distal gastric adenocarcinoma in the United States, and no recommendations are widely accepted for the screening of immigrants from high-risk areas. Screening for proximal gastric or GE junction cancer is probably warranted in people with long-standing reflux symptoms.

LYMPHOMA OF THE STOMACH

24. **What is a mucosal-associated lymphoid tissue (MALT) lymphoma?**
    MALT lymphomas are also referred to as *extranodal marginal zone B cell lymphomas*. They can occur in any mucosal location, both within and outside the gastrointestinal tract, but are most common in the stomach. MALT lymphomas are often low-grade B cell lymphomas (Fig. 10.5) but may also be high-grade aggressive tumors.

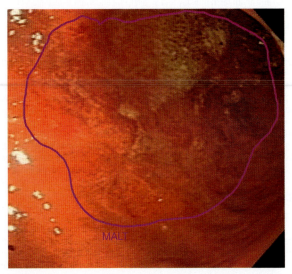

Fig. 10.5 Endoscopic view of superficial low-grade mucosal-associated lymphoid tissue (MALT) lymphoma.

25. **What is unique about gastric MALT lymphomas?**

    Gastric MALT lymphomas, unlike MALT lymphomas in other locations, are often associated with infection by *H. pylori*. Lymphoid tissue is not a normal part of the gastric epithelium, and infection with *H. pylori* seems to drive lymphoid proliferation and tumor development.

26. **What is the role of antibiotic therapy in gastric MALT lymphomas?**

    Treatment of *H. pylori* infection usually leads to regression and cure of low-grade B cell gastric MALT lymphomas. It is believed that the low-grade tumors retain responsiveness to *H. pylori* antigen stimulation. Complete responses can take up to 18 months after antibiotic therapy. In general, high-grade gastric MALT lymphomas and those with more advanced chromosomal abnormalities do not respond well to antibacterial therapy.

27. **What is the staging scheme for gastric lymphoma?**

    Several staging systems are used for gastric lymphoma, including TNM staging. A clinical staging system used for non-Hodgkin lymphoma, the Ann Arbor classification, identifies the primary site of lymphoma as nodal or extranodal and assesses the extent of disease based on the number of sites involved, the relation of the tumor to the diaphragm, and whether the disease has metastasized to non-lymphoid organs. In the Ann Arbor system, a lymphoma involving both the stomach and a lymph node may be stage IIE (two sites with extranodal primary) or stage IV (nodal primary with metastasis to the stomach). A new staging system that combines TNM staging with Ann Arbor criteria has recently been recommended for gastric lymphomas.

28. **What is the best therapy for high-grade gastric lymphoma?**

    Therapy is somewhat determined by stage. For most cases of Ann Arbor stages I and II, surgery can be curative. Data suggest that chemotherapy with or without radiation therapy can be equally effective. T stage may be important in the decision of whether to use a surgical approach because of the possibility of perforation when chemotherapy is used for T3 or T4 tumors. The trend is moving away from surgery for all stages.

NEUROENDOCRINE TUMORS

29. **What are gastric carcinoid tumors?**

    Gastric carcinoid tumors are growths of neuroendocrine cells that may be benign or malignant; they stain for chromogranin. As a rule, even malignant tumors are slow growing. Tumors greater than 1 cm in diameter are generally more dangerous, whereas smaller tumors are not and may represent enterochromaffin cell hyperplasia. Tumors larger than 2 cm have often metastasized. As a rule, large tumors often require partial gastrectomy, whereas smaller tumors can be managed endoscopically or with localized surgery (Fig. 10.6).

30. **What are the different types of gastric carcinoid tumors?**

    Two processes appear to lead to gastric carcinoid—de novo malignant transformation and loss of normal growth regulation in response to chronic elevation of serum gastrin levels. Tumors arising from de novo malignant (type III) (Fig. 10.7) transformation are usually single, larger, and more aggressive, whereas those arising from elevated gastrin levels (types I and II) are often multiple and smaller. It is important to distinguish between those with and without elevated gastrin levels. If the gastrin level is elevated, evaluation for atrophic gastritis should be carried out with an assessment for vitamin B_{12} levels and consideration of gastric biopsies to look for the presence of parietal cells.

31. **How do you differentiate gastric carcinoids from autoimmune gastritis versus Zollinger-Ellison syndrome?**

    Serum antiparietal cell antibodies can be obtained to demonstrate autoimmune atrophic gastritis. If gastrin is elevated and the patient does not appear to have atrophic gastritis, an evaluation for Zollinger-Ellison syndrome (gastrinoma) should be conducted.

32. **How are gastric carcinoid tumors staged?**

    TNM staging for gastric carcinoid tumors differs from gastric adenocarcinoma in that the diameter of the primary tumor and the depth of invasion are considered to separate early stages of the disease. Superficial tumors more than 1 cm in size are T2 lesions, which is the same stage as smaller tumors that penetrate the muscularis propria.

GASTROINTESTINAL STROMAL TUMORS

33. **What is a GIST?**

    A GIST is a tumor, benign or malignant, that develops in the gastric wall from the interstitial cells of Cajal (Fig. 10.8). Generally, malignancy correlates with the size (greater than 3–5 cm in cross-section) and histologic features, such as the number of mitoses per 10 high-power fields. Histologically, these tumors resemble leiomyomas, and the distinction between gastric leiomyomas and GIST can be difficult without histocytochemistry. Most

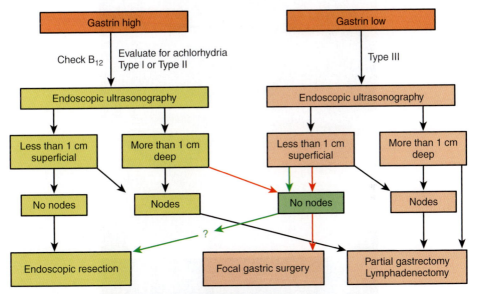

Fig. 10.6 Algorithm for the management of gastric carcinoid tumors.

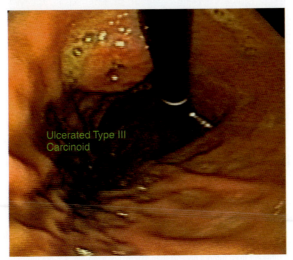

Fig. 10.7 Endoscopic view of ulcerated type III gastric carcinoid. (This patient is described in the video for the Clinical Vignette.)

GISTs (70%–80%) stain for an antibody against surface KIT (CD117), a tyrosine kinase. Another 10% have mutations in the platelet-derived growth factor receptor alpha (*PDGFRα*) gene.

34. What is a wild-type GIST?

GISTs without mutations in KIT or *PDGFRα* are known as *wild-type GISTs*. They express high levels of KIT and occur throughout the gastrointestinal tract. Like GISTs with common mutations, wild-type GISTs do not highlight with neural or muscle stains. These tumors are heterogeneous and may have mutations in RAS, BRAF, or succinate dehydrogenase.

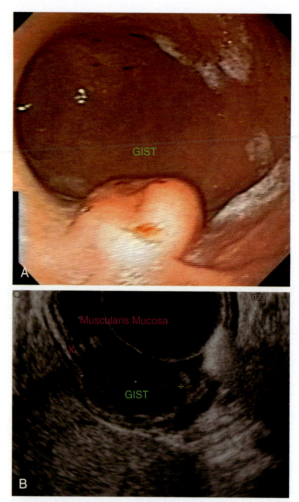

Fig. 10.8 (A) Endoscopic view of a gastrointestinal stromal tumor (GIST). (B) Endoscopic ultrasound image of the same GIST, arising from the muscularis mucosa.

35. How are gastric GISTs staged?

The staging system for gastric GIST is unusual in that tumor size and histologic findings (mitoses per 50 high-powered fields) play major roles in staging. Tumors smaller than 5 cm are staged differently than tumors from 5 to 10 cm and are different from tumors greater than 10 cm. For example, a 1-cm tumor with a high mitotic rate is at the same stage as a 12-cm tumor with a low mitotic rate. Furthermore, nodal metastases are quite rare with GISTs, and if no nodes are identified, the stage is considered N0 rather than Nx.

36. How are gastric GISTs treated?

Smaller gastric GISTs, such as those smaller than 3 cm, without ulcerations and normal homogeneous internal echoes, can be followed. Larger GISTs are removed surgically. High-risk GISTs that have been removed, those that cannot be removed, or those that have metastasized can be treated with drugs that bind to KIT and place it into the inactive conformation. The prototype drug is imatinib mesylate. Other drugs are used in imatinib-resistant patients.

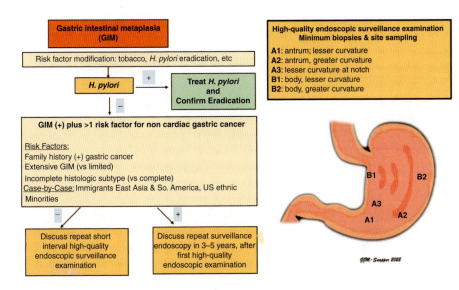

Fig. 10.9 Decision algorithm for gastric intestinal metaplasia (GIM) and components of high-quality endoscopic surveillance examination.

GASTRIC INTESTINAL METAPLASIA

37. **What is gastric intestinal metaplasia (GIM)?**
    GIM may be the precursor to dysplasia and is associated with an increased risk of gastric cancer. The American Gastroenterological Association recommends testing for *H. pylori* followed by eradication in patients with GIM.

38. **Does GIM require surveillance endoscopy?**
    No. Routine endoscopic surveillance is not recommended in patients with limited GIM. Indications for high-quality endoscopic surveillance of GIM are outlined in Fig. 10.9.

ACKNOWLEDGMENT

I thank Dr. John C. Deutsch for the work he did on this chapter for the previous edition.

CLINICAL VIGNETTE

Available Online.

BIBLIOGRAPHY

Available Online.

CHAPTER 11

THICKENED GASTRIC FOLDS

Andrew T. Mertz, MD, MAJ, MC, Sarah Zimmer, MD and
Patrick E. Young, MD, MACP, FACG, FASGE

 Additional content available online.

1. What are thickened gastric folds?

Although *thickened gastric folds* is a somewhat ambiguous term, it generally refers to abnormally large gastric folds (generally >1 cm) that do not flatten on insufflation at upper endoscopy (Fig. 11.1).

2. Describe the differential diagnosis for thickened gastric folds.

The differential diagnosis includes Ménétrier disease (MD), chronic gastritis (*Helicobacter pylori*–associated, eosinophilic, etc.), gastric malignancy (lymphoma and scirrhous gastric adenocarcinoma), and Zollinger-Ellison syndrome.

3. What are the clinical features of MD?

Patients with MD may present with a combination of local and systemic symptoms. Local symptoms include epigastric pain, nausea, vomiting, postprandial fullness, and diarrhea. Systemic symptoms generally stem from substantial protein loss and include weight loss and peripheral edema. Of note, a recent case-control study showed that patients with MD had a markedly lower 5- and 10-year survival (73% and 65%, respectively) when compared with matched controls.

4. How do you diagnose MD?

Full-thickness mucosal biopsy, via suction technique or snare resection, will reveal the characteristic foveolar hyperplasia, tortuous and dilated glands, inversion of the pit-gland ratio, and marked parietal cell loss. The lack of inflammatory cells in MD is a key differentiating factor between MD and its mimics (*Helicobacter*-associated hypertrophy and allergic hypertrophic gastritis). Laboratory findings that support the diagnosis include low basal and stimulated acid output and low albumin. Serologic testing for cytomegalovirus (CMV) is also a reasonable test to obtain, particularly in pediatric cases in which up to one-third of cases are CMV-associated.

5. List the treatment options for MD.

Historically, supportive care, including a high-protein diet, albumin infusions, and pain medications, was the cornerstone of therapy. When these conservative options failed, gastrectomy was required. We now know that MD in adults often relates to local overproduction of transforming growth factor–alpha, leading to an increase in epidermal growth factor (EGF), which acts on the tyrosine kinase receptor. Cetuximab, a monoclonal antibody that blocks EGF receptor binding, has proven an effective treatment for MD in recent small trials. Case reports and small series suggest that octreotide, a somatostatin analog that modulates the same pathway, may also have therapeutic benefits.

6. What are the key features of gastric mucosa–associated lymphoid tissue (MALT) lymphoma?

MALT lymphoma is a type of non-Hodgkin lymphoma that represents 3% of gastric malignancies. Like gastric adenocarcinoma, MALT is highly associated with *H. pylori* infection. Diagnosis is made via tissue histologic

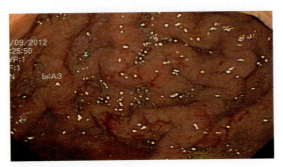

Fig. 11.1 Thickened gastric folds in a patient with Ménétrier disease.

examination in conjunction with immunohistochemical testing of B lymphocyte markers. Tumors with more than 20% large blast cells are high grade.

7. Describe the treatment of gastric MALT lymphoma.

First-line therapy for gastric MALT lymphoma is antibiotic therapy directed at *H. pylori*, followed by the documentation of eradication. The success of this regimen to induce remission correlates with the disease stage, with 80% of low-grade lymphomas regressing compared to only 50% of high-grade lymphomas. Even after successful bacterial eradication, complete remission may take more than 1 year. Several studies show residual clonal B cells, even after histologic regression. You should watchfully wait in these cases, withholding further treatment unless evidence of histologic recurrence arises. In cases in which antibiotic therapy fails to induce remission, external beam radiation (with or without systemic chemotherapy) is indicated.

8. Should you still treat gastric MALT lymphoma with antibiotics in *H. pylori*–negative cases?

Yes. There are data showing that even *H. pylori*–negative cases of MALT lymphoma may respond to antibiotic therapy. This is, at least in part, due to the presence of *Helicobacter* species other than *H. pylori* in these cases.

GASTRIC POLYPS

9. What are the types of gastric polyps, and what is the relative prevalence of each type?

There are essentially three types of gastric polyps: fundic gland (77%), hyperplastic (17%), and adenomatous (1%). In geographic areas with higher *H. pylori* infection rates, hyperplastic polyps (HPs) and adenomas are correspondingly more prevalent.

10. Describe the relationship of proton pump inhibitors (PPIs) to fundic gland polyps (FGPs).

Prolonged PPI therapy is associated with the formation of FGPs. A meta-analysis including over 40,000 subjects showed that patients on PPI for at least 12 months were at a fivefold increased risk of FGP formation when compared to controls. The regression of FGPs after PPI cessation also supports their role in polyp formation.

11. What is the relationship between medical conditions and the occurrence of FGPs?

FGPs can occur in association with polyposis syndromes, including familial adenomatous polyposis (FAP), Gardner syndrome, MUTYH-associated polyposis (MAP), and gastric adenocarcinoma and proximal polyposis of the stomach (GAPPS). One study of 102 asymptomatic patients with FAP found that 72% had FGPs when including micro- and macroscopic assessment. Additionally, 11% of patients with MAP have FGPs. GAPPS is an autosomal-dominant syndrome characterized by dysplastic FGP formation in the proximal stomach and an increased risk of invasive gastric adenocarcinoma. You should consider surveillance with upper endoscopy in these patients due to their higher risk of progression to adenocarcinoma.

12. How likely is it that a gastric adenoma will progress to adenocarcinoma?

It depends. Much like adenomas of the colon, gastric adenomas are precursors of adenocarcinoma. Both size and histologic characteristics influence the malignancy potential of a given lesion. For instance, progression occurs in 30%–40% of adenomas with villous features and in adenomas larger than 2 cm. The overall incidence of gastric adenomas progressing to adenocarcinoma is approximately 5%. As such, you should completely remove them whenever possible.

13. Describe the management of gastric HPs.

HPs have a lower risk of malignant transformation than adenomas but often occur in settings where the overall risk of malignancy in the gastric mucosa is elevated (pernicious anemia, *H. pylori*–associated gastritis, chronic gastritis, etc.). Reported rates of adenocarcinoma arising in an HP range from 0.6% to 2.1%, but between 1% and 20% of HPs harbor foci of dysplasia. As the cancer risk increases with size, most experts recommend removing HPs greater than 0.5–1 cm in diameter. In addition, you should take multiple biopsies from the antrum and corpus to rule out autoimmune gastritis and *H. pylori*. Treatment of *H. pylori* has been associated with regression of HPs. For patients with HPs and chronic atrophic gastritis, you can perform risk stratification for gastric cancer histologically using the Operative Link for Gastritis Assessment or the Operative Link on Gastritis/Intestinal Metaplasia Assessment staging systems.

SUBEPITHELIAL TUMORS

14. What are the endosonographic layers of the stomach?

The stomach has five distinct endosonographic layers. The first and innermost layer is hyperechoic (white on endoscopic ultrasound [EUS]) and represents the interface between the ultrasound probe and the superficial mucosa. The second layer is hypoechoic (dark on EUS) and represents the deep mucosa, which contains the

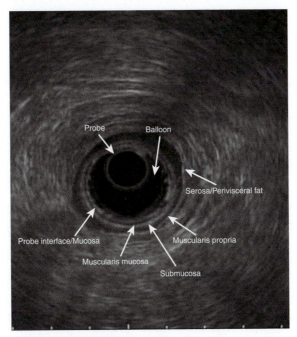

Fig. 11.2 Endosonographic image of the gastric wall layers.

muscularis mucosa. Lesions that penetrate through to this layer are ulcerations, whereas superficial mucosal lesions are erosions. The third layer is hyperechoic and corresponds to the submucosa. Layer four is hypoechoic and corresponds to the muscularis propria (MP), from which most subepithelial gastric tumors arise. Layer five is the serosa, which is typically indistinguishable from the perivisceral fat since both are hyperechoic (Fig. 11.2).

15. What is the differential diagnosis for gastric subepithelial tumor (SET) (Table 11.1)?

We first divide the differential diagnosis for a SET into intrinsic versus extramural lesions. Table 11.2 provides descriptions for each potential intrinsic lesion. Extramural lesions most often result from the spleen and its associated vessels but can less commonly be a result of extrinsic compression from the gallbladder, left hepatic lobe, and pancreas. Abscesses, enlarged lymph nodes, or renal cysts are less common causes of extramural lesions.

16. Describe the common methods of making a tissue diagnosis of a SET.

Symptomatic or large SETs often can be resected without prior sampling. When a tissue diagnosis is required, stacked or "bite-on-bite" forceps biopsies are technically simple but with a diagnostic yield inferior to other methods. EUS-guided fine-needle aspiration (FNA) is the gold standard for tissue sampling as it evaluates the SET, locoregional lymph nodes, and extramural lesions. Single-incision needle-knife electrocautery (or other unroofing methods) followed by cold forceps biopsy is an alternative if EUS-FNA is not readily available or technically challenging due to size or location. EUS-guided fine-needle biopsy (FNB) with a core needle provides a larger core tissue sample and thus better tissue architecture. See the diagnostic and treatment algorithm in Fig. 11.3.

17. What are the roles of endoscopic mucosal resection (EMR), endoscopic submucosal dissection (ESD), and endoscopic full-thickness resection (EFTR) in the management of SET?

You may resect small SETs (1–2 cm) with EMR with snare electrocautery or EMR with ligating device as long as lesions do not penetrate the submucosa. Only endoscopists with significant ESD experience should perform this procedure as inconsistent complete resections with relatively high perforation rates occur when SETs originate from the MP layer. EFTR has a complication profile similar to ESD but allows for en bloc resections of SETs that originate from or are tightly adherent to the MP layer. One may employ novel laparoscopic-assisted EFTR techniques to remove larger tumors and may decrease the risk of perforation due to the addition of direct peritoneal visualization.

Table 11.1 Types of Gastric Subepithelial Tumors and Their Characteristics.

SUBEPITHELIAL LESION	EUS LAYER	MALIGNANT POTENTIAL	ENDOSONOGRAPHIC FEATURES	IMPORTANT FACTS
Leiomyoma	2, 3, or 4 (fourth is most common)	None	Hypoechoic	Rare in the stomach CD117 (–), smooth muscle actin (+)
Neural origin tumors (schwannoma, neuroma, neurofibroma)	3 or 4	None	Hypoechoic	Schwannoma = fourth layer, S100 (+)
Lipoma	3	None	Intensely hyperechoic	Yellow hue "pillow sign" when probed with closed forceps
Duplication cyst	Any/extramural	None	Anechoic	Embryonic remnant lined with GI epithelium that can enlarge and lead to mass effect, rupture, or bleeding
Pancreatic rest	2 or 3		Hypoechoic/mixed	Endoscopy = characteristic central umbilication or "volcano sign"
Inflammatory fibroid polyp	3 or 4		Hyperechoic	Histologic findings = unencapsulated fibrous tissue, eosinophilic infiltrate, and small blood vessels
Granular cell tumor	2 or 3		Hypoechoic	
Varices	2 or 3		Hypo- or anechoic	Blue hue Suspect with findings of portal vs. sinistral hypertension (e.g., splenic vein thrombosis)
GIST	4 (rarely 2)	See Question 20	Hypoechoic, homogenous	GIST = fourth layer + CD117 (+)/c-kit protein/ DOG1 (+) and most CD34 (+)
Lymphoma	2, 3, or 4		Hypoechoic	Usually DLBCL or B cell–associated MALT lymphoma Typically require deep-tissue sampling for diagnosis
Carcinoid	2 or 3	See subtypes below[a]	Hypoechoic	Arise from ECL cells
Metastatic carcinoma	Any		Hypoechoic	Rare Associated with melanoma, breast, lung, kidney, ovaries
Glomus tumor	3 or 4	Typically benign, but can have malignant potential	Hypoechoic	CD117 (–), vimentin (+), smooth muscle actin (+)

DLBCL, Diffuse large B cell lymphoma; *ECL*, enterochromaffin-like; *EUS*, endoscopic ultrasound; *GI*, gastrointestinal; *GIST*, gastrointestinal stromal tumor; *MALT*, mucosa-associated lymphoid tissue.
[a]Types of carcinoid tumors: type 1: associated with hypergastrinemia from chronic atrophic gastritis; type 2: associated with Zollinger-Ellison syndrome; and type 3: sporadic, associated with normal gastrin levels, can become malignant or metastatic and should be resected irrespective of size.

Table 11.2 Characteristics of Gastric Spindle Cell Tumors.

TYPE	CD117	CD34	SMA	S100 PROTEIN	DESMIN
GISTs	+ (95%)	+ (70%)	± (20%-30%)	− (10%+)	Very rare
Leiomyoma	−	+ (10%-15%)	+	−	+
Leiomyosarcoma	−	−	+	−	+
Schwannoma	−	−	−	+	−

GIST, Gastrointestinal stromal tumor; *SMA,* smooth muscle actin.
From Liu X, Chu KM. Molecular biomarkers for prognosis of gastrointestinal stromal tumor. Clin Transl Oncol. 2019;21(2):145-151;
Miettinen M, Lasota J. Gastrointestinal stromal tumors – definition, clinical, histological, immunohistochemical, and molecular genetic
features and differential diagnosis. Virchows Arch. 2001;438(1):1-12.

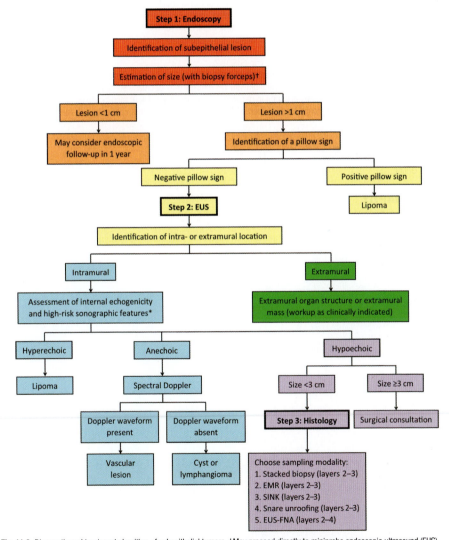

Fig. 11.3 Diagnostic and treatment algorithm of subepithelial tumors. †May proceed directly to miniprobe endoscopic ultrasound (EUS) or conventional EUS evaluation depending on availability and expertise. *Endoscopic and sonographic features deemed high risk for malignancy include irregular borders, cystic space, ulceration, echogenic foci, and heterogeneity. *EMR,* Endoscopic mucosal resection; *FNA,* fine-needle aspiration; *SINK,* single-incision needle-knife. (Adapted from Eckardt AJ, Wassef W. Diagnosis of subepithelial tumors in the GI tract. Endoscopy, EUS, and histology: bronze, silver, and gold standard? Gastrointest Endosc. 2005;62(2):209-212; Cho JW, Korean ESD Study Group. Current guidelines in the management of upper gastrointestinal subepithelial tumors. Clin Endosc. 2016;49(3):235-240.)

18. **How is a GI stromal tumor (GIST) differentiated from other spindle cell mesenchymal SETs?**
    GI spindle cell mesenchymal SETs include leiomyoma, leiomyosarcoma, schwannoma, and GIST. While there are histologically distinct subtypes of GIST, mesenchymal spindle cells are generally difficult to distinguish based on histologic examination alone, so immunohistochemical stains are vital to distinguish among them (Table 11.2).

19. **What is the cell of origin for a GIST?**
    The cells of origin for GISTs are the interstitial cells of Cajal. These cells serve as "pacemakers" for the gut by providing the stimulus for smooth muscle contraction.

20. **What is the role for surgery in the management of gastric GISTs?**
    GISTs have malignant potential making risk stratification crucial in management. Tumor size combined with mitotic rate provides the most accurate prediction of metastatic potential. Tumors <2 cm have exceedingly low metastatic risk regardless of the mitotic index. Therefore guidelines suggest resecting any GIST ≥2 cm if possible. There are no consensus data regarding the management of GISTs smaller than 2 cm in size. Consider surgical resection when worrisome EUS features (irregular borders, cystic space, ulceration, echogenic foci, or adjacent pathologically enlarged lymph nodes) are present. Some experts perform EUS surveillance in patients with small GISTs, although no guideline-directed interval exists.

21. **What medical options are available for GISTs?**
    Tyrosine kinase inhibitors (TKIs), such as imatinib mesylate, can be used as neoadjuvant, adjuvant, or medical monotherapy for the treatment of GISTs. Neoadjuvant TKI therapy may decrease surgical morbidity via downsizing the tumor. Adjuvant TKI therapy is useful in patients with a significant risk of recurrence as predicted by the mitotic index and size at diagnosis. Medical therapy with TKI alone is common in patients with metastases or disease recurrence.

CLINICAL VIGNETTE

Available Online.

BIBLIOGRAPHY

Available Online.

CHAPTER 12

GASTROPARESIS

Peter R. McNally, DO, MSRF, MACG

 Additional content available online.

1. **What is gastroparesis?**

   Gastroparesis is defined by symptomatic delay in gastric emptying (GE) in the absence of mechanical obstruction.

2. **What are the typical symptoms of gastroparesis?**

   Nausea is the most common symptom seen in 95% of patients with gastroparesis. Other cardinal symptoms of gastroparesis include vomiting, early satiety, bloating, postprandial fullness, and/or weight loss.

   Abdominal pain is a less common symptom associated with gastroparesis (22%), when it is present, one should consider other organic causes (peptic ulcer, ischemia, biliary and pancreatic diseases) or functional dyspepsia (FD).

3. **How should gastroparesis be diagnosed?**

   Scintigraphic GE is the current gold standard test for gastroparesis. An anteroposterior gamma-camera recording of the gastric area for 4 hours after ingestion of a Tc-99m labeled low-fat Egg Beaters meal is the standardized procedure that has been internationally validated. Due to radiation exposure, it should be avoided in females of childbearing potential.

   Recently, several breath tests have been developed and demonstrated to reliably quantify GE. Both octanoic acid, a medium-chain fatty acid, and *Spirulina platensis,* an edible algae, can be tagged with a non-radioactive carbon isotope (^{13}C) and incorporated into the solid component of a low caloric test meal. After being emptied from the stomach the substrates are digested and absorbed in the proximal small intestine and metabolized by the liver so that ^{13}C is expired by the lungs, and its rise over baseline in breath samples can be measured by mass spectrometry. The rate-limiting step is GE and therefore the appearance of ^{13}C in the breath correlates with GE. ^{13}C breath testing GE shows a strong correlation with simultaneously obtained scintigraphy.

4. **Can and should gastroparesis be quantified?**

   Yes.

   Scintigraphic GE is the current gold standard.

   Most tertiary motility centers utilize the percentage of meal retained at 4 hours on scintigraphy to define the severity of gastroparesis.

5. **What are the most common causes of gastroparesis?**

   A recent US national claims database study identified diabetes mellitus type 2 to be the most common cause (Fig. 12.1). It is estimated that ~5 million US adults suffer from gastroparesis, with a prevalence of 37.8 per 10,000 for adult females and 9.6 per 10,000 for adult males.

6. **What are some of the more common reversible causes of gastroparesis?**

   For reversible causes of gastroparesis, see Table 12.1.

7. **What are some of the mimics of gastroparesis?**
   - FD
   - Celiac artery compression syndrome
   - Superior mesenteric artery syndrome
   - Cannabinoid hyperemesis syndrome
   - Cyclic vomiting syndrome
   - Intestinal pseudo-obstruction
   - Narcotic bowel syndrome
   - Rumination syndrome
   - Medications: opioids and glucagon-like peptide-1 receptor agonists

8. **Describe the normal physiology of the stomach.**

   The main motor functions of the stomach are accommodation, which allows the delivery and storage of food, followed by trituration (grinding of food into fragments) and emptying of solid food. Ingestion of a meal converts the stomach from a relatively inactive fasting state into an active motor and secretory state. There are three

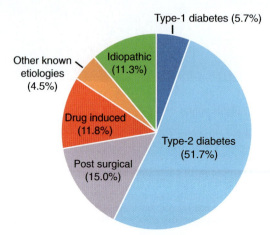

Fig. 12.1 Etiology of gastroparesis in overall cohort. (From Ye Y, Yin Y, Huh SY, Almansa C, Bennett D, Camilleri M. Epidemiology, etiology, and treatment of gastroparesis: real-world evidence from a large US National Claims Database. Gastroenterology. 2022;162:109-121.)

Table 12.1 Reversible Causes of Gastroparesis.

CAUSES	EXAMPLES	TREATMENTS
CNS disorders	Multiple sclerosis, Parkinson disease	Specific Rx CNS disorder
Endocrine	DM type 1/2, hypoadrenalism, and hypothyroidism	Glycemic control, corticosteroids, and levothyroxine
Mechanical	Celiac artery syndrome, superior mesenteric artery syndrome, and median arcuate ligament syndrome	Surgery and interventional radiology
Metabolic	Neuromyelitis optica with antibodies to astrocytic aquaporin-4 water channel	Corticosteroids
Paraneoplastic	ANNA-1 sometimes called anti-Hu	Immunomodulators and plasmapheresis
Pharmacologic	Anticholinergics, proton pump inhibitors, calcium channel blockers, cyclosporine, exenatide, pramlintide, semaglutide, lithium, and octreotide	Stop the Rx

ANNA-1, Antineuronal nuclear antibodies type 1; *CNS*, central nervous system; *DM*, diabetes mellitus; *Rx*, prescription.

distinct neuromuscular compartments of the stomach involved in GE: fundus, antrum, and pylorus. Swallowing triggers active relaxation of the gastric fundus so that it can accommodate large volumes of ingesta without "discomfort" or significant increases in intragastric pressure. Subsequently, a steady increase in the fundic tone compresses gastric contents toward the antrum, which are captured by phasic contractions and pushed toward an oscillating pylorus so that digestible solids are ground together with gastric secretions and buoyed backward into the proximal part of the stomach. The frequency of antral contractions is driven by interstitial cells of Cajal (ICC, "gastric pacemaker") located at the upper part of the greater curvature with a frequency of ~3 cycles per minute. This process continues until all digestible solids are reduced to particles of 1–2 mm before exiting the stomach in small volumes of liquid and homogenized food (chyme).

9. What tests should be performed to evaluate gastroparesis?
- Physical examination
  - Succussion splash—suggestive for delayed GE or outlet obstruction
  - Upper abdominal bruit—celiac artery compression syndrome
  - Digital ulcers and telangiectasia—scleroderma
  - Ascites, a mass or enlarged lymph nodes—malignancy

- Labs: electrolytes, thyroid-stimulating hormone, and fasting cortisol (if suggestions for adrenal insufficiency)
- Upper endoscopy

10. What are the pathophysiologic characteristics of gastroparesis?

Gastroparesis is defined by delay in GE, but there are multiple possible defining motor/sensory abnormalities.

- Impaired accommodation
- Electrical dysrhythmias
- Antro-duodenal dyscoordination
- Pyloric dysfunction
- Antral hypomotility
- Vagal nerve injury
- Disorders of visceral sensation

Gastroparesis in diabetes is thought to be a manifestation of autonomic neuropathy. Other factors that predispose to gastroparesis include impaired release of gastrointestinal hormones, such as pancreatic polypeptide, motilin, and ghrelin (Fig. 12.2).

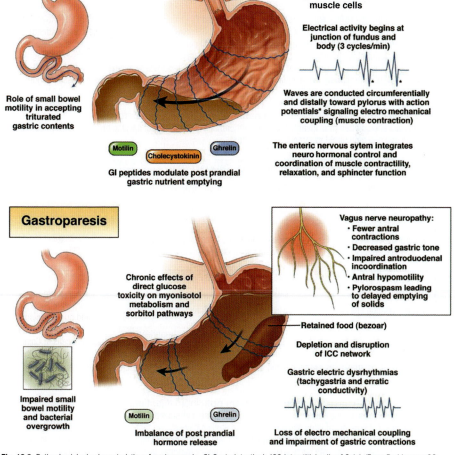

Fig. 12.2 Pathophysiologic characteristics of gastroparesis. *GI,* Gastrointestinal; *ICC,* interstitial cells of Cajal. (From Reddymasu SC. Severe gastroparesis: medical therapy or gastric electrical stimulation. Clin Gastroenterol Hepatol. 2010;8:117-124.)

11. **What are the ICCs in health and in gastroparesis?**
    The molecular understanding of gastroparesis has significantly evolved over the last decade.
       We have gone from a disorder of unknown etiology to enteric neuropathy to myopathy to an established role in the loss or dysfunction of the ICCs. The emerging bench research suggests the role of an innate immune dysregulation in gastroparesis and immune interactions that may be driving the injury to the enteric nervous system and ICCs.

12. **How can bloating be explained in gastroparesis?**
    The degree of bloating has not been shown to correlate with the severity of gastroparesis. Small intestinal dysmotility is more commonly seen in patients with gastroparesis, and a secondary complication is bacterial overgrowth, which can be diagnosed by hydrogen breath test (HBT).

13. **What prokinetic medications are approved by the US Food and Drug Administration (FDA) and available for the treatment of gastroparesis in the United States?**
    Endogenous dopamine inhibits the release of acetylcholine, and this results in decreased motility of the stomach and proximal small intestine. Dopamine (D_2) receptor antagonists block the inhibitory effects of endogenous dopamine, thereby inducing a prokinetic effect. Metoclopramide and domperidone are both dopamine (D_2) receptor antagonists, equally effective in inducing a prokinetic effect on the stomach. Cardiac and central nervous system (CNS) side effects limit the utility of both agents. Domperidone is only available for physician prescription through the FDA's program for Expanded Access to Investigational Drugs (https://www.fda.gov/drugs/investigational-new-drug-ind-application/how-request-domperidone-expanded-access-use). Domperidone has been associated with cardiac dysrhythmias. It should not be used if the QTc interval on a patient's electrocardiogram is >470 ms in males and >450 ms in females.

14. **How is medically refractory gastroparesis defined?**
    Persistent symptoms in the context of objectively confirmed GE delay, despite the use of dietary adjustment and metoclopramide. Formal dietary instruction on a low-fat, small particle size should be used instituted with a trial of metoclopramide (the only FDA-approved medication for gastroparesis) at a minimum dose of 10 mg tid before meals and at hour of sleep for at least 4 weeks. Clinicians should warn patients of potential side effects associated with metoclopramide use to include tardive dyskinesia (black box warning), restlessness, fatigue, and lassitude.

15. **How should treatment be directed in patients with refractory gastroparesis?**
    The clinician should attempt to identify the dominant pathophysiologic defect causing predominant symptoms of gastroparesis and then target treatment for this defect.

PHYSIOLOGIC DEFECTS	DIRECTED TREATMENT	
Antral hypomotility	Prokinetic (metoclopramide and domperidone)	
Pyloric dysfunction	Endoscopic (gastric per oral endoscopic myotomy [G-POEM] and stent) or surgical outlet procedures	
Visceral dysesthesia (pain)	Neuromodulators (tricyclic antidepressants and serotonin-norepinephrine reuptake inhibitors)	**Never opioids!
Eating/psychologic disorders	Cognitive and behavioral therapy/hypnotherapy	
Vomiting	Antiemetic	
Accommodation failure	5-Hydroxytryptaine 1A receptor antagonist	
Bloating	Bacterial overgrowth (+HBT) treatment	

Often, the gastroparesis symptoms and even the pathophysiologic abnormalities will overlap, making successful treatment even more difficult.

16. **Can patients with gastroparesis benefit from botulinum injections into the pylorus?**
    Early studies of intra-pyloric botulinum toxin injection suggested improved gastroparesis symptoms in patients with diabetes, but two recent large placebo-controlled studies have shown that there is no benefit over placebo.
       Functional lumen imaging probe impedance planimetry of the pylorus has identified a potential subgroup of patients with gastroparesis with decreased pyloric distensibility that may benefit from this treatment.

17. When should G-POEM be used in gastroparesis?

Two multicenter trials or G-POEM in patients with gastroparesis have noted improvement in symptoms and reduction in GE times. At this time, G-POEM should be reserved for select, refractory cases of gastroparesis with appropriate selection criteria (obstructive pyloric physiology), and only performed at a tertiary-level motility center with advanced endoscopists.

18. What is the role of gastric electrical stimulation (GES) for gastroparesis?

GES (Enterra Therapy) uses high frequency (12 cycles per minute), low-energy stimuli for the treatment of refractory nausea and vomiting due to gastroparesis. The GES does NOT improve GE but has been shown to improve refractory nausea and vomiting in some and may improve glycemic control, nutritional status, and quality of life. Gastroparesis associated with pain is not an indication for GES device, and chronic opioid use is a contraindication to GES placement.

19. How does GES work?

The precise mechanism of action for GES remains unknown; beneficial effects may occur via modulation of ICCs, increased vagal activity, better fundic relaxation/accommodation, sensory afferents to CNS nausea and vomiting control centers, and/or release of local peptides (Fig. 12.3).

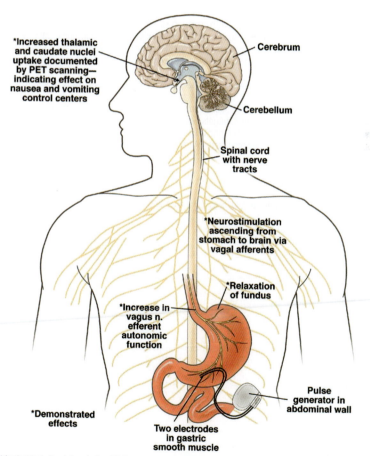

Proposed mechanisms of action of the gastric neurostimulator

*Increased thalamic and caudate nuclei uptake documented by PET scanning—indicating effect on nausea and vomiting control centers

Cerebrum

Cerebellum

Spinal cord with nerve tracts

*Neurostimulation ascending from stomach to brain via vagal afferents

*Relaxation of fundus

*Increase in vagus n. efferent autonomic function

Pulse generator in abdominal wall

*Demonstrated effects

Two electrodes in gastric smooth muscle

Fig. 12.3 Gastric electrical stimulation device. *ED,* Emergency department; *PET,* positron emission tomography. (From Reddymasu SC. Severe gastroparesis: medical therapy or gastric electrical stimulation. Clin Gastroenterol Hepatol. 2010;8:117-124.)

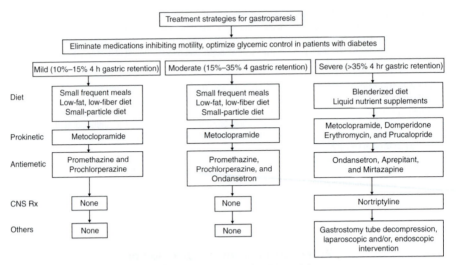

Fig. 12.4 Treatment strategy for gastroparesis. *CNS*, Central nervous system; *Rx*, prescription.

20. **Describe the strategy for escalating therapy in gastroparesis.**

Once again, the clinician should attempt to identify the dominant pathophysiologic defect causing predominant symptoms of gastroparesis and then target treatment for this defect. The algorithm in Fig. 12.4 is a systematic approach to the treatment of gastroparesis, based on the severity of GE delay (mild, moderate, or severe).

21. **What investigational medications are in the pipeline for the treatment of gastric motility disorders?**

Recent advances in the mechanistic understanding of diverse motor dysfunctions evident in gastroparesis have provided multiple potential pharmacologic targets. Some have shown research potential in the treatment of FD, idiopathic, and/or diabetic gastroparesis (IG and DG, respectively). These potential pharmacologic agents have variable impacts on GE, gastric accommodation (GA); and fundal, antral, and/or pyloric contractions.

5-HT4 receptor agonists:
- Prucalopride (IG and DG) ↑GE
- Tegaserod (FD) ↑GA

D2/D3 receptor antagonist:
- Trazpiroben (IG and DG) ↑ volume to fullness, no change in GE

Ghrelin receptor agonist:
- Relamorelin (DG) ↑ GE and ↑ antral contractions

Muscarinic M1/M2 receptor antagonist
- Acotiamide (FD) ↑GE and GA

Motilin receptor agonist:
- Erythromycin (IG & DG) ↑GE, ↑ fundic and antral contractions, ↓ pyloric contractions

NK1 receptor agonist:
- Aprepitant (IG and DG) ↑ GA, no Δ in GE.

ACKNOWLEDGMENT

The author acknowledges the previous contributions of Drs Richard W. McCallum and Joseph K. Sunny, authors of this chapter in the fifth edition of *GI/Liver Secrets*.

BIBLIOGRAPHY

Available Online.

EVALUATION OF ABNORMAL LIVER TESTS

William Carey, MD, MACG, FAASLD

CHAPTER 13

 Additional content available online.

1.   What are liver tests?

Broadly, liver tests encompass serum-based testing, imaging, elastography, and liver biopsy that identify the presence, type, and etiology of liver disorders. Most often the term refers to the routine chemistry panel that includes alanine aminotransferase (ALT), aspartate aminotransferase (AST), γ-glutamyl transpeptidase (GGT), alkaline phosphatase (AP), bilirubin, albumin, and protein. Other terms for the same tests are *liver function tests* and *liver-associated enzymes*, but neither is totally accurate. Only the first four are properly called *enzymes*, and only the last two provide a measure of liver function. These initial tests help to characterize injury patterns and provide a crude measure of the synthetic function of the liver. Individually none are diagnostic of any specific condition.

2.   What are serum transaminases?

The three serum transaminases commonly assayed in clinical practice are ALT (previously called serum glutamic pyruvate transaminase), AST (formerly serum glutamic oxaloacetic transaminase), and GGT (gamma-glutamyl transferase).

Elevation of ALT or AST usually reflects the presence of hepatocellular (HC) injury. Acute elevations are most commonly related to hepatitis A, hepatitis B, drugs, alcohol, or ischemia. Elevations of more than 1000 are usually related to viruses or drugs. Levels of more than 5000 are related to acetaminophen toxicity, ischemia, or unusual viruses. Alcoholic hepatitis has enzyme elevations usually less than 400 with the AST/ALT ratio greater than 2:1. Chronic elevations (6 months or more) in ALT and AST are often due to hepatitis B, hepatitis C, nonalcoholic fatty liver disease (NAFLD), alcohol, and autoimmune hepatitis (AH) (Fig. 13.1).

3.   What is the most specific liver enzyme for HC damage?

GGT is a liver-specific enzyme that is elevated in most cases of HC and cholestatic (CS) liver disease. Both AST and ALT reside in other organs, so elevated levels do not always reflect liver injury. ALT is somewhat more liver

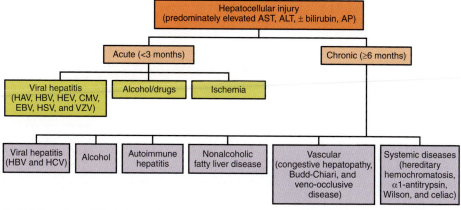

Fig. 13.1 Diagnostic possibilities for hepatocellular pattern liver injury depend on the context and duration of injury. *ALT,* Alanine aminotransferase; *AP,* alkaline phosphatase; *AST,* aspartate aminotransferase; *CMV,* cytomegalovirus; *EBV,* Epstein-Barr virus; *HAV,* hepatitis A virus; *HBV,* hepatitis B virus; *HCV,* hepatitis C virus; *HEV,* hepatitis E virus; *HSV,* herpes simplex virus; *VZV,* varicella zoster virus.

specific than AST but both may be elevated in, for example, acute muscle injury. Both enzymes are released into the circulation when liver tissue is damaged or destroyed.

4. What is a normal value for ALT?

Studies, surprisingly, arrive at different conclusions about normal ALT values. Most often, normal ranges are derived by measuring values in an apparently normal population, defining normal as those that fall within 2 standard deviations of the mean. This approach is subject to error if those deemed normal actually have an undiagnosed liver problem, for example, fatty liver. Another approach is to determine the threshold below which excessive liver morbidity or mortality is not seen. The National Health and Nutrition Examination Survey demonstrated ALT values >30 U/L for adult males and >19 U/L for adult females were associated with increases in liver (and cardiovascular) mortality. These thresholds are considerably lower than the "normal range" reported by most laboratories.

5. How is CS injury best diagnosed?

In the standard panel of liver tests, CS injury is suggested by an elevated AP level, an enzyme bound in the hepatic canalicular membrane. Because AP can be derived from other body tissues (e.g., bone, intestine, and placenta), a concurrent elevation of GGT (an enzyme of intrahepatic biliary canaliculi) or 5′-nucleotidase helps to support a CS mechanism.

6. What makes the AP level rise?

AP is a group of enzymes that catalyze the transfer of phosphate groups. Different isoenzymes can be identified from multiple sites in the body, including liver, bone, and intestine. Most hospital laboratories can determine the isoenzyme responsible for the elevated AP level. In one large study, elevated AP was caused by the liver in only approximately 65% of hospitalized patients. When the source is the liver, the mechanism appears to be related to the stimulation of enzyme synthesis associated with local increases in bile acids. Common causes of CS injury include primary biliary cirrhosis, primary sclerosing cirrhosis, large bile duct obstruction, drug-induced injury, infiltrative disease, and inflammation-associated injury (Fig. 13.2). Serum AP levels may be modestly increased in HC disease; this increase is due to the release of cellular enzymes without excessive stimulation of new enzymes.

7. Does my patient have HC or CS liver injury and why does it matter?

Most liver insults leave a characteristic imprint in that the injury is centered on the hepatocyte or bile duct. Diagnostic tests to determine the cause will be influenced to a great degree on which type of liver injury is likely. It makes little sense, for example, to perform cholangiography in a patient who presents with a normal AP and very high transaminases typical for viral hepatitis. Figs. 13.1 and 13.2 provide more detail. The first task then is to determine whether the enzyme elevation is predominately that of ALT and AST (HC) or AP (CS).

The much lower upper limit of normal (ULN) for ALT and AST compared to that for AP needs to be taken into account. For example, a female with ALT of 200 and AP of 415 should not be considered to have CS liver injury. In this case, the ALT is more than 10 times the ULN, whereas the AP is less than 3 times the ULN. Note that the bilirubin level plays no role in distinguishing HC from CS liver injury.

R-Factor is a tool to help distinguish HC for CS liver injury. Online tools are available, for example, <https://www.mdcalc.com/calc/4064/r-factor-liver-injury>. The R-Factor was developed to help distinguish HS from CS drug liver injury; its use in other types of liver injury has not been validated. This tool is built to take into account the differences in ULN for ALT and AP.

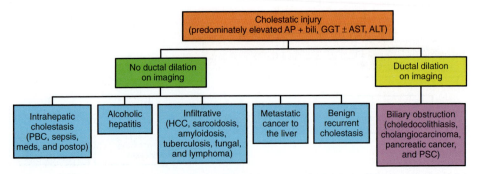

Fig. 13.2 Cholestatic liver injury can be caused by large- or small-bile duct injury or by infiltrative liver disorders. Imaging studies frequently serve as the best early test to distinguish causes. *ALT*, Alanine aminotransferase; *AP*, alkaline phosphatase; *AST*, aspartate aminotransferase; *bili*, bilirubin; *GGT*, γ-glutamyl transpeptidase; *HCC*, hepatocellular carcinoma; *PBC*, primary biliary cirrhosis; *PSC*, primary sclerosing cholangitis.

8. **What does an elevated bilirubin mean?**

Bilirubin, a breakdown product of red blood cells, exists in two forms: conjugated (direct) and unconjugated (indirect). Unconjugated bilirubin is water insoluble, exists in the circulation tightly bound to albumin, is taken up by the hepatocyte, and conjugated with glucuronic acid, making it water soluble and allowing it to be excreted in bile. Jaundice occurs when the bilirubin level is greater than 2.5 mg/dL. Unconjugated bilirubin appears in the serum when blood is broken down at a rate that overwhelms the processing ability of the liver found commonly in patients with hemolysis or reabsorption of a hematoma. Because unconjugated bilirubin is tightly albumin bound, it does not appear in urine. Accordingly, an elevated serum bilirubin with a negative urine bilirubin implies indirect hyperbilirubinemia and suggests the absence of liver injury. Conversely, bilirubinuria means the elevated serum bilirubin reflects the presence of liver disease.

Certain genetic enzyme deficiencies result in improper or incomplete bilirubin conjugation in the liver. The most common is Gilbert syndrome, characterized by a relative deficiency of uridine diphosphate–glucuronyltransferase (UDPGT). More profound deficiencies in UDPGT may be seen in neonates. Babies with Crigler-Najjar I and II rarely reach adulthood.

Conjugated hyperbilirubinemia can result from HC dysfunction (viral-, chemical-, drug-, or alcohol-induced hepatitis; cirrhosis or metabolic disorders), cholestasis (intrahepatic or extrahepatic biliary obstruction), or genetic disorders of excretion of bilirubin (Dubin-Johnson syndrome, Rotor syndrome). It is a common misperception that an elevated bilirubin implies CS liver injury. It is just as often seen in severe acute HC damage.

9. **Is Gilbert syndrome a disease?**

An inherited modest reduction of the UDPGT, seen in 5% of the US population, may result in a modestly high level of indirect bilirubin. UDPGT enzyme production is genetically controlled by the *UGT1A1* gene. The UGT1A1*28 variant is associated with Gilbert syndrome. Elevated indirect bilirubin levels usually first become manifest in adolescence or early adulthood. Gilbert syndrome is not associated with hepatic inflammation, fibrosis, chronic liver disease, liver failure, or altered life expectancy. As such, Gilbert syndrome is not a disease, or condition, but a normal variant.

Diminished UDPGT does have consequences for drug metabolism; however, irinotecan, a cancer drug commonly used in colorectal, gynecologic, lung, and gastric cancers, relies on UDPGT for the metabolism of a toxic intermediary. Increased drug toxicity has been observed in those with UGT1A*28. Drugs that may increase indirect bilirubin (without causing liver injury) in Gilbert syndrome include atazanavir, gemfibrozil, and nilotinib.

10. **What tests should be ordered to evaluate acute viral hepatitis?**

Hepatitis A: Three commonly available lab tests are (1) total hepatitis A virus (HAV) (measures the presence of both immunoglobulin M [IgM] and IgG), (2) HAV IgM, and (3) HAV IgG. If hepatitis A is suspected in the setting of acute liver disease, HAV IgM should be measured, as this is the only one that will be diagnostic.

Hepatitis B: In acute hepatitis B, the hepatitis B surface antigen (HBsAg) emerges within 2 weeks of exposure and is the test of choice. However, if testing is delayed, HBsAg may become undetectable. In this case detection of anti-HB core antigen (HBc) IgM can be used to make a confident diagnosis of hepatitis B. Hepatitis B virus (HBV) DNA determination is not necessary in most cases of acute hepatitis B.

Acute hepatitis C is an uncommon cause of symptoms and so is uncommonly identified. The best diagnostic tool is serum hepatitis C virus (HCV) RNA.

Many clinical laboratories provide testing for acute viral hepatitis (A, B, and C) in a single test, often called acute hepatitis panel.

Dozens of viruses may cause acute hepatitis. It is not practical or necessary to test for all in every patient. Keep in mind that Epstein-Barr virus, cytomegalovirus, hepatitis E, herpes simplex virus, and others may cause acute hepatitis.

11. **What tests detect chronic viral hepatitis?**

Hepatitis not resolved after 6 months is termed chronic. The most common causes of chronic viral hepatitis in the United States are hepatitis C and hepatitis B (with or without hepatitis D). A confident diagnosis of hepatitis C requires the demonstration of HCV RNA in serum. The presence of anti-HCV is insufficient as this antibody will persist even if the infection is cleared.

The diagnosis of chronic hepatitis B requires the detection of HBsAg, typically with anti-HBc (IgG) but without the development of anti-HBs. The classification of chronic hepatitis B is complicated and discussed in more detail in Chapter 16.

12. **Are there tests to diagnose NAFLD?**

NAFLD is now the most common chronic liver disease in the United States and many other parts of the world. No specific blood test diagnoses NAFLD. The diagnosis is based on evidence of hepatic steatosis (imaging or biopsy), and the absence of competing etiologic factors for hepatic steatosis (e.g., alcohol, calcium channel blockers, amiodarone, corticosteroid, and methotrexate) and other chronic liver disease. Distinguishing simple steatosis (usually benign) from nonalcoholic steatohepatitis (NASH), which often leads to fibrosis and cirrhosis, is difficult except by liver biopsy. However, liver biopsy is unattractive for a number of reasons, including the very high prevalence of NAFLD, cost, and morbidity.

Noninvasive tests (NITs) are helpful but imperfect. They usually estimate the likelihood of hepatic fibrosis, a consequence of NASH, but not simple steatosis. A number of formula-based serum tests (NITs) are available. Proprietary tests are send-out tests, take time to be resulted, and are costly. Nonproprietary tests perform just as well and can be instantly calculated without added cost, using readily available parameters. AST-to-platelet ratio index incorporates AST, ALT, and platelet count (https://www.mdcalc.com/calc/3094/ast-platelet-ratio-index-apri). NAFLD fibrosis score uses age, blood glucose, body mass index (BMI), platelet count, albumin level, and AST/ALT ratio (https://www.mdcalc.com/calc/3081/nafld-non-alcoholic-fatty-liver-disease-fibrosis-score). Finally, Fib 4 uses age, platelet count, and ALT and AST levels (https://www.mdcalc.com/calc/2200/fibrosis-4-fib-4-index-liver-fibrosis).

Hepatic vibration–controlled transient elastography (VCTE) measures liver stiffness, reported in kilopascals (kPa), and has become an integral part in the evaluation of chronic liver disease including NAFLD. VCTE can be measured by magnetic resonance imaging, ultrasound, or with a stand-alone FibroScan. Unfortunately, the results from each technology are not interchangeable. All guidelines and consensus statements refer to FibroScan-derived transient elastography and will be used here. An additional feature of FibroScan is the measurement of ultrasonic attenuation of the echo wave, termed the controlled attenuation parameter (CAP), that provides an estimate of the percentage of hepatocytes containing fat. There is a moderate correlation between findings by FibroScan and liver biopsy.

Signal-to-noise is a consideration in all testing systems including FibroScan. This is especially true in the context of NAFLD. A report of <8–10 kPa provides a clear signal that significant fibrosis is absent. A value >20 reliably denotes cirrhosis. Values between 10 and 20, particularly in NAFLD, provide a low signal and should be considered indeterminate with respect to the level of fibrosis.

Practice guidelines suggest elastography (usually FibroScan) plus one NIT be used to distinguish steatosis from NASH.

13. **What tests are used to evaluate hemochromatosis?**
Hemochromatosis, a disease of iron overload in the liver and other organs, may be hereditary or acquired. In the former, the defect is in a regulatory mechanism for iron absorption in the duodenum. The most common screening test for hemochromatosis is serum ferritin; an elevated level suggests the possibility of iron overload. Ferritin is also an acute-phase reactant and may be falsely elevated in various inflammatory processes (including alcohol use). If ferritin is elevated (greater than 300 µg/L in adult males and 200 µg/L in adult females), serum iron and total iron-binding capacity (TIBC) should be assessed. If the fasting serum iron divided by the TIBC (serum transferrin saturation) is ≥45%, the diagnosis of hemochromatosis should be further pursued. If the ferritin is chronically greater than 1000, there is a heightened risk of cirrhosis.

The definitive diagnosis rests on a quantitative assessment of hepatic iron from a liver biopsy specimen. A modest increase in hepatic iron is normal with aging. Thus a calculation based on the patient's age and iron content in the liver is used to create the iron-age index to determine the presence or absence of iron overload (>1.9 is suggestive of hemochromatosis). Chapter 31 provides more detail.

14. **What is the role of genetic testing in hemochromatosis?**
Many individuals with iron overload have a genetic disorder. Two major *HFE* gene defects have been described. They involve single amino acid mutations, which result in altered iron absorption. Hereditary hemochromatosis is an autosomal recessive disorder. Therefore two aberrant genes must be present. Table 13.1 defines the possible combinations and the association of each with iron overload. Detection of *HFE* abnormalities provides the clinician a powerful tool for screening relatives.

Table 13.1 Likelihood of Hereditary Hemochromatosis Based on Genetic Defects.

HFE PROTEINS	PROBABILITY OF IRON OVERLOAD
C282Y:C282Y	High
C282Y:H63D	Moderate
H63D:H63D	Low
H63D:wild type	Low
C282Y:wild type	Low
Wild-type:wild type	None

It must be borne in mind that genetic susceptibility does not establish the presence of iron overload. It is also apparent that the currently available genetic testing does not capture all cases. More than 95% of cases in Australia but only 50% of Mediterranean cases will be uncovered by the currently available genetic tests.

Novel gene proteins are being studied for hereditary hemochromatosis, including ferroportin, transferrin receptor 2, hemojuvelin, and hepcidin.

15. Describe the role of α1-antitrypsin.
The liver enzyme α1-antitrypsin helps break down trypsin and other tissue proteases. Multiple gene variants are described. The most common is termed *MM* (indicating one allele from each parent) and this is considered normal (or wild-type). One variant, called *Z*, is the product of a single amino acid gene mutation from the wild-type protein. The Z protein is difficult to excrete from the liver cell and causes local damage that may result in hepatitis and cirrhosis.

16. What tests are used to diagnose α1-antitrypsin deficiency?
Deficiency of α1-antitrypsin is most often associated with chronic obstructive pulmonary disease at an early age. Hepatic manifestations include neonatal jaundice. Adults with no prior history of neonatal jaundice and no lung disease may develop otherwise unexplained cirrhosis. The ZZ phenotype is most commonly associated with liver disease, although MZ may also cause cirrhosis. Available tests include as follows:
1. Quantitative α1-antitrypsin: Subnormal levels suggest the possibility of disease.
2. α1-Antitrypsin phenotype: This test designates the allelic protein types in the serum (e.g., MM, ZZ, MZ, FZ). Patients with protein of the ZZ type are said to be homozygotic for Z-type α1-antitrypsin deficiency. This is the form most frequently associated with significant liver disease.
3. Liver biopsy. If α1-antitrypsin is trapped in hepatocytes, it can be seen in liver tissue as small globules that stain with the periodic acid-Schiff reaction and resist subsequent digestion with an enzyme called *diastase*. An immunostain is also available in some institutions.

17. What is the relationship of α1-antitrypsin abnormal phenotypes to disease?
Deficiency of α1-antitrypsin is most often associated with chronic obstructive pulmonary disease at an early age. Hepatic manifestations include neonatal jaundice. Adults with no prior history of neonatal jaundice and no lung disease may develop otherwise unexplained cirrhosis. The ZZ phenotype is most commonly associated with liver disease, although MZ may also cause cirrhosis.

18. What is Wilson disease?
Wilson disease, a rare disorder of copper storage, is caused by a deficiency in the enzyme responsible for copper excretion. The enzyme is under the control of the *ATP7B* gene.

Copper deposition may be seen in the eye (Kayser-Fleischer rings) and parts of the brain (basal ganglia). Many chronic CS diseases (e.g., primary biliary cholangitis [PBC]) also result in aberrant copper storage but not to the degree seen in true Wilson disease.

19. How is Wilson disease diagnosed?
The initial screening test is the serum ceruloplasmin level, which is low in more than 95% of patients with Wilson disease. Conditions in which the ceruloplasmin may be low include massive liver failure or terminal cirrhosis of any cause. Some individuals have idiopathic hypoceruloplasminemia without Wilson disease.

Total serum copper levels are not useful in diagnosis because most circulates bound to ceruloplasmin. However, measurement of serum-free copper is possible in many laboratories. A value greater than 25 mcg/dL suggests copper overload. Twenty-four-hour urine copper levels higher than 40 mcg/24 hours also suggest copper overload.

Kayser-Fleischer rings are virtually always present when there are neurologic features of Wilson disease. Demonstration most often requires a slit lamp examination. The absence of Kayser-Fleischer rings does not exclude Wilson liver disease. Kayser-Fleischer rings have rarely been reported in other conditions (e.g., PBC).

Quantitative assessment of copper in liver tissue from liver biopsy provides a definitive diagnosis. Copper stains (e.g., rhodamine stain) are often falsely negative in those with Wilson disease so quantitative copper levels in liver tissue are needed. As mentioned, chronic CS liver disease may also result in hepatic copper accumulation, usually to a moderate degree. Hepatic copper levels of greater than 250 mcg/g dry weight are diagnostic of Wilson disease.

Gene testing: *ATP7B* is the gene responsible for copper homeostasis. More than 900 deleterious gene variants have been described. Genetic testing may be indicated for confirmation of diagnosis, family screening, and in unclear cases. Gene testing is not a first-order screening test for Wilson disease.

20. Summarize the tests for common metabolic disorders of the liver.
See Table 13.2 for testing for common metabolic disorders of the liver. Numerous other rare hereditary diseases of the liver, including Gaucher disease, Niemann-Pick disease, and hereditary tyrosinemia usually diagnosed in children, are beyond the scope of this chapter.

Table 13.2 Tests for Common Metabolic Disorders of the Liver.

DISEASE	PRIMARY TEST	SUPPORTIVE TEST	DEFINITIVE TEST
Hemochromatosis	Serum ferritin >300 mcg/L in adult males and 200 mcg/L in adult females	Iron saturation ≥45% Iron age index >2 Positive *HFE* testing	Liver biopsy with iron stain and quantitative iron content—hepatic iron index
α-Antitrypsin	SPEP or α-antitrypsin level	Phenotype (Pi ZZ type)	Liver biopsy with PAS-positive diastase-resistant granules
Wilson disease	Ceruloplasmin <20 mg/dL	Urine copper >40 mcg/24 hr, Kayser-Fleischer rings *ATP7B* genetic testing	Liver biopsy with quantitative copper >250 mcg/g dry weight

PAS, Periodic acid-Schiff test; *SPEP*, serum protein electrophoresis.

21. What autoimmune tests are useful in liver disease?

Two liver diseases most directly proven to be immune mediated are AH and PBC. Each is discussed elsewhere (Chapters 17–19). Autoantibodies are typically present but not required to make a diagnosis of either AH or PBC. Moreover, autoantibodies are frequently seen in normal individuals.

Autoimmune markers include antinuclear antibody (ANA), anti–smooth muscle antibody (ASMA; also called *antiactin antibody*), liver-kidney microsomal antibody type 1 (LKM-1), antimitochondrial antibody (AMA), soluble liver antigen, and antiasialoglycoprotein receptor antibody. ANA, ASMA, and AMA are the most readily available tests and help to define the probability of the more common classes of autoimmune liver disease.

AH: AH is suspected especially in a female with significant elevation of AST and ALT (>5 times ULN) and in the absence of competing etiologies such as alcohol, viral hepatitis, and hepatotoxic drugs. Typical antibodies found include ANA, smooth muscle antibody, and anti-LKM, usually in titers >1:80. Gamma globulin elevations more than 1.5 times ULN are frequent. The absence of autoantibodies does not exclude this diagnosis.

PBC: PBC is typically seen in females, with liver enzymes demonstrating predominant elevation of AP. AMA is typically present in PBC, usually in a high titer. The absence of AMA does not exclude the diagnosis.

Intermix syndrome: Features of AH and PBC may each be present. For example, an individual with predominant elevation of AST and ALT, with a negative SMA but high titer AMA, may be considered to have AH/PBC intermix.

22. The tortoise and the hare—sequential versus simultaneous testing?

The cost of testing is not inconsequential. A recent simulation study of an adult with persistently elevated ALT attempted to determine the cost and benefit of ordering a batch of diagnostic testing (the hare), or a more measured approach (the tortoise). Each approach provided a definitive diagnosis in 53%–54% of simulated cases. The cost per diagnosis was higher taking the sequential approach, even more so when taking into account the higher number of patient visits. There was a swing toward the superiority of the tortoise approach when assuming more alcoholic liver disease, NAFLD, and drug-induced liver injury and when information from prior evaluations were included.

23. What are other uses of noninvasive markers of fibrosis?

Noninvasive markers of fibrosis have already been discussed in the context of NAFLD. Their role is rapidly expanding. Current guidelines on cirrhosis rely heavily on the following non-invasive makers: FibroScan, platelet count, BMI, and etiology of cirrhosis to define risk and guide management.

Transient elastography (especially Fibrosan) is currently a central measure in staging cirrhosis of all etiologies. Conventionally, cirrhosis is staged as mild (portal pressure 5–10 mm Hg); clinically significant (portal pressure 10–12 mm Hg, no bleeding varices, ascites, and encephalopathy); early-decompensated (portal pressure >12 mm Hg, and bleeding from varices, ascites, or encephalopathy); or late-decompensated with refractory complications.

It is impractical to measure portal pressure invasively on multiple occasions over time. Noninvasive markers, especially FibroScan and platelet count, are now recommended for clinical decision-making.

Recommendations of 2021 Portal Hypertension Consensus Conference have recently been published [1]. The current use of FibroScan, including the "5-10-15-20-25" demarcation boundaries, is shown in Fig. 13.3.

Baveno VII–Renewing consensus in portal hypertension

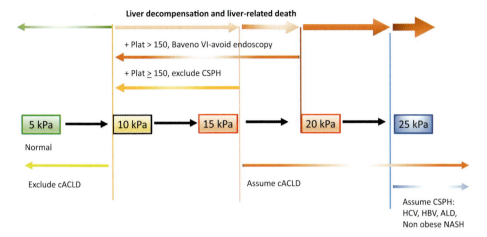

Fig. 13.3 Algorithm for the noninvasive determination of compensated advanced chronic liver disease (cACLD) and clinically significant portal hypertension (CSPH). Liver stiffness is expressed in kilopascals (kPa). *ALD*, Alcohol-related liver disease; *HBV*, hepatitis B virus; *HCV*, hepatitis C virus; *NASH*, nonalcoholic steatohepatitis; *Plat*, platelets. (Adapted from de Franchis R, Bosch J, Garcia-Tsao G, Reiberger T, Ripoll C, on behalf of the Baveno VII Faculty. Baveno VII – renewing consensus in portal hypertension. J Hepatol. 2022;76:959-974.)

For example,
1. Clinically significant portal hypertension is excluded if FibroScan reveals <10 kPa or if <15 kPa and platelet count ≥150k.
2. Endoscopic screening for varices is not needed if FibroScan reveals <20 kPa and platelet count >150k.
3. Noncardioselective beta-blocker therapy is recommended regardless of the presence or absence of varices if elastography indicated clinically significant portal hypertension.

24. **What is the role of liver biopsy?**
    Liver biopsy is much less frequently used since the development of precise diagnostic tests and noninvasive markers of fibrosis. Liver biopsy is now done most often when there are competing etiologies for liver disease, or when testing yields conflicting or ambiguous results. Many academic centers perform liver biopsy in those with suspected acute alcoholic hepatitis. The value of the biopsy depends on two factors—provision of an adequate specimen, defined as an intact liver slice containing more than 11 portal areas, and review by a qualified pathologist or hepatologist. Liver biopsy provides important prognostic information in many patients with various chronic liver diseases.

CLINICAL VIGNETTE
Available Online.

BIBLIOGRAPHY
Available Online.

CHAPTER 14

MICROBIOME IN HEALTH AND DISEASE

Gerald Dryden, Jr., MD, PhD, MSPH

 Additional content available online.

1. What is the scope of the gastrointestinal (GI) microbiome?

Millions of years of coevolution between man and the environment have led to the complex colonization of microbes on every human surface exposed to the environment. Perhaps the greatest microbial diversity exists in the digestive tract. The gut microbiome is composed of trillions of bacteria, archaea, viruses, fungi, and eukaryotic microbes that make up over 50% of the cells found within the human body and weigh up to 2 kg in an adult. The number of organisms is limited in the stomach by its acid milieu and the small intestine by the presence of bile and pancreatic juice. The complex and active peristalsis seen in the small intestine further inhibits microbial colonization. Thus the colon is where the overwhelming majority (10^{14}) of the microbiota live and interact with the human host.

2. What are the benefits of being colonized by microbes?

Microbes living within the confines of the GI tract provide incredible benefits to the host, including the release of nutrients from ingested food, the stimulation of GI immune function and control of barrier physiology, and the protection of the host from pathogens. However, the balance of microbial diversity that contributes to health can easily flip to a population that contributes to disease of the host. The delicate balance between health and disease (symbiosis and dysbiosis) can be altered by food intake, environmental conditions, or host factors.

3. Where has our knowledge of the microbiome come from?

The Human Microbiome Project began in 2008 to characterize the human microbiome. Utilizing advanced molecular sequencing techniques, over 1300 reference strains were identified. Microbiota profiling derived from genetic information contained within the 16S/18S rRNA (ribosomal RNA) sequencing of both highly conserved and hypervariable regions allows precise identification of bacterial species and a fingerprint of the gut microbiome. Bacteria constitute the predominant species colonizing the human digestive tract, which spans the mouth to the anus. Historical estimates peg the number of total nonhuman organisms residing in the GI tract at 10^{14}, an order of magnitude higher than the estimated number of mammalian cells present in the body. The term microbiota refers to the sum of microorganisms harbored in specific organs or tissues of an organism, which contribute mostly commensal or symbiotic functions to their host.

4. Is the human GI tract sterile at birth?

Until recently, dogma maintained that the newborn digestive tract remained sterile until delivery. Recent animal and human studies raise the possibility of in utero translocation of bacteria, based on 16S rRNA analysis of amniotic fluid, meconium, and oropharyngeal swabs. Furthermore, the effects that dietary and lifestyle factors confer on maternal GI flora mirror the patterns seen in infants born to those mothers under study, suggesting that maternal factors influence prenatal development. Animal studies now offer some evidence for placental transfer of microbiota, as evidenced by the presence of genetically altered bacteria administered to the mother showing up in the fetal GI tract and the presence of effector memory T cells in the GI tract of second-trimester fetal tissue, which challenges the concept of a completely sterile GI tract during fetal development.

5. How do microorganisms populate the GI tract?

GI tract seeding occurs most profoundly during delivery, strongly influencing the microbiota in the earliest stages of life after birth. Infants delivered by vaginal delivery (VD) take on the microbiota of their mother, but infants born by cesarian delivery (CS) exhibit vastly different microbiota that increases their risk of multiple problems, including neonatal infections, immune disorders, and obesity. Maternal vaginal gauze seeding partially normalized the trajectory for microbiota development between CS and VD compared to nonswabbed neonates. After delivery, infants exhibit low species diversity and elevated levels of composition flux. Actinobacteria (*Bifidobacterium* sp.) anchor infant intestinal microbial profiles in general, followed by Firmicutes (*Lactobacillus* sp.) in breastfed infants or Bacteroidetes in formula-fed infants. Microbiologists now recognize Bacteroidetes as specialists in degrading high-molecular-weight organic matter, such as proteins and carbohydrates.

6. **Is there a difference between breastfed and formula-fed bacterial population?**
   Yes. Variations in infant microbiome composition reflect substrate differences between breast milk and formula, with a formula containing high concentrations of the prebiotics galacto-oligosaccharide (GOS) and fructo-oligosaccharide likely accounting for the high levels of *Bifidobacterium* found in many formula-fed infants. Breastfeeding, regardless of duration, continues to heavily influence microbiota. After weaning and the first or second year of life, the adult microbiome begins to emerge and depends on solid food dietary influences and other microbial factors from that point on. By 3 years of age, the child's microbiota cannot be distinguished from an adult's microbiota.

7. **How does the mucosal immune system tolerate all those bacteria?**
   In constant contact with resident microbiota, animal hosts coevolved an immune system to prevent microbial invasion of the interior tissues of the body. These immune systems exhibited complex methods for identifying and destroying invading bacteria, including commensals and primary pathogens seeking entry into the body. Immune molecules evolved more than 500 million years ago in simple single-cell organisms, while innate immune antimicrobial peptides and pattern recognition receptors arose later to maintain order at the major sites of bacteria-facing epithelial surfaces. These processes provide contextual cues allowing the host to catalog resident microbes and initiate defensive action against invading pathogens. The eventual development of an adaptive immune system provided even more protection and an ability to shape the microbiota through secreted antibodies and antibacterial proteins. In fact, the intestinal microbiota serves a crucial role in shaping the host immune system. Germ-free (axenic or gnotobiotic) mice exhibit less-developed intestinal epithelia, smaller organs and lymphoid tissue, less skeletal muscle and adiposity, and underdeveloped immune systems. Enhanced lethality upon exposure to pathogens is another consequence of being born germ-free. The presence of an established microbial population provides the host with a buffer against pathogens. As a consequence of these entanglements, the presence of a healthy bacterial population provides irrefutable benefits to the host.

8. **How does the microbiota assist in the nutritional health of human host?**
   The bacterial population of the gut drives the metabolic capacity of the microbiota; major substrates include bile acid and short-chain fatty acids. By-products of the microbial metabolic pathways of food items fuel important aspects of immune function, inflammation, and even cancer susceptibility or resistance. Other food components also provide a direct impact on microbial function, including plant-derived exosomes. The microbial population of the gut depends on a steady stream of nutrients to maintain normal function. Changes in diet can cause day-to-day variations in the microbiome, but the adult population remains relatively stable with approximately 60%–70% of bacterial strains present in the GI tract remaining unchanged over a 5-year period of study.

9. **Are there other important components of the microbiome besides bacteria?**
   Yes—viruses and fungi.
   Viruses.
   Viruses co-colonize the human gut more heavily than bacteria by a 1–10× multiple, collectively referred to as the intestinal virome. The human virome is composed of eukaryotic and prokaryotic viruses (capable of infecting human cells and microbes such as bacteria, fungi, and archaea) plus plant viruses that are primarily sourced from the environment and diet. Virome development following birth through early childhood differs from the trajectory of the microbiome, as bacteriophage diversity is highest in the earliest years but decreases as the complexity of the bacterial component increases beyond the first years of life. This finding supports the concept that the virome can help shape the microbiome. As infants mature, the number of phages decreases and eukaryotic viruses become outnumbered by prokaryotic viruses by 9:1 and remain fairly stable through adulthood. Much in the same way that bacteria can be associated with certain disease phenotypes and that microbial transfer can ameliorate or reproduce those conditions, phage populations can be associated with certain phenotypes such as diabetes, inflammatory bowel disease (IBD), liver disease, or cancer. Furthermore, certain outcomes influenced by bacterial transfer such as resolution of *Clostridium difficile* infection by fecal matter transfer can be completely recapitulated with cell-free phage transfer. Detection efforts have been hampered by the complexity of nonbacterial DNA/RNA signal in stool, lack of sentinel viral genes, and relative paucity of genetic material compared to other larger organisms. Much needs to be learned about the interactions between the virome and bacterial microbiome.
   Fungi.
   Knowledge of fungal elements of the microbiome have generally been limited to those species amendable to isolation and culture techniques available, limiting the diversity detected and overestimating the contribution of *Candida* and *Saccharomyces*. Advances in DNA reading technology that benefited bacterial research have also increased our knowledge of the mycobiome. Mucosal biopsy and stool studies found that the gut mycobiome includes many genera of fungi, including *Alternaria, Aspergillus, Candida, Cladosporium, Cryptococcus, Debaryomyces, Fusarium, Galactomyces, Malassezia, Penicillium, Pichia, Rhodotorula, Saccharomyces,* and *Trichosporon*, with a predominance by species from the family Saccharomycetaceae. While the mycobiome varies considerably by age, food intake, and environmental considerations, fungal dysbiosis has also been detected in IBD. In particular, elevated levels of *Candida tropicalis* have been found in the stool of patients with Crohn disease (CD), *Debaryomyces hansenii* in

the inflamed mucosa of these patients, *Aspergillus* in colon biopsies taken from patients with ulcerative colitis (UC), and even in patients with flaring, as evidenced by an increased stool counts of *Candida albicans* and decreased counts of both *Malassezia sympodialis* and *Saccharomyces cerevisiae*. Although incorporation of the mycobiome into predictive models integrating the microbiome, biomarkers, and demographic data together accurately predicted IBD flares and differentiated between CD and UC phenotypes, considerable research needs to be pursued to fully appreciate the contribution of the mycobiome to the field of IBD.

10. Does a core microbiome exist that can apply across the human experience?

While contributions of the microbiome to particular disease states have been heavily researched, the definition of a normal or core microbiome has been difficult to define. The general trend has been to look for differences that define a particular disease state. Using an opposite approach, many researchers have been pursuing the concept of a core microbiome. Loosely defined, the core microbiome can be defined as any set of microbial taxa, as well as the associated genomic or functional attributes characteristic of a specific host or environment. The identification of core microbiome components has been hypothesized to be a key to maintaining long-term human oral and gut health. One challenge in defining a "core microbiome" has been standardizing testing methodology as heterogeneity of the results led to multiple different hypotheses about the core microbiome, including that (1) cores may exist within certain human populations but not globally, (2) a core may be discernible only at a higher taxonomic level such as genera, or that (3) the core may be wholly functional, comprised of functional gene clusters rather than individual taxa. However, most healthy adults harbor similar microbiota, where 99% of the organisms include Firmicutes, Bacteroidetes, Proteobacteria, and Actinobacteria. Of those organisms, Firmicutes and Bacteroidetes make up the bulk, accounting for approximately 90% of the microbiota.

11. If there is no core microbiome, how do we know an abnormal microbiome when we see one?

Gut dysbiosis occurs whenever a host or environmental factor alters the composition, diversity, and/or function of the baseline microbiome. Typically, this disturbance creates stress on the host organism harboring the microbiome. Dysbiotic states may perturb the normal function of any organ system present in the host, causing dysfunction in the GI tract or distant organ systems. Gut dysbiosis occurs in association with many disease states but discerning whether the dysbiosis is cause or effect can be challenging.

12. The GI tract is packed with bacteria and other organisms. What impact could the microbiome have on IBD?

The study of the microbiome in association with IBD ushered in the modern era of microbiome research. While Samuel Wilks first postulated a microbial basis for IBD, researchers have failed to implicate a single causative microbial organism in the pathogenesis of IBD. The concept of microbial etiology has morphed into an understanding that the imbalance of organisms in a susceptible human host likely initiates the onset of IBD. Reduced biodiversity characterizes patients with IBD associated with an abundance of Firmicutes and an expansion of Proteobacteria such as *Enterobacteriaceae*, *Bilophila*, and Bacteroidetes. Lower biodiversity may set the host up for altered metabolic output from the microbial community, alter immune tolerance, or increase susceptibility to pathogens. Dysbiosis can also lead to increased mucolytic bacteria capable of degrading the mucosal barrier and enhancing exposure of immune structures microbiome constituents. From both cultural and serologic evidence, variations in fungal populations have accompanied IBD diagnoses. Patients with CD exhibit greater fungal diversity than controls, implicating the mycobiota in the pathogenesis of IBD. In fact, the anti-*S. cerevisiae* antibody stands as the most robust biomarker identified with the diagnosis of CD. The phage populations have been least studied, but patients with IBD have demonstrated an increased abundance of phages of the order *Caudovirales*, a finding with unclear clinical implications. The difficult task consists of linking these characteristic changes to causality.

13. How does the gut microbiome affect skin diseases?

Several dermatologic conditions, such as acne, atopic dermatitis, psoriasis, and rosacea, are linked with intestinal dysbiosis. Members of the gut microbiome can influence skin conditions through their metabolic activity and immunologic impact. Gut–skin communication occurs when elements of the immune system conduct crosstalk between the gut and the skin. Intestinal dysbiosis can lead to elevated levels of phenol, a bacterial metabolite that causes dry skin and affects keratinization. Administration of the probiotic *Bifidobacterium breve* with GOS reduced phenol levels and restored skin condition. The presence of circulating DNA from intestinal microbes in peripheral blood coincides with elevated levels of inflammatory cytokines compared to nonpsoriatic normal controls. A strong connection between CD and psoriasis exists, further linking the concept of intestinal injury leading to peripheral skin disorders. Limited within-sample (alpha) diversity in infants increases the risk of atopic dermatitis later in life. Similarly, acne has been tied to reductions in the prevalence of *Actinobacteria, Bifidobacterium, Butyricicoccus, Coprobacillus*, and *Lactobacillus* in the setting of increased Proteobacteria.

14. **What is the role of the gut microbiome in the risk of cardiovascular (CV) disease?**

Plant-based diets (PBDs) foster reduced risks of metabolic disorders, including type 2 diabetes, CV disease, and obesity, while meat-based diets increase cardiometabolic risk. To investigate the role of the microbiome in this risk pattern, a large cohort study evaluated short- and long-term adherence to PBD intake by the Food Frequency Questionnaire and 16S rRNA analysis of stool microbiome. After 3 years, PBD yielded higher alpha diversity, associated with lower serum triglycerides, fasting insulin, and C-reactive protein (CRP). A lower abundance of *Peptostreptococcus* on PBD correlated with a lower CRP and higher high-density lipoprotein cholesterol. Short-term PBD made no impact on CV risk factors. While many other studies have highlighted the benefit of PBD for CV risk, this study highlights the impact of PBD on CV risk factors while tying the alterations to specific changes in the microbiota.

15. **Can the microbiome alter the risk for cancer or alter the response to treatment?**

Helicobacter pylori's impact on gastric cancer stands as a prominent example of a single-species role in GI cancer development. More recently, microbiome implication in colorectal cancer (CRC) susceptibility includes higher proportions of *Fusobacterium nucleatum*, *Bacteroides fragilis*, *Escherichia coli*, *Enterococcus*, *Campylobacter*, *Peptostreptococcus*, *Shigella*, *Klebsiella*, and *Akkermansia* in patients with CRC, and lower levels of *Ruminococcus*, *Bifidobacterium*, *Eubacteria*, and *Lachnospira* compared with healthy subjects. *F. nucleatum* normally resides in the mouth only in normal controls, but it has frequently been detected in tumors and stools of patients with CRC. *F. nucleatum* activates a Th17 inflammatory response in the tissue, increasing the likelihood of a neoplastic transformation according to animal studies. Enterotoxigenic *B. fragilis* similarly demonstrates a propensity to induce inflammation and facilitate tumor transformation, especially in conjunction with *E. coli*. *E. coli* itself has been implicated as a microbial factor involved in CRC development, although other data implicate a form of *E. coli* that expresses polyketide synthetase (*pks*), a gene responsible for synthesizing colibactin (a genotoxin involved in DNA damage and cell cycle abnormalities) as the source of tumor susceptibility and chromosomal instability in human cells. Yet other data support the role of bacterial metabolites as factors involved in CRC susceptibility, as well as response to cancer therapies. To this point, *Bifidobacterium* enhanced anticancer immune responses by increasing dendritic cell activation and subsequent CD8+ effector T cell priming, driving subsequent tumor microenvironment invasion. Anti-PD-1 monoclonal antibody effects on a mouse model of melanoma also benefited outcomes based on inhibitory effects of the *Bifidobacterium* metabolite hippurate. Similar effects have been seen with other probiotics, such as *Lactobacillus rhamnosus* GG. The use of probiotics or even fecal matter transplant has been applied to clinical practice with varying results. However, numerous studies have demonstrated detrimental effects of antibiotics on cancer treatment outcomes.

16. **How can the study of the human metabolome define the complex interactions of the human host and the microbiome?**

The final frontier in microbiome research likely lies in the field of metabolomics. This form of "omics" research encompasses all the permutations mentioned previously and measures the output of the sum total of the organisms and the host. This avoids confusion regarding the meaning of diversity changes or loss of individual components and their impact on the system. For example, under the wrong environmental conditions, a perfectly normal microbiome may metabolize something from the environment (highly processed food, simple sugars, and chemical toxin), and the metabolic output puts a strain on the host that creates a disease state. Conversely, a dysbiotic microbiome resulting from some exogenous factor may be fed a healthy, noninflammatory diet and not produce the toxic output that would be required to incite a state of impaired health. Investigating the metabolome with a comprehensive analysis of the various biomolecules produced in a system's microbiome will provide researchers with data to assess how microbes interact with each other and the cells of the adjacent host system. These findings will then provide the ultimate tool for measuring how external interventions can alter a microbiota's metabolic output in a quantitative way. This technique will usher in an era where scientists and clinicians will be able to measure the outcome of pharmacologic, biologic, or dietary therapies on the underlying microbial population, profile the response, and predict the impact on the disease process of interest.

BIBLIOGRAPHY

Available Online.

CHAPTER 15

ANTIVIRAL THERAPY FOR HEPATITIS C

Gabriel A. Bolaños Guzmán, MD and Jorge L. Herrera, MD

 Additional content available online.

1. How is hepatitis C virus (HCV) infection diagnosed?

All people for whom HCV screening is recommended should initially be tested for HCV antibody. A positive HCV antibody test indicates either a current HCV infection, a past infection that has resolved, or a false positive. A test to detect HCV viremia (HCV-RNA by polymerase chain reaction [PCR]) is, therefore, necessary to confirm active HCV infection and guide clinical management. To expedite diagnosis, it is recommended that whenever possible, the initial diagnostic test ordered should be "HCV antibody with reflex to HCV-RNA PCR." This will automatically alert the laboratory to run a viral quantitation if the antibody test is positive, avoiding a second visit and blood draw. HCV-RNA testing should also be performed in people with a negative HCV antibody test who are either immunocompromised (e.g., people receiving chronic hemodialysis or cancer chemotherapy) or might have been exposed to HCV within the last 6 months because these people may be HCV antibody negative despite being viremic with the HCV. People who have a positive HCV antibody test and negative results for HCV-RNA by PCR should be informed that they do not have laboratory evidence of current HCV infection, although it is possible that they may have had a previous exposure. Additional HCV testing is typically unnecessary. The HCV-RNA test can be repeated when there is a high index of suspicion for recent infection or in patients with ongoing HCV infection risk.

2. Can HCV be cured?

Yes. HCV is an RNA virus that does not integrate into the host's genome and can be permanently eradicated with a finite course of direct-acting antiviral (DAA) therapy. It is essential to test for HCV-RNA 12 weeks (or longer) after treatment completion. A negative HCV-RNA at that point is defined as a sustained virologic response (SVR), which is consistent with a cure for chronic HCV infection. Patients who achieve SVR can have HCV recurrence due to reinfection or late relapse which is very rare (<1%). HCV antibody remains positive in most patients after achieving SVR; thus testing for HCV recurrence using an assay that detects HCV-RNA is recommended if reinfection or relapse is suspected.

3. What are the indications for antiviral therapy in patients with chronic HCV?

Treatment is recommended for all individuals with active HCV infection (acute or chronic) to prevent the development of complications from cirrhosis, decompensation, hepatocellular carcinoma (HCC), and extrahepatic manifestations. Additionally, treatment is recommended to prevent transmission of HCV infection to others, including children born to mothers with HCV infection. The only exception would be people with a short life expectancy that cannot be remediated by HCV therapy, liver transplantation, or another directed therapy.

4. What is the recommended evaluation of patients with chronic HCV before antiviral therapy is started?

A pretreatment evaluation is necessary to assess the severity of fibrosis and other baseline factors that may impact HCV treatment and to determine if a patient should be comanaged with specialist support.

During the initial assessment, a physical examination and detailed patient history should be obtained, which should include the risk of HCV acquisition, prior HCV therapies, the presence of other liver diseases, and the stigmata of cirrhosis. Patients should be assessed for alcohol consumption, injection drug use (IDU), body mass index, diabetes, and metabolic syndrome, which often may coexist with HCV infection.

Recommended pretreatment assessments and blood tests are shown in Fig. 15.1. These tests are important to assess hepatic and renal function, exclude viral coinfection, and assess the need for hepatitis A and/or B immunizations. Females of childbearing age should be tested for pregnancy. Patients should be referred to a specialist if they have been previously treated for HCV infection but not cured, have coinfection with hepatitis B virus (HBV) (positive for hepatitis B surface antigen [HBsAg]) or human immunodeficiency virus (HIV), severe renal impairment (renal replacement therapy or an estimated glomerular filtration rate <30 mL/min/1.73 m²), or have uncontrolled comorbidities. Fibrosis assessment is recommended for all patients with chronic HCV infection. The primary purpose of fibrosis assessment is to detect advanced fibrosis that may require referral to a specialist.

5. How is fibrosis assessed in patients with HCV infection?

In most cases, a liver biopsy is not required to assess fibrosis. Noninvasive methods have been developed and validated to assess liver fibrosis. These include serum-based tests using the aspartate aminotransferase

Laboratory tests recommended within 6 months prior to starting DAA therapy:
• Complete blood count
• Hepatic function panel (i.e., serum albumin, total and direct bilirubin, alanine aminotransferase (ALT), aspartate aminotransferase (AST), and alkaline phosphatase levels)
• Estimated glomerular filtration rate (eGFR)

Laboratory tests recommended any time prior to starting DAA therapy:
• Quantitative HCV RNA (HCV viral load)
• HCV genotype test (optional for patients treated with pangenotypic regimens)
• HIV antibody test

Complete list of prescription and non-prescription medications for assessment of possible drug-drug interactions.

Assessment for active hepatitis B virus (HBV) coinfection with HBV surface antigen (HBsAg), and for evidence of prior infection with HBV core antibody (anti-HBc) and HBV surface antibody (anti-HBs) testing. Immunity against hepatitis A virus (HAV) should be assessed with anti-HAV-Ab total titer.

Patients found or known to be HBsAg-positive should be referred to specialty care.

All patients should be assessed for HIV coinfection prior to initiating DAA therapy.

All patients should be assessed for liver fibrosis prior to starting therapy.

Fig. 15.1 Recommended Assessments Prior to Starting Direct-Acting Antiviral (DAA) Therapy.
DAA, Direct acting antiviral; *HAV-Ab*, hepatitis A virus antibody; *HBsAg*, hepatitis B surface antigen; *HBV*, hepatitis B virus; *HCV*, hepatitis C virus; *HIV*, human immunodeficiency virus.

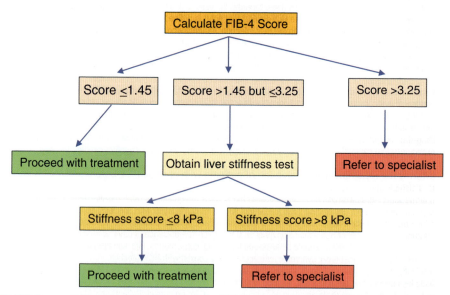

Fig. 15.2 Assessment of fibrosis in patients with hepatitis C virus (HCV) infection. *FIB-4*, Fibrosis four-factor index.

(AST)-to-platelet ratio index or the fibrosis index based on a four-factor (FIB-4) score. Anatomical tests to assess for liver stiffness (which reflects fibrosis) include elastography (FibroScan) or abdominal ultrasound with acoustic radiation force impulse imaging. Magnetic resonance elastography is probably the most accurate noninvasive method to assess fibrosis but is not widely available and is expensive. It is important to recognize that noninvasive tests are best to exclude fibrosis. These tests tend to overestimate fibrosis; thus when negative, it is fairly certain that fibrosis is absent. In case of disagreement between tests, a liver biopsy may be necessary to fully assess fibrosis. The approach to assessing fibrosis in patients with HCV is shown in Fig. 15.2.

6. **What is the importance of genotype testing in HCV?**
Based on viral sequencing, HCV has six different genotypes. Current antiviral regimens for hepatitis C are considered pangenotypic—they are equally effective regardless of the genotype causing the infection. For this reason, HCV genotyping is no longer necessary prior to treatment initiation in treatment-naive patients. In those with evidence of cirrhosis and/or past unsuccessful HCV treatment, treatment regimens may differ by genotype, and thus pretreatment genotyping is recommended in those circumstances.

7. **What are the treatment options for HCV infection?**
Treatment-naive patients with HCV should receive a regimen that is effective for all genotypes (pangenotypic). The pangenotypic therapies glecaprevir/pibrentasvir (GLE/PIB) and sofosbuvir/velpatasvir (SOF/VEL) are currently approved in the United States for the initial treatment of HCV. Both regimens have generally comparable efficacy and safety profiles with one exception. SOF/VEL can be used in patients at all stages of liver fibrosis, including decompensated liver disease (Child-Pugh B and C cirrhosis), whereas GLE/PIB is contraindicated in Child-Pugh B and C cirrhosis. The reason for this is that GLE/PIB contains a protease inhibitor which can be hepatotoxic in patients with decompensated cirrhosis. Both regimens have cure rates exceeding 95% among patients without cirrhosis or with compensated cirrhosis. SOF/VEL therapy consists of a single pill taken once a day for 12 weeks. GLE/PIB consists of three tablets taken together once a day for 8 weeks.

8. **What are the side effects of antiviral therapy?**
Minimal side effects occur with these therapies, and most are mild. Common side effects include headache, fatigue, and nausea with both GLE/PIB and SOF/VEL, as well as asthenia and insomnia with SOF/VEL. Laboratory abnormalities such as elevated lipase and creatine kinase with SOF/VEL, and alanine aminotransferase (ALT) and bilirubin levels with GLE/PIB are extremely rare. The treatment is well tolerated with discontinuation rates due to adverse events of <1%.

9. **How should patients on antiviral therapy be monitored?**
Treatment with GLE/PIB or SOF/VEL requires minimal monitoring due to the high efficacy and favorable safety profile of these therapies. For otherwise healthy and reliable patients in whom compliance is not a concern, the only recommended laboratory testing consists of a liver function panel (AST, ALT, alkaline phosphatase, bilirubin, and albumin) 12 or more weeks after completion of therapy to confirm cure. A clinic visit or telephone encounter at 4 weeks of therapy is recommended to ensure adherence and assess for adverse events. Additional monitoring may be needed for patients with diabetes and those on warfarin-based anticoagulation. Eradication of HCV may enhance insulin sensitivity in patients with diabetes. Patients taking drugs that can cause hypoglycemia need to monitor their blood glucose and reduce the dose if necessary to prevent hypoglycemia. Those taking warfarin should have a more frequent international normalized ratio (INR) monitoring to detect potential subtherapeutic anticoagulation as a result of enhanced liver function from viral eradication.

10. **What are the main drug-drug interactions of antiviral therapies?**
Drug-drug interactions may impact the treatment choice between GLE/PIB and SOF/VEL. The presence of a protease inhibitor in GLE/PIB increases the likelihood of drug-drug interactions compared to SOF/VEL, which does not contain a protease inhibitor. Common drug classes that may interact with these products include statins, antiseizure drugs, HIV antiretroviral therapies (ARTs), oral contraceptives, and proton pump inhibitors. There may also be interactions with herbal supplements such as St. John's wort. It is recommended that providers or pharmacists consult with one of the several web-based drug interaction sites such as the University of Liverpool drug interaction checker (https://www.hep-druginteractions.org/) prior to prescribing these regimens to patients taking multiple drugs. In addition, patients should discontinue all herbal and nutritional supplements for the duration of the therapy.

11. **Is antiviral therapy recommended for HCV infection in people who inject drugs (PWID)?**
IDU is the most common risk factor for HCV infection in the United States and Europe. The term PWID includes individuals who are actively using drugs and those who have previously used injection drugs. IDU accounts for most new HCV infections (approximately 70%) and is the driving force in the perpetuation of the epidemic. All individuals who currently inject drugs or have previously used injection drugs should be tested for HCV infection and offered treatment if positive. Among people with a negative HCV antibody test who are at high risk for a new HCV infection due to current IDU, testing for HCV-RNA or follow-up testing for HCV antibody is recommended if HCV exposure may have occurred within the past 6 months. Once an infection is diagnosed, treatment is indicated. Studies have shown that among PWID, the safety and efficacy of pangenotypic regimens are similar to that of people that do not use drugs. Treatment of HCV-infected PWID should ideally be delivered in a multidisciplinary care setting with services to reduce reinfection risk and manage the common social and psychiatric comorbidities in this population. Recent and active IDUs are not contraindications to HCV therapy. People cured of chronic HCV no longer transmit the virus to others but if actively using drugs should be monitored for possible reinfection with HCV-RNA testing every 6–12 months.

12. **Are there any specific considerations regarding antiviral therapy in females of childbearing age?**

All pregnant patients should be tested for HCV infection to allow for appropriate assessment of liver disease status and facilitate linkage to HCV care after delivery. In addition, prenatal HCV diagnosis is a prerequisite for appropriate screening and care for exposed children. HCV-infected pregnant females should be linked to care so that antiviral treatment can be initiated at the appropriate time, treatment during pregnancy is not currently recommended. Females of reproductive age with HCV should be counseled about the benefit of antiviral treatment prior to pregnancy to improve the health of the mother and eliminate the low risk of mother-to-child transmission (<5%). Females who become pregnant while on DAA therapy should discuss the risks versus benefits of continuing treatment with their physicians. Currently, there are no available data on the safety of pangenotypic regimens during pregnancy, and these regimens are not US Food and Drug Administration (FDA) approved for use during pregnancy.

13. **Should patients with decompensated cirrhosis secondary to HCV infection be treated with antiviral therapy?**

Clinical trial data demonstrate that in the population of people with decompensated cirrhosis, most patients receiving DAA therapy experience improvement in clinical and biochemical indicators of liver disease between baseline and post-treatment week 12, including patients with Child-Turcotte-Pugh class C cirrhosis. Improvements, however, may be insufficient to avoid liver-related mortality, the need for liver transplantation, or achieve a meaningful improvement in quality of life. The decision to treat or not is complex and must be made in conjunction with the liver transplant center. For this reason, treatment of patients with advanced fibrosis and decompensated disease should be performed by hepatologists or gastroenterologists.

14. **Should patients with HCV/HIV coinfection receive antiviral therapy for HCV infection?**

Patients with HIV/HCV coinfection suffer from more liver-related morbidity and mortality, nonhepatic organ dysfunction, and overall mortality than those infected with HCV monoinfection. Even in the potent HIV ART era, HIV infection remains independently associated with advanced liver fibrosis and cirrhosis in patients with HIV/HCV coinfection. As such, HCV treatment in patients with HIV infection should be a priority. With the availability of HCV DAAs, efficacy and adverse event rates among people with HIV/HCV coinfection are similar to those observed with HCV monoinfection and the treatment regimens are the same as for monoinfected patients. Treatment of patients with HIV/HCV coinfection, however, requires attention to the complex drug-drug interactions that can occur between DAAs and antiretroviral medications. For this reason, it is best to start HCV antiviral therapy once the patient is on a stable and well-tolerated HIV drug regimen.

15. **How should patients with HCV/HBV coinfection be managed and treated?**

HCV/HBV coinfection is diagnosed in patients who tested positive for HCV-RNA and for HBsAg. In most cases, the HCV is dominant (high HCV-RNA) and hepatitis B is suppressed (low or undetectable HBV-DNA). As hepatitis C is controlled with therapy, HBV reactivation, occasionally fulminant, during or after DAA therapy has been reported. Therefore all patients initiating DAA therapy should be assessed for HBV coinfection with HBsAg testing and for evidence of prior infection with anti-HBc.

HBsAg patients with low or undetectable HBV viral load should start prophylactic antiviral therapy for HBV, if the patient remains HBV-DNA negative at 12 weeks, or longer after completing DAA therapy, the HBV antiviral therapy may be discontinued. Patients need close monitoring for the next year to assess for post–antiviral therapy reactivation of HBV. Prophylactic therapy for HBV may be initiated at the time of HCV therapy initiation or 1–2 weeks before initiating HCV therapy.

For the rare patient who has active HBV (high HBV-DNA) and active HCV (high HCV-RNA), antiviral therapy against hepatitis B is recommended and should be continued after completion of DAA therapy until the patient achieves the treatment goal for chronic hepatitis B (See Question 7, Chapter 16). In this situation, initiation of hepatitis B therapy 1–4 weeks prior to DAA therapy is recommended, but if not possible, both therapies can be started simultaneously.

Reactivation of hepatitis B during DAA therapy in patients who are HBsAg (−), hepatitis B core antibody–positive is exceedingly rare, and antiviral therapy for HBV is not recommended. At SVR assessment (12 weeks or later after completion of DAA therapy) liver enzymes should be tested. If elevated, test for HBsAg and HBV-DNA to assess for possible HBV reactivation.

16. **How should patients with HCV and renal impairment be treated?**

Chronic hepatitis C is independently associated with the development of chronic kidney disease (CKD). There is also a higher risk of progression to end-stage renal disease in individuals with chronic HCV infection and CKD, and an increased risk of all-cause mortality in individuals on dialysis. Successful HCV antiviral treatment improves clinical outcomes. No dose adjustment in DAAs is required when using current pangenotypic regimens even in patients on hemodialysis. The efficacy of pangenotypic regimens is similar in patients with CKD compared to those with normal renal function. Due to their comorbidities, these patients should be monitored carefully during treatment and are best treated by a hepatologist or gastroenterologist in conjunction with a nephrologist.

17. How should patients who cleared HCV be monitored?

Patients with undetectable serum HCV-RNA, as assessed by a sensitive PCR assay ≥12 weeks after treatment completion, are deemed to have achieved SVR (i.e., cure). SVR typically aborts the progression of liver injury with regression of liver fibrosis in most (but not all) treated patients. Liver fibrosis and liver function test results improve in most patients who achieve SVR. Because of the lack of progression, noncirrhotic patients who achieve SVR should receive standard medical care that is recommended for patients who were never infected with HCV unless they remain at risk for non-HCV-related liver disease, such as nonalcoholic fatty liver disease or alcoholic liver disease.

Among patients with cirrhosis who achieve SVR, decompensated liver disease rarely develops during follow-up and overall survival is prolonged. Importantly, these patients remain at risk for developing HCC and should therefore undergo lifelong surveillance for HCC every 6 months utilizing ultrasound and alpha-fetoprotein testing despite the lowered risk that results after viral eradication. Patients in whom SVR is achieved but who have another potential cause of liver disease (e.g., excessive alcohol use, metabolic syndrome with or without proven fatty liver disease, or iron overload) remain at risk for hepatic fibrosis progression. It is recommended that such patients be educated about the risk of liver disease and monitored for liver disease progression with blood tests and noninvasive liver fibrosis assessment. Patients who achieve SVR can have HCV recurrence due to reinfection. Annual or biannual testing for HCV reinfection among patients with ongoing risk for HCV infection (e.g., IDU or high-risk sexual exposure) is recommended. Because HCV antibody remains positive in most patients after achieving SVR, testing for HCV recurrence using an assay that detects HCV-RNA (i.e., quantitative HCV-RNA test) is recommended.

18. How should patients with acute HCV infection be managed and treated?

Patients with acute HCV infection should be treated upon initial diagnosis without awaiting spontaneous resolution. Individuals with acute HCV should be counseled to reduce behaviors that could result in virus transmission, such as sharing injection equipment and engaging in high-risk sexual practices. Patients with acute hepatitis C are often asymptomatic or have nonspecific symptoms (e.g., fatigue, anorexia, mild or moderate abdominal pain, low-grade fever, nausea, and/or vomiting) that are frequently not recognized as being associated with acute HCV infection. A small proportion of patients with acute HCV develop jaundice. Patients diagnosed with acute HCV should initially be monitored with hepatic panels (ALT, AST, bilirubin, and INR). With treatment, a rapid improvement of laboratory parameters is expected.

To date, there is insufficient data to support a particular regimen or treatment duration for acute hepatitis C infection outside of a clinical trial. The same regimens that are recommended for chronic HCV infection are recommended for acute infection, cure rates are similar or superior to those of people with chronic infection. Using the same regimens to treat acute/recent HCV as for chronic HCV infection also simplifies management, as defining acute HCV may be clinically challenging because specific tests to diagnose acute hepatitis C infection are not available.

19. How should patients who do not achieve a virologic cure after initial therapy for HCV be managed?

Although rare, a small minority of patients do not clear HCV infection after initial treatment. Patients who do not achieve SVR retain the possibility of continued liver injury, progression of hepatic fibrosis, and the potential to transmit HCV infection to others. There are FDA-approved options for retreatment of initial failures. The decision to retreat and which antiviral agents to use is complex and should be done by a hepatologist or gastroenterologist with an interest in treating liver disease.

CLINICAL VIGNETTE

Available Online.

BIBLIOGRAPHY

Available Online.

WEBSITES

Available Online.

CHAPTER 16

ANTIVIRAL THERAPY FOR HEPATITIS B

Chad M. Spencer, MD and Jorge L. Herrera, MD

 Additional content available online.

1. Is antiviral therapy recommended for acute hepatitis B?

In the majority of cases, no. Acute hepatitis B, defined as a positive test for hepatitis B surface antigen (HBsAg) and the presence of hepatitis B core antibody-immunoglobulin M (HBcAb-IgM; Table 16.1), is a self-limited disease in more than 95% of adults and resolves without specific antiviral therapy within 3–6 months after the onset of clinical symptoms. For this reason, only supportive care is offered to the majority of patients with acute hepatitis B infection. Antiviral therapy is then considered only for patients with chronic hepatitis B (positive HBsAg test for longer than 6 months).

However, antiviral treatment is recommended in those with acute hepatitis B resulting in acute liver failure (defined as at least two of the following: international normalized ratio [INR] >1.6, encephalopathy, and total bilirubin >10.0 mg/dL) or in those with severe, protracted liver injury (total bilirubin >3.0 mg/dL or direct bilirubin >1.5 mg/dL, INR >1.5, encephalopathy, or ascites) lasting at least 4 weeks.

2. Do all patients with chronic hepatitis B benefit from therapy?

No. Only patients with detectable viremia and evidence of ongoing hepatic necrosis, such as elevated liver enzymes or liver biopsy demonstrating active inflammation or fibrosis, are likely to benefit from therapy. Patients with chronic hepatitis B who do not meet treatment criteria still need to be closely monitored to detect spontaneous conversion to a phase of the disease that would benefit from treatment (Table 16.1).

Table 16.1 Antiviral Therapy for Patients With Hepatitis B Infection.

SEROLOGIC PATTERN	INTERPRETATION	COURSE OF ACTION
HBsAg-positive and HBcAb-IgM-positive	Acute hepatitis B	Observe; resolution likely in 90%–95% of adults.
HBsAg-positive >6 months, HBeAg-positive, HBeAb-negative, HBV DNA >20,000 IU/mL, and elevated ALT level	Immune-active chronic hepatitis B	Initiate antiviral therapy if ALT >2× ULN.[a] Assess with elastography or liver biopsy if ALT > ULN but <2× ULN; treat for F2 or greater fibrosis or if elevated ALT persists for at least 6 months without other cause.
HBsAg-positive >6 months, HBeAg-negative, HBeAb-positive, ALT normal, and HBV DNA negative or <2000 IU/mL	Inactive chronic hepatitis B	Monitor ALT and HBV DNA every 3–6 months and HBsAg annually.
HBsAg-positive >6 months, HBeAg-negative, HBeAb-positive, HBV DNA >2000 IU/mL, elevated ALT level	Chronic infection with HBeAg/precore mutant	Initiate antiviral therapy if ALT >2× ULN. Assess with elastography or liver biopsy if ALT >ULN but <2× ULN; treat for F2 or greater fibrosis or if elevated ALT persists for at least 6 months without other cause.
HBsAg-positive >6 months, HBeAg-positive, HBeAb-negative, HBV DNA levels >200,000 IU/mL, normal ALT levels, no inflammation or fibrosis on biopsy, and age <30 years	Immune-tolerant phase of chronic hepatitis B	Monitor ALT and HBV DNA every 3–6 months and HBeAg every 6–12 months.

ALT, Alanine aminotransferase; *HBcAb-IgM,* hepatitis B core antibody-immunoglobulin M; *HBeAb,* hepatitis B e-antibody; *HBeAg,* hepatitis B e-antigen; *HBsAg,* hepatitis B surface antigen; *HBV DNA,* hepatitis B virus DNA by polymerase chain reaction; *IU,* international units; *ULN,* upper limit of normal.
[a]ULN ALT in adults: 35 U/L for males and 25 U/L for females.

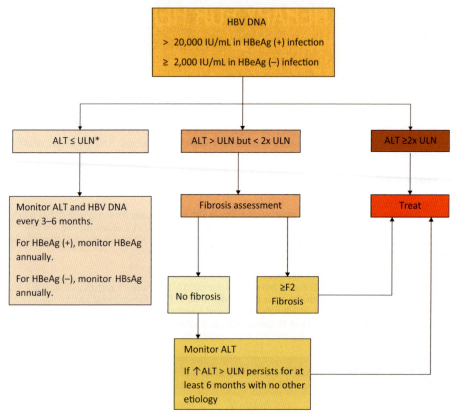

Fig. 16.1 Algorithm for the treatment of hepatitis B infection. *Upper limit of normal (ULN) ALT (alanine aminotransferase) in adults: 35 U/L for males, 25 U/L for females. *HBeAg*, hepatitis B e-antigen; *HBsAg*, hepatitis B surface antigen; *HBV DNA*, hepatitis B DNA by polymerase chain reaction; *IU*, international units.

Established thresholds for treatment are dependent on hepatitis B e-antigen (HBeAg)-positivity, the degree of alanine aminotransferase (ALT) elevation, hepatitis B virus (HBV) DNA levels, and the presence of cirrhosis or advanced fibrosis. A chronic hepatitis B treatment algorithm is illustrated in Fig. 16.1.

3. How should the HBV DNA by polymerase chain reaction assay results be used to make therapy decisions?

Unlike hepatitis C, hepatitis B infection is almost never totally eradicated. Instead, it can be controlled with medications. Treatment is indicated when the viral load is high, and there is evidence of ongoing liver damage. Low levels of HBV DNA in the absence of inflammation are not associated with progressive liver disease and do not require therapy. The upper limit of HBV DNA levels that are consistently associated with inactive disease has not been clearly established, but it is generally agreed that treatment is not necessary when viral levels are undetectable or consistently less than 2000 IU/mL and associated with normal ALT levels or a liver biopsy showing no inflammation. It is important to note that in some cases, particularly in HBeAg-negative disease, viral DNA levels can fluctuate over time and multiple measurements may be necessary to confirm that levels remain at less than 2000 IU/mL.

Most importantly, a decision to initiate therapy should not only be based on viral load but also requires evidence of ongoing hepatic damage (elevated ALT or liver biopsy showing inflammation or fibrosis). In patients with compensated cirrhosis and any detectable hepatitis B viral load, no matter how low, treatment should be initiated regardless of ALT levels. All patients with decompensated cirrhosis who are positive for HBsAg should be treated, even those without a detectable HBV DNA level and normal ALT levels. On the other extreme, young patients (<30 years old) in the immune-tolerant stage of hepatitis B infection, characterized by very high viral loads (>200,000 IU/mL), HBeAg-positivity, normal levels of ALT, and a normal liver biopsy, are typically not treated with antiviral agents despite high levels of HBV DNA as histologic progression of disease is not observed in this situation (see Table 16.1).

4. Is liver biopsy required before therapy is started?

A liver biopsy is not needed to establish the diagnosis of hepatitis B infection; however, it is an important tool to determine severity and activity of disease. Liver biopsy is the only method currently available that detects both fibrosis and inflammation. Treatment decisions are different for patients with advanced fibrosis and cirrhosis compared with those with mild histologic disease. The risk of liver cancer and the intensity of surveillance for liver cancer would be greater for those patients with cirrhosis. The detection of cirrhosis on liver biopsy selects a group of patients who require closer observation as well as screening for esophageal varices. A liver biopsy is also important for patients who have high viral loads (>2000 IU/mL) but normal liver enzymes. The presence of inflammation or fibrosis on biopsy is a strong indication that therapy should be considered.

While liver biopsy remains the gold standard, it is an invasive procedure that is not without risk. As a result, several noninvasive tests for fibrosis have been developed. The main noninvasive methods for assessing fibrosis involve the use of serum fibrosis biomarkers or elastography. Several tests, such as the aspartate aminotransferase (AST)-to-platelet ratio index (APRI) and fibrosis index based on four factors (FIB-4) scores, have been developed using such markers as AST and platelets (the FIB-4 score also includes age and ALT) to predict fibrosis. Elastography, using either ultrasound or magnetic resonance imaging (MRI) technology, can also help to determine the degree of fibrosis by measuring liver stiffness and is generally considered to be more accurate than serum biomarker tests. One important limitation of noninvasive tests is that they tend to overestimate fibrosis when necroinflammation (usually presenting as elevated ALT) is present. Therefore, when interpreting liver stiffness measurements, it is important to consider the degree of ALT elevation at the time of the test (Fig. 16.2).

5. What is the role of the HBeAg in determining the need for treatment?

HBeAg has traditionally been considered to be a marker of high viral replication. Although this is true for the "wild" HBV, a large number of patients are infected with mutated forms of HBV that do not produce e-antigen despite high levels of viral replication. Thus, although a positive HBeAg is a marker of high viral load, a negative HBeAg does not always indicate a low viral load. HBeAg mutant viruses do not replicate as efficiently as the HBeAg-positive wild strain; for this reason, viral levels in HBeAg-negative patients are typically lower and fluctuate more than in HBeAg-positive infections. Because of these differences, the level of HBV DNA, and not the HBeAg status, is used to determine the need for therapy. However, because HBeAg-negative mutants replicate less efficiently, a lower threshold of HBV DNA is used to determine treatment according to some guidelines. For HBeAg-positive infections, an HBV DNA level of more than 20,000 IU/mL is considered high; in contrast, for HBeAg-negative mutant infections, a level of more than 2000 IU/mL is considered high. The duration of treatment with antivirals is also influenced by HBeAg-positivity. An algorithm for the treatment of hepatitis B infection is outlined in Fig. 16.1.

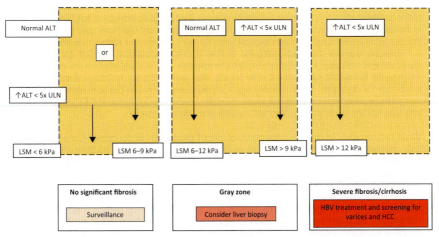

Fig. 16.2 Fibrosis assessment in hepatitis B infection. *ALT,* Alanine aminotransferase; *HBV,* hepatitis B virus; *HCC,* hepatocellular carcinoma; *kPa,* kilopascals; *LSM,* liver stiffness measurement; *ULN,* upper limit of normal.

Table 16.2 Hepatitis B Treatment Endpoints.

Viral response	Decrease in HBV DNA to nondetectable levels during antiviral treatment
Functional cure	Clearance of serum HBsAg ± seroconversion to anti-HBs
Complete cure	Clearance of serum HBsAg ± seroconversion to anti-HBs with complete eradication of HBV intrahepatic covalently ccDNA and integrated HBV DNA

Anti-HBs, Hepatitis B surface antibody; *ccDNA*, closed circular DNA; *HBsAg*, hepatitis B surface antigen; *HBV DNA*, hepatitis B virus DNA by polymerase chain reaction.

6. **What are the endpoints of HBV therapy?**
The main endpoint of current HBV therapies is functional cure. Patients who achieve a functional cure have cleared their serum HBsAg, and some may have developed anti-HBs. This reflects long-standing suppression of HBV replication. It is important to note that in cases of functional cure, HBV DNA still persists in the liver and remains integrated into the cellular genome. Current therapies have been unable to achieve a complete cure, which requires the eradication of all retained HBV DNA. Several novel therapies are being investigated with the goal of complete cure. Endpoints of HBV therapy are demonstrated in Table 16.2.

7. **What is the duration of treatment in HBV?**
The duration of HBV therapy is largely dependent on HBeAg-positivity as well as the presence of cirrhosis.
   In patients with cirrhosis and positive HBsAg, treatment should be continued lifelong or until HBsAg clearance, regardless of HBeAg seroconversion, ALT levels, or HBV DNA levels, to reduce the risk of clinical decompensation from viral relapse.
   In patients without cirrhosis who are HBeAg-positive and meet treatment criteria, treatment should be continued with a goal of achieving a negative HBeAg and positive hepatitis B e-antibody (HBeAb), confirmed on two different tests at least 2 months apart. In the majority of patients, this will require treatment for greater than 5 years. However, even in those who reach HBeAg negativity, it is recommended to continue treatment for at least 1 more year after HBeAg seroconversion to reduce the rate of viral relapse. These patients should then have monitoring of ALT levels, HBV DNA, and HBeAg every 3 months for at least 1 year due to the continued risk for relapse off therapy. Serologic monitoring is particularly important in those of Asian descent and in those over 40 years old, as these groups carry the highest risk of relapse. Alternatively, it is not unreasonable to continue treatment until clearance of HBsAg, although this often requires lifelong therapy due to very low annual rates of HBsAg clearance. In patients without cirrhosis who are HBeAg-negative and meet treatment criteria, treatment should be continued lifelong or until HBsAg clearance.

8. **What are the available options for treating chronic hepatitis B infection?**
One of the prior mainstays of hepatitis B treatment, pegylated interferon, is now rarely used due to its side effect profile and lower efficacy in achieving a virologic response. Another agent, lamivudine, has fallen out of favor due to the emergence of viral resistance to the drug. Therefore the drugs most commonly used to treat hepatitis B infection today are entecavir, tenofovir disoproxil fumarate (TDF), and tenofovir alafenamide (TAF) (Table 16.3).
   Entecavir is an oral *nucleoside* analog and tenofovir is an oral *nucleotide* analog. Both are dosed once a day and inhibit viral replication without enhancing immune response. Entecavir and tenofovir are very potent and have a high barrier to resistance in treatment-naive patients. After years of therapy, resistance to entecavir is observed in less than 1% of patients, and no clinically significant resistance to tenofovir has been reported.
   The side effect profile of these oral agents is excellent and similar to placebo in the short term, although long-term TDF use has been associated with possible renal and bone toxicity.

9. **What factors should decide between the use of entecavir- or tenofovir-based therapy?**
Both entecavir and tenofovir are excellent options for the treatment of hepatitis B, but there are several differences that need to be considered. The main difference is that there is a significant risk of drug resistance (up to 40% after 4 years of treatment) with entecavir in lamivudine-resistant patients. Resistance has not been demonstrated to tenofovir in any subset of patients.
   Entecavir has not been widely studied in pregnancy, but due to teratogenic effects observed in some animal studies, its use is not recommended in pregnant patients or patients who may become pregnant during therapy. TDF has been found safe in pregnancy based on registry studies, and it is the preferred agent for hepatitis B treatment in pregnant patients, with data also supporting its use to prevent mother-to-child transmission. TAF has not been studied in this patient population, and due to the lack of data, its use is not advised.
   While both entecavir and TDF require dose reduction for renal impairment with glomerular filtration rate (GFR) <50 mL/min, entecavir does not carry any risk of renal or bone toxicity. TDF carries the risk of kidney injury

Table 16.3 Preferred Drugs for the Treatment of Hepatitis B Infection.

	ENTECAVIR	TENOFOVIR DISO-PROXIL FUMARATE	TENOFOVIR ALAFENAMIDE
Potency	++++	++++	++++
e-Antigen seroconversion (1 year)	~15%–25%	~15%–25%	~15%–25%
Duration of treatment HBeAg (+) chronic hepatitis	≥1 year (until e-antigen seroconversion)	≥1 year (until e-antigen seroconversion)	≥1 year (until e-antigen seroconversion)
HBeAg (−) chronic hepatitis	Until HBsAg loss	Until HBsAg loss	Until HBsAg loss
Dose	0.5 mg daily[a] on an empty stomach	300 mg daily without regard to food	25 mg daily with food
Safety in patients with cirrhosis	Safe	Safe	Avoid in Child-Pugh class B or C cirrhosis (lack of data)
Safety in chronic kidney disease	Reduce dose for GFR <50 mL/min	Reduce dose for GFR <50 mL/min	No dose adjustment for renal insufficiency. Avoid if GFR <15 mL/min and not on hemodialysis. Safe in patients on hemodialysis.
Safety in pregnancy	Avoid	Safe	Avoid (lack of data)
Side effects	Uncommon, similar to placebo	Uncommon, renal and bone toxicity possible	Uncommon, similar to placebo
Drug resistance	<1% by 5 years in naive patients; up to 40% after 4 years in lamivudine-resistant patients	No clinically significant resistance reported in naive or lamivudine-resistant patients	No clinically significant resistance reported in naive or lamivudine-resistant patients

GFR, Glomerular filtration rate; *HBeAg*, hepatitis B e-antigen; *HBsAg,* hepatitis B surface antigen.
[a]1 mg daily for lamivudine-resistant infection or prior nonresponse to the 0.5 mg dose.

and decreased bone mineral density. In rare cases, it has also been implicated in the development of Fanconi syndrome, which impairs mineral absorption by proximal convoluted tubule of the kidney. Because TAF requires lower doses of the drug with less systemic exposure, it is felt to have a lower risk of renal and bone toxicity than TDF, thus allowing its use at full dose in patients with GFR ≥15 mL/min as well as those in hemodialysis.

10. What factors should decide between the use of TDF and tenofovir alafenamide (TAF)?

TAF is a prodrug of TDF and was approved for use by the Food and Drug Administration in 2016. Because of the higher bioavailability of TAF, the same therapeutic benefit can be achieved at a much lower dosage of the drug (300 mg for TDF vs 25 mg for TAF). While TDF can be taken with or without food, it is advised that TAF be taken with a meal, as this improves absorption of the drug.

As a result of the lower drug concentration, TAF has 90% decreased systemic exposure compared to TDF and, therefore, less toxicity on the kidneys and bones. Less than 1% of TAF is excreted by the kidneys, thus dose reduction is not needed for those with renal impairment. However, because TAF has not been studied in patients with GFR <15 mL/min who are not on hemodialysis, its use is not recommended in these patients. In patients on hemodialysis, TAF can be safely administered at full dosage on dialysis days after dialysis has been completed.

TAF has not been extensively studied in pregnancy and so TDF remains the therapy of choice in pregnant patients. Additionally, TAF has not been thoroughly investigated in those with decompensated cirrhosis (Child-Pugh class B or C) and so should be avoided in these patients until more data become available regarding its safety and efficacy.

11. **What is the expected response to oral nucleoside or nucleotide therapy?**
In most patients the HBV DNA serum level decreases dramatically or becomes undetectable within the first year after initiating therapy. This decrease is associated with the normalization of liver enzyme levels. For patients who tested positive for HBeAg prior to therapy, seroconversion from HBeAg-positive to HBeAg-negative status may occur after prolonged therapy and represents an important milestone. In selected patients, HBeAg seroconversion may be considered a therapy-stopping point. Confirmed loss of HBsAg rarely occurs, but when achieved and sustained for 1 year or longer, it is considered functional cure and therapy may be discontinued.

Response to therapy should be monitored with HBV DNA levels and liver enzymes. When treated with entecavir or tenofovir, the majority of patients will see a substantial decrease in HBV DNA levels by 6 months and achieve undetectable levels of HBV DNA within 24–48 months. Because these agents have a high barrier to resistance (with the exception of entecavir in lamivudine-resistant patients), lack of response or increase in HBV DNA is usually due to medication noncompliance.

12. **Should patients with advanced, decompensated cirrhosis secondary to hepatitis B receive antiviral therapy or be referred for liver transplantation without a trial of therapy?**
Those with severe liver disease from hepatitis B, in addition to being evaluated for liver transplant, should be treated with oral antivirals as soon as possible. All patients with decompensated cirrhosis and a positive HBsAg should be treated promptly with antiviral therapy, regardless of HBV DNA level, ALT levels, or liver transplant candidacy. In this population, treatment with nucleoside or nucleotide analogs is beneficial and often lifesaving. In many patients with decompensated cirrhosis from hepatitis B, treatment with an antiviral agent reverses hepatic decompensation and improves survival outcomes, thus precluding the need for transplant. Antiviral therapy, when continued after transplantation in conjunction with hepatitis B immune globulin, is associated with a decreased chance of recurrence of infection in the graft. Once a response is achieved, lifelong therapy is recommended, as flares induced by discontinuation of antiviral therapy could be fatal in these patients.

13. **How should response to therapy be monitored?**
After initiation of therapy, repeat viral load should be performed at 3-month intervals. After achieving an undetectable viral load, testing should be repeated at least every 6 months for the duration of therapy to document sustained response and evaluate for virological breakthrough. Because the development of resistance is very rare, a rise in viral load of more than 1 log10 (10-fold increase) during therapy most often occurs when patients are not compliant with the medication regimen. Entecavir and TDF are renally excreted, and dosing should be adjusted when renal function is compromised. For that reason, renal function should be assessed prior to therapy and monitored at least once a year and the dose of oral antiviral agent adjusted if renal insufficiency is present. Once a year, patients who were positive for HBeAg at the start of therapy should be tested for HBeAg and HBeAb to assess for seroconversion. All patients should also be tested once a year for HBsAg to assess for treatment induced HBsAg clearance.

14. **Can therapy reverse fibrosis or cirrhosis?**
Yes, continued viral suppression with oral nucleotide or nucleoside therapy has been shown to reverse fibrosis and improve liver histologic findings in a substantial number of patients. After 5 years of tenofovir therapy in HBeAg-negative and HBeAg-positive patients, histologic improvement was noted in 87% and regression of fibrosis in 51%. Of the patients with cirrhosis at baseline, 74% no longer had cirrhosis after 5 years of therapy with tenofovir. Similar results have been shown in a smaller number of patients with prolonged entecavir therapy.

15. **Are treatment decisions for hepatitis B infection different if patients are immune suppressed?**
The immune system plays a pivotal role in the control of hepatitis B infection. Patients who are HBsAg-positive but have no detectable viremia or low level of virus can promptly reactivate if immunosuppressed. If immunosuppression is planned (i.e., cancer chemotherapy, biologic disease–modifying antirheumatic drugs [anti-TNF$\geq\alpha$ {anti–tumor necrosis factor α}, interleukin 12/23, signal transducers and activators of transcription/Janus kinase, sphingosine 1-phosphate therapy, etc.], high-dose corticosteroid therapy [>20 mg daily]), patients should be screened for HBsAg and HBcAb.

For patients positive for HBsAg who are about to start therapy with biologics or cancer chemotherapy, initiation of antiviral therapy with a nucleoside or nucleotide analog is indicated even if HBV DNA is undetectable and the ALT is normal. Ideally, antiviral therapy should be started 2–4 weeks before or simultaneously with the introduction of the immunosuppressant and continued for at least 6–12 months after the completion of the immunosuppression. For those experiencing profound immunosuppression, such as from rituximab or other anti-CD20 agents, the 12-month post immune suppression duration is preferred.

For patients who are negative for HBsAg but who have a positive HBcAb the risk of reactivation is lower and depends on the immunosuppressant agent used. All patients with a positive HBcAb who are receiving profound immunosuppression with agents such as anti-CD20 therapy or undergoing stem cell transplantation should receive hepatitis B prophylaxis regardless of ALT, HBV DNA, or HBsAg and continue therapy for at least 12 months after completion. For patients receiving other, less potent immunosuppressants including anti-TNFα, monitoring of ALT, HBV DNA, and HBsAg every 2–3 months during the first year of therapy is recommended. Treatment should be initiated if viral reactivation occurs (i.e., HBV DNA becomes detectable or there is reverse HBsAg seroconversion from a negative HBsAg to a positive HBsAg) or if ALT increases. However, if monitoring is not possible, initiation of antiviral therapy at the time of immunosuppression initiation is an optional approach. Agents associated with a low risk of reactivation include azathioprine, 6-mercaptopurine, methotrexate, short-term low-dose corticosteroids (<20 mg for <6 weeks), and intra-articular steroid injections. The use of these agents does not require prophylaxis against hepatitis B reactivation.

Patients who would have met the criteria for hepatitis B therapy before immunosuppression (i.e., high viral load, elevated ALT) should continue on long-term antiviral therapy even after immunosuppression ceases until traditional endpoints of treatment are achieved.

16. **How should HBV infection be treated in patients coinfected with the human immunodeficiency virus (HIV)?**
Most of the antiviral agents currently available for the treatment of hepatitis B have activity against HIV. Initiation of monotherapy for HBV in patients with known or undiagnosed HIV can lead to emergence of HIV-resistant mutants. All patients infected with HBV should be tested for HIV. If coinfected with HIV, they should be evaluated for highly active antiretroviral therapy (HAART). Current HIV treatment guidelines consider the presence of hepatitis B infection an indication to initiate HAART. Selection of a HAART regimen that includes at least two drugs active against HBV (i.e., tenofovir and emtricitabine or lamivudine) is recommended. Patients coinfected with HBV and HIV should not receive lamivudine as the only HBV-active drug in the HAART regimen, as HBV resistance to lamivudine develops rapidly. Tenofovir alafenamide is approved for HIV (in combination with emtricitabine) and is generally preferred over TDF due to its more favorable safety profile.

17. **Should hepatitis B be treated during pregnancy?**
Hepatitis B infection is vertically transmitted. The introduction of the hepatitis B vaccine and hepatitis B immune globulin injection for babies born to HBsAg-positive mothers has markedly decreased vertical transmission of HBV but has not eliminated the risk. A high maternal viral load (>200,000 IU/mL) has been associated with an increased risk of vertical transmission. Even when appropriate passive and active immunization is used at birth, 7%–9% of children born to mothers with high viral load will develop chronic hepatitis B infection. Limited clinical research suggests that lowering the viral load during the last trimester of pregnancy decreases the risk of vertical transmission.

All pregnant females should be screened for hepatitis B (Fig. 16.3). TDF is the agent of choice for hepatitis B treatment in pregnancy. Entecavir is not safe in pregnancy and its use should be avoided. While tenofovir

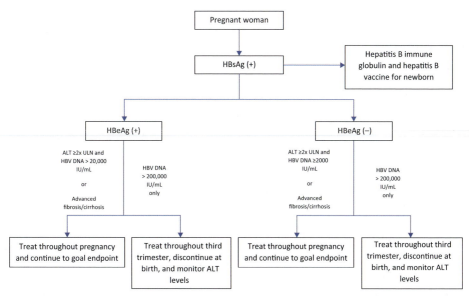

Fig. 16.3 Treatment of hepatitis B in pregnancy. *ALT*, Alanine aminotransferase; *HBeAg*, hepatitis B e-antigen; *HBsAg*, hepatitis B surface antigen; *HBV DNA*, hepatitis B virus DNA by polymerase chain reaction; *IU*, international units; *ULN*, upper limit of normal.

Table 16.4 Recommendations for Hepatocellular Carcinoma (HCC) Screening Among Patients With Chronic Hepatitis B Infection.
All patients with cirrhosis
Asian or Black males over the age of 40 years
Asian females over the age of 50 years
First-degree relatives with a history of HCC
Coinfection with HDV

HDV, Hepatitis delta virus.

alafenamide is likely safe in pregnancy, it has not been extensively studied in this patient population. Therefore its use in pregnancy *is not currently recommended* until more data become available regarding its safety profile.

In general, all infants of hepatitis B–infected mothers should receive the hepatitis B immune globulin and hepatitis B vaccine immediately after birth. Pregnant females with immune-active hepatitis or cirrhosis should be treated using the same guidelines as nonpregnant patients. Pregnant females with a positive HBsAg who otherwise would not meet the criteria for treatment but who have an HBV DNA level >200,000 should receive treatment with TDF throughout the third trimester to decrease the risk of perinatal transmission. Tenofovir may be discontinued at birth, but ALT levels should be monitored every 3 months for 6 months after discontinuation to evaluate for hepatitis B flare.

18. **Should patients with chronic hepatitis B be screened for hepatocellular carcinoma (HCC)?**
Yes. HBV is an oncogenic virus. In the majority of patients, HCC develops as a result of years of inflammation, fibrosis, and development of cirrhosis, but in a significant minority genetic predisposition increases the risk of HCC at a younger age and before fibrosis and cirrhosis develop. For these reasons, screening for HCC is recommended for subgroups of patients with chronic hepatitis B, as shown in Table 16.4. Recommended screening for HCC consists of an ultrasound examination of the liver and an alpha-fetoprotein level every 6 months. For patients in whom the ultrasound exam is suboptimal or a possible lesion is noted, evaluation with triple-phase MRI or computed tomography is recommended.

CLINICAL VIGNETTE

Available Online.

BIBLIOGRAPHY

Available Online.

CHAPTER 17

AUTOIMMUNE HEPATITIS—DIAGNOSIS

James F. Trotter, MD

 Additional content available online.

1. **What is autoimmune hepatitis (AIH)?**

   AIH is an unresolving inflammatory hepatic disease of unknown cause that is characterized histologically by interface hepatitis along with autoantibodies and hypergammaglobulinemia. There are no disease-specific features and the diagnosis requires exclusion of other conditions including viral hepatitis, drug-induced liver injury (DILI), alcoholic and nonalcoholic fatty liver disease, as well as the immune-mediated cholangiopathies of primary sclerosing cholangitis (PSC) and primary biliary cholangitis (PBC) (Table 17.1).

2. **What are its principal clinical and laboratory features?**

   AIH primarily affects females (about three-fourths of all cases) and can occur at any age, most commonly before the age of 40 years. Smooth muscle antibodies (SMAs) and antinuclear antibodies (ANAs) are the primary serologic features. Antibodies to liver-kidney microsome type 1 (anti-LKM1) occur in about a quarter of children and are present in <5% of adults. Serum aspartate aminotransferase (AST) and alanine aminotransferase (ALT) elevations are typically present as is hypergammaglobulinemia especially an increase in immunoglobulin G (IgG).

Table 17.1 Differential Diagnosis of Autoimmune Hepatitis and Discriminative Tests.

DIFFERENTIAL DIAGNOSIS	DIAGNOSTIC ASSESSMENTS	DIAGNOSTIC FINDINGS	LIVER BIOPSY
α_1-Antitrypsin deficiency	Phenotyping	ZZ (strongest association) MZ, MS, and SZ (probably comorbid factors)	Diastase-resistant PAS-positive intrahepatocyte globules (see Fig. 32.5C)
Chronic viral hepatitis B and C	Serologic tests	HBsAg, HBV-DNA anti-HCV, and HCV RNA	Ground-glass hepatocytes Viral inclusions Portal lymphoid aggregates Steatosis (see Fig. 32.4A)
Acute viral hepatitis E	Serologic tests	Anti-HEV IgM	Immunohistochemistry for HEV pORF2 protein
Drug-induced hepatitis	Clinical history	Recent exposure to medication, nutritional supplements, or herbal agents (especially minocycline or nitrofurantoin)	Little or no hepatic fibrosis Portal neutrophils Intracellular cholestasis
	Clinical behavior	Acute idiosyncratic reaction Resolves after drug withdrawal No recurrence	
Hemochromatosis	Genetic testing	C282Y and H63D mutations Positive family history	Increased iron by stain Hepatic iron index > 1.9 (see Fig. 32.5D)
	Iron studies	Transferrin saturation index >45%	

Continued

Table 17.1 Differential Diagnosis of Autoimmune Hepatitis and Discriminative Tests.—cont'd

DIFFERENTIAL DIAGNOSIS	DIAGNOSTIC ASSESSMENTS	DIAGNOSTIC FINDINGS	LIVER BIOPSY
Nonalcoholic steatohepatitis	Clinical findings	Obesity (BMI >30 kg/m²) Type 2 diabetes Hyperlipidemia	Macrosteatosis Mallory-Denk bodies Megamitochondria Absent apoptotic bodies Ballooned hepatocytes (see Fig. 32.2A–D)
	Hepatic ultrasonography	Hyperechogenicity	
	Genetic tests	*PNPLAS3* gene (investigational)	
Primary biliary cirrhosis	Serologic tests	AMA titer ≥ 1:40 Antipyruvate dehydrogenase-E2	Destructive cholangitis (florid duct lesion) (see Figs. 17.6 and 32.7A and B) Increased hepatic copper concentration
Primary sclerosing cholangitis	Cholangiography (Fig. 17.7)	Focal biliary strictures and dilations	Ductopenia Portal fibrosis and edema Fibrous obliterative cholangitis (rare) (see Figs. 17.8 and 32.7C and D)
Wilson disease	Copper studies	Low ceruloplasmin Low serum copper level High urinary copper excretion	Increased hepatic copper concentration
	Slit-lamp eye examination	Kayser-Fleischer rings	
	Genetic tests	*ATP7B* gene (chromosome 13q14.3) ≥200 disease-causing mutations *H1069Q* mutation	

AMA, Antimitochondrial antibody; *ATP7B*, ATPase copper transporting beta polypeptide; *BMI*, body mass index; *C282Y*, mutation within *HFE* gene associated with substitution of tyrosine for cysteine at amino acid position 282 in α₃ loop; *H1069Q*, mutation within *ATP7B* gene of Wilson disease in which histidine is replaced by glutamic acid at position 1069; *H63D*, mutation within *HFE* gene associated with substitution of histidine for aspartate at amino acid position 63 in α₁ loop; *HBsAg*, hepatitis B surface antigen; *HBV*, hepatitis B virus; *HCV*, hepatitis C virus; *HEV*, hepatitis E virus; *HFE*, high iron Fe gene; *IgM*, immunoglobulin M; *PAS*, periodic acid-Schiff; *PNPLAS3*, adiponutrin/patatin-like phospholipase domain–containing protein 3 gene associated with hepatic fat accumulation; *ZZ, MZ, MS,* and *SZ*, major protease inhibitor deficiency phenotypes associated with α₁-antitrypsin deficiency.

Concurrent immune diseases are present in about one-third of patients, including thyroid disease, ulcerative colitis, or rheumatoid arthritis (Table 17.2).

3. What are the symptoms of AIH?

Many patients are asymptomatic, but the major symptoms of AIH are fatigue and arthralgias. Jaundice is usually indicative of acute severe disease or a chronic indolent process with advanced fibrosis. While many patients with AIH may be asymptomatic at presentation, a third of patients may have symptoms that emerge later.

4. What are the characteristic histologic features in AIH?

Interface hepatitis is the sine qua non for the diagnosis of AIH. The limiting plate of the portal tract is disrupted by a lymphocytic infiltrate that extends into the lobule (Fig. 17.1). Plasma cells are present in two-thirds of the

Table 17.2 Concurrent Immune-Mediated Diseases Associated With Autoimmune Hepatitis.

Autoimmune sclerosing cholangitis	Lichen planus
Autoimmune thyroiditis[a]	Myasthenia gravis
Celiac disease	Neutropenia
Coombs-positive hemolytic anemia	Pericarditis
Cryoglobulinemia	Peripheral neuropathy
Dermatitis herpetiformis	Pernicious anemia
Erythema nodosum	Pleuritis
Fibrosing alveolitis	Pyoderma gangrenosum
Focal myositis	Rheumatoid arthritis[a]
Gingivitis	Sjögren syndrome
Glomerulonephritis	Synovitis[a]
Grave disease[a]	Systemic lupus erythematosus
Idiopathic thrombocytopenic purpura	Ulcerative colitis[a]
Insulin-dependent diabetes	Urticaria
Intestinal villous atrophy	Vitiligo
Iritis	

[a]Most common association.

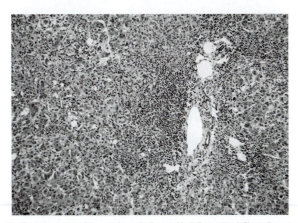

Fig. 17.1 Interface hepatitis. The limiting plate of the portal tract is disrupted by inflammatory infiltrate (hematoxylin and eosin, original magnification ×100).

inflammatory infiltrates, but they are neither specific nor required for the diagnosis (Fig. 17.2). Hepatocyte rosettes are also characteristic histologic features. Centrilobular necrosis probably represents an early stage or an acute injury of chronic disease (Fig. 17.3). Most patients with centrilobular necrosis have interface hepatitis and cirrhosis may be present.

5. **Can AIH have an acute or severe acute (fulminant) presentation?**
   Yes. AIH has an acute presentation, defined as the abrupt onset of symptoms coincident with the onset or discovery of disease. An acute severe or fulminant presentation, defined as the development of hepatic encephalopathy within 26 weeks of disease discovery, occurs in about 5% of patients.

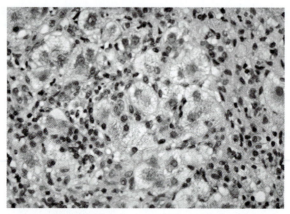

Fig. 17.2 Plasma cell infiltration. Plasma cells, identified by the cytoplasmic haloes about their nucleus, infiltrate the periportal region (hematoxylin and eosin, original magnification ×400).

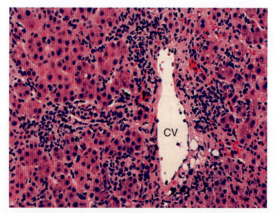

Fig. 17.3 Centrilobular (zone 3) necrosis. Inflammatory and degenerative changes concentrate around the central vein (CV) and involve the centrilobular or Rappaport zone 3 region of the liver tissue (hematoxylin and eosin, original magnification ×200).

6. What are the clinical features of an acute or fulminant presentation?

Symptoms may resemble acute viral or toxic hepatitis and the classical phenotype of AIH may be unrecognizable. Serum IgG level is normal and ANA may be absent in up to a third of patients. The histologic features are reflective of the severe presentation with intense lymphoplasmacytic infiltration spilling out of the portal tracts, often leading to bridging necrosis.

7. Which patients are the most difficult to diagnose?

Infants, older adults, and patients with acute or fulminant presentations may have AIH that can be unsuspected, confused with other diseases, or atypical. Patients over 60 years of age are frequently taking medications or have other chronic illnesses (heart disease) so their presentation may be mistakenly attributed to DILI or congestive heart failure. An algorithmic approach for acute severe hepatitis with possible AIH versus DILI etiology is demonstrated in Fig. 17.4.

8. What are the different types of AIH?

Two types predominate in the clinical jargon based on distinctive serologic markers (Table 17.3). However, their identification has limited clinical relevance. These types do not define subtypes of different etiologic factors or prognoses. Instead, they are clinical descriptors that denote a clinical phenotype and maintain homogeneity of study populations. Type 1, the most common form of AIH, is characterized by SMA or ANA. Antibodies to actin (anti-actin) also support the diagnosis. Type 2 AIH is characterized by anti-LKM and denotes mainly young

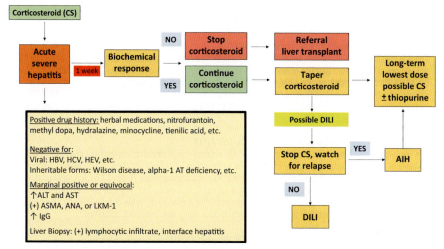

Fig. 17.4 Algorithmic approach for acute severe hepatitis: autoimmune hepatitis (AIH) versus drug-induced liver injury (DILI). *ALT*, Alanine aminotransferase; *ANA*, antinuclear antibody; *ASMA*, anti-smooth muscle antibody; *AST*, aspartate aminotransferase; *AT*, antitrypsin; *CS*, corticosteroid; *HBV*, hepatitis B virus; *HCV*, hepatitis C virus; *HEV*, hepatitis E virus; *LKM*, liver kidney microsome.

Table 17.3 Types of Autoimmune Hepatitis.

FEATURES	TYPE 1	TYPE 2
Autoantibodies	Smooth muscle Nucleus Actin α-Actinin (investigational) Soluble liver antigen	Liver/kidney microsome type 1 Liver cytosol type 1 Liver/kidney microsome type 3
	Atypical pANCA	
Organ-specific antibodies	Thyroid	Thyroid Parietal cells Islets of Langerhans
Target autoantigen	Unknown	CYP2D6 (P450 IID6)
HLA associations	B8, DRB1*03, and DRB1*04	DQB1*02, DRB1*07, DRB1*03, and B14
Susceptibility alleles	DRB1*0301, DRB1*0401 (North American and Northern Europe) DRB1*04 alleles (Japan, China, and Mexico) DRB1*1301 (South America)	DQB1*0201 (principal) DRB1*0701 DRB1*03 C4A-Q0
Predominant age	Adult	Childhood (2–14 years)
Acute onset	25%–75%	Possible
Acute severe (fulminant) onset	6% (North American patients)	Possible
Concurrent immune disease	38%	34% Autoimmune sclerosing cholangitis (children)
Progression to cirrhosis	36%	82%
Corticosteroid responsive	Yes	Yes

HLA, Human leukocyte antigen; *pANCA*, perinuclear antineutrophil cytoplasmic antibodies.

(pediatric) White European patients. Antibodies to liver cytosol type 1 (anti-LC1) also support this diagnosis. Anti-LKM and anti-LC1 typically do not coexist with SMA and ANA.

9. **What are the clinical criteria for diagnosis?**
   There is no single test to confirm the diagnosis. The definitive diagnosis requires a combination of serum AST or ALT abnormalities, serum gamma globulin or IgG levels greater than 1.5 of the upper limit of normal (ULN), and the presence of SMA, ANA, or anti-LKM greater than 1:80 along with the histologic features of interface hepatitis with or without plasma cell infiltration (Table 17.4). Of course, other causes of liver disease (viral, hereditary, drug-induced, alcohol-related, and metabolic disorders) must be excluded. The probable diagnosis is based on similar but less pronounced or certain findings.

10. **What are the diagnostic scoring systems for AIH?**
    The comprehensive diagnostic scoring system for AIH ensures the systematic assessment of all the clinical features of AIH. It evaluates 12 clinical components and renders 27 possible scores. Response to corticosteroid therapy is scored in the treatment and the outcome influences the diagnosis (Table 17.5). A simplified diagnostic scoring system has been developed for easy clinical application. It evaluates only four clinical components and renders seven possible grades (Table 17.6). It is based on the presence of levels of autoantibody, serum IgG concentration, histologic features, and viral markers. It does not grade treatment outcomes.

11. **What are the performance parameters of the diagnostic scoring systems?**
    The comprehensive scoring system has greater sensitivity for the diagnosis of AIH than the simplified scoring system, but the simplified scoring system has superior specificity and predictability. Clinical judgment has been the gold standard against which performance has been measured and it always supersedes the results of the scoring systems. The comprehensive scoring system is useful in evaluating patients with absent or atypical features in which every component must be assessed. The simplified scoring system is useful in excluding AIH in patients who have concurrent immune features. The scoring systems have not been validated prospectively and they should be used mainly to support clinical judgment.

Table 17.4 Codified Diagnostic Criteria for Autoimmune Hepatitis.

DIAGNOSTIC TESTS	DEFINITE DIAGNOSIS	PROBABLE DIAGNOSIS
Autoantibodies	Serum ANA, SMA, or anti-LKM1 ≥1:80 titer (confident EIA level uncertain) Absent AMA	Titers ≥1:40 Titers negative but anti-SLA, anti-LC1, or atypical pANCA positive
Biochemical tests	Increased serum AST and ALT levels ULN Serum AP level ≤ twofold ULN Normal serum ceruloplasmin level Normal α_1-antitrypsin phenotype	Same as for definite
Immunoglobulin levels	Serum γ-globulin or IgG levels ≥1.5 ULN	Any abnormal value
Liver tissue examination	Interface hepatitis No biliary lesions or granulomata No changes indicating alternative diagnosis	Same as for definite
Toxic exposures	No hepatotoxic drugs Alcohol consumption <25 g daily	Previous but not recent drugs or alcohol Alcohol consumption <50 g daily
Viral markers	No serologic markers for hepatitis A, B, and C	Same as definite

ALT, Alanine aminotransferase; *AMA*, antimitochondrial antibody; *ANA*, antinuclear antibodies; *AP*, alkaline phosphatase; *AST*, aspartate aminotransferase; *EIA*, enzyme immunoassay; *IgG*, immunoglobulin G; *LC1*, liver cytosol type 1; *LKM1*, liver-kidney microsome type 1; *pANCA*, perinuclear antineutrophil cytoplasmic antibodies; *SLA*, soluble liver antigen; *SMA*, smooth muscle antibodies; ULN, upper limit of the normal range.
Adapted from Alvarez F, Berg PA, Bianchi, FB, Burroughs AK, Cancado EL, Chapman RW, et al. International Autoimmune Hepatitis Group report: review of criteria for diagnosis of autoimmune hepatitis. J Hepatol. 1999;31:929-938. https://doi.org/10.1016/s0168-8278(99)80297-9.

Table 17.5 Revised Original Scoring System for the Diagnosis of Autoimmune Hepatitis.

CLINICAL FEATURES	SCORE	CLINICAL FEATURES	SCORE
Female	+2	Average alcohol intake	
		<25 g/day	+2
		>60 g/day	−2
AP:AST (or ALT) ratio		Histologic findings	
<1.5	+2	Interface hepatitis	+3
1.5–3.0	0	Lymphoplasmacytic infiltrate	+1
>3.0	−2	Rosette formation	+1
		Biliary changes	−3
		Other atypical changes	−3
		None of above	−5
Serum γ-globulin or IgG		Concurrent immune disease	+2
level ULN	+3	Other AIH-related autoantibodies	+2
>2.0	+2	HLA DRB1*03 or DRB1*04	+1
1.5–2.0	+1		
1.0–1.5	0		
<1.0			
ANA, SMA, or anti-LKM1		Response to corticosteroids	+2
>1:80	+3	Complete	+3
1:80	+2	Relapse after drug withdrawal	
1:40	+1		
<1:40	0		
AMA positive	−4	Aggregate score posttreatment	
		Definite AIH	>15
		Probable AIH	10–15
Hepatitis markers		Aggregate score pretreatment	
Positive	−3	Definite AIH	>17
Negative	+3	Probable AIH	12–17
Hepatotoxic drug exposure			
Positive	−4		
Negative	+1		

AIH, Autoimmune hepatitis; *ALT*, alanine aminotransferase; *AMA*, antimitochondrial antibody; *ANA*, antinuclear antibodies; *AP*, alkaline phosphatase; *AST*, aspartate aminotransferase; *HLA*, human leukocyte antigen; *IgG*, immunoglobulin G; *LKM1*, liver/kidney microsome type 1; *SMA*, smooth muscle antibodies; *ULN*, upper limit of the normal range.
Adapted from Alvarez F, Berg PA, Bianchi, FB, Burroughs AK, Cancado EL, Chapman RW, et al. International Autoimmune Hepatitis Group report: review of criteria for diagnosis of autoimmune hepatitis. J Hepatol. 1999;31:929-938. https://doi.org/10.1016/s0168-8278(99)80297-9.

12. What is the standard serologic battery for diagnosis?

ANA and SMA (and for some clinicians anti-LKM1) are the standard diagnostic markers of AIH (Table 17.7). They do not connote prognosis and they cannot be used to monitor treatment response. The combination of ANA and SMA at presentation has superior sensitivity and diagnostic accuracy than each marker alone. Serum titers of 1:320 or more have high diagnostic specificity (>90%) but low sensitivity (<50%). Weak positivity (titer 1:40) cannot be ignored and some patients with AIH may lack the conventional markers.

13. What other autoantibodies may have diagnostic and prognostic implications?

Multiple autoantibodies have been described in AIH, but none have been incorporated into a codified diagnostic algorithm. These serologic markers are ancillary diagnostic tools (Table 17.7). Antibodies to soluble liver antigen (anti-SLA) have high specificity for AIH but low sensitivity. They identify individuals with severe disease who are treatment dependent and they have a strong association with DRB1*0301 and antibodies to ribonucleoprotein/Sjögren syndrome A antigen. Antiactins are a subset of SMAs that react against filamentous (F) actin and they have greater specificity for AIH than SMA. Anti-LC1s occur mainly in young patients and they are detected in

Table 17.6 Simplified Scoring System of the International Autoimmune Hepatitis Group.

FEATURES	CUTOFF	POINTS
ANA or SMA	≥1:40	1
ANA or SMA	≥1:80	2[a]
or LKM	≥1:40	2[a]
or SLA	Positive	2[a]
IgG	>ULN	1
	>1.10 × ULN	2
Liver histology (must demonstrate hepatitis)	Compatible with AIH	1
	Typical of AIH	2
Absence of viral hepatitis	Yes	2

Interpretation of aggregate simplified score:

0 ≠ AIH

>6: probable AIH

>7: definite AIH

AIH, Autoimmune hepatitis; *ANA*, antinuclear antibody; *IgG*, immunoglobulin G; *LKM*, liver-kidney microsomal antibody; *SLA*, soluble liver antigen; *SMA*, smooth muscle antibody; *ULN*, upper limit of the normal range.
[a]Addition of points for all autoantibodies (maximum of 2 points).
Adapted from Alvarez F, Berg PA, Bianchi, FB, Burroughs AK, Cancado EL, Chapman RW, et al. International Autoimmune Hepatitis Group report: review of criteria for diagnosis of autoimmune hepatitis. J Hepatol. 1999;31:929-938. https://doi.org/10.1016/s0168-8278(99)80297-9.

one-third of patients with anti-LKM1. They have been associated with severe disease and they may be the sole maker in European patients with AIH.

14. What autoantibodies should be sought if the usual markers are absent?

Atypical perinuclear antineutrophil cytoplasmic antibodies (pANCAs) are present in many patients with AIH who lack anti-LKM1 (Table 17.7). They are also common in patients with chronic ulcerative colitis or PSC. Atypical pANCA can indicate the possibility of AIH in patients who lack other autoantibodies. IgA antibodies to tissue transglutaminase (tTG) or endomysium are valuable in excluding celiac disease, which can coexist with AIH or be associated with a liver disease that resembles AIH. Since AIH mimics celiac disease, this diagnosis must be considered in seronegative patients that otherwise resemble AIH.

15. What investigational autoantibodies have promise as diagnostic and prognostic markers?

Antibodies to asialoglycoprotein receptor (anti-ASGPR) are present in three-fourths of patients with SMA or ANA (Table 17.7). They are associated with histologic activity and the propensity to relapse after corticosteroid withdrawal. The ASGPR is composed of two subunits (H1 and H2) and an enzyme immunoassay based on recombinant H1 may prove useful in monitoring the treatment response.

16. What is the significance of antimitochondrial antibody (AMA) on AIH?

AMA can be present in a small fraction of patients with AIH, about 10% or less. Histologic features may be similar to those of patients without AMA, and the AMA can persist or disappear in the absence of cholestatic clinical or laboratory features. The occurrence of AMA does not necessarily require a change of diagnosis or treatment in these patients. However, the possibility of PBC or transition to PBC over time must always be considered and may represent patients with "overlap syndrome" with features of both AIH and PBC.

17. Is there an autoantibody-negative AIH?

Yes. About 10% of adults with chronic cryptogenic hepatitis satisfy the diagnostic criteria for AIH but lack the conventional autoantibodies. These patients are otherwise similar by age, sex, human leukocyte antigen (HLA) phenotype, laboratory findings, and histologic features to patients with classic AIH. They may also respond to corticosteroid therapy. Because other causes of chronic liver function tests elevation such as nonalcoholic steatohepatitis must be ruled out, the comprehensive diagnostic scoring system (Table 17.5) can be useful in diagnosis and clinical treatment decisions.

Table 17.7 Autoantibodies Associated With Autoimmune Hepatitis.

AUTOANTIBODY SPECIES	FEATURES
Standard Serologic Battery	
Antinuclear antibodies	Type 1 AIH Reactive to multiple nuclear antigens Lacks disease or organ specificity
Smooth muscle antibodies	Type 1 AIH Reactive to actin (mainly) and nonactin components Frequently associated with ANA Lacks disease or organ specificity
Antibodies to liver/kidney microsome type 1	Type 2 AIH Target antigen, CYP2D6 Typically unassociated with ANA and SMA May occur in chronic hepatitis C
Ancillary Serologic Battery	
Antibodies to soluble liver antigen	Antigenic target is Sep (*O*-phosphoserine) tRNA:Sec (selenocysteine) tRNA synthase High specificity (99%) but low sensitivity (16%) for AIH Associated with DRB1*0301 Can indicate severe disease and relapse after treatment Frequently coexists with anti-Ro/SSA
Antibodies to actin	Diagnostic specificity better than SMA Associated with SMA Commonly young patients Immune reactive region, α-actinin Aggressive disease (if antibodies to α-actinin present) Nonstandardized assay
Antibodies to liver cytosol type 1	Type 2 AIH Young patients Possibly worse prognosis May be a sole serologic marker of AIH Directed against formiminotransferase cyclodeaminase
Atypical perinuclear antineutrophil cytoplasm	Common in type 1 AIH Absent in type 2 AIH Common in CUC and PSC Atypical because reactive against nuclear membrane May be useful in otherwise seronegative patients
Investigational Serologic Markers	
Antibodies to ASGPR	Generic marker of AIH Correlates with histologic activity Disappears with resolution of AIH during treatment Associated with relapse after drug withdrawal Promising EIA based on recombinant subunit (H1) of ASGPR

AIH, Autoimmune hepatitis; *ANA*, antinuclear antibody; *anti-Ro/SSA*, antibodies to ribonucleoprotein/Sjögren syndrome A antigen; *ASGPR*, asialoglycoprotein receptor; *CUC*, chronic ulcerative colitis; *EIA*, enzyme immunoassay; *PSC*, primary sclerosing cholangitis; *SMA*, smooth muscle antibody.

18. **What is the appropriate testing sequence for autoantibodies?**

All patients with acute and chronic hepatitis of undetermined cause should be assessed for ANA and SMA. Adults with chronic hepatitis of undetermined cause should also be assessed for AMA (Fig. 17.5). Although almost never used in clinical practice, patients who lack these markers may undergo a second battery of tests that include determinations of atypical pANCA, anti-SLA, and IgA antibodies to tTG or endomysium. The conventional testing

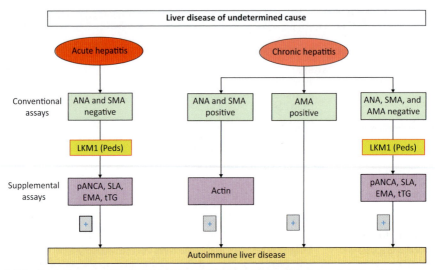

Fig. 17.5 Serologic testing sequence for diagnosing autoimmune liver disease in patients with acute or chronic hepatitis of undetermined cause. The conventional serologic battery includes antinuclear antibody (ANA), smooth muscle antibody (SMA) and antimitochondrial antibody (AMA). Supplemental serologic tests to confirm or further direct the diagnosis include atypical perinuclear antineutrophil cytoplasmic antibodies (pANCA), antibody to soluble liver antigen (SLA), and antibody for celiac disease, including immunoglobulin A endomysial antibodies (EMA) and tissue transglutaminase (tTG). *LKM1*, Liver-kidney microsome type 1.

battery of ANA and SMA should be repeated in seronegative patients because these autoantibodies may be expressed later. Once detected, autoantibodies do not need to be reassessed.

19. **When should AIH be considered?**
    AIH should be considered in any patient with acute, fulminant, or chronic hepatitis or in liver transplant recipients with graft dysfunction. AIH recurs in about 20% of patients after liver transplantation and may develop de novo in 5% of children and adults transplanted for non-autoimmune liver disease. The frequency of recurrence increases with time after transplantation. The aggressiveness of untreated AIH and responsiveness to conventional corticosteroid treatment mandate that it be considered in all patients with acute or chronic liver disease of undetermined nature.

20. **What are the overlap syndromes of AIH?**
    The overlap syndromes of AIH are popular designations for patients with predominant features of AIH and ancillary cholestatic features that may resemble PBC or PSC. Patients with AIH may have AMA and histologic findings of bile duct injury or loss that suggest PBC (Fig. 17.6). They may have an absence of AMA and a cholangiogram that suggests PSC (Fig. 17.7), or they may have a cholestatic syndrome characterized by the absence of AMA, normal cholangiogram, and histologic features of bile duct injury or loss (Fig. 17.8). Such patients are characterized as "small duct" PSC or AMA-negative PBC, respectively. The major value of this clinical designation is that such patients may respond to conventional corticosteroid therapy.

21. **What is the frequency of the overlap syndromes of AIH?**
    The estimated frequency of overlap syndromes of AIH is about 15%, although this estimate may be high because of the absence of codified diagnostic criteria.

22. **What are the Paris criteria for the overlap syndrome with PBC?**
    The Paris criteria characterize patients with PBC and overlapping features of AIH. All patients must have interface hepatitis and they must also have a serum ALT level fivefold or more of the ULN, serum IgG level twofold or more of the ULN, or SMAs. The PBC component must have two of the three features including serum alkaline phosphatase level twofold or more of the ULN or gamma-glutamyl transferase level fivefold or more of the ULN, and AMA and florid duct lesions on histologic examination. Only 1% of patients with PBC satisfy these criteria and individuals with less pronounced features are not accommodated by these criteria.

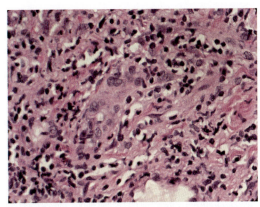

Fig. 17.6 Destructive cholangitis (florid duct lesion). Lymphocytic and histiocytic inflammatory cells destroy the bile duct. The histologic pattern suggests the possibility of primary biliary cirrhosis (hematoxylin and eosin, original magnification ×400).

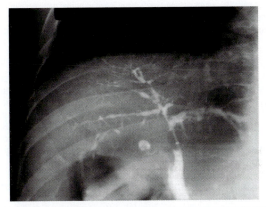

Fig. 17.7 Endoscopic retrograde cholangiogram showing features of primary sclerosing cholangitis. Focal biliary strictures and dilations are demonstrated.

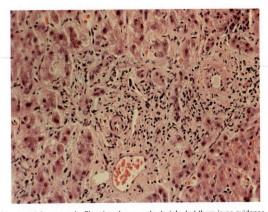

Fig. 17.8 Ductopenia. Portal tract contains a venule, fibrosis, edema, and arteriole, but there is no evidence of a bile duct. Cholangioles proliferate at the periphery of the portal tract. The histologic pattern suggests the possibility of primary sclerosing cholangitis (hematoxylin and eosin, original magnification ×200).

23. **What are the caveats in diagnosing the overlap syndromes?**

The major caveat is to recognize that patients with AIH and features of PBC or PSC have different phenotypes and outcomes than patients with PBC or PSC and features of AIH. Each syndrome should be designated by its predominant component. The diagnostic scoring systems for AIH should not be used to define AIH in patients with PBC or PSC as they have not been validated for this purpose. The rarity of an overlap syndrome between PBC and PSC suggests that most overlap syndromes constitute a classical disease with nonspecific inflammatory features that resemble AIH.

24. **Is the diagnosis of AIH more difficult in children?**

Yes. Children with AIH are commonly asymptomatic, their serologic markers may be weakly expressed, and AIH may not be suspected. ANA, SMA, or anti-LKM in any titer or level is pathologic in children and children are more likely to express anti-LKM than adults (25% vs. 4%). Testing for only ANA and SMA in children may misdirect the diagnosis. Children may also have concurrent autoimmune sclerosis cholangitis in the absence of inflammatory bowel disease or cholestatic clinical features, and this consideration lowers the threshold for cholangiography.

25. **How is AIH clinical presentation different in children versus adults?**

Two-thirds of pediatric AIH cases are AIH-1 (typically presenting during adolescence), whereas AIH-2 typically affects younger children, including infants. The same female preponderance seen in adults is encountered in children. However, acute onset is more common in children, seen in over 60% of the cases. A fulminant presentation is more frequent in AIH-2, affecting up to one-quarter of the cases; some 40% of AIH-1 children and 25% of AIH-2 children present mild, nonspecific symptoms, similar to adults.

Pediatric patients with AIH, whether type 1 or 2, have isolated partial deficiency of the HLA class III complement component C4, which is genetically determined. AIH-2 can be part of the autoimmune polyendocrinopathy-candidiasis-ectodermal dystrophy syndrome, in which AIH is present in some 20%–30% of cases.

26. **Can drugs cause an autoimmune-like hepatitis?**

Yes. Minocycline and nitrofurantoin are the principal drugs that have been implicated in current practice, accounting for 90% of all drug-induced autoimmune-like hepatitis (Table 17.8). Other drugs that have been well documented to cause liver injury indistinguishable from classic AIH are rarely used (dihydralazine, halothane, and methyldopa). Numerous other drugs, nutritional supplements, herbal medicines, and environmental pollutants have been proposed and the possibility of DILI must be considered in all patients with AIH. One new and important class of drug causing autoimmune-like hepatitis is the checkpoint inhibitor used in cancer treatment. While occurring in <5% of treated patients, autoimmune liver disease in this setting is typically severe and difficult to treat and may persist for many weeks or even months after the last dose of the drug.

27. **How is drug-induced autoimmune-like hepatitis distinguished from classical disease?**

Drug-induced autoimmune-like hepatitis is typically an acute idiosyncratic reaction with a low frequency of cirrhosis at presentation. It fully resolves after discontinuation of the drug and it does not recur unless rechallenged. Suppositions that the drug unleashes or potentiates latent AIH cannot be discounted, but such occurrences must be rare. In contrast, classical AIH is self-perpetuating and may not resolve after drug

Table 17.8 Implicated Causes of Drug-Induced Autoimmune-Like Hepatitis.

DEFINITE DRUG ASSOCIATION	PROBABLE DRUG ASSOCIATION	NUTRITIONAL AND HERBAL SUPPLEMENTS
Minocycline[a]	Atorvastatin	Black cohosh
Nitrofurantoin[a]	Clometacine	Dai-saiko-to
Dihydralazine	Diclofenac	Germander
Halothane[b]	Infliximab	Hydroxycut
Methyldopa[b]	Isoniazid	Ma huang
Oxiphenisatin[c]	Propylthiouracil	
Tienilic acid[c]		

[a]Most commonly implicated in current clinical practice.
[b]Largely replaced by alternative medications.
[c]Removed from marketplace.

withdrawal. Classical AIH (non-drug induced) has a low frequency of acute onset (20%), high occurrence of advanced fibrosis or cirrhosis at presentation (20%), and a high frequency of relapse after corticosteroid withdrawal (over 50%).

28. **What are the genetic predispositions for AIH?**
Susceptibility to AIH in White northern European and North American populations relates mainly to the presence of HLA DRB1*03 and DRB1*04. HLA DRB1*03 is the principal risk factor and HLA DRB1*04 is a secondary but an independent risk factor. Eighty-five percent of White North American patients with type 1 AIH have HLADRB1*03, DRB1*04, or both. HLA DQB1*02 is probably the principal susceptibility factor for type 2 AIH, and it is in close association with HLA DRB1*07 and DRB1*03. HLA DRB1*13 is associated with AIH in South America, especially in children. The HLA phenotype identifies individuals with a predisposition for AIH, but it does not predict the disease or familiar occurrence.

29. **How do susceptibility alleles produce AIH?**
Each susceptibility allele for AIH encodes an amino acid sequence in the antigen-binding groove of the HLA DR molecule, and this sequence influences recognition of the displayed antigen by the T cell antigen receptor of CD4+ T-helper cells. The sequence encoded by DRB1*0301 and DRB1*0401 in White northern Europeans and North Americans consists of six amino acids at positions 67 through 72 or the DR-beta polypeptide chain. Different susceptibility alleles that encode the same or similar short amino acid sequence in this critical location carry the same risk for AIH. AIH associated with alleles that encode dissimilar amino acid sequences is probably triggered by different antigens that may be region and ethnic specific.

30. **Should HLA typing be part of the standard diagnostic algorithm?**
No. HLA typing does not change clinical management and is expensive and should not be assessed routinely.

ACKNOWLEDGMENT

The author acknowledges the previous contributions to this chapter by Dr. Albert J. Czaja.

BIBLIOGRAPHY

Available Online.

WEBSITE

Available Online.

CHAPTER 18

AUTOIMMUNE HEPATITIS—TREATMENT

James F. Trotter, MD

 Additional content available online.

1. What is the preferred treatment for autoimmune hepatitis (AIH)?

In general, prednisone or prednisolone at a dose of 20–40 mg daily tapered to 5–10 mg daily is the preferred treatment (Table 18.1). Many clinicians will treat in combination with azathioprine 50 mg daily. In patients with acute severe or fulminant presentation, higher doses of corticosteroids may be indicated (80–120 mg daily). Mild cases may respond to initial doses as little as prednisone 10 mg daily and clinical judgment is the best determinant for dosing. Azathioprine may not be indicated for patients with severe cytopenia or known azathioprine intolerance.

2. Can budesonide be used in place of prednisone as frontline therapy?

Yes, but the appropriate target population is uncertain, the durability of the response is unclear, and the frequency of histologic resolution is unknown (Fig. 18.1). Budesonide 6–9 mg daily in combination with azathioprine 1–2 mg/kg daily normalized serum aminotransferase levels more commonly (47% vs. 18%) and with fewer side effects (28% vs. 53%) than prednisone (40 mg daily tapered to 10 mg daily) and azathioprine (1–2 mg/kg daily) when administered as frontline therapy for 6 months in a large randomized European trial. The strongest rationale may be in patients with medical conditions worsened by prednisone (osteoporosis, diabetes, and hypertension). In the United States, most experienced hepatologists still use prednisone as the preferred first therapy and budesonide as a secondary therapy primarily for patients nonresponsive to prednisone or at high risk for or who have developed complications related to corticosteroid therapy.

3. What are the caveats of using budesonide in place of prednisone as frontline therapy?

There are many uncertainties besides the durability of response and the frequency of histologic resolution. Budesonide has low systemic bioavailability because of its high hepatic first-pass clearance. Therefore concurrent immune-mediated diseases such as vasculitis and arthritis may not be managed effectively. Patients with cirrhosis and decreased hepatic clearance can develop side effects similar to those of prednisone. The effectiveness of budesonide in patients with severe, rapidly progressive, or life-threatening disease is uncertain. The appropriate target population may be patients with mild, noncirrhotic, uncomplicated AIH or individuals with preexisting comorbid conditions that could be worsened by conventional corticosteroid therapy.

4. What are the indications for treatment?

All patients with active AIH are candidates for treatment regardless of symptoms or disease severity (Table 18.2). Patients requiring immediate therapy have an acute severe or fulminant presentation and incapacitating symptoms or severe inflammatory activity as assessed by serum aspartate aminotransferase (AST) or alanine aminotransferase (ALT) level, gamma-globulin concentration, and histologic findings of bridging necrosis. The mortality of these patients

Table 18.1 Recommended Treatment Regimens.

INTERVAL DOSE ADJUSTMENTS	SINGLE-DRUG THERAPY (MG DAILY)	COMBINATION THERAPY (MG DAILY)	
	Prednisone (or prednisolone)	Prednisone (or prednisolone)	Azathioprine
Week 1	60	30	50
Week 2	40	20	50
Week 3	30	15	50
Week 4	30	15	50
Daily maintenance dose until endpoint	20	10	50

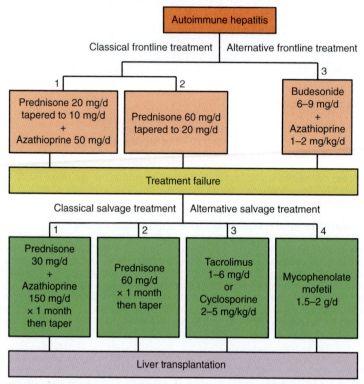

Fig. 18.1 Frontline and salvage therapies for autoimmune hepatitis. Prednisone in combination with azathioprine is the preferred classical frontline treatment and a higher dose of prednisone alone is appropriate for patients with severe pretreatment cytopenia, absent thiopurine methyltransferase activity, or azathioprine intolerance. Budesonide in combination with azathioprine can be considered for selected patients (mild disease, no cirrhosis, no concurrent immune disease, or premorbid conditions for therapy with prednisone). The possible salvage therapies for treatment failure include high-dose corticosteroids, calcineurin inhibitors, and mycophenolate mofetil.

Table 18.2 Indications for Therapy and Criteria for Treatment Selection.

INDICATIONS FOR TREATMENT	CRITERIA FOR TREATMENT SELECTION
Urgent	**Prednisone or prednisolone regimen**
Acute severe (fulminant) presentation AST or ALT ≥10-fold normal AST or ALT ≥5-fold normal and γ-globulin ≥2-fold ULN Histologic findings of bridging or multilobular necrosis Incapacitating symptoms Disease progression	Acute severe (fulminant) presentation Severe cytopenia Little or no thiopurine methyltransferase activity Pregnancy or contemplation of pregnancy Known azathioprine intolerance Short-term (≤6 months) treatment trial
Nonurgent	**Prednisone or prednisolone and azathioprine regimen**
Asymptomatic mild disease Mild symptoms Mild–moderate laboratory changes	Preferred therapy (fewer side effects) Postmenopausal women Obesity Osteopenia Brittle diabetes Labile hypertension Long-term (>6 months) treatment
None	
Inactive or minimally active cirrhosis	

ALT, Alanine aminotransferase; *AST*, aspartate aminotransferase; *ULN*, upper limit of the normal range.

if untreated is as high as 40% within 6 months. Treatment is less urgent but still important in patients with fewer/no symptoms and less severe inflammatory activity. Treatment is not indicated in patients with inactive or minimally active disease with cirrhosis. In such patients the treatment may create more problems than the inactive or minimally active disease.

5. Can some patients improve without therapy?

Yes. Controlled trials and retrospective studies have indicated spontaneous improvement in 10%–15% of patients with AIH and these remissions can be long-lasting. Furthermore, patients may have inactive AIH with or without cirrhosis at presentation. These patients have had an indolent, unsuspected AIH that has become inactive spontaneously (albeit with cirrhosis as a consequence). Such patients do not require treatment as they may have more risk than benefit from the medications (Table 18.2). Unfortunately, the patients who resolve spontaneously cannot be reliably identified at presentation.

6. Do asymptomatic patients require treatment?

Yes. Asymptomatic patients have the same frequency of moderate–severe lobular hepatitis, periportal fibrosis, and bridging fibrosis on histologic examination as asymptomatic patients. Furthermore, untreated asymptomatic patients improve less commonly than treated symptomatic patients and they have a lower 10-year survival (67% vs. 98%). The fluctuating and unpredictable nature of disease activity in AIH compels the institution of treatment of all patients with active disease (Table 18.2).

7. How does prednisone work?

Prednisone is a prodrug that is converted within the liver to prednisolone (Figs. 18.1 and 18.2). Prednisolone binds to the glucocorticoid receptor within the cytosol. The complex translocates to the nucleus, interacts with the glucocorticoid-responsive genes, reduces cytokine production, and inhibits the proliferation of activated lymphocytes. Prednisolone also inhibits nuclear factor kappa B and the cytokine pathways necessary for the expansion of plasma cells in the production of immunoglobulin. Anti-inflammatory actions include impaired

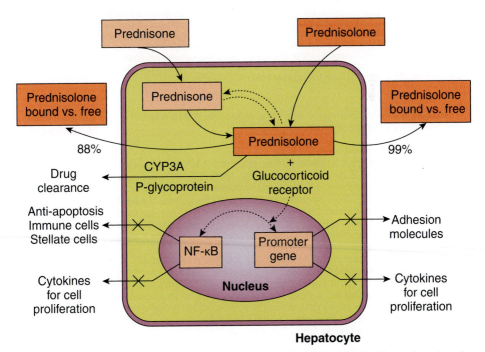

Fig. 18.2 Metabolic pathways of prednisone and prednisolone and the putative actions of prednisolone. Prednisone is the prodrug and prednisolone is the active metabolite. Prednisolone that is not protein-bound (unbound or free) is responsible for treatment efficacy and toxicity. Prednisolone blocks (X) antiapoptotic factors and cytokines required for lymphocyte proliferation by inhibiting NF-κB. It also blocks (X) the production of adhesion molecules needed for the trafficking of inflammatory cells and cytokines that modulate cell proliferation by inhibiting promoter genes. *CYP3a*, Cytochrome P4503a; *NF-κB*, nuclear factor kappa B. (Reproduced with permission of Future Drugs, Ltd, London, UK, from Czaja AJ. Drug choices in autoimmune hepatitis: part A – steroids. Expert Rev Gastroenterol Hepatol. 2012;6(5):603-615.)

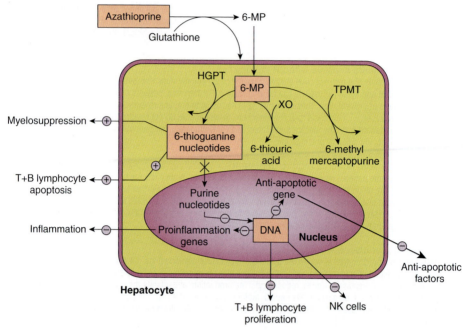

Fig. 18.3 Metabolic pathways of azathioprine and its putative actions. Azathioprine is a prodrug that is converted to 6-mercaptopurine (6-MP) which in turn is converted to 6-thioguanine nucleotides via a pathway mediated by hypoxanthine guanine phosphoribosyl transferase (HGPT). Detoxification pathways are mediated by xanthine oxidase (XO) and thiopurine methyltransferase (TPMT). The 6-thioguanine nucleotides can cause myelosuppression (+), apoptosis, and T and B lymphocytes (+) as well as inhibit (–) the creation of new DNA necessary for the proliferation of immune cells, including natural killer cells (NK), anti-apoptoptic factors, and inflammatory activity. (Reproduced with permission of Future Drugs, Ltd, London, UK, from Czaja AJ. Drug choices in autoimmune hepatitis: part B—nonsteroids. Expert Rev Gastroenterol Hepatol. 2012;6(5):617-635.)

production of adhesion molecules that attract inflammatory cells, increase apoptosis of lymphocytes and hepatic stellate cells, and decrease hepatic collagen production.

8. How does azathioprine work?

Azathioprine is a prodrug that is converted to 6-mercaptopurine (6-MP) in blood by nonenzymatic, glutathione-based pathways (Fig. 18.3). The 6-MP is converted in the liver to either thioguanine nucleotides by hypoxanthine guanine phosphoribosyl transferase, 6-thiouric acid by xanthine oxidase, or 6-methylmercaptopurine by thiopurine methyltransferase (TPMT). The 6-thioguanine nucleotides block the synthesis of purine-based nucleotides and limit the proliferation of activated lymphocytes. The 6-thioguanine nucleotides can also inhibit the expression of genes affecting inflammatory reactivity, and they can promote the apoptosis of activated T- and B cells and reduce the number of natural killer cells in blood and tissue.

9. What are the important points to remember at the start of therapy?

Azathioprine is a corticosteroid-sparing agent with a slow onset of action (>3 months), and it is not an essential drug for treatment. Azathioprine should not be given if there is drug intolerance, severe cytopenia, or severe TPMT deficiency. Prednisone and prednisolone are equally effective, but prednisolone does not require intrahepatic conversion. Its faster peak plasma concentration (1.3 vs. 2.6 hours) and greater systemic bioavailability (99% vs. 84%) justify its preference for prednisone in treating severe or fulminant cases. Corticosteroids have a short half-life and must be administered daily.

10. What are the side effects of therapy with prednisone?

Prednisone induces cosmetic changes, including facial rounding, dorsal hump formation, striae, weight gain, acne, alopecia, and facial hirsutism (Table 18.3). Severe side effects including osteopenia, vertebral compression, diabetes, cataracts, emotional instability, pancreatitis, opportunistic infection, and hypertension necessitate drug withdrawal in some patients. Patients with cirrhosis develop side effects more commonly than noncirrhotics, 25% versus 8%.

Table 18.3 Side Effects Associated With Prednisone and Azathioprine Therapy.

PREDNISONE-RELATED SIDE EFFECTS		AZATHIOPRINE-RELATED SIDE EFFECTS	
Type	Frequency (%)	Type	Frequency (%)
Cosmetic Facial rounding Acne Weight gain Dorsal hump Striae Hirsutism Alopecia	80	Hematologic cytopenia	50 (especially with cirrhosis)
Somatic Osteopenia Vertebral compression Cataracts Diabetes Emotional instability Hypertension	13 (treatment ending)	Hematologic (severe) Leukopenia Thrombocytopenia Bone marrow failure (rare)	6 (treatment ending)
Inflammatory/neoplastic Pancreatitis Opportunistic infection Malignancy	Rare	Somatic (variable severity) Cholestatic hepatitis Pancreatitis Opportunistic infection Nausea Emesis Rash Fever Arthralgias Villous atrophy and malabsorption	5
		Neoplastic Diverse cell types	3 (after 10 years)

11. What are the side effects of therapy with azathioprine?

Azathioprine can induce cholestatic liver injury, nausea, emesis, rash, pancreatitis, opportunistic infection, arthralgias, and cytopenia including severe myelosuppression (Table 18.3). Five percent develop early-onset adverse reactions including nausea, vomiting, fever, skin rash, or pancreatitis that warrant drug withdrawal. The frequency of side effects in patients treated with 50 mg daily is 10% and side effects typically improve after dose reduction or withdrawal. Cytopenia occurs in 50% and occurrence of severe hematologic abnormalities in 5%. The risk of malignancy is 1.4-fold greater than normal.

12. What are the factors contributing to prednisone toxicity?

The dose and duration of treatment are most important. Age and preexisting comorbidities, especially obesity, osteoporosis, and cirrhosis, also contribute. Doses of prednisone of less than 5–10 mg daily can be well tolerated for long term, whereas higher doses for longer than 18 months cannot. Postmenopausal women have a higher cumulative frequency of drug-related complications, 77% versus 48%, and greater occurrence of multiple complications, 44% versus 13%, than premenopausal women, probably because of age-related comorbidities. Cirrhosis can be associated with protracted hyperbilirubinemia and hypoalbuminemia and therefore increase the risk of side effects.

13. What are the factors contributing to azathioprine toxicity?

Azathioprine toxicity relates to the integrity of its detoxification pathways which in turn influence the erythrocyte concentration of the 6-thioguanine nucleotides. Competing enzymatic pathways convert 6-MP to the inactive metabolites of 6-thiouric acid via the xanthine oxidase pathway or 6-methylmercaptopurine by the TPMT pathway (Fig. 18.3). Drugs that inhibit xanthine oxidase (allopurinol) or people with deficiencies in TPMT activity, can increase the production of 6-thioguanine metabolites and predispose to toxicity over drug efficacy. At least 10 variant alleles are associated with low TPMT activity, and inheritance of these deficiency alleles can result in lower or absent TPMT activity.

14. **Can drug toxicity be predicted?**

No. Old age and the presence of comorbid conditions are not predictors of corticosteroid intolerance, but they are precautionary indices that compel an individualized treatment strategy. Similarly, the occurrence of azathioprine-induced side effects cannot be reliably predicted by measuring TPMT activity or determining the TPMT genotype. Patients with azathioprine intolerance do have lower TPMT activities than patients with azathioprine tolerance, but most patients with azathioprine intolerance have normal TPMT activity. Similarly, alleles associated with low TPMT activity are present in only 50% of patients with azathioprine intolerance. Pretreatment cytopenia is the most common precautionary index affecting azathioprine tolerance.

15. **Should TPMT activity be measured before azathioprine therapy?**

There is insufficient evidence to promulgate a formal recommendation. Routine pretreatment TPMT testing can be considered (Table 18.4). The assay for TPMT activity is readily available, and patients with the near-zero TPMT activity are at risk for life-threatening myelosuppression. TPMT activity is absent in only 0.3% and not all completely deficient develop bone marrow failure. Nevertheless, pretreatment TPMT testing provides the greatest level of reassurance about the likelihood of a serious hematologic consequence. Moderate reductions in TPMT activity are present in about 10% of normal individuals, and they have not been associated with severe azathioprine-induced toxicity. However, TPMT does not reduce the frequency of other common azathioprine or 6-MP side effects such as nausea, rash, and arthralgias, and dose-dependent toxicities including cytopenia may occur with normal TPMT activity.

16. **What adjuvant measure should be undertaken before and after therapy?**

All susceptible patients should be vaccinated against the hepatitis A and B virus prior to treatment (Table 18.4). A bone maintenance regimen, consisting of calcium, vitamin D, and a regular weight-bearing exercise program, should be recommended in all corticosteroid-treated patients. Bone density should be determined pretreatment in all postmenopausal females and in males 60 years or older, and it should be reassessed after 1 year of corticosteroid treatment. Bisphosphonate therapy should be instituted in patients with osteopenia and bone status

Table 18.4 Management Strategies to Reduce Treatment-Related Side Effects.

CLINICAL SITUATION	MANAGEMENT STRATEGY
No protective antibodies against hepatitis A virus or hepatitis B virus infection	Vaccinate against hepatitis A and B viruses before treatment
Never taken azathioprine previously	Assess thiopurine methyltransferase activity and avoid azathioprine if near-zero enzyme activity
Preexistent cytopenia	Assess thiopurine methyltransferase activity and avoid azathioprine if near-zero enzyme activity Avoid azathioprine treatment if leukocyte counts below 2.5×10^9/L or platelet counts below 50×10^9/L regardless of thiopurine methyltransferase activity Monitor leukocyte and platelet counts at 6-month intervals while on treatment Discontinue azathioprine if leukocyte counts decrease below 2.5×10^9/L or platelet counts below 50×10^9/L
Pregnancy	Provide early counseling about potential hazards to mother and fetus Avoid mycophenolate Anticipate flare in disease activity after delivery and treat accordingly
Osteopenia or its possibility	Institute bone maintenance regimen in all patients on long-term corticosteroid treatment ($\geq$12 months) Encourage calcium supplements, 1–1.5 g daily, vitamin D, and an active exercise program daily Assess bone density pretreatment in postmenopausal females and in older males ($\geq$60 years) and repeat after 12 months on corticosteroid treatment Initiate therapy with bisphosphonates if pretreatment osteopenia Perform bone density assessment every 2–3 years on corticosteroid treatment in all patients

monitored every 2–3 years and all patients during treatment. Leukocyte and platelet count should be determined at 6-month intervals in all patients receiving azathioprine.

17. Can azathioprine be used during pregnancy?

Yes. A meta-analysis of 3000 patients with inflammatory bowel disease found no increased risk of low birth weight or birth defects in mothers taking azathioprine, although preterm birth was increased. Mycophenolate is associated with birth defects and therefore is not to be used during pregnancy. Ideally, pregnancy should be planned so the patients may be on stable treatment with controlled disease for at least 1 year and mycophenolate should be avoided in the treatment regimen. In addition, patients with cirrhosis should be screened for varices as portal hypertension can worsen during pregnancy. Finally, liver tests should be monitored carefully during the pregnancy, especially during the final trimester and even a few months postpartum, as flares of AIH may occur during this time period.

18. What are the endpoints of treatment?

Standard corticosteroid treatment should be continued until normalization of all laboratory indices of active inflammation (AST and ALT) and/or until the occurrence of drug toxicity, treatment failure, or incomplete response. Treatment failure connotes progressive worsening of laboratory tests, persistent or recurrent symptoms, ascites formation, or encephalopathy despite compliance with therapy. An incomplete response connotes clinical and laboratory improvement that is insufficient to satisfy remission criteria. An alternative treatment is warranted in these patients after 3 years of continuous therapy because the risk of serious drug toxicity exceeds the likelihood of remission.

19. When should a liver biopsy be performed during therapy?

For patients with noncirrhosis with evidence of clinical resolution (normalization of AST and ALT) on minimal therapy, treatment withdrawal may be considered. Prior to treatment withdrawal a liver biopsy may be performed but is not required. Typically, histologic improvement lags behind clinical and laboratory resolution by 3–8 months. Histologic activity is present in one-third to half of liver specimens from patients with normal liver tests during treatment and tissue examination is the only method to document disease resolution before drug withdrawal. A liver biopsy is particularly beneficial to evaluate treatment failure especially to exclude corticosteroid-related fatty liver disease or previously unrecognized or emerging cholestatic syndrome such as primary biliary cholangitis or primary sclerosing cholangitis.

20. What are the results of therapy?

Normal liver tests are achieved in up to 90% of treated patients within 2 years, and the average duration of treatment until normalization of tests is 18 months. Clinical, laboratory, and histologic remission is achieved within 2 years in two-thirds of patients, and improvements are usually sufficient to attempt drug withdrawal after 2 years. About 10% of patients develop drug-related side effects that prematurely limit treatment and intolerable obesity or cosmetic change in osteoporosis with vertebral compression are the most common reasons for premature drug withdrawal. Treatment failure occurs in about 10% of patients, and improvement, but not resolution, occurs in another 10%.

21. Is survival improved?

Yes. Three control clinical trials have established this benefit. The 10-year survival rate of treated patients with and without cirrhosis is 90%. The overall 10-year survival rate is 93%, and it is comparable to that of matched normal patients from the same geographic region. Survival rates in liver-related death or liver transplantation are 91% and 70% after 10 and 20 years, respectively, and the standard mortality ratio for all-cause death is 1.63.

22. Does corticosteroid treatment prevent reverse fibrosis?

Yes. Corticosteroid therapy reduces hepatic fibrosis in 50% of patients and prevents its progression in 25% during a mean observation period of 5 years. By suppressing inflammatory activity, corticosteroids stimulate the degradation of fibrotic liver matrix and enhance the apoptosis of hepatic stellate cells. Corticosteroids have been reported to reverse cirrhosis in AIH, but this outcome is infrequent and uncertain. Cirrhosis still develops in about a third, usually during the early most active stages of the disease. The mean annual incidence of cirrhosis is 10% during the first 3 years of illness and 1% thereafter.

23. Are there any predictors of outcome prior to treatment?

Yes, but they have limited accuracy (Table 18.5). A Model for End-stage Liver Disease (MELD) score of at least 12 points at presentation has a sensitivity of 97% and specificity of 68% for treatment failure, death from liver failure, or need for liver transplantation. Patients with human leukocyte antigen (HLA) DRB1*03 have a higher frequency of treatment failure than patients with other HLAs, and individuals with antibodies to soluble liver antigen frequently have severe disease, relapse after drug withdrawal, and have treatment dependence. These findings do not alter the initial management strategy. Histologic cirrhosis at presentation is not a predictor of the treatment response.

Table 18.5 Clinical Indices Associated With Treatment Outcomes.

CLINICAL INDEX	FINDING	IMPLICATION
MELD	Score ≥12 points at presentation	Sensitivity of 97% and specificity of 68% for treatment failure
UKELD	Failure to improve pretreatment score by ≥2 points within 7 days of therapy in patients with icterus	Sensitivity of 85% and specificity of 68% for a poor outcome
Laboratory changes	Unimproved hyperbilirubinemia after 2 weeks of therapy in patients with multilobular necrosis	Sensitivity of 60%, specificity of 96%, and positive predictability of 43% for death within 4 months
Rapidity of clinical, laboratory, and histologic resolution	Failure to achieve resolution within 12 months of treatment	Progression to cirrhosis, 54%, need for liver transplantation, 15%
HLA phenotype (White patients)	HLA DRB1*03 or DRB1*04	HLA DRB1*03: young age and frequent treatment failure; HLA DRB1*04: concurrent immune diseases, female sex, and treatment responsiveness
Antibodies to soluble liver antigen	Pretreatment seropositivity	Relapse after drug withdrawal, 100%, associated with HLA DRB1*03, 83%

HLA, Human leukocyte antigen; *MELD*, Model of End-stage Liver Disease; *UKELD*, United Kingdom End-stage Liver Disease.

24. **Does the rapidity of the response to treatment have prognostic value?**
    Yes. Dynamic indices measured during therapy have a greater prognostic value than indices measured at presentation (Table 18.5). Failure to improve a pretreatment hyperbilirubinemia or the worsening of any liver test within 2 weeks of therapy in patients with multilobular necrosis predicts death within 4 months. In addition, failure to induce resolution of AIH within 2 years of treatment is associated with increased frequency of progression to cirrhosis or liver transplant.

25. **What are the factors that influence the rapidity of treatment response?**
    Disease severity and the age of the patient are important factors. Patients with mild disease respond more quickly to corticosteroid therapy than patients with severe disease, and older patients (over age 60 years) respond more rapidly than younger patients (age less than 40 years).

26. **What is the most common treatment problem?**
    Relapse after drug withdrawal is the most common treatment problem. Fifty percent of patients relapse within 6 months after termination of treatment and 75%–80% relapse within 3 years. The frequency of relapse increases after each subsequent retreatment and drug withdrawal and it decreases with the duration of sustained remission. The frequency of relapse after sustained remission of 6 months or more is 10%, but the risk never disappears. Relapse has occurred more than 20 years after drug withdrawal and the unpredictable propensity for relapse warrants lifelong surveillance for this possibility. Liver tissue examination is not necessary to diagnose relapse if it occurs within 6 months of drug withdrawal and if the serum AST level has increased from normal to at least threefold the upper limit of the normal range.

27. **What are the consequences of relapse and retreatment?**
    The consequences of relapse and retreatment are progression to cirrhosis, death from liver failure, requirement for liver transplantation, and drug-induced side effects. Repeated relapse and retreatment have cumulative morbidity and mortality. The frequency of each complication increases with each subsequent relapse and retreatment. The optimal time to interrupt this sequence is after the first treatment and relapse.

28. **How should relapse be managed?**
    Relapse is managed by maximizing efforts of prevention and by instituting long-term maintenance therapy immediately after the first relapse. The frequency of relapse can be reduced from 80% to as low as 25% by treating patients until normal AST and gamma-globulin levels and normal liver tissue are present before drug

withdrawal. If relapse occurs, long-term maintenance regimen is justified, preferably with azathioprine (Fig. 18.4). The treatment of relapse depends on its severity. For mild cases of relapse with small AST/ALT elevation (<2 times the upper limit of normal [ULN]), incremental increases in treatment may accomplish remission. Careful monitoring of therapy may prevent a severe relapse (AST/ALT >5 times the ULN), but such recurrence may require prednisone and azathioprine doses for initial treatment (Fig. 18.1). Eighty percent of patients can sustain remission over 10 years. Low-dose prednisone at about 5 mg daily can be used for azathioprine intolerance.

29. How should treatment failure be managed?

Treatment failure, the reappearance of hepatic inflammation through abnormal liver tests or histology, requires therapy; either reinstitution of treatment in patients after withdrawal or increased treatment in patients on therapy. The intensity of treatment is based on the severity of recurrence. In patients with mild liver test elevations (AST/ALT twofold the ULN), small doses of prednisone (5–10 mg) may be sufficient. For severe recurrences (AST/ALT >fivefold the ULN), high-dose prednisone (60 mg daily) or prednisone (30 mg daily) in conjunction with azathioprine (150 mg daily) induces clinical and laboratory remission in 75% of patients within 2 years (Fig. 18.1). The doses of medication reduced each month of clinical laboratory improvement by 10 mg of prednisone and 50 mg of azathioprine (if patients are receiving combination therapy) until conventional doses are achieved (prednisone 10 mg daily and azathioprine 50 mg daily or prednisone 20 mg daily). Histologic resolution occurs in 20% or less and most patients are treatment-dependent and at risk for disease progression and drug-related complications. Progression to liver failure is an indication of liver transplantation.

30. Can calcineurin inhibitors be used for treatment failure?

Yes (Fig. 18.1). The compilation of experiences with cyclosporine and tacrolimus as a salvage therapy have indicated a positive response of any degree in up to 90% of patients. The problems with calcineurin inhibitors are a higher degree of immunosuppression, lack of dosing guidelines, and the risk of serious side effects, especially nephrotoxicity.

31. Can mycophenolate mofetil be used for treatment failure?

Yes (Fig. 18.1). Mycophenolate mofetil has been effective as a salvage agent in about 50% of patients. The drug seems to be more effective in rescuing patients from azathioprine intolerance than from corticosteroid-refractory AIH. Its side effect profile is very similar to azathioprine, although some patients intolerant to azathioprine will tolerate mycophenolate without difficulty.

32. Is liver transplantation effective in AIH?

Ten percent of patients with AIH who fail conventional treatment require transplantation and steroid-refractory patients with a MELD score over 15 or symptoms of decompensation or liver cancer are candidates for the procedure. Liver transplantation is effective in patients with AIH (Fig. 18.1). The 5-year survival after transplant is about 80%. Patients transplanted for AIH experience acute rejection more frequently than patients transplanted for other diseases and AIH recurs in about a third of patients depending on the length of follow-up after the procedure. Disease recurrence can lead to graft failure requiring retransplantation.

33. What strategy is best for patients with drug toxicity or incomplete response?

For drug toxicity the dose of the implicated medication is reduced to the lowest possible level or withdrawn (Fig. 18.4). Disease activity is controlled by the medication (prednisone or azathioprine) that has been tolerated and doses adjusted to suppress inflammation. Mycophenolate mofetil has been used for azathioprine intolerance, but its side effects are similar to those of azathioprine. It should be avoided in patients with marked cytopenia or pregnancy. For an incomplete response, the medication is reduced to the lowest level possible to prevent symptoms and suppress histologic activity as reflected by a serum AST level maintained threefold or more below the ULN. Inadequately controlled patients may require liver transplantation.

34. Does hepatocellular carcinoma occur?

Yes. The frequency of hepatocellular carcinoma in AIH and cirrhosis is about 2% per year. Cirrhosis is typically a requisite for hepatocellular carcinoma in AIH.

35. Should patients undergo surveillance for hepatocellular carcinoma?

Yes. Surveillance is recommended in the guidelines for managing AIH in otherwise healthy individuals. Patients with cirrhosis for 10 years or more, immunosuppressive therapy for 3 years or more, and worsening laboratory tests during corticosteroid treatment have the greatest risk, but surveillance should include all patients with AIH and cirrhosis. Hepatic ultrasonography every 6 months is the cornerstone of surveillance. Determination of the serum alpha-fetoprotein level increases the frequency of tumor detection but also increases the frequency of false-positive findings and decreases the positive predictive value. Its additive value remains controversial.

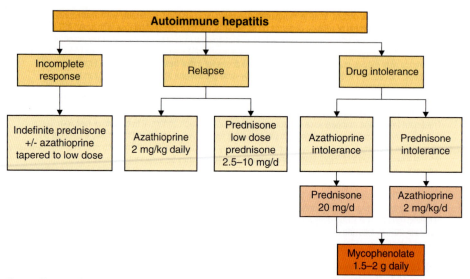

Fig. 18.4 Management of incomplete response, relapse, and drug toxicity. The preferred treatments for relapse are shown. Indefinite low-dose prednisone (range 2.5–10 mg daily; median dose 7.5 mg daily) can be considered after initial relapse in patients with severe cytopenia or azathioprine intolerance.

36. How are the overlap syndromes of AIH managed?

Conventional corticosteroid therapy in combination with ursodeoxycholic acid has been endorsed for patients who satisfy the Paris criteria for AIH with overlapping features of primary biliary cholangitis and for patients with overlap findings of primary sclerosing cholangitis (Fig. 18.5). Patients with AIH and an undetermined cholestatic syndrome can be treated with corticosteroids in combination with ursodeoxycholic acid or ursodeoxycholic acid alone or conventional corticosteroid therapy depending on the strength of the cholestatic component. All therapies are empiric and recommendations are not strongly evidence-based.

37. What new therapies are promising?

Molecular and cell-directed interventions have promise in AIH mainly because of successes already achieved in animal models and humans with other immune-mediated diseases (Table 18.6). They constitute investigation opportunities in AIH that have not yet emerged in clinical practice. Monoclonal antibodies against key components of the cytokine pathways and recombinant molecules that dampen immune activity and manipulations of regulatory T cells and natural killer cells in a disease-specific fashion are examples of these promising new interventions.

38. What is the role of serum-based biomarkers and elastography in patients with AIH?

Serum-based biomarker panels for hepatic fibrosis have emerged as a noninvasive measure of chronic fibrosis in some types of liver disease. These tests include serum AST/platelet ratio index, the Fibrosis-4 index, the enhanced liver fibrosis score, as well as proprietary tests. However, serum-based biomarkers for hepatic fibrosis are not established in AIH and their use should generally be discouraged. Hepatic elastography is a noninvasive test to estimate the degree of chronic fibrosis. Platforms are available through magnetic resonance imaging or more commonly ultrasonography which is available in many hepatology clinics. Elastography provides a reasonably accurate assessment of the general degree of fibrosis and can be helpful in the assessment of patients with AIH

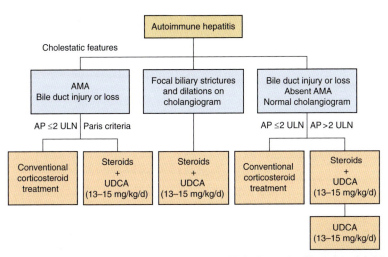

Fig. 18.5 Treatment algorithm for the overlap syndromes of autoimmune hepatitis. Autoimmune hepatitis may have cholestatic features that can resemble the clinical phenotypes of primary biliary cholangitis (PBC) or primary sclerosing cholangitis (PSC). In patients with antimitochondrial antibody (AMA), histologic evidence of bile duct injury or loss, and a serum alkaline phosphatase (AP) level, the upper limit of the normal (ULN) range may respond to conventional corticosteroid therapy, whereas in patients who satisfy the Paris criteria with florid duct lesions and serum AP >twofold, the ULN are candidates for corticosteroid therapy combined with ursodeoxycholic acid (UDCA) (13–15 mg/kg/d). This combination regimen has also been recommended for patients with focal biliary strictures and dilations on cholangiogram that resemble PSC. Individuals with an indeterminate cholestatic syndrome lack formal recommendations and their empiric therapy must be directed by the strength and nature of the cholestatic features and resemblances to PBC or PSC.

Table 18.6 Emerging New Therapies for Autoimmune Hepatitis.

THERAPY	PRINCIPLE ACTION	EXPERIENCE
Rituximab	CD20 monoclonal antibody	Limited efficacy in small series of AIH
Infliximab	TNF-α	Limited efficacy in small series of AIH
Interleukin-2	Regulatory T cell promoter	Limited efficacy in small case series of AIH
Belimumab	B cell activating factor monoclonal antibody	Efficacy in randomized controlled trial in lupus nephritis
Zetomipzomib	Selective immunoproteasome inhibitor	Efficacy in small series of lupus

AIH, autoimmune hepatitis; *TNF-α*, tumor necrosis factor–α.

to determine the likelihood of advanced fibrosis or cirrhosis. However, because intense hepatic inflammation can increase hepatic stiffness independent of the presence of fibrosis, elastography measurement should be deferred for up to 6 months until the disease is brought under long-term control with therapy to obtain the most accurate measure of fibrosis.

BIBLIOGRAPHY

Available Online.

WEBSITE

Available Online.

PRIMARY BILIARY CHOLANGITIS AND PRIMARY SCLEROSING CHOLANGITIS

John E. Eaton, MD

 Additional content available online.

1. Define primary biliary cholangitis (PBC) and primary sclerosing cholangitis (PSC).

PBC and PSC are chronic cholangiopathies. PBC mainly affects females in the sixth decade of life and is characterized by the destruction of interlobular and septal bile ducts. PSC mainly affects males in the fifth decade of life. Classic (large-duct) PSC is characterized by diffuse inflammation and fibrosis of the intrahepatic and/or extrahepatic bile ducts. Both PBC and PSC may eventually progress to end-stage liver disease requiring consideration for liver transplantation.

2. What are the clinical features of PBC and PSC?

The clinical presentations of both PBC and PSC may be similar, although some demographic and clinical characteristics differ. From 85% to 90% of patients with PBC are females presenting in the fourth to sixth decade of life, whereas up to 70% of patients with PSC are males with an approximate age of 40 years at diagnosis. Despite an increasing frequency of asymptomatic or subclinical disease greater than 40%, affected patients with either condition generally present with the gradual onset of fatigue and pruritus. Fatigue can be problematic and it is important to evaluate for other causes of this symptom such as medication side effects, hypothyroidism, or depression. Right upper quadrant pain and anorexia also may be observed at diagnosis. Although uncommon, steatorrhea in PBC and PSC is usually due to bile salt malabsorption. However, other etiologies of malabsorption can include pancreatic exocrine insufficiency, coexisting celiac disease, or bacterial overgrowth. Jaundice can occur in either condition though it is typically a manifestation of advanced disease. In PSC, the development of bacterial cholangitis is characterized by recurrent fever (abdominal pain and jaundice may or may not be present). The symptoms of end-stage liver disease, such as gastrointestinal bleeding, ascites, and encephalopathy, occur late in the course of both diseases.

3. What are the common findings on physical examination?

Physical examination may reveal jaundice and excoriations from pruritus in both disorders. Xanthelasmas (raised lesions over the eyelids from cholesterol deposition) and xanthomas (lesions over the extensor surfaces) are occasionally seen in the late stages of both diseases, particularly PBC. Hyperpigmentation, especially in sun-exposed areas, and vitiligo may be present. The liver is often enlarged and firm to palpation. The spleen may also be palpable if portal hypertension from advanced disease has developed. Characteristics of end-stage liver disease, including muscle wasting and spider angiomata, appear in the advanced stages of both diseases.

4. What diseases are associated with PBC?

Up to 80% of patients with PBC also have coexistent extrahepatic autoimmune diseases. The most common extrahepatic autoimmune disease is the sicca (Sjögren) syndrome. Other conditions described in association with PBC include autoimmune thyroiditis, scleroderma/calcinosis, Raynaud's phenomenon, esophageal dysmotility, sclerodactyly, and telangiectasia, rheumatoid arthritis, dermatomyositis, mixed connective tissue disease, systemic lupus erythematosus, renal tubular acidosis, and idiopathic pulmonary fibrosis.

5. What diseases are associated with PSC?

Chronic ulcerative colitis (CUC) and, less frequently, Crohn colitis are present in at least 70%–80% of patients with PSC. In contrast, only 5%–8% of patients with inflammatory bowel disease will have concurrent PSC. Consequently, patients with known inflammatory bowel disease should be evaluated for PSC if liver test abnormalities are detected. In addition, patients with PSC should undergo a colonoscopy at the time of diagnosis regardless of the presence of concurrent inflammatory bowel disease or symptoms of inflammatory bowel disease. CUC can develop even after a liver transplant just as PSC can develop following a colectomy.

6. How does CUC associated with PSC differ from CUC not associated with PSC?

Several observations have suggested that PSC-CUC is a different phenotype compared to those with CUC alone. For example, patients with PSC-CUC tend to have pancolitis with minimal endoscopic inflammation. A higher risk of colorectal cancer, pouchitis, peristomal varices following a proctocolectomy with ileostomy, rectal sparing, and backwash ileitis has also been observed in PSC-CUC.

7. **What important biochemical abnormalities are associated with PBC and PSC?**

   In both disorders, serum alkaline phosphatase elevations can fluctuate through the disease course and normalize in those with PSC and in those with treated PBC. Mild-to-moderate increases in alanine aminotransferase (ALT) and aspartate aminotransferase (AST) may be observed in either condition, though elevations greater than four to five times the upper limit of normal are unusual but can be seen if a concurrent process is present (autoimmune hepatitis [AIH] and acute biliary obstruction). For either disease, serum bilirubin may be elevated in individuals with advanced disease or in the presence of a flow-limiting biliary stricture among those with PSC. Tests reflective of synthetic liver function, including serum albumin and prothrombin time (PT), remain normal unless advanced liver disease is present. Serum immunoglobulin M levels are elevated in 90% of patients with PBC. Based on the widespread use of automated blood chemistries, an increasing number of asymptomatic patients with PBC and PSC are being diagnosed.

8. **How is PBC diagnosed?**

   Elevated alkaline phosphatase plus one of the following criteria: (1) positive antimitochondrial antibody (AMA) or the presence of PBC-specific autoantibodies (sp100 or gp210) if AMA is negative or (2) compatible histology.

9. **How is PSC diagnosed?**

   Multifocal biliary strictures on cholangiography after exclusion of secondary causes of sclerosing cholangitis. Alkaline phosphatase is not required to be abnormal.

10. **What is the lipid profile in patients with PBC? Are they at increased risk for developing coronary artery disease?**

    Serum cholesterol levels are usually elevated in PBC. In the early stages of disease, increases in high-density lipoprotein (HDL) cholesterol exceed those of low-density lipoprotein (LDL) and very-low-density lipoprotein. With liver disease progression, the concentration of HDL decreases while LDL concentrations become markedly elevated. An increased risk for atherosclerotic disease has not been demonstrated among patients with persistent hyperlipidemia in association with PBC.

11. **What serum autoantibodies are associated with PBC?**

    Serum AMA is found in up to 95% of patients with PBC. Although considered nonorgan-specific as well as nonspecies-specific, serum AMA usually is detected by an enzyme-linked immunosorbent assay. However, antibodies directed against a specific group of antigens on the inner mitochondrial membrane (M2 antigens) are present in 95% of patients with PBC. This subtyping of serum AMA increases the sensitivity and specificity for disease detection. AMA can be detected in the general population without PBC. It is estimated that 1 per 6250 adults without a diagnosis of PBC will have a positive AMA and only a minority will develop PBC in the future.

    Antinuclear antibodies (ANAs) may be present in PBC including two that recognize gp210 and sp100 nuclear pore membrane proteins. Anti-gp210 and sp100 antibodies have a high specificity (>95%) but a low sensitivity (<30%) to detect PBC and can be used for diagnostic purposes when AMA is negative. The presence of gp210 and sp100 antibodies may be associated with an increased severity of disease.

12. **What serum autoantibodies are associated with PSC?**

    In PSC, serum AMA is rare and if present, is usually seen in very low titers. However, detectable titers of serum ANA, anti–smooth muscle antibodies, and anti–thyroperoxidase antibodies have been found in up to 70% of patients with PSC. Perinuclear antineutrophil cytoplasmic antibodies have been observed in up to 65% of patients with PSC. The lack of specificity of autoantibodies limits their use in the diagnostic evaluation of PSC and their use for diagnosis is not routinely recommended. A small subset of patients diagnosed with PSC based on biliary strictures seen on cholangiography may indeed have immune-associated cholangitis or autoimmune pancreatitis with concurrent biliary strictures. Therefore it is recommended that all patients with PSC have a serum IgG4 measured.

13. **What are the cholangiographic features of the biliary tree in PSC?**

    Evaluation of the biliary tree in PSC by cholangiography may reveal multifocal stricturing of both intrahepatic and extrahepatic ducts with saccular dilatation of intervening areas. These abnormalities result in the characteristic beads-on-a-string appearance seen with PSC. Intrahepatic involvement alone occurs frequently while isolated extrahepatic involvement is unusual. In some patients, particularly those with mild disease, the strictures can be subtle and limited to the peripheral intrahepatic branches. Secondary causes of sclerosing cholangitis such as ischemic cholangitis or portal hypertensive bilopathy can mimic the cholangiographic findings of PSC. Magnetic resonance cholangiography (MRC) is the diagnostic test of choice. It has an excellent diagnostic performance, is more cost-effective, and safer than endoscopic retrograde cholangiography (ERC). Hence, MRC is the preferred diagnostic imaging modality (Fig. 19.1).

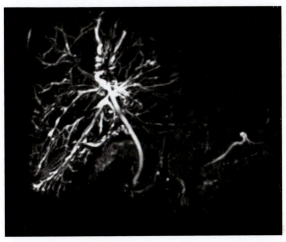

Fig. 19.1 Magnetic resonance cholangiogram exhibiting classic features of primary sclerosing cholangitis, including diffuse intrahepatic stricturing and dilation.

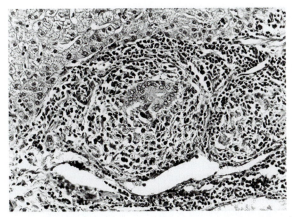

Fig. 19.2 Florid duct lesion (granulomatous bile duct destruction) in primary biliary cholangitis. A poorly formed granuloma surrounds and destroys the bile duct in an eccentric fashion.

14. Is it important to evaluate the biliary tree in PBC?

In PBC, an ultrasound examination of the biliary tree is usually adequate to exclude the presence of extrahepatic biliary obstruction. However, in patients with atypical features, such as male sex, AMA seronegativity, or associated inflammatory bowel disease, an MRC should be considered to distinguish PBC from PSC and other disorders causing biliary obstruction.

15. What are the hepatic histologic features of PBC and PSC?

Histologic abnormalities on liver biopsy are highly characteristic of both PBC and PSC in the early stages of disease. In PBC, the classic diagnostic finding is described as a florid duct lesion, which reveals bile duct destruction and granuloma formation. A severe lymphoplasmacytic inflammatory cell infiltrate in the portal tracts is accompanied by the segmental degeneration of interlobular bile ducts (also termed chronic nonsuppurative destructive cholangitis) (Fig. 19.2).

Early histologic changes in PSC include enlargement of portal tracts by edema, increased portal and periportal fibrosis, and proliferation of interlobular bile ducts. The diagnostic morphologic abnormality in PSC is termed fibrous obliterative cholangitis, which leads to the complete loss of interlobular and adjacent septal bile ducts from fibrous chord and connective tissue deposition. This histologic feature, however, occurs in only 10% of

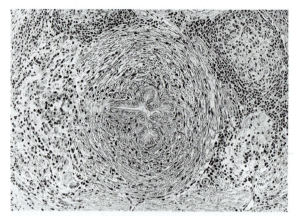

Fig. 19.3 Fibrous obliterative cholangitis in primary sclerosing cholangitis. The interlobular bile duct shows a typical fibrous collar, and the epithelium seems undamaged.

known cases. The histologic findings of end-stage liver disease for PBC and PSC are characterized by a paucity of bile ducts and biliary cirrhosis (Fig. 19.3).

16. Do asymptomatic patients with PBC have a normal life expectancy?
Most patients with PBC experience a progressive clinical course resulting in eventual cirrhosis. Asymptomatic patients have a longer median survival than symptomatic patients. However, a reduced median survival in asymptomatic patients with PBC compared with age- and sex-matched healthy populations is observed. Estimates of overall median survival without liver transplantation range between 10 and 12 years from the time of diagnosis; advanced histologic disease imparts a median survival approaching 8 years.

17. Do asymptomatic patients with PSC have a normal life expectancy?
Asymptomatic patients will have a reduced survival compared to normal controls. Indeed, nearly a quarter of patients who were asymptomatic at the time of diagnosis will develop clinical symptoms after 5 years. The median time of survival until death or liver transplant is 12–20 years for all patients with PSC, regardless of symptoms, and approximately 9 years for those with symptoms upon presentation.

18. What is the role of mathematical models in estimating survival for PBC and PSC?
The development of mathematical models for both PBC and PSC has improved the ability to predict rates of disease progression and survival without liver transplantation. They are useful for developing endpoints of treatment failure and designing therapeutic trials. There are a number of binary predictors that suggest responsiveness to ursodeoxycholic acid (UDCA) that involve alkaline phosphatase reductions for those with PBC and varied alkaline phosphatase cutoff values associated with improved outcomes in those with PSC.

The GLOBE PBC risk score and the UK-PBC score are both highly accurate in their ability to predict patient survival. The Mayo Clinic PSC risk score uses patient age, serum total bilirubin, albumin, AST, and history of variceal bleeding to predict patient survival. The PRESTO score uses artificial intelligence to predict the development of hepatic decompensation in those with PSC. Model for End-stage Liver Disease-sodium (MELD-Na) is utilized to allocate patients for liver transplantation.

19. Describe the relationship between alkaline phosphatase and the natural history of PSC.
Several studies have suggested that improvements in serum alkaline phosphatase over time are associated with improved outcomes. For example, the persistent improvement of alkaline phosphatase to less than or equal to 1.5 times the upper limit of normal (either spontaneously or with treatment) was associated with a reduction in the development of cholangiocarcinoma and liver-related endpoints, including liver-related deaths. These observations seem to occur most often in patients with intrahepatic PSC alone but can occur with diffuse PSC. Additional studies are required to verify these initial observations.

20. What vitamin deficiencies are associated with PBC and PSC?
Patients with PBC and PSC are susceptible to fat-soluble vitamin deficiencies, especially in the advanced stages of disease. The occurrence of diminished visual acuity at night can be attributed to vitamin A deficiency. Vitamin D deficiency occurs commonly in association with marked steatorrhea, which is related to a decrease in small bowel bile acid concentration. Other factors that may contribute to malabsorption include pancreatic insufficiency,

bacterial overgrowth, or celiac disease. Prolongation of serum PT is associated with vitamin K deficiency (or worsening hepatic synthetic function). If the bilirubin is greater than 2 mg/dL, vitamins A, D, and K should be checked annually. Finally, vitamin E deficiency infrequently occurs but when present results in neurologic abnormalities affecting the posterior spinal columns, leading to areflexia, loss of proprioception, and ataxia.

21. What bone disease is associated with PBC and PSC?

Metabolic bone disease (i.e., hepatic osteodystrophy), which may lead to disabling pathologic fractures, is a serious complication of both PBC and PSC. Clinical manifestations include osteopenia, osteoporosis, and fracture. Severe bone pain in an acute or chronic setting related to avascular necrosis may occur in PBC and PSC.

22. Describe the risk factors for osteoporosis in PBC and PSC?

Patients with PBC are eight times more likely to develop osteoporosis compared to sex-matched controls. Risk factors for osteoporosis include advancing age, low body mass index, previous history of fractures, and advanced histologic disease. Both vitamin D deficiency and smoking have been implicated as risk factors for metabolic bone disease. Additional risk factors that have been described in the general population include glucocorticoid use, excessive alcohol intake, smoking, or having a parent who sustained a fracture. Elevations in serum bilirubin have also been correlated with the rate of bone loss in patients with PBC. Osteoporosis has been reported in up to 15% of patients with PSC, which is a 24-fold increase compared to a matched control population. In addition to advanced age and a lower body mass index, a duration of inflammatory bowel disease of 19 years or greater has been identified as a risk factor for osteoporosis in patients with PSC. At the present time, baseline testing and regular follow-up screening with bone density scans every 2–3 years should be performed among patients with PBC and PSC.

23. What are the nonmalignant hepatobiliary complications related to PSC?

- Cholangitis which may occur in 15% of individuals with PSC. This can be related to malignant or benign strictures or intraluminal obstruction (hepatolithiasis/choledocholithiasis) or develop following an ERC.
- Pruritus is reported by more than 40% of patients. Among those with pruritus, 20% may experience itching that is refractory to multiple medications.
- Dominant strictures are defined as stenosis ≤1 mm in the hepatic duct or ≤1.5 mm in the common bile duct. They have been reported in up to 20%–50% of patients with PSC and are associated with symptoms in 10%–30% of individuals. When encountered, it should raise a suspicion for the presence of cholangiocarcinoma. When encountered, fluorescence in situ hybridization (FISH) may detect chromosomal abnormalities (such as polysomy) from biliary brushings and can aid in the diagnosis of cholangiocarcinoma. Conventional biliary cytologic analysis is also routinely performed.
- Cholelithiasis, choledocholithiasis, and hepatolithiasis are common among patients with PSC. For example, nearly 25% of patients with PSC have been found to have concurrent cholelithiasis and hepatolithiasis is observed in 10%–20% of cases.
- Cirrhosis and portal hypertension may ultimately develop as a result of progressive cholestasis and fibrosis. The 10-year incidence of the development of ascites, encephalopathy, or variceal hemorrhage is approximately 13%.

24. What malignancies are associated with PSC and how should patients be screened?

- Cholangiocarcinoma may occur in 5%–10% of patients with PSC. The risk of this malignancy is nearly 400-fold higher in PSC compared to the general population. Nearly one-quarter of cases are diagnosed within the first 2 years of the PSC diagnosis. It is rare in patients with small-duct PSC and pediatric patients. Most experts advocate screening for cholangiocarcinoma by an annual magnetic resonance cholangiopancreatography (MRCP) and serum CA 19-9 among adults with large-duct PSC. Compared to ultrasound, MRCP is superior for the detection of early-stage cholangiocarcinoma. The presence of a perihilar mass or periductal thickening with progressive enhancement on delayed phase imaging is highly specific for cholangiocarcinoma. Similarly, a stricture with periductal thickening without delayed enhancement, a progressive stricture observed over time, or an ill-defined delayed enhancement of the ductal wall without a mass are also concerning for cholangiocarcinoma and should prompt an ERC with biliary brushings for routine cytology and FISH testing. Early detection of cancer with MRC through an annual surveillance program has translated into improved patient survival.
- Gallbladder cancer may occur in PSC. In large multicenter cohort studies, 1.3% of patients with PSC were diagnosed with gallbladder cancer. This risk increases with age and if there is an underlying polyp or mass on imaging. Screening with annual ultrasound or MRC can be performed. Features of gallbladder polyps that are suggestive of a neoplastic origin include size greater than 8 mm or interval growth, sessile or mass-like morphology, and an arterial signal on Doppler. Patients who have gallbladder polyps with concerning features should be considered for a cholecystectomy.
- Hepatocellular carcinoma (HCC) may develop in individuals with cirrhosis. Generally, this is infrequent in those with PSC with a prevalence ranging from 0.8% to 1.8% of large multicenter cohorts. When HCC is detected in

those with PSC, it is often found incidentally on explant. When cirrhosis is present, some have advocated imaging every 6 months, alternating ultrasound and MRC. However, the benefit of this approach is unclear.
- Colorectal cancer is strongly associated with PSC and concurrent inflammatory bowel disease. Compared to patients with CUC alone, those with PSC-CUC have a 4- to 10-fold increased risk of colorectal cancer. In addition, patients with colonic Crohn disease may also have an increased risk. Importantly, colorectal neoplasia can develop soon after the two conditions are diagnosed. In addition, patients remain at risk following a liver transplant. Therefore after a diagnosis of PSC, individuals should undergo a surveillance colonoscopy and if inflammatory bowel disease is detected they should continue colonoscopy with surveillance biopsies every 1–2 years. Surveillance should continue after liver transplantation. Regular surveillance is associated with improved survival.

25. How can you establish the diagnosis of cholangiocarcinoma in patients with PSC?
The presence of a mass or periductal stricture with thickening that shows delayed venous enhancement is specific for cholangiocarcinoma. Biliary cytology is highly specific when adenocarcinoma is detected but is hampered by poor sensitivity (50%). More frequent passes with the cytology brush, repeated sampling, and the use of FISH testing can increase the diagnostic yield. In patients without a malignant mass, polysomy detected on FISH testing from biliary brushings has a sensitivity and specificity of 65% and 90%, respectively, for cholangiocarcinoma. The presence of suspicious cytology, multifocal polysomy, polysomy on repeated samples, or polysomy in the setting of an elevated CA 19-9 or malignant stricture all increase the likelihood of biliary cancer being present even when a mass is absent. One-third of CA 19-9 elevations beyond 129 U/mL are unrelated to malignancies and 7% of the population are unable to express CA 19-9. Hence, CA 19-9 elevations should be interpreted in the context of the individual patient and other testing.

26. What is AMA-negative PBC?
Patients may have the typical clinical features of PBC but have a negative AMA. This can occur in approximately 5% of patients with PBC. When AMA-negative PBC is suspected, gp210 and sp100 antibody testing should be performed where available. If negative, this does not exclude AMA-negative PBC and a liver biopsy is required to confirm the diagnosis. The natural history and response to UDCA are similar to patients with AMA-positive PBC.

27. What is meant by an overlap or a variant syndrome in PBC and PSC?
The presence of features consistent with both AIH and PBC is defined as an overlap or a variant syndrome. It occurs in approximately 5%–10% of patients with PBC and PSC. This should be suspected when the aminotransferases are elevated more than four to five times the upper limit of normal. Histologic features of AIH and excluding other causes for elevations in the aminotransferases (drug-induced liver injury, viral hepatitis, alcohol, etc.) are required to substantiate the diagnosis. Smooth muscle antibody titers may be normal or elevated. In those with PBC, they appear to benefit from UDCA and standard AIH therapies. The prognosis of AIH-PSC appears to be more favorable than classic PSC but worse when compared to the prognosis of pure AIH. Patients with AIH-PSC overlap syndrome may benefit from immunosuppressive therapy.

28. What is meant by small-duct PSC?
Small-duct PSC is defined by the presence of chronic cholestatic liver test abnormalities, liver histology compatible with PSC, and a normal biliary tree by cholangiography. Most patients also have a concurrent diagnosis of inflammatory bowel disease. Approximately 20% of patients will progress to classic PSC over a 10-year period. Compared to classic PSC, small-duct PSC is associated with a longer survival and decreased risk of cholangiocarcinoma.

29. Describe the treatment of pruritus in patients with PBC and PSC.
An ERC can be performed in those with PSC who have a worsening flow-limiting stricture resulting in pruritus. Cholestyramine relieves the itching associated with PBC and PSC by reducing serum bile acid levels in patients with cholestasis. In addition, it increases the intestinal excretion of bile acids by preventing their absorption. It is administered in 4-g doses (mixed with liquids) with meals or after breakfast for a total daily dose of 12–16 g. Cholestyramine should be given 1½ hours before or after other medications to avoid nonspecific binding and diminished intestinal absorption. Once the itching remits, the dosage should be reduced to the minimal amount that maintains relief.

Rifampin at a dosage of 300–600 mg/day also has been effective in relieving pruritus due to either p450 enzyme induction or inhibition of bile acid uptake.

For refractory cases, sertraline 100 mg a day or naltrexone 50 mg a day could be considered. Ultraviolet phototherapy can be employed with variable success. Molecular adsorbent recirculating system, which is an extracorporeal hemofiltration system that uses an albumin-enriched dialysate, can remove pruritogens and provide temporary relief for patients with refractory itching. Debilitating and intractable pruritus is an indication for liver transplantation, which results in symptomatic relief.

30. **How is osteoporosis treated in patients with PBC and PSC?**

Treatment of osteoporosis includes exercise, adequate supplementation of calcium and vitamin D, and bisphosphonates. Bisphosphonates are considered a first-line agent for the treatment of osteoporosis. Most suggest that parenteral (compared to oral) bisphosphonates are preferred when varices are present.

31. **Describe the treatment of fat-soluble vitamin deficiency in PBC and PSC.**

Problems with night vision due to vitamin A deficiency may be alleviated by oral replacement therapy. Decreased serum levels can be corrected with the oral administration of vitamin A (25,000–50,000 U/day) two or three times per week. Because excessive vitamin A intake has been associated with hepatotoxicity, serum levels should be frequently monitored. In patients with low vitamin E levels, oral replacement therapy with 400 IU/day can be instituted. If PT levels improve after a trial of water-soluble vitamin K (5–10 mg/day for 1 week), patients should be maintained on this regimen indefinitely. Prolongation of PT may be associated with hepatic failure in treatment-unresponsive cases. Severe vitamin D deficiency (less than 20 ng/mL) should be substituted with vitamin D 50,000 IU/day one to three times a week. A repeat vitamin D level should be obtained after 8 weeks of high-dose therapy, and if repleted, patients should be maintained on 800–1000 IU/day thereafter.

32. **Describe the treatment of bacterial cholangitis in PSC.**

Bacterial cholangitis in PSC should be treated with broad-spectrum parenteral antibiotics. The administration of ciprofloxacin results in high biliary concentrations and has broad Gram-negative and Gram-positive coverage. Similar results can be observed with other fluoroquinolones, such as norfloxacin and levofloxacin. MRC should be performed to investigate for a possible flow-limiting benign or malignant stricture. When an actionable stricture that may be contributing to cholangitis is detected, proceeding to ERC is appropriate. Often, cholangitis can reoccur in the absence of a stricture amenable to endoscopic therapy. Such cases are managed with antibiotics. Recurrent use of antibiotics and prophylactic antibiotics may be required in some instances. In highly select cases, patients may be considered for liver transplantation particularly when they have experienced recurrent episodes of cholangitis with bloodstream infections that are not otherwise amenable to other therapies.

33. **What are the therapeutic options for biliary strictures in PSC?**

Balloon dilation of dominant strictures by either transhepatic or endoscopic approaches can relieve biliary obstruction in PSC. Balloon dilation is most effective in patients with acute elevations of serum total bilirubin level or recent onset of bacterial cholangitis. It appears less effective in patients with long-standing jaundice. Some studies have suggested an increased risk of complications following biliary stenting and their use should be reserved for clinically significant strictures refractory to dilation. A short course (5–7 days) of oral antibiotics following dilation and/or stenting can reduce the risk of postprocedural cholangitis as well.

There are several endoscopic options for patients with advanced cholangiocarcinoma or gallbladder cancer who are ineligible for curative therapies. Palliative self-expanding metal stents can be considered when technically feasible and when life expectancy is greater than 3–6 months. In nonoperative candidates with a symptomatic cystic duct obstruction, endoscopic cystic duct stent placement or endoscopic ultrasound–guided cholecystogastrostomy and cholecystoduodenostomy can be employed. When ERC has failed to alleviate a nonoperative advanced malignant biliary obstruction, an endoscopic ultrasound–guided hepaticogastrostomy or choledochoduodenostomy can be performed.

34. **What medical therapies are available for those with PBC?**

UDCA in dosages of 13–15 mg/kg/day is the first-line treatment for PBC. It has been associated with an improved transplant-free survival and a reduction in the development of portal hypertension. Individuals who have an adequate biochemical response to UDCA have a similar survival to the general population. Large national registries have indicated that the proportion of patients with PBC requiring liver transplantation has decreased over time since the introduction of UDCA. In addition to initiating UDCA, the cornerstone of managing patients with PBC involves the early recognition and treatment of comorbid conditions (Fig. 19.4).

Approximately 30% of patients have an inadequate response to UDCA. Obeticholic acid is a farnesoid X receptor agonist that is conditionally approved for use in those who are intolerant to UDCA or have an incomplete response. It has been shown to improve liver tests in 50% of individuals but its ability to improve clinical outcomes is continuing to be studied. Obeticholic acid may cause or worsen pruritus and it should be avoided in individuals with cirrhosis with signs of portal hypertension. Bezafibrate has been shown to normalize alkaline phosphatase in two-thirds of patients who had an incomplete response to UDCA while also improving pruritus. Bezafibrate is not available in the United States. Several smaller studies have observed that fenofibrate can also lead to improvement in liver tests.

35. **Which patients with PBC are less likely to respond to UDCA?**

Age and sex have been associated with the response to UDCA. For example, males are less likely to respond than females (72% vs. 80%, respectively). In addition, those who present at an older age (greater than 70 years) have a response rate of 90% compared to a response rate of 50% among patients who were diagnosed at a younger age (less than 30 years). In addition, patients with cirrhosis are less likely to benefit from UDCA. Individuals who have

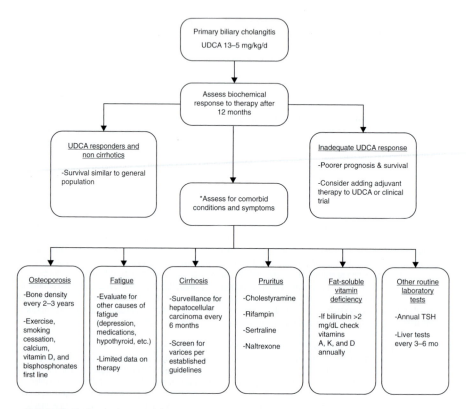

Fig. 19.4 Overview of the management of primary biliary cholangitis. TSH, Thyroid stimulating hormone; UDCA, ursodeoxycholic acid.

improvements in their liver biochemistries are also more likely to be UDCA responders and have the most benefit from this therapy. Indeed, there are several criteria that are largely based on alkaline phosphatase to assess the response to UDCA. One such criterion that has been widely validated is the Paris criteria. After 1 year of treatment, individuals who met the Paris criteria (alkaline phosphatase level ≤3× the upper limit of normal, together with AST level ≤2× the upper limit of normal and a normal bilirubin level) had a 10-year transplant-free survival of 90%. More recently, large international registries have suggested that the goal of therapy should be normalization of alkaline phosphatase and bilirubin.

36. **Is there a role for UDCA in PSC?**
Effective medical therapy for PSC is lacking. UDCA in standard doses (13–15 mg/kg/day) appears to improve biochemical parameters, but no significant effect on histology or survival has been observed. While higher doses of UDCA (20–30 mg/kg/day) were observed to improve biochemical, cholangiographic, and Mayo risk scores in two pilot investigations, a large prospective randomized, double-blind controlled trial in Europe failed to confirm these initial results. Results from a North American trial using even higher doses of UDCA also failed to demonstrate a survival benefit and raised concerns about safety in this population.

.37. **What is the role of liver transplantation in PBC and PSC?**
The treatment of choice for patients with end-stage PBC and PSC is liver transplantation and is associated with 5-year patient survival rates between 85% and 90%. In addition to increased survival, improvements in health-related quality of life after liver transplantation for patients with PBC and PSC have been documented.

Factors that influence the consideration for liver transplantation are deteriorating hepatic synthetic function, the development of comorbid conditions (e.g., HCC), intractable symptoms, and diminished quality of life. A specialized protocol involving neoadjuvant chemoradiation, brachytherapy, followed by liver transplantation has produced excellent results for selected patients with early-stage, perihilar cholangiocarcinoma associated with PSC.

The MELD-Na score helps prioritize patients on the deceased donor transplant list. However, patients with intractable symptoms and diminished quality of life may have a relatively low MELD-Na score. Therefore patients may pursue living-related donor transplantation. Indeed, PSC is a leading indication for living donor-related liver transplantation for intractable symptoms such as recurrent cholangitis. However, recurrent cholangitis has not been associated with an increase in waitlist mortality.

38. Do PBC and PSC recur after liver transplantation?

Recurrence rates are estimated to be approximately 30% 10 years after transplant. Recurrent PBC is diagnosed based on an elevated alkaline phosphatase and compatible histology (serum AMA levels may remain elevated after transplantation regardless of disease recurrence). Recurrent PSC is diagnosed with either compatible histologic or cholangiographic feature occurring at least 90 days after transplant following the exclusion of other causes of post-transplant biliary strictures. Recurrence of either disease may lead to reduced patient survival though recurrent PSC is associated with a larger reduction in 5-year survival compared to recurrent PBC (80% vs. 90%). Among those with recurrent PBC, UDCA may improve outcomes. Some centers start UDCA shortly after transplantation for all patients with a history of PBC. Repeat transplantation, particularly for recurrent PSC, may be required. Repeat liver transplantation for recurrent PSC is associated with a 5-year survival of 80% which is higher than other indications for repeat transplantation (primary nonfunction, vascular complications, etc.).

CLINICAL VIGNETTE

Available Online.

BIBLIOGRAPHY

Available Online.

WEBSITES

Available Online.

VACCINATIONS AND IMMUNOPROPHYLAXIS IN GASTROINTESTINAL AND LIVER DISORDERS

CHAPTER 20

Yoo Jin Lee, MD and Gil Y. Melmed, MD, MS

 Additional content available online.

1. What is immunization?

The body's immune system is stimulated by pathogens (bacteria or viruses). This in turn causes an immunologic response through the generation of memory B cells that produce antibodies (humoral response) and cytotoxic T cells (cellular response). Immunizations allow for controlled exposure to pathogens or proteins that induce these protective humoral and cellular responses so the body can respond immunologically upon subsequent exposure to the pathogen proteins.

2. What are the main types of vaccines?

- Inactivated vaccines, also known as killed vaccines, are those in which the pathogen stimulates antibody production by triggering an immunologic response. Killed vaccines do not reproduce and thus cannot cause infection in the host.
- Attenuated vaccines, also known as live vaccines, are made from pathogens that have been disabled from causing active disease. They are still able to stimulate antibody production resulting in protection from the disease, but in patients with compromised immunity this may theoretically result in infection with the pathogen being introduced in the vaccine.
- Messenger RNA (mRNA) vaccines (see, Q4).
- Viral vector vaccines, in which live attenuated adenoviruses deliver the antigen(s) of interest into the host; this is then used to induce humoral and cellular immunity.

3. Compare the recommended immunization schedule by vaccine per the Centers for Disease Control and Prevention (CDC) guidelines in adults based on medical conditions.

The recommended immunization schedule by vaccine per the CDC guidelines can be seen in Fig. 20.1.

4. What is a mRNA vaccine? How is this different from what we have known in the past?

mRNA vaccines are approved for use against severe acute respiratory syndrome coronavirus 2 (SARS-CoV-2, the virus that causes coronavirus disease [COVID-19]). Microbial mRNA is delivered within lipid bubbles (nanoparticles) and incorporated into host cell DNA to create proteins (antigens) taken up by antigen-presenting cells and used to stimulate the immune response. Since mRNA cannot enter the nucleus where the DNA is, it does not alter our genes.

Although conventional vaccines, such as inactivated vaccines, live-attenuated vaccines, and protein subunit vaccines, have shown favorable results for a variety of diseases, the demand for improved safety, faster and easier manufacturing, and lower production costs remains unmet. Advantages of mRNA vaccines are that they can be made quickly, with standardized and simple manufacturing and low production costs, and have demonstrated excellent safety.

5. Who should receive immunization against hepatitis A?

1. All children aged 12–23 months, unvaccinated children, and adolescents aged 2–18 years.
2. Individuals who are at increased risk for hepatitis A (hepatitis A virus [HAV]) infection including international travelers, men who have sex with men, users of illicit drugs whether injectable or not, individuals with occupational risk, individuals who anticipate close personal contact with an international adoptee, and individuals experiencing homelessness.
3. Individuals who are at increased risk for severe disease from HAV infection including chronic liver disease and HIV infection.
4. Pregnant women at risk for HAV infection.

Vaccine	Pregnancy	Immuno-compromised (excluding HIV infection)	HIV infection CD4 percentage and count: <15% or <200 mm³	HIV infection CD4 percentage and count: ≥15% and ≥200 mm³	Asplenia, complement deficiencies	End-stage renal disease, or on hemodialysis	Heart or lung disease; alcoholism[a]	Chronic liver disease	Diabetes	Health care personnel[b]	Men who have sex with men
COVID-19		See Notes									
IIV4 or RIV4	1 dose annually										
or LAIV4	Contraindicated					Precaution				1 dose annually	
Tdap or Td	1 dose Tdap each pregnancy	1 dose Tdap, then Td or Tdap booster every 10 years									
MMR	Contraindicated*	Contraindicated		1 or 2 doses depending on indication							
VAR	Contraindicated*	Contraindicated			2 doses						
RZV		2 doses at age ≥19 years			2 doses at age ≥50 years						
HPV	Not Recommended*	3 doses through age 26 years			2 or 3 doses through age 26 years depending on age at initial vaccination or condition						
Pneumococcal (PCV15, PCV20, PPSV23)		1 dose PCV15 followed by PPSV23 OR 1 dose PCV20 (see notes)									
HepA	2 or 3 doses depending on vaccine										
HepB	3 doses (see notes)	2, 3, or 4 doses depending on vaccine or condition									
MenACWY	1 or 2 doses depending on indication, see notes for booster recommendations										
MenB	Precaution	2 or 3 doses depending on vaccine and indication, see notes for booster recommendations									
Hib		3 doses HSCT[c] recipients only			1 dose						

- Recommended vaccination for adults who meet age requirement, lack documentation of vaccination, or lack evidence of past infection
- Recommended vaccination for adults with an additional risk factor or another indication
- Recommended vaccination based on shared clinical decision-making
- Precaution–vaccination might be indicated if benefit of protection outweighs risk of adverse reaction
- Contraindicated or not recommended–vaccine should not be administered. *Vaccinate after pregnancy.
- No recommendation/ Not applicable

a. Precaution for LAIV4 does not apply to alcoholism. b. See notes for influenza; hepatitis B; measles, mumps, and rubella; and varicella vaccinations. c. Hematopoietic stem cell transplant.

Fig. 20.1 Recommended adult immunization schedule by a medical condition or other indication, United States. (From www.cdc.gov/vaccines/schedules/hcp/adult.html.)

5. Any unvaccinated adults who request vaccination.
6. Unvaccinated individuals during outbreaks who are at risk for HAV infection or at risk for severe disease from HAV.
7. Individuals who provide services to adults in which a high proportion of those persons have risk factors for HAV infection.

6. **If someone naive to HAV is traveling to an endemic area and has not previously received the vaccine, what should they do?**
   - Healthy individuals between the ages of 12 months and 40 years should receive a single dose of HAV vaccine as soon as they plan to travel and complete their routine series.
   - Healthy individuals over 40 years of age, patients with immunocompromised and chronic liver disease, and those planning to travel within 2 weeks are recommended to receive anti-HAV immune globulin (IG) in addition to HAV vaccine.
   - Because IG provides short-term protection against hepatitis A through passive transfer of antibody, IG also applies to those who are unwilling or unable to receive HAV vaccination.

7. **What are the recommendations for postexposure prophylaxis for hepatitis A?**
   - Younger than 12 months of age: IG within 2 weeks of exposure to hepatitis A.
   - Healthy individuals aged 12 months to 40 years: A single dose of HAV vaccine.
   - Healthy individuals older than 40 years of age: Both IG and HAV vaccine should be considered.
   - Immunocompromised/chronic liver disease: Both IG and HAV vaccine.
   - Those with vaccine allergy: IG is recommended.

8. **Who should receive hepatitis B vaccination?**
   - All infants, children, and adolescence.
   - All adults through age 59 years.
   - Adults older than 60 years with risk factors for hepatitis B.
   - Persons at risk for infection by sexual exposure such as sexual contact with hepatitis B virus (HBV)–infected person, sexually active persons who are not in a mutually monogamous relationship, persons seeking workup or therapy for a sexually transmitted disease, and men who have sex with men.
   - Persons at risk for infection by percutaneous or mucosal exposure to blood such as injection drug user, household contacts with HBV-infected person, residents and workers of facilities for persons with developmental disabilities, health care worker, patients undergoing dialysis, and patients with diabetes.
   - International travelers where hepatitis B is endemic (hepatitis B surface antigen [HBsAg] prevalence rates exceed 2%).
   - Persons with hepatitis C infection, chronic liver disease, or HIV infection.
   - Persons who are incarcerated.
   - Adults older than 60 years without risk factors for hepatitis B should be offered HBV vaccination.

9. **How to interpret serologic markers for HBV infection?**
   Typical interpretation of test results for hepatitis B virus infection can be seen in Table 20.1.

11. **What should be done after exposure to HBV?**
   If a person that has not received full HBV vaccination is exposed to HBV, then they should be treated with a single dose of hepatitis B IG (HBIG) and three doses of hepatitis B vaccine over 6 months. However, if the exposed person has previously been vaccinated for hepatitis B and had a blood test documenting a response to the vaccine, then no treatment is necessary. The mainstay of postexposure immunoprophylaxis is the hepatitis B vaccine, but in certain circumstances the addition of HBIG will provide increased protection and should be given as soon as possible, within 7 days for percutaneous exposure and 14 days for sexual exposure.

12. **What is the recommended strategy for infants born to mothers with HBV?**
   - Infants whose mothers are HBsAg-positive should receive HBIG and the first dose of hepatitis B vaccine within 12 hours of birth. They should also complete a routine hepatitis B vaccine series. This strategy can prevent up to 94% of perinatal transmission.
   - If the mother's hepatitis B status is unknown but there is other evidence suggesting maternal hepatitis B infection, the infant should be managed the same as infants born to an infected mother.
   - All infants born to mothers infected with hepatitis B should have postvaccination serologic testing consisting of HBsAg and hepatitis B surface antibody (anti-HBs) between 9 and 12 months of age (or 1–2 months after completion of hepatitis B vaccine series).

Table 20.1 Typical Interpretation of Test Results for Hepatitis B Virus Infection.

HBSAG	TOTAL ANTI-HBC	IGM ANTI-HBC	ANTI-HBS	HBV DNA	INTERPRETATION
−	−	−	−	−	Never infected
+	−	−	−	+ or −	Early acute infection: transient (up to 18 days) after vaccination
+	+	+	−	+	Acute infection
−	+	+	+ or −	+ or −	Acute resolving infection
−	+	−	+	−	Recovered from past infection and immune
+	+	−	−	+	Chronic infection
−	+	−	−	+ or −	False-positive (i.e., susceptible); past infection; "low level" chronic infection; or passive transfer of anti-HBc to an infant born to HBsAg-positive mother
	−	−	−	−	Immune if anti-HBs concentration is >10 mIU/mL after vaccine series completion; passive transfer after hepatitis B immune globulin administration

−, Negative; +, positive; *anti-HBc*, antibody to hepatitis B core antigen; *anti-HBs*, antibody to hepatitis B surface antigen; *HBsAg*, hepatitis B surface antigen; *HBV DNA*, hepatitis B virus deoxyribonucleic acid; *IgM*, immunoglobulin class M.
Adapted from Schillie S, Vellozzi C, Reingold A, Harris A, Haber P, Ward JW, et al. Prevention of hepatitis B virus infection in the United States: recommendations of the Advisory Committee on Immunization Practices. MMWR Recomm Rep. 2018;67(No. RR-1):1-31.

13. **Are booster doses of hepatitis B vaccine recommended?**
Booster doses of hepatitis B vaccine are recommended only in patients on dialysis with anti-HBs levels less than 10 mIU/mL. For other immunocompromised persons (e.g., HIV infected, hematopoietic stem-cell transplant recipients, and those receiving chemotherapy), the need for booster doses has not been determined. For a person with a normal immune system who has received previous vaccination, booster doses are not recommended.

14. **Why are patients with liver cirrhosis susceptible to infection?**
The liver plays a key role in the innate immune response because it encounters ingested pathogens from the gut via circulation from the portal vein system. Patients with cirrhosis have a fibrotic and poorly functioning liver with dysfunction of the reticuloendothelial system (Kupffer cells in the liver, macrophages, and monocytes) as well as granulocytes (neutrophils, eosinophils, and basophils). There have been studies demonstrating increased gut permeability of bacteria and associated toxins in patients with cirrhosis leading to spontaneous infections. There is frequently extensive shunting of venous circulation away from the liver in patients with cirrhosis, thus impairing clearing capacity following infections.

15. **Why is vaccination against hepatitis A and B strongly recommended in patients with cirrhosis?**
- A cirrhotic liver cannot sustain any more injury (i.e., infection) without serious risk of decompensation and liver failure!
  - Patients with cirrhosis with superimposed acute hepatitis A infection are at significantly increased risk for liver failure and death compared to those patients without liver disease.
  - When a patient with cirrhosis develops acute hepatitis B infections, they more frequently have severe manifestations including encephalopathy, ascites, hypoprothrombinemia, and acute liver failure. Furthermore, coinfection with hepatitis B and hepatitis C in patients with chronic liver disease is associated with an increased risk of hepatocellular carcinoma.

16. **When is the optimal timing for vaccination in patients with liver cirrhosis?**
Vaccinations for patients with chronic liver disease (e.g., persons with hepatitis C, cirrhosis, fatty liver disease, alcoholic liver disease, autoimmune hepatitis, and alanine aminotransferase or aspartate aminotransferase level greater than twice the upper limit of normal) are recommended as soon as possible, as immunologic responses to vaccinations are known to be suboptimal in advanced liver disease such as cirrhosis. Patients planning liver

transplantation (LT) should be vaccinated prior to transplantation if possible, to achieve higher vaccine efficacy. Since immunocompromised LT recipients have a lower immunologic response to the vaccines, patients planning LT should be vaccinated before transplantation if possible or wait up to 3–6 months after transplantation. Note that live vaccines are contraindicated after transplantation and should not be given at least 4 months prior to transplantation.

17. Should patients with cirrhosis receive vaccination against the influenza virus?

Yes! The influenza vaccine is recommended for patients with chronic liver disease including cirrhosis. Furthermore, studies have demonstrated increased hepatic decompensation in those patients with advanced cirrhosis who develop influenza infections and administration of the influenza vaccine can reduce the complication. The live-attenuated influenza vaccine is not indicated for patients with chronic liver disease.

18. Should patients with cirrhosis or LT recipients receive COVID-19 vaccine?

Yes! The CDC has classified people with chronic liver disease including cirrhosis and solid organ transplant recipients including LT recipients as high-risk groups for severe COVID-19. Therefore patients with cirrhosis or LT candidates are advised to obtain primary series and booster doses of COVID-19 vaccine.

19. What other vaccinations should patients with cirrhosis receive?

They should receive standard immunizations that are applicable to an otherwise healthy population. This includes routine diphtheria and tetanus booster immunizations every 10 years, and other age-appropriate vaccines. In general, killed/non-live vaccines are preferred to live vaccines, when possible.

20. Are patients with inflammatory bowel disease (IBD; Crohn's and ulcerative colitis) more susceptible to vaccine-preventable infections? If so, why?

- Yes. Several infections including herpes zoster, human papillomavirus (HPV), pneumonia, and acute HBV infection are more common in patients with IBD and can be particularly dangerous among those who are on immunosuppressive therapies.
- There are two primary reasons why patients with IBD are more susceptible to infections, including vaccine-preventable ones. First, IBD is characterized by dysregulation of the immune system which is activated inappropriately by commensal gut bacteria, resulting in an inadequate intestinal immune response. Second, patients are frequently treated with short- and long-term immunosuppressive medications, namely, glucocorticoids, immune modulators (including azathioprine, 6-mercaptopurine, and methotrexate), and tumor necrosis factor–α [TNF-α] inhibitors such as infliximab, adalimumab, golimumab, and certolizumab, and small molecules including Janus kinase (JAK) inhibitors and sphingosine 1-phosphate (S1P) receptor modulators. Infections are among the most common serious adverse events associated with these therapies. The risk for serious infections is higher among those on combination therapy with TNF-α inhibitors and immunosuppressants and/or corticosteroids, as well as kinase (JAK) inhibitors and S1P receptor modulators, while antitrafficking and anti-IL-12/23 mechanisms have lower risk. JAK inhibitors have been associated with increased risks of herpes zoster, and both JAK inhibitors and S1P receptor modulators are associated with lymphopenia, which can increase infection risk.

21. When is the best time to address issues regarding vaccination status in patients with IBD?

As soon as the diagnosis is made, ideally before starting immunosuppressive medications which may blunt immune responses to vaccines. Most vaccines can be given whenever possible but should be timed ideally before the initiation of immunosuppressive therapy to obtain a maximum immune response.

22. Is there an increased risk of IBD exacerbation after vaccination?

No, currently used vaccines including influenza and pneumococcal vaccines are not known to be associated with an increase in the risk of IBD relapse. Recent data also support that vaccination against COVID-19 is not associated with significant flare risk in patients with IBD.

23. Which vaccines are recommended for IBD regardless of immunosuppression?

In general, all killed/non-live vaccines should be given as per routine guidelines. These include the following:
- Inactivated influenza vaccine (ideally before immunosuppression)
- Tetanus vaccine/booster (as part of Td, Tdap, or DTap)
- HPV vaccine
- Meningococcus vaccine
- Hepatitis A vaccine
- Hepatitis B vaccine
- Pneumococcus (pneumococcal conjugate vaccine 15 [PCV15], PSSV23, or PCV20, ideally before immunosuppression)
- Pertussis (ideally before immunosuppression)

- Inactivated/recombinant zoster vaccine
- COVID-19 vaccine (mRNA and adenovirus vector vaccines)

24. **Which vaccines are contraindicated in patients with IBD who are on immunosuppressive therapies such as corticosteroids, immunomodulators, and biologics and small molecular agents?**
    - In general, all live vaccines. These include the following:
      - Live, attenuated influenza vaccine (intranasal vaccine)
      - Varicella zoster vaccine (generally)
      - Zoster live vaccine (no longer used in the United States)
      - Yellow fever vaccine
      - Measles-mumps-rubella vaccine
      - Typhoid live oral vaccine
      - Bacillus Calmette-Guérin (BCG) vaccine (not given in the United States)
      - Polio live oral vaccine (no longer used in the United States)
      - Anthrax vaccine
      - Smallpox vaccine

25. **Which live vaccines might be considered in patients with IBD on immunosuppressive therapies in special circumstance? In what immune conditions?**
    Although generally contraindicated, live vaccines such as varicella (chicken pox) vaccine might be considered in patients on a case-by-case basis. Circumstances that warrant these special considerations are when the risk of natural infection outweighs the risks of the vaccine, such as in occupations at high risk of exposure such as preschool teachers and health care workers.

    Patients with significant immunocompromised status include those on high-dose steroids $\geq$20 mg per day of oral prednisone for $\geq$14 days, use of immunosuppressive medications (azathioprine $\geq$3 mg/kg/d, 6-mercaptopurine $\geq$1.5 mg/kg/d, or $\geq$0.4 mg/kg/wk), use of necrosis factor-α inhibitors, ustekinumab, or transplant-related immunosuppressive medications (cyclosporine, tacrolimus, and mycophenolate).

    Per Food and Drug Administration labeling, live vaccines may be administered concurrently with vedolizumab, if the benefits outweigh the risks.

    Adults and children with IBD who may be immunosuppressed that acquire varicella infection can develop widespread dissemination of varicella zoster virus which can be fatal. Varicella is a live-attenuated virus vaccine, it is generally considered contraindicated in immunocompromised patients.

26. **Should the yellow fever vaccine be given to a patient with IBD on immunosuppression who will be traveling to an endemic area?**
    No! It is a live, attenuated vaccine and serious adverse effects have been noted such as encephalitis and multiorgan system failure. Travel to these endemic areas (including sub-Saharan Africa and parts of South America) should ideally be avoided among patients who cannot receive the vaccine safely. If travel to these areas is necessary, patients should be counseled on the risks of the disease and prevention of mosquito bites, the transmission vector for the disease. They will also require a formal vaccination waiver from a travel medicine specialist. For patients with IBD planning to travel to an endemic area in the future, a yellow fever vaccine can be recommended before starting immunosuppressive therapies (at least 4 weeks, but not less than 2 weeks prior to immunosuppression).

27. **Do patients with IBD on immune suppression have an adequate immune response to vaccinations?**
    Not to all. Several studies have demonstrated that patients who are on combination therapy (azathioprine or 6-mercaptopurine together with a TNF inhibitor) have significantly decreased immunologic responses to several vaccines compared to those not on combinations of immunosuppressants. Therefore patients should be targeted for vaccination soon after diagnosis, before immunosuppression is initiated, whenever possible.

    Although COVID-19 vaccines are highly effective in patients with IBD, the immunologic response to COVID-19 vaccination is blunted in patients receiving combination therapy or high-dose systemic corticosteroid therapy. However, as partially blunted protection is considered better than no protection, all patients with IBD should receive primary series and booster vaccine against COVID-19, regardless of their treatment regimen.

28. **Should patients with IBD receive the HPV vaccine? If so, why?**
    Yes. Patients with IBD have an increased risk for cervical dysplasia and cancer-causing HPV serotypes including cervical, vulvar, vaginal, penile, anal, and oropharyngeal cancers, particularly if on immunosuppression for greater than 6 months. Recombinant HPV 9-valent vaccine (Gardasil 9) is indicated for all women and men aged 9–45 years, and the Advisory Committee on Immunization Practices (AICP) recommends shared decision-making based on risk for the acquisition of HPV for those aged 27–45 years.

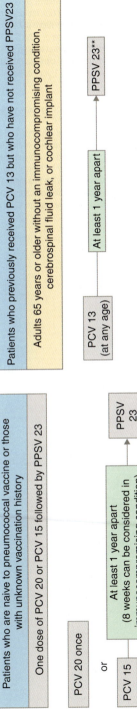

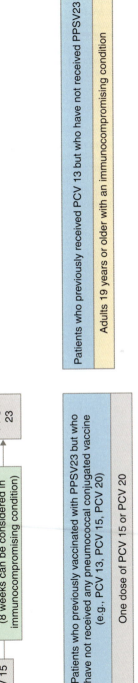

Fig. 20.2 October 2021, the Advisory Committee on Immunization Practices recommended two new pneumococcal conjugate vaccines (PCV15 and PCV20) for PCV-naive adults aged 65 and older and for adults aged 19-64 years who have certain medical conditions or other risk factors. **For adults who have received PCV13 but have not completed their recommended pneumococcal vaccine series with PPSV23, one dose of PCV20 may be used if PPSV23 is not available. If PCV20 is used, their pneumococcal vaccinations are complete.

29. **Could you briefly summarize the pneumococcal vaccination recommendations for patients with chronic liver disease and IBD?**

    In October 2021, the AICP recommended two new PCVs (PCV15 and PCV20) for PCV-naive adults aged 65 and older and for adults aged 19–64 years who have certain medical conditions or other risk factors. Pneumococcal vaccination is recommended for patients with chronic liver disease and IBD. Vaccine-naive patients or those with unknown vaccination history aged 19 and older should be administered a single dose of PCV15 or PCV20. When PCV15 is used, PPSV23 should be administered at least 8 weeks later in immunocompromised individuals. For adults who have previously received PPSV23 but have not received a pneumococcal conjugated vaccine (e.g., PCV13, PCV15, and PCV20), a single dose of PCV15 or PCV20 may be given at least 1 year later.
    See Fig. 20.2.

30. **Can babies born to mothers who received biologic therapy during pregnancy receive their usual childhood vaccinations?**

    For the most part—yes, with the notable exception that **live** vaccines should **NOT** be administered during the first 6 months of life in newborns whose mothers received any biologic therapy during the third trimester of pregnancy. Many anti-TNF therapies are monoclonal antibodies that may be actively transported across the placenta, particularly during the third trimester, such that the drug concentrations at birth may be higher in the newborn than in the mother. In the United States the only live vaccine offered to newborns during this initial 6-month period is the rotavirus vaccine, although in other countries there may be additional live vaccines (such as the BCG vaccine) that should be withheld due to concerns for disseminated infection from live vaccines.

BIBLIOGRAPHY

Available Online

CHAPTER 21

PREGNANCY AND LIVER DISEASE

Devina Bhasin, MD and Roshan Shrestha, MD

 Additional content available online.

NORMAL ANATOMIC AND PHYSIOLOGIC CHANGES DURING PREGNANCY

1. **What are the structural and functional hepatic adaptations during pregnancy?**
   Liver size and histologic characteristics do not change during pregnancy. Maternal blood volume and cardiac output increase significantly, without a corresponding increase in hepatic blood flow, with a net decrease in fractional blood flow to the liver. An enlarging uterus makes venous return via the inferior vena cava progressively more difficult toward term. Blood is shunted via the azygous system with possible development of esophageal varices.

2. **Does liver function change during pregnancy?**
   Hepatic function remains normal during pregnancy, but the normal range of laboratory values changes because of hormonal changes and an increase in blood volume with subsequent hemodilution. Aspartate aminotransferase (AST), alanine aminotransferase (ALT), γ-glutamyl transpeptidase (GGTP), bilirubin, and prothrombin remain within normal limits. Total alkaline phosphatase (AP) is elevated. The placenta is a major source of AP; levels return to normal within 20 days after delivery. Estrogen increases the synthesis of fibrinogen, as well as other coagulation proteins (factors VII, VIII, IX, and X). Also attributed to estrogen's effects are significant increases in serum concentrations of major lipid classes (triglycerides, cholesterol, and low- and very-low-density lipoproteins). These levels may be twice the normal limit of nonpregnant females of the same age. Serum albumin decreases slightly, contributing to the approximately 20% decline in serum protein concentration. Plasma concentrations of other serum proteins (ceruloplasmin, corticosteroids, testosterone, and serum-binding protein for thyroxine), as well as vitamin D and folate also increase during pregnancy.

DISEASES DURING PREGNANCY

- Coincident occurrence of liver disease (viral hepatitis, alcoholic hepatitis, gallstone disease, and autoimmune hepatitis)
- Intrahepatic cholestasis of pregnancy (IHCP)
- Acute fatty liver of pregnancy (AFLP)
- Hemolysis, elevated liver enzymes, and low platelet count (HELLP syndrome)

3. **Can gestational age differentiate between different liver diseases in pregnancy?**
   Yes. Hyperemesis gravidarum presents in the first trimester of pregnancy. Patients have severe nausea and vomiting, and approximately one-half have associated elevations of bilirubin, AST, or ALT. Cholestasis of pregnancy, viral hepatitis, and abnormal liver chemistries caused by cholelithiasis may present at any point in gestation, from the first to the third trimester. AFLP and preeclamptic liver disease (HELLP, hepatic infarct, and hepatic rupture) are specifically encountered in the third trimester of pregnancy. Both herpes simplex virus and hepatitis E virus are exacerbated in pregnancy and usually present in the third trimester. The presentation may be a mild elevation in transaminases or severe hepatic failure. Budd-Chiari syndrome presents from the second half of pregnancy to 3 months postpartum.

COINCIDENT OCCURRENCE

4. **Can we assume the presence of chronic liver disease in a pregnant patient with angiomas and palmar erythema on physical examination and small esophageal varices detected endoscopically?**
   No. Spider angiomas and palmar erythema are common and appear in approximately two-thirds of pregnant females without liver disease. Small esophageal varices are present in approximately 50% of healthy pregnant females without liver disease because of the increased flow in the azygous system.

5. **What is the most common cause of jaundice in pregnancy?**
   Viral hepatitis is the most common cause of jaundice during pregnancy.

6. **How severe is the course of viral hepatitis acquired during pregnancy?**
   - Hepatitis A, B, and C run a similar course in pregnant and nonpregnant patients.
   - Hepatitis E runs a different course in pregnancy. It is fulminant in up to 20% of patients, compared with less than 1% of nonpregnant females. The fatality rate is 1.5% during the first trimester, 8.5% during the second trimester, and up to 21% during the third trimester compared with 0.5%–4% in nonpregnant females. Fetal complications and neonatal deaths are increased if the infection is acquired in the third trimester of pregnancy.
   - Herpes simplex hepatitis can be fulminant in pregnancy and associated with high mortality rates. Patients may present in the third trimester with fever, systemic symptoms, and possibly vesicular cutaneous rash. Associated pneumonitis or encephalitis may be present. Liver biopsy is characteristic, showing necrosis and inclusion bodies in viable hepatocytes, along with few or no inflammatory infiltrates. Response to acyclovir therapy is prompt; there is no need for immediate delivery of the baby.

7. **What signs and symptoms suggest the diagnosis of Budd-Chiari syndrome?**
   The clinical triad of sudden onset of abdominal pain, hepatomegaly, and ascites, near-term or shortly after delivery. Ascitic fluid shows a high protein content in approximately one-half of cases. Biopsy typically shows centrilobular hemorrhage and necrosis, along with sinusoidal dilation and erythrocyte extravasation into the space of Disse. Hepatic scintigraphy and computed tomography (CT) typically show compensatory hypertrophy of the caudate lobe resulting from its separate drainage into the inferior vena cava. Doppler analysis of portal and hepatic vessels and magnetic resonance imaging (MRI) establish hepatic vein occlusion.

8. **Is the serum ceruloplasmin level a good diagnostic marker in pregnant females at term who are suspected of having Wilson disease?**
   No. Ceruloplasmin levels increase gradually during pregnancy, reaching the maximum at term. Because of this, in a patient with Wilson disease who usually has a low level of ceruloplasmin, the level may increase misleadingly into the normal range (greater than 20 mg/dL) during pregnancy.

9. **Can we maintain a female with Wilson disease on therapy during pregnancy?**
   Absolutely. Therapy must continue during pregnancy; otherwise, the mother is at risk for hemolytic episodes associated with fulminant hepatic failure. Agents approved by the US Food and Drug Administration (FDA) are D-penicillamine, trientine, and zinc. Evidence indicates that penicillamine and trientine (tissue copper-chelating agents) are teratogenic in animal studies, and there are reports of penicillamine effects in humans, including cutis laxis syndrome or micrognathia, low-set ears, and other abnormalities. According to the current consensus, penicillamine and trientine are safe in doses of 0.75–1 g/day during the first two trimesters; the dosage should be reduced to 0.5 g/day during the last trimester and in nursing mothers. Zinc therapy is an attractive alternative with a different mechanism of action; it induces the synthesis of metallothionein, which sequesters copper in enterocytes, blocking its absorption. No teratogenic effects with zinc have been reported in animals or humans. The recommended doses are 50 mg three times/day for patients with 24-hour urinary copper values greater than 0.1 and 25 mg three times/day for patients with lower urinary copper values. Close monitoring of urinary copper and zinc levels is suggested; the zinc dose should be adjusted accordingly.

INTRAHEPATIC CHOLESTASIS OF PREGNANCY

10. **What is the most common liver disorder unique to pregnancy?**
    IHCP is the most common disorder unique to pregnancy.

11. **What is the major clinical manifestation of IHCP?**
    Severe pruritus with onset in the second or, more commonly, third trimester (more than 70% of cases).

12. **What biochemical changes are noted in IHCP?**
    Serum bile acids, often measured as cholylglycine, increase by 10- to 100-fold. Serum levels of AP rise by 7- to 10-fold, along with a modest rise in serum levels of 5'-nucleotidase (confirming the hepatic source of AP). AST, ALT, and direct bilirubin also rise. No evidence of hemolysis is found. GGTP is usually normal, as is prothrombin time (PT) and international normalized ratio (INR).

13. **What is the expected clinical and biochemical course after delivery for patients with IHCP?**
    Pruritus should improve promptly after delivery (within 24 hours). Jaundice is rare and, if present, may persist for days. Biochemical abnormalities may persist for months.

14. **What is a possible cause for abnormal bleeding in a postpartum female previously diagnosed with IHCP? What is the treatment?**
    Malabsorption of liposoluble vitamins, including vitamin K, especially in patients treated with cholestyramine for pruritus. The INR corrects with parenteral administration of vitamin K.

15. **What is the effect of IHCP on the fetus?**

Fetal distress requiring cesarean section develops in approximately 30%–60% of cases. Prematurity occurs in approximately 50% of cases and fetal death in up to 9% of affected pregnancies. All of these effects are more likely if the disorder begins early in pregnancy.

16. **What is the therapy for IHCP?**

Alleviating pruritus is the main goal. Therapeutic agents include:

Vitamin K before delivery is highly recommended to minimize the risk of postpartum hemorrhage. Mother and fetus should be observed closely. Elective induction is recommended at 36 weeks (severe cases) or 38 weeks (average cases) if the fetal lungs have matured.

- Ursodeoxycholic acid, 15 mg/kg/day; up to 24 mg/kg/day studied with good results
- Cholestyramine, 4 g four or five times/day (bile acid–binding resin)
- Hydroxyzine hydrochloride (Atarax) 25–50 mg every 6 hours as needed, or pamoate (Vistaril, antihistamines) 15–30 mg every 6 hours as needed
- Phenobarbital, 100 mg/day (choleretic and centrally acting sedative)
- Phototherapy with ultraviolet B light as directed by a dermatologist

17. **Can IHCP recur?**

Yes. Approximately 40%–70% of subsequent pregnancies show evidence of mild intrahepatic cholestasis. The same pattern can be seen with the use of estrogen-containing contraceptives.

18. **What atypical signs and symptoms make the diagnosis of IHCP doubtful?**

Fever, hepatosplenomegaly, pain, jaundice preceding or without pruritus, and pruritus after delivery or before 21 weeks of pregnancy, especially with a singleton pregnancy, should prompt the search for an alternate diagnosis.

19. **What biochemical changes suggest an alternate diagnosis?**

- Normal AST and ALT levels
- Elevated AP and GGTP (i.e., biliary disease)
- Predominantly unconjugated hyperbilirubinemia (i.e., hemolysis)

ACUTE FATTY LIVER OF PREGNANCY

20. **What are the clinical and laboratory features of AFLP?**

AFLP is a rare disorder with an incidence of 1 in 13,000 to 1 in 16,000 pregnancies. Onset occurs in the second half of pregnancy, usually during the third trimester, although occasionally postpartum onset is reported. Clinical manifestations include nausea and vomiting, jaundice, malaise, thirst, and altered mental status. Severe cases progress rapidly to hypoglycemia, disseminated intravascular coagulation (DIC), renal insufficiency, coma, and death. Signs of coexistent preeclampsia may be present, such as moderately increased arterial blood pressure, proteinuria, and hyperuricemia. Laboratory abnormalities consist of moderate AST and ALT elevations (usually less than 1000), conjugated hyperbilirubinemia, elevated PT, fibrin split products, and DD-dimers, along with low platelet count, elevated levels of ammonia and serum uric acid, and leukocytosis. Hypoglycemia is a sign of extreme severity; blood glucose levels must be monitored closely.

21. **How do we diagnose and treat AFLP?**

High clinical suspicion is crucial for early recognition and appropriate management. AFLP is suggested by hepatic failure at or near-term or shortly after delivery in the absence of risk factors or serologic findings suggesting viral hepatitis. Thirst, a symptom of underlying vasopressin-resistant diabetes insipidus, is characteristic of AFLP and HELLP syndrome. Liver biopsy, if feasible, is diagnostic in the appropriate clinical context. Treatment consists of admission to the hospital, close monitoring by a multidisciplinary team (hepatologist, maternal-fetal medicine specialist, and intensive care specialist), and immediate delivery. Recovery is usually complete, although it may be delayed in patients with significant clinical complications before delivery (e.g., DIC, renal failure, and infections).

22. **Is biopsy pathognomonic for AFLP?**

Biopsy is confirmatory but not pathognomonic or indispensable in making the diagnosis. Histologic findings are characterized by microvesicular fatty infiltration, mostly in centrilobular zones. In general, lobular and trabecular architecture is preserved, and inflammatory infiltrates and cell necrosis are mild, if present at all. AFLP is a systemic disorder. Similar fatty changes have been noted in pancreatic acinar cells and tubular epithelial cells of the kidneys. The same prominent microvesicular steatosis is seen in other conditions such as Reye syndrome, sodium valproate toxicity, Jamaican vomiting sickness, and congenital defects of urea cycle enzymes or beta-oxidation of fatty acids.

23. **Describe the pathogenesis of AFLP.**

Pathogenesis remains somewhat unclear. In some cases the fetus has an isolated deficiency of long-chain 3-hydroxyacyl-CoA dehydrogenase (LCHAD), which leads to a disorder of mitochondrial fatty acid oxidation. The inheritance pattern is recessive and involves a mutation from glutamic acid to glutamine at amino acid residue 474 (Glu474Gln) on at least one allele. It is hypothesized that in the presence of this mutation in homozygous or compound heterozygote fetuses, long-chain fatty acid metabolites produced by the fetus or placenta accumulate in the mother and are highly toxic to the maternal liver. The mother is phenotypically normal; her genotype does not correlate with the development of AFLP.

24. **What is the outcome of a child whose mother has AFLP?**

Previously reported fetal mortality rates of 75%–90% have been significantly reduced by better awareness, earlier diagnosis, availability of neonatal intensive care units, and institution of close monitoring and dietary treatment through childhood. In pregnancies associated with LCHAD defects, children present at a mean age of 7.6 months (range, 0–60 months) with acute hepatic dysfunction (incidence of 79%). They may experience hypoketotic hypoglycemia, hypotonia, hepatomegaly, hepatic encephalopathy, high transaminase levels, and fatty liver. The condition may progress rapidly to coma and death. Frequent feedings of a low-fat diet in which the fats are medium-chain triglycerides prevent hypoketotic hypoglycemic liver dysfunction. According to recent studies, 67% of children treated with dietary modification are alive, and most attend school.

25. **Does AFLP recur in subsequent pregnancies?**

In the cases associated with LCHAD defects, the disorder is recessive, affecting one in four fetuses. The rate of recurrence of maternal liver disease is 15%–25%.

26. **Is genetic testing indicated in females diagnosed with AFLP?**

All females with AFLP, as well as their partners and children, should be advised to undergo molecular diagnostic testing. Testing for Glu474Gln only in the mother is not sufficient to rule out LCHAD deficiency in the fetus or other family members.

HEMOLYSIS, ELEVATED LIVER ENZYMES, AND LOW PLATELETS

27. **What is the spectrum of liver involvement in preeclampsia?**

Liver involvement in preeclampsia ranges from subclinical, with biopsy evidence of fibrinogen deposition along hepatic sinusoids, to several, possibly severe disorders. In patients with HELLP syndrome the chief complaint is abdominal pain, which usually presents in the second half of gestation but may occur up to 7 days after delivery (almost 30% of affected females). Hepatic infarction is another rare manifestation of liver involvement in preeclampsia. Patients present in the third trimester or early after delivery with unexplained fever, leukocytosis, abdominal or chest pain, and extremely elevated aminotransferases (greater than 3000 U/L). The diagnosis depends on the visualization of hepatic infarcts on CT contrast images or MRI. Subcapsular hematomas and hepatic rupture are life-threatening complications with high morbidity and mortality rates. A high index of suspicion and early CT imaging allow diagnosis and prompt intervention.

28. **How common is HELLP syndrome?**

The incidence of HELLP syndrome is 0.2%–0.6% in all pregnancies and 4%–12% in patients with preeclampsia. The incidence is higher in multiparous, White, and older females, but the mean age of occurrence is around 25 years.

29. **Describe the incidence and prognosis of spontaneous intrahepatic hemorrhage.**

Spontaneous intrahepatic and subcapsular hemorrhage occurs in approximately 1%–2% of patients with preeclampsia, with an estimated incidence of 1 in 45,000 live births. Prognosis improves with awareness, early diagnosis by imaging studies, and aggressive surgical management. Recent reported maternal mortality rates range from 33% to 49%. Fetal mortality remains high (60%).

30. **What findings typically lead to the diagnosis of HELLP syndrome?**

Diagnosis relies on typical laboratory evidence of liver involvement with associated thrombocytopenia. Not all patients have clinical hypertension or proteinuria at presentation. Liver test abnormalities are hepatocellular. Liver function is normal. Thrombocytopenia is present, usually less than 100,000/mm^3. Hemolysis is mild, with microangiopathic findings on peripheral smear. Biopsy is characteristic but may be extremely risky and is not needed for diagnosis. It shows periportal hemorrhage, fibrin deposition, and necrosis, possibly with steatosis or deposition of fibrinogen along sinusoids with focal parenchymal necrosis. A normal biopsy does not exclude the diagnosis, because involvement may be patchy.

31. **What is the treatment for severe preeclamptic liver disease?**

The initial priority is to stabilize the mother by administering intravenous fluids, correcting any concurrent coagulopathy, administering magnesium for seizure prophylaxis, and treating severe hypertension. Early hepatic imaging is indicated to rule out infarcts or hematomas. Fetal functional status should be determined. Fetal outcome is related mostly to gestational age. Beyond 34 weeks of gestation with evidence of fetal lung maturity, delivery is the recommended therapy. If fetal lungs are immature, the fetus can be delivered 48 hours after the administration of two doses of steroids. Delivery should be attempted immediately with evidence of fetal or maternal distress. In cases of ruptured subcapsular hematoma, massive transfusions and immediate surgical intervention are required. In cases where surgical intervention is not possible and there are signs and symptoms of acute liver failure, liver transplantation should be considered for survival. Liver transplantation is usually done under the urgent category "status 1," thus giving top priority for organ offers, and both graft and patient survival outcomes have been excellent.

32. **Does HELLP recur in subsequent pregnancies?**

Possibly. Studies report recurrence risks as low as 3.4% and as high as 25%.

33. **What information helps to differentiate AFLP from HELLP?**

At presentation, AFLP and HELLP may be difficult to differentiate. Hypertension is usually but not invariably associated with HELLP syndrome. Patients with HELLP have mild, predominantly unconjugated hyperbilirubinemia caused by hemolysis, along with severe thrombocytopenia, but no laboratory values suggestive of hepatic failure. Laboratory abnormalities are significantly more severe in AFLP; evidence of hepatic synthetic failure manifests as prolonged PT and significant hypoglycemia in advanced stages. Fibrinogen is low, and ammonia is elevated. Biopsy shows microvesicular steatosis, predominantly in the central zone, in patients with AFLP, whereas patients with HELLP show predominantly periportal fibrin deposition, necrosis, and hemorrhage.

34. **Is prospective screening necessary in pregnancies complicated by AFLP or HELLP?**

From 15% to 20% of pregnancies complicated by AFLP and less than 2% of pregnancies complicated by HELLP syndrome are associated with fetal LCHAD deficiency. Newborns should be screened prospectively at birth in all pregnancies complicated by AFLP. Homozygosity and heterozygosity for Glu474Gln would indicate the need for avoidance of prolonged fasting and replacement of dietary long-chain fatty acids with medium-chain fatty acids. Parents and physicians should be educated on the risk of metabolic crises and sudden death and instructed on the need for early intervention with intravenous glucose during episodes of vomiting, lethargy, and even minor illnesses.

Recent results do not justify routine screening of newborns in pregnancies complicated by HELLP syndrome. Molecular diagnostic testing should, however, be considered in females with recurrent HELLP syndrome in multiple pregnancies.

CARE OF PATIENTS WITH PREEXISTING LIVER DISEASE

BEFORE AND DURING PREGNANCY

- Contraception
- Management of underlying liver disease
- Management of portal hypertension
- Management in the setting of transplantation
- Prevention of vertical transmission

CONTRACEPTION

35. **What methods of contraception are available for patients with liver disease?**

Patients with advanced or untreated liver disease commonly experience amenorrhea and infertility. If clinical improvement leads to restoration of fertility, multiple methods of contraception are available, including barrier methods and intrauterine devices. Tubal ligation may be used in females who have completed their families. Estrogen-based contraceptive agents are generally contraindicated, especially for patients with acute liver disease, but progestin contraceptives are safe alternatives. Combination contraceptives are absolutely contraindicated in patients with cholestatic jaundice of pregnancy or jaundice with prior use, and the World Health Organization has listed them as category 4 type drugs for patients with decompensated cirrhosis of any cause. Numerous formulations and delivery systems are available.

MANAGEMENT OF UNDERLYING LIVER DISEASE

36. **How should patients with preexisting liver disease be managed if pregnancy occurs?**
Patients are best managed by a multidisciplinary team that includes a maternal-fetal medicine specialist, perinatologist, and hepatologist. They have an increased risk for maternal complications along with a higher incidence of fetal loss and prematurity. In general, patients should be maintained on the previous therapy that was successful in controlling liver disease and restoring fertility. Females with autoimmune hepatitis should be continued on corticosteroids alone or in combination with azathioprine, which is not teratogenic at standard doses. Patients with Wilson disease should be continued on the anticopper agent. Patients with portal hypertension should have a baseline endoscopy. If they have never bled and medium or large varices are present, they are at increased risk for variceal hemorrhage during pregnancy. Primary prophylaxis with a nonselective beta-blocker or isosorbide mononitrate should be instituted. The fetus should be monitored for bradycardia or growth retardation if the mother is maintained on beta-blockers. Variceal bleeding is safely managed with variceal band ligation or sclerotherapy. Octreotide in customary doses is safe in pregnancy if needed. Performing surgical portacaval shunts for patients with well-preserved liver function is possible. Placement of a transjugular intrahepatic portosystemic shunt and splenectomy (in patients with massive splenomegaly, varices, and thrombocytopenia) also have been reported.

MANAGEMENT OF PORTAL HYPERTENSION

37. **What are the effects of pregnancy on the mother with portal hypertension?**
The morbidity rate is 30%–50% because of the possible onset of hepatic encephalopathy, spontaneous bacterial peritonitis, and progressive liver failure. The incidence of variceal hemorrhage is 19%–45%, especially in the second trimester and during labor. Postpartum hemorrhage is seen in 7%–10% of females, most frequently in those with cirrhotic portal hypertension; thrombocytopenia plays a major role. The mortality rate of these complication is 4%–7% in patients with noncirrhotic and 10%–18% in patients with cirrhotic portal hypertension. Data regarding this topic originate mostly from case series and prospectively acquired data are few.

38. **What is the effect of maternal portal hypertension on pregnancy?**
Spontaneous abortion rates for patients with cirrhosis range from 15% to 20%. Most cases occur in the first trimester. Of interest, patients with extrahepatic portal hypertension and patients with well-compensated cirrhosis who underwent surgical shunting before conception have abortion rates similar to the general population. The incidence of premature termination of pregnancy in the second and third trimesters is similar in all previously mentioned groups. Fetal mortality rates are approximately 50% if the mother requires emergent surgical intervention for variceal hemorrhage. Perinatal mortality rates in mothers with cirrhosis are as high as 11%–18% because of premature delivery, stillbirth, and neonatal death, but they are similar to those for the general population in patients with noncirrhotic portal hypertension and patients who underwent previous portal surgical decompressive procedures.

MANAGEMENT IN THE SETTING OF ORTHOTOPIC LIVER TRANSPLANTATION

39. **When can a liver transplant recipient actively seek conception?**

At least a 1-year waiting period is advisable. Case reports suggest that conception close to the transplant date may result in increased maternal and fetal morbidity and mortality. Contraception should be instituted before resuming sexual relations, preferably with barrier methods.

40. **Is pregnancy possible after liver transplantation?**
Pregnancy will become possible once normal menstrual cycles resume. In females with chronic liver disease, most pretransplant amenorrhea resolves in approximately 3–10 months following liver transplantation.

41. **What are the possible complications of pregnancies occurring after liver transplantation?**
Hypertensive complications, preterm delivery, infection, and fetal growth restriction are possible complications. Immunosuppressive agents used such as cyclosporine and tacrolimus cause hypertension and renal insufficiency, as well as impairment of placental amino acid transport systems, leading to fetal growth restriction. Cytomegalovirus (CMV) infection can cause congenital anomalies and liver disease if the mother was infected early in the pregnancy. Risk for CMV infection is greatest immediately after transplant or in case of increased immunosuppression caused by rejection episodes. Rejection is a rare complication; only approximately 10% of the reported pregnancies have been complicated by biopsy-proved rejection.

42. **What is recommended in the management of a pregnancy occurring following liver transplantation?**
Management as high-risk pregnancy by a specialist in maternal-fetal medicine is preferred. Immunosuppression should be continued with close monitoring of blood levels. Abnormal liver function tests should be evaluated aggressively. Percutaneous liver biopsy is not contraindicated but should be performed under ultrasound guidance. Monitoring for maternal and fetal CMV infection is indicated. Quantitative CMV immunoglobulins or detection of CMV viremia and viruria in the mother are adequate tests, and even amniotic fluid analysis could be used if there is suspicion of fetal infection. Deliveries should be via cesarean section if there are active herpes simplex lesions present. Prophylactic antibiotics should be used for deliveries in general.

43. **What are pregnancy safety data regarding maintenance immunosuppressive agents used in orthotopic liver transplantation?**
- Category B (no evidence of risk in humans): prednisone
- Category C (risks cannot be ruled out): cyclosporine, tacrolimus (FK506), rapamycin (sirolimus), OKT3, antithymocyte globulin, and antilymphocyte globulin
- Category D (evidence of risk): azathioprine
- Category D with black box warning (high risk: mutagenic/teratogenic): mycophenolate mofetil (CellCept and Myfortic). It is advised that anyone pregnant or wishing to become pregnant be changed to azathioprine.

44. **Is breastfeeding permitted after delivery in a liver transplant recipient?**
Prior recommendations had been to not breastfeed while on immunosuppressive drugs. More recent data have supported the safety of breastfeeding while on prednisone, azathioprine, cyclosporine, and tacrolimus. There is inadequate information on m-Tor inhibitors (sirolimus, everolimus), mycophenolate, and belatacept. Manufacturer recommends against breastfeeding in mothers administered interferon therapy, ribavirin, and ganciclovir. No specific recommendation can be made regarding foscarnet. No data are available regarding ursodeoxycholic acid excretion in breast milk. LACTMED database can be a resource for information to discuss the risk and benefits of female transplant recipients wishing to breastfeed.

45. **Are immunosuppressive agents safe during pregnancy?**
Corticosteroids, azathioprine, cyclosporine, tacrolimus, and OKT3 have no apparent teratogenic potential. All may contribute to low birth weights and fetal prematurity. Tacrolimus crosses the placenta and may contribute to transient perinatal hyperkalemia and mild, reversible renal impairment. There are no reports of allograft loss as a result of pregnancy in the tacrolimus-treated group of 35 patients at the University of Pittsburgh. The Philadelphia-based cyclosporine registry reports an allograft rejection rate of 17% and a graft loss rate of 5.7% in 35 patients taking cyclosporine during gestation and the postpartum period. Mycophenolate mofetil should not be used during pregnancy because of increased risks of birth defects and miscarriage. Patients should have one pregnancy test immediately before starting mycophenolate mofetil and another pregnancy test 8–10 days later. Pregnancy tests should be repeated during routine follow-up visits. Patients should be counseled about acceptable birth control during mycophenolate mofetil therapy, and continue birth control for 6 weeks after it is discontinued. A risk evaluation and mitigation strategy was mandated by the FDA to minimize the risks associated with mycophenolate mofetil use in the childbearing population.

PREVENTION OF VERTICAL TRANSMISSION

46. **How may vertical transmission of viral hepatitis A be prevented?**
Maternal infection with the hepatitis A virus (HAV) is not associated with fetal loss or teratogenic effects. Vertical transmission of HAV is rare. There are no restrictions concerning breastfeeding. Passive immunization can be performed with immunoglobulin for urgent postexposure prophylaxis. HAV vaccine is safe and recommended for pregnant females who are at the risk of acquiring the disease, such as females traveling to endemic areas.

47. **How may vertical transmission of viral hepatitis B be prevented?**
The hepatitis B virus (HBV) may be transmitted vertically. If the mother acquires HBV in the first trimester of pregnancy, there is a 10% risk that the infant will test positive for hepatitis B surface antigen (HBsAg) at birth. The percentage dramatically increases to 80%–90% if the acute maternal infection develops during the third trimester. In mothers who have chronic hepatitis B and test positive for the hepatitis B e-antigen (HBeAg), 90% of neonates develop chronic hepatitis B without prophylaxis. If the mother has HBeAg- and hepatitis B e-antibody (HBeAb)-negative chronic hepatitis B, 40% of neonates develop chronic hepatitis B infection without prophylaxis. The rate decreases to less than 5% if the mother is HBeAg-negative and HBeAb-positive. Antepartum serum HBsAg testing is mandatory. Neonates of HBsAg-positive mothers or HBsAg status–unknown mothers are treated with HBV human hyperimmunoglobulin, 0.5 mL intramuscularly, at delivery. At the same time, they are given the

first dose of HBV vaccine within 12 hours of delivery. The second dose is administered at 1 month of age, and the third dose at 6 months of age. If the mother is HBsAg-negative, the child should be vaccinated only with the three-dose regimen, with the first inoculation at birth. The regimen is approximately 85% effective in preventing chronic hepatitis B in neonates and is ineffective in cases of hematogenous transplacental transmission, which are seen in approximately 15% of pregnancies as a result of small placental tears. Active and passive immunization at birth also reduces the possibility of viral transmission by breastfeeding. Hepatitis B vaccination is safe in pregnant females. Lamivudine, telbivudine, and tenofovir have been studied and have no associated teratogenicity. Tenofovir disoproxil fumarate (TDF) has a higher barrier to resistance and is the recommended option for antiviral therapy at this time. General recommendations are to offer antiviral therapy with TDF at 28–32 weeks of gestation if HBV DNA is greater than 200,000 IU/mL as prophylaxis against vertical transmission, if HBV DNA is greater than 7-log IU/mL then treatment should be initiated early to allow time for an adequate decline in the HBV viral load.

48. **What is the risk of vertical transmission of viral hepatitis C?**
The risk of perinatal transmission is approximately 2% for infants of anti–hepatitis C virus (HCV) seropositive females. When a pregnant female is HCV RNA–positive at delivery, this risk increases to 4%–7%. Higher HCV RNA levels appear to be associated with a greater risk. Levels of RNA of 1 million copies/mL are reportedly associated with vertical transmission rates as high as 50%. HCV transmission increases up to 20% in females coinfected with HCV and human immunodeficiency virus (HIV). There are currently no data to determine whether antiviral therapy reduces perinatal transmission. Immunoglobulin therapy is ineffective. The rate of infection is similar among first- and second-born children.

49. **Is it possible to prevent vertical transmission of viral hepatitis D and G?**
Perinatal transmission of the hepatitis D virus (HDV) is rare. There are no documented cases of vertical transmission of HDV in the United States. No clinical data about hepatitis G infection during pregnancy are available, and no studies of vertical transmission have been done. Because of the lack of data on HDV, recommendations regarding breastfeeding are unknown.

50. **Are HCV-infected females allowed to breastfeed?**
Current available studies show that the average rate of infection is 4%, similar for breastfed and bottle-fed infants. According to the Centers for Disease Control and Prevention and a 1997 consensus statement from the National Institutes of Health (NIH) and the American Association for the Study of Liver Diseases guidelines, breastfeeding is not contraindicated for HCV-positive mothers. The risk of transmission by breastfeeding was not found to be significant unless coinfection with HIV was present. There are general recommendations to temporarily hold breastfeeding if there is significant skin breakdown.

51. **Does the mode of delivery influence hepatitis C transmission?**
Current data are limited but indicate that infection rates are similar in infants delivered vaginally and cesarean-delivered infants. There are no prospective studies evaluating the use of elective cesarean section for the prevention of mother-to-infant transmission of HCV. However, avoiding fetal scalp monitoring and prolonged labor after rupture of membranes may reduce the risk of transmission to the infant.

52. **How can perinatal HCV infection be diagnosed?**
Infants passively acquire maternal antibodies that can persist for months. Anti-HCV antibodies after 15 months of age or positive HCV RNA, which can be detected as early as 1 or 2 months, are diagnostic of perinatal transmission of HCV. A recent NIH consensus conference recommends that infants born to HCV-positive mothers be tested for HCV infection by HCV RNA tests on two occasions between the ages of 2 and 6 months and/or have tests for anti-HCV after 15 months of age. Positive anti-HCV in infants prior to 15 months of age may be due to transplacental transfer of maternal anti-HCV antibody.

CLINICAL VIGNETTE

Available Online

BIBLIOGRAPHY

Available Online

WEBSITES

Available Online

CHAPTER 22

RHEUMATOLOGIC MANIFESTATIONS OF HEPATOBILIARY DISEASES

Kristine A. Kuhn, MD, PhD, FACR

 Additional content available online.

VIRAL HEPATITIS

1. **How often is viral hepatitis associated with rheumatic manifestations?**
   Approximately 25% of patients with hepatitis B and up to 50% of patients with hepatitis C develop a rheumatic syndrome. Transient arthralgias can occur in 10% of patients during acute hepatitis A viral infection.

2. **What are the most common extrahepatic rheumatologic manifestations of hepatitis B infection?**
   - Acute polyarthritis: dermatitis syndrome
   - Polyarteritis nodosa (PAN)
   - Membranous or membranoproliferative glomerulonephritis
   - Cryoglobulinemia: usually associated with hepatitis C; only 5% of all essential mixed cryoglobulinemia is due to hepatitis B alone

3. **Describe the clinical characteristics of the polyarthritis-dermatitis syndrome associated with hepatitis B infection.**
   In the preicteric prodromal period of acute hepatitis B infection, 10%–25% of patients develop a polyarthritis that is acute, severe, and symmetric, involving both small (fingers) and large (knees and ankles) joints. Classically, an urticarial rash frequently (40%) accompanies the arthritis. Both arthritis and rash can precede the onset of jaundice or transaminitis by several days. Arthritis improves with nonsteroidal anti-inflammatory drugs and usually subsides soon after the onset of jaundice. Patients who develop chronic hepatitis B viremia may subsequently have recurrent arthralgias or arthritis. This syndrome is caused by the deposition of circulating hepatitis B surface antigen-hepatitis B surface antibody immune complexes in the joints and skin.

4. **What is the typical presentation of hepatitis B–associated PAN?**
   Up to 10% of all patients with PAN have positive hepatitis B serologic findings and evidence of viral replication (hepatitis B e-antigen and hepatitis B virus DNA). They may present with a combination of fever, arthritis, mononeuritis multiplex, abdominal pain, renal disease, or cardiac disease. Although liver-associated enzymes may be abnormal, symptomatic hepatitis is not a prominent feature.

5. **How is PAN associated with hepatitis B antigenemia diagnosed?**
   The diagnosis is made on the basis of a consistent clinical presentation coupled with an abdominal or renal angiogram showing vascular aneurysms and corkscrewing of blood vessels, often referred to as "beads on a string" (Fig. 22.1). The gold standard is a tissue biopsy showing medium-vessel vasculitis.

6. **What is the treatment of hepatitis B–associated PAN?**
   Patients are typically very ill and will die without aggressive therapy. Antiviral agents and plasmapheresis for the removal of immune complexes are used early to control acute symptoms and antigenemia. Corticosteroids (1 mg/kg/d) are also used early to control inflammation. Once the acute process is controlled, corticosteroids are tapered (usually over 2–3 weeks) because they, alone or in combination with cytotoxic drugs, can enhance viral replication. Cyclophosphamide should be avoided. Patients older than 50 years of age and those with renal insufficiency or cardiac, gastrointestinal, or central nervous system involvement have the worst prognosis. The overall 5-year survival rate is 50%–70%.

7. **What are the most common hepatitis C virus (HCV)–related autoimmune disorders?**
   - Mixed (types II and III) cryoglobulinemia (40%–60% of patients with HCV have cryoglobulins but only ~10% develop vasculitis). Older age and longer duration of HCV infection increase the likelihood of cryoglobulins.
   - Systemic PAN–like vasculitis (<1% of patients with HCV).

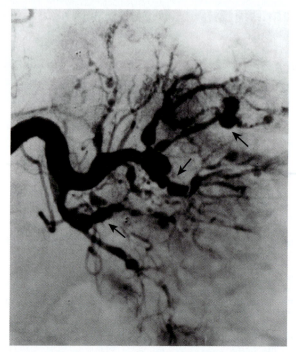

Fig. 22.1 Renal angiogram showing vascular aneurysms in a patient with hepatitis B–associated polyarteritis nodosa (*arrows*).

- Membranoproliferative glomerulonephritis.
- Nonerosive polyarthritis (2%–20%): patients with acute hepatitis C infection can have an acute (usually transient) polyarthritis resembling rheumatoid arthritis (RA) with involvement of hands, wrists, shoulders, knees, and hips symmetrically. Although these patients are frequently rheumatoid factor (RF)-positive because of cryoglobulinemia, they do not have anti-cyclic citrullinated peptide antibodies. Other patients have intermittent monoarthritis or oligoarthritis affecting large- and medium-sized joints.
- Autoantibody production (40%–65%): RF, antinuclear antibodies (ANAs), anticardiolipin antibodies, anti-smooth muscle antibodies, anti-liver kidney microsomal antibody 1, and antithyroid antibodies.
- Sjögren-like syndrome with dry eyes and dry mouth (5%–19%): caused by lymphocytic sialadenitis. Anti-SS-A(Ro) and anti-SS-B(La) antibodies are negative.
- Autoimmune thrombocytopenia, myasthenia gravis, and sarcoidosis have been rarely associated with HCV infection or its therapy.

8. **What is the relationship between viral hepatitis and cryoglobulinemia?**
   Approximately 80%–90% of patients with essential mixed cryoglobulinemia (types II and III) are positive for hepatitis C. Hepatitis C viral RNA and anti-HCV antibodies are found within the cryoprecipitate. Cryoglobulins are thought to form because of HCV's predilection to bind to B lymphocytes via CD81, which lowers the activation threshold for these cells, facilitating autoantibody production and cryoglobulinemia. Also, HCV can infect B cells, causing proto-oncogene *bcl-2* recombination, which inhibits apoptosis, leading to extended B cell survival. This results in cryoglobulinemia and neoplastic transformation (non-Hodgkin B cell lymphomas). Antiviral therapy reduces cryoglobulins and their clinical manifestations in most cases.

9. **Describe the typical clinical features of cryoglobulinemia associated with hepatitis C infection.**
   A cryoglobulin is an immunoglobulin that precipitates at temperatures of less than 37°C and redissolves with rewarming. They precipitate in blood vessels in patients, causing inflammation and a variety of symptoms. Patients present with a combination of fever, arthritis (which can be confused with RA), renal disease, paresthesias from peripheral neuropathy, and a predominantly lower extremity petechial rash, positive RF, and low complement levels (especially C4). Hepatitis is not a prominent feature. Patients have been successfully treated with combined corticosteroids, peginterferon α-2b/ribavirin/protease inhibitor combination, and plasmapheresis. Refractory or severe cases are treated with rituximab (anti-CD20) to deplete the B cell population making the cryoglobulins.

AUTOIMMUNE AND OTHER LIVER DISEASES

10. What is autoimmune hepatitis (AIH)?

AIH (formerly called lupoid hepatitis) can occur in all age groups, but most patients are young (bimodal peak 10–20 and 45–70 years old) and predominantly females (~70%). Many patients have clinical (arthralgias and rashes) and laboratory (e.g., ANA) manifestations that may resemble systemic lupus erythematosus (SLE). Patients commonly have positive ANAs (40%–60%), antibodies against smooth muscle antigen (90%) frequently with specificity against F-actin, anti-soluble liver antigen/liver pancreas antibodies, antineutrophil cytoplasmic antibodies (atypical p-ANCA), antimitochondrial antibodies (AMAs), anti-DNA antibodies, anti-liver-kidney microsomal-1 and -3 antibodies, and anti-liver cytosol antibodies. Hypergammaglobulinemia (immunoglobulin G) is usually present (~70%). Type I AIH often overlaps with other autoimmune diseases and has been described in patients with SLE, Sjögren syndrome, mixed connective tissue disease, and limited systemic sclerosis.

11. To what degree is type I AIH similar to SLE?

See Table 22.1 for the comparison of type I AIH and SLE.

Table 22.1 Comparison of Type I Autoimmune Hepatitis (AIH) and Systemic Lupus Erythematosus (SLE).

	SLE	TYPE I AIH
Young females	+	+
Polyarthritis	+	+
Fever	+	+
Rash	+	+
Nephritis	+	−
Central nervous system disease	+	−
Photosensitivity	+	−
Oral ulcers	+	−
ANA	99%	70%
Polyclonal gammopathy	+	+
Anti-Smith antibodies	25%	−
Anti-dsDNA	70%	25%–35%
Anti-F-actin	Rare	60%–95%
ASMA	−	65%
Anti-SLA/LP antibodies	−	10%–30%

ANA, Antinuclear antibody; *ASMA*, anti-smooth muscle antibody; *dsDNA*, double-stranded deoxyribonucleic acid; *SLA/LP*, soluble liver antigen/liver pancreas.

12. What is the difference between anti-Sm and anti-SM antibodies?

Anti-Sm antibodies are antibodies against the Smith antigen, which is an epitope on small ribonuclear proteins. It is highly diagnostic of SLE. The anti-SM antibody is an antibody against the smooth muscle antigen (which is frequently F-actin). It is highly diagnostic of type I AIH (Table 22.2).

Table 22.2 Anti-Smith (Anti-Sm) Versus Anti-Smooth Muscle (Anti-SM) Antibodies.

	SLE	TYPE I AIH
Anti-Sm antibodies	Yes	No
Anti-SM antibodies	No	Yes

AIH, Autoimmune hepatitis; *SLE*, systemic lupus erythematosus.

13. **List the common autoimmune diseases associated with primary biliary cirrhosis (PBC).**
Approximately 50% of patients with PBC have one or more additional autoimmune diseases. The following disorders are most commonly seen:
    - Keratoconjunctivitis sicca (mostly secondary Sjögren syndrome): 40%–60%.
    - Autoimmune thyroiditis (Hashimoto disease): 10–15%.
    - Raynaud phenomenon: 20%.
    - RA: 5%–10%.
    - Limited systemic sclerosis (calcinosis, Raynaud phenomenon, esophageal, telangiectasia [CREST]) occurs in 5%–15% of patients with PBC and antedates PBC by an average of 14 years. Most have anticentromere antibodies.
    - Others: pernicious anemia (4%), celiac disease, SLE (1.5%), and polymyositis.

14. **Compare and contrast the arthritis that may occur with PBC and RA.**
See Table 22.3 for the comparison and contrast between PBC and RA.

Table 22.3 Primary Biliary Cirrhosis (PBC) Arthritis Versus Rheumatoid Arthritis (RA).

	PBC ARTHRITIS	RA
Frequency in patients	10% develop RA	1%–10% develop PBC
No. of joints[a]	Polyarticular	Polyarticular
Symmetry	Symmetric	Symmetric
Inflammatory	Yes	Yes
Rheumatoid factor	Sometimes	Yes (85%)
Anti-CCP antibodies	Rare	Yes (~80%)
Erosions on radiograph	Rare	Common

CCP, Cyclic citrullinated peptide.
[a]PBC can involve distal interphalangeal joints of fingers, whereas RA does not involve these joints.

15. **What other musculoskeletal manifestations may occur in patients with PBC?**
    - Osteomalacia caused by fat-soluble vitamin D malabsorption (low 25-OH vitamin D level).
    - Osteoporosis caused by renal tubular acidosis.
    - Hypertrophic osteoarthropathy.

16. **What autoantibodies commonly occur in patients with PBC?**
The most common and diagnostic antibody is the AMA seen in 80%–90% of patients with PBC. This antibody is directed against various mitochondrial enzymes, most commonly the E2 component of the pyruvate dehydrogenase complex. Approximately 60% of patients have one or more autoantibodies other than AMA including:
    - ANAs: 20%–50%.
    - Antiphospholipid antibodies (usually immunoglobulin M): 15%–20%.
    - Anticentromere antibodies: 15%–20%.
    - Most patients also have manifestations of the CREST variant of limited systemic sclerosis.

17. **How commonly does arthritis occur in patients with hereditary hemochromatosis (HHC)?**
Approximately 40%–75% of patients have a noninflammatory degenerative arthritis, most commonly involving the second and third metacarpophalangeal (MCP) joints, proximal interphalangeal joints, wrists, hips, knees, and ankles. Of importance, this arthropathy may be the presenting complaint (30%–50%) of patients with hemochromatosis and is frequently misdiagnosed in young males as seronegative RA.

18. **Describe the radiographic features suggestive of hemochromatotic arthropathy (HA).**
Suggestive radiographic features include subchondral sclerosis, cyst formation, irregular joint space narrowing, chondrocalcinosis, and osteophyte formation consistent with degenerative arthritis of involved joints. The key finding is degenerative changes in the MCP joints (typically second and third) with hook-like osteophytes (Fig. 22.2). This finding is important, because the MCP joints and wrists rarely develop degenerative joint disease without an underlying cause such as hemochromatosis.

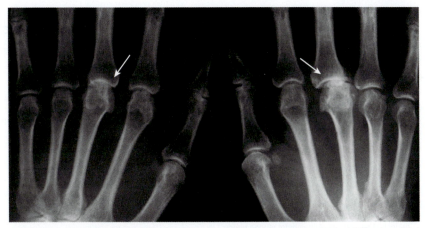

Fig. 22.2 Radiographs of hands showing degenerative arthritis with hook-like osteophytes of the second and third metacarpophalangeal joints in a patient with hemochromatosis (*arrows*).

19. **What is the relationship between calcium pyrophosphate disease and hemochromatosis?**

Chondrocalcinosis of the triangular fibrocartilage at the ulnar side of the wrist and the hyaline cartilage of the knees is seen in 20%–50% of patients with hemochromatosis. Crystals of calcium pyrophosphate may shed into the joints, causing superimposed flares of inflammatory arthritis (i.e., pseudogout).

20. **Discuss the genetics of HHC.**

HHC is among the most common genetic disorders in Whites of northern European descent. There are four types of HHC, and all are related to genetic mutations. Classic HHC (type 1) is the most common type (80%). It is autosomal recessive and associated with a mutation of the *HFE* gene on chromosome 6 that encodes for a protein involved in the regulation of iron absorption. Between 80% and 90% of patients are homozygous for the same mutation (C282Y) of this gene. The homozygote frequency in the White population is 0.3%–0.5%, and the carrier frequency is 7%–10% (i.e., heterozygotes). However, not all patients homozygous for this *HFE* mutation develop clinical manifestations of iron overload (28% of male and 1% of female homozygotes over 12 years). Therefore other genes as well as environmental factors (alcohol, etc.) may play a role in modifying the phenotypic expression of iron overload.

21. **Compare and contrast the features of HA and RA.**

See Table 22.4 for the comparison and contrast between HA and RA.

Table 22.4 Comparison of Hemochromatotic Arthropathy and Rheumatoid Arthritis.

	HEMOCHROMATOTIC ARTHROPATHY	RHEUMATOID ARTHRITIS
Sex	M > F (10:1)	F > M (3:1)
Age of onset	>35 years	All ages
Joints	Polyarticular	Polyarticular
Symmetry	Symmetric	Symmetric
Inflammatory signs and symptoms	Only if pseudogout attack	Yes
Rheumatoid factor	Negative	Positive (85%)
Anti-CCP antibody	Negative	Positive (~80%)
Gene	*HFE* (90%)	HLA DR4 (70%)
Synovial fluid	Noninflammatory	Inflammatory
Radiographs	Degenerative changes	Inflammatory and erosive disease

CCP, Cyclic citrullinated peptide; *F*, female; *HFE*, hemochromatosis gene; *HLA*, human leukocyte antigen; *M*, male.

22. **How effective is phlebotomy in halting the progression of HA?**
Phlebotomy does not halt the progression of arthropathy.

23. **What is the correlation between the severity of arthropathy and severity of liver disease in hemochromatosis?**
There is no correlation.

24. **Why does hemochromatosis cause a degenerative arthritis?**
Arthropathy is characterized by hemosiderin deposition in synovium and chondrocytes. The presence of iron in these cells may lead to increased production of destructive enzymes (e.g., matrix metalloproteinases), free radical generation, or crystal deposition that causes cartilage damage. Other mechanisms also may be possible; the precise pathway by which chronic iron overload leads to tissue injury has not been fully established.

25. **What other musculoskeletal problems may occur in patients with hemochromatosis?**
   - Osteoporosis caused by gonadal dysfunction from pituitary insufficiency caused by the iron overload state (low follicle-stimulating hormone, luteinizing hormone, and testosterone).
   - Osteomalacia caused by vitamin D deficiency resulting from liver disease (low 25-OH vitamin D level).
   - Hypertrophic osteoarthropathy—cirrhosis of any cause including hemochromatosis can be associated with periosteal reaction involving shafts of long bones.

CLINICAL VIGNETTE

Available Online

BIBLIOGRAPHY

Available Online

WEBSITES

Available Online

CHAPTER 23

EVALUATION OF FOCAL LIVER MASSES

Mark W. Russo, MD, MPH and Roshan Shrestha, MD

 Additional content available online

1. Describe the initial workup for a patient with a liver mass.

When evaluating a patient with a liver mass one of the key issues is determining if the mass is benign or malignant. This can frequently be determined by obtaining an accurate history and physical examination. Important historical questions include a previous history of malignancy, particularly breast and colon, which commonly metastasize to the liver. In patients with cirrhosis who have a liver mass a primary hepatic malignancy must be excluded. Risk factors for chronic viral hepatitis B or C, nonalcoholic fatty liver disease, or a history of heavy alcohol use raise the possibility of a primary malignant process, particularly hepatocellular carcinoma (HCC). Physical exam findings of abdominal distension and ascites, splenomegaly, or stigmata of chronic liver disease, such as palmar erythema, spider angiomata, or gynecomastia, may be present. Hepatic adenoma may be associated with oral contraceptives or anabolic steroids.

Liver enzymes, with the exception of gamma-glutamyl transpeptidase, are usually normal with benign liver tumors. Serum alkaline phosphatase levels may be elevated with hepatic metastases, but not in all cases, and total bilirubin may be elevated if the mass is causing obstruction of the biliary system, such as cholangiocarcinoma or pancreatic adenocarcinoma. An increase in serum transaminases may signify chronic hepatitis or cirrhosis. Positive hepatitis B surface antigen or hepatitis C viral load or iron saturation may identify an underlying cause of liver dysfunction or cirrhosis. See Table 23.1.

Table 23.1 Differential Diagnosis of Focal Liver Masses in Adults.

BENIGN	MALIGNANT
Epithelial Tumors	
Hepatic adenoma	Hepatocellular carcinoma
Bile duct adenoma	Cholangiocarcinoma
Biliary cystadenoma	Biliary cystadenocarcinoma
	Fibrolamellar
	Hepatocellular carcinoma
Mesenchymal Tumors	
Cavernous hemangioma	Angiosarcoma
	Primary hepatic lymphoma
Other Lesions	
Focal nodular hyperplasia	Metastatic tumors
Liver abscess	
Macroregenerative nodules in cirrhosis	
Focal fatty infiltration	
Simple hepatic cyst	

Modified from Kew MC. Tumors of the liver. In Zakim, D, Boyer, TD, eds. Hepatology: A Textbook of Liver Disease. 2nd ed. Philadelphia, PA: W.B. Saunders; 1990:1206-1239.

2. What tumor markers are useful in the evaluation of focal liver lesions?

Serum alpha-fetoprotein (AFP) and carbohydrate-associated antigen CA 19-9 (cholangiocarcinoma carbohydrate antigen 19) are markers of primary hepatic malignancy and are used when radiographic studies indicate a focal neoplasm originating in the liver. Mild elevations in AFP are sensitive for detecting HCC, while higher elevations are more specific. Carcinoembryonic antigen is used to measure adenocarcinomas, particularly colon cancer.

Although it has its limitations, AFP is the best widely available diagnostic marker for HCC and also plays a role in screening programs for at-risk populations. AFP levels above 200 ng/mL are highly suggestive of HCC, whereas lesser elevations may be due to benign chronic hepatitis and may not indicate the presence of HCC. A universally accepted cutoff value for AFP in the diagnosis of HCC has not been established, and levels of >200 ng/mL have greater than 90% specificity for HCC. Not all hepatomas secrete AFP, and approximately one-third of patients have a normal AFP value, especially when the tumor is smaller than 2 cm. AFP levels are useful to follow after treatment for HCC and should decrease or normalize with successful treatment. Other tumor markers that have been studied for the detection of hepatocellular include AFP-L3% (lens culinaris agglutinin-reactive fraction of AFP) and des-gamma-carboxy prothrombin (DCP). The sensitivity and specificity of AFP-L3% and DCP for HCC have been reported to be 56% and 90% and 87% and 85%, respectively. The American Association for the Study of Liver Diseases guidelines recommend AFP and right upper quadrant ultrasound for HCC surveillance.

CA 19-9 is used in the diagnosis of cholangiocarcinoma, a malignancy originating in the bile ducts. CA 19-9 levels >100 U/mL are found in over 50% of patients and values >1000 suggest unresectability. This marker is more sensitive in patients with primary sclerosing cholangitis (PSC), a risk factor for cholangiocarcinoma. Significant false-positive elevations in CA 19-9 can occur with bacterial cholangitis or nonmalignant obstruction, such as benign strictures or gallstones. CA 19-9 also serves as a tumor marker for pancreatic carcinoma. Although widely used, CA 19-9 has no proven benefit for screening of cholangiocarcinoma and may create undue anxiety when elevated because it is nonspecific.

3. **What imaging modalities are used in the detection and characterization of focal liver masses?**

Recent advances in computed tomography (CT) and magnetic resonance imaging (MRI) allow detailed assessment of focal liver lesions. These imaging studies with advances in contrast agents for MRI have largely supplanted previously used nuclear medicine–based protocols for the characterization of liver masses.

Triphasic CT, which is now widely available, offers a substantial improvement in hepatic imaging because of its rapid scan time within a single breath-hold. This feature eliminates respiratory motion and allows contrast injection to be viewed in unenhanced, arterial (early or late), portal venous phases of perfusion, and delayed phases after portal venous perfusion. Lesions that derive their vascular supply from the hepatic artery, such as HCC and hypervascular metastases, are prominent during the arterial phase. The venous or portal phase of helical CT provides maximal enhancement of normal liver parenchyma and optimizes the detection of hypovascular lesions, such as colon, gastric, and pancreatic metastases. CT may be preferred in patients with cirrhosis who are claustrophobic or cannot hold their breath for MRI or in patients with ascites which creates motion of the liver and artifact on MRI.

MRI scanning has undergone refinements to reduce motion artifact, with breath-hold T1-weighted images and fast (turbo) spin-echo T2-weighted sequences, and makes use of contrast agents to differentiate hepatocytes from cholangiocytes. Gadolinium-enhanced MRI should be considered in patients with contraindications to iodine-based CT, such as contrast allergies or renal insufficiency if the estimated glomerular filtration rate (eGFR) is greater than 30 mL/min/1.73 m². Nephrogenic systemic fibrosis (NSF) is a rare serious condition associated with gadolinium-based contrast agents associated with eGFR less than 30 mL/min/1.73 m². Thus, although MRI may be preferred to CT in patients with renal failure, caution should be taken to avoid NSF which can be fatal. MRI also has the benefit of obtaining images of the biliary tree (magnetic resonance cholangiopancreatography [MRCP]) in patients with suspected biliary tract tumors or biliary obstruction. Despite refinements in image acquisition MR images may be degraded in patients who cannot hold their breath or move due to claustrophobia.

Liver Imaging Reporting and Data System (LI-RADS) was developed by the American College of Radiology as a standardized method to report liver lesions and imaging findings. In many cases a biopsy of a liver mass does not need to be obtained in patients with cirrhosis if the mass meets LI-RADS-5 imaging characteristics. LI-RADS categories range from 1 to 5 with an increasing probability that a liver mass is malignant. For example, a patient with cirrhosis of the liver who has a mass that meets LI-RADS-5 criteria then it is >95% certainty the mass is HCC even if the AFP is normal.

Contrast-enhanced ultrasonography has been studied outside of the United States as a modality to distinguish benign from malignant lesions. This modality may decrease costs and exposure to radiation but is not widely available in the United States because the contrast agents for ultrasound are not US Food and Drug Administration approved.

Many focal liver masses are found incidentally on ultrasound examination of the abdomen. Although liver ultrasound often cannot fully characterize the lesion, it has a role in verifying simple hepatic cysts, which may have nonspecific radiographic patterns on CT or MRI. Hepatic cysts are common and present in up to 10% of the population. More than five hepatic cysts or cysts with septations warrant further investigation because the patient may have polycystic liver disease or biliary cystadenoma. See Chapter 69 for a comprehensive discussion of imaging options and examples for the evaluation of liver lesions. See Table 23.2.

Table 23.2 Computed Tomography (CT) Versus Magnetic Resonance Imaging (MRI) for Evaluating a Liver Mass.

WHICH TEST SHOULD BE ORDERED CT OR MRI TO EVALUATE A LIVER MASS?		
	CT	**MRI**
Claustrophobic	X	
Estimated GFR 30–40 mL/min		X
Ascites	X	
Magnetized foreign body	X	
Distinguish adenoma from FNH		X
Suspect bile leak		X (with MRCP)[a]

FNH, Focal nodular hyperplasia; *GFR*, glomerular filtration rate; *HIDA*, hepatobiliary iminodiacetic acid; *MRCP*, magnetic resonance cholangiopancreatography.
[a]HIDA scan is a nuclear imaging study that is also an excellent diagnostic test if bile leak is strongly suspected but does not evaluate hepatic parenchyma.

4. **What is the most common benign cause of a focal liver lesion?**
   Cavernous hemangiomas are the most common benign hepatic tumor, occurring in up to 20% of the population. They occur in all age groups, more commonly in women, as solitary (60%) or multiple asymptomatic masses. Most are <3 cm and usually occur in the posterior segment of the right hepatic lobe. The term giant hemangioma is sometimes used when the size exceeds 5 cm. Rarely, hemangiomas are large enough to cause abdominal pain and if compressing the suspect or other organs may require resection. However, even for giant hemangioma, the risk of tumor growth or bleeding is minimal and does not justify surgical removal unless the patient is significantly symptomatic. Microscopically, hemangiomas consist of blood-filled vascular sinusoids separated by connective tissue septae. Kasabach-Merritt syndrome is a rare condition associated with hepatic hemangioma, consumption coagulopathy, and thrombocytopenia that can be treated surgically.

5. **Why is oral contraceptive use important in the differential diagnosis of focal liver masses?**
   Most cases of hepatic adenomas are associated with long-term use of oral contraceptive pills. This benign tumor was rarely seen before oral contraceptive agents came into common usage in the 1960s. Risk correlates with the duration of use and age >30 years. Hepatic adenomas most commonly occur in young and middle-aged women, with an incidence of 3–4 per 100,000. Men infrequently develop adenomas, although cases have been reported with anabolic steroid use.
   Hepatic adenomas are well-demarcated, fleshy tumors with prominent surface vasculature. Microscopically, they consist of monotonous sheets of normal or small hepatocytes with no bile ducts, portal tracts, or central veins. MRI is the imaging modality of choice to determine if a liver mass is a hepatic adenoma because the contrast agent gadoxetate disodium (Eovist) is excreted by the biliary system. Because adenomas do not have bile duct gadoxetate disodium will not uptake the contrast and adenomas will not enhance the biliary phase of imaging. This is particularly useful in differentiating adenomas from focal nodular hyperplasia (FNH).

6. **Why is surgical resection of hepatic adenomas recommended?**
   Spontaneous rupture and intraabdominal hemorrhage can occur in up to 30% of patients with hepatic adenoma, especially during menstruation or pregnancy or with larger lesions. HCC also can develop within adenomas, especially adenomas larger than 10 cm. In most cases adenomas are asymptomatic, but adenoma hemorrhage abdominal pain is a presenting symptom. Adenomas have been known to regress with discontinuation of birth control pills, which should be recommended, but surgical resection remains the management of choice. Ablation is another modality used to treat adenoma particularly in patients who are not good surgical candidates or have small lesions (<3 cm).

7. **What is FNH?**
   FNH is a round, nonencapsulated mass, usually exhibiting a vascular central scar. Fibrous septae radiate from the scar in a spoke-like fashion. Hepatocytes are arranged in nodules or cords between the septae, and the mass includes bile ductules, Kupffer cells, and chronic inflammatory cells. FNHs are considered the result of a hyperplastic response to increased blood flow secondary to vascular malformations.

FNH is the second most common benign liver tumor. Over 90% occurs in women and usually is diagnosed between 20 and 60 years of age. Oral contraceptives are not directly linked as a causative agent of FNH and do not need to be discontinued in patients with FNH.

8. **List the differences between hepatic adenomas and FNH.**
See Table 23.3 for the differences between hepatic adenomas and FNH.

Table 23.3 Characteristics of Hepatic Adenoma and Focal Nodular Hyperplasia.

	HEPATIC ADENOMA	FOCAL NODULAR HYPERPLASIA
Size (mean, cm)	10	<5
Kupffer cells	No	Yes
Central scar	Rare	Common
Symptoms	Common	Rare (only with large lesions)
Complications	Bleeding, malignancy	Rare, lesions may grow in size
Treatment	Surgical resection	Resection not necessary
	Ablation	
	Stop OCPs	
Sulfur colloid liver scan	Cold defect	Positive uptake in 60%–70%

OCPs, Oral contraceptive pills.

9. **What is the most frequent malignancy in the liver?**
Metastatic disease of the liver is much more common than primary hepatic tumors in the United States and Europe. Cancers arising in the colon, stomach, pancreas, breast, and lung and melanoma are the most likely to metastasize to the liver. Esophageal, renal, and genitourinary neoplasms also should be considered when searching for the primary site. Neuroendocrine tumors may metastasize to the liver. Multiple defects in the liver suggest a metastatic process: only 2% present as solitary lesions. The involvement of both lobes is most common; 20% are confined to the right lobe alone and 3% to the left lobe.

10. **What is the most common primary liver cancer?**
HCC is by far the most common malignancy originating in the liver, accounting for approximately 80% of primary liver cancers. The incidence in the United States ranges from 2 to 3 cases per 100,000 and has doubled over the past two decades. The recent increase in HCC in the United States over the past decade is directly attributable to the rising incidence of nonalcoholic fatty liver disease. Geographic location influences both the age of peak occurrence (>55 years in the United States) and male-to-female incidence ratios. High-incidence areas in Asia and Africa, related to hepatitis B, have a much younger average age of onset and a higher male predominance. Worldwide, men are more likely than women to develop HCC by a factor of 4:1. In the United States most cases of HCC occur in patients with cirrhosis. See Box 23.1.

11. **Describe the various presenting forms of HCC.**
Nodular: Most common; multiple nodules of varying size scattered throughout the liver.
Solitary (or massive): Occurs in younger patients; large, solitary mass, often in the right lobe.
Diffuse: Rare; difficult to detect on imaging; widespread infiltration of minute tumor foci.
Fibrolamellar HCC is a rare histologic variant that rarely occurs in young women in the absence of cirrhosis. This variant is characterized by increased stromal fibrosis, eosinophilic glass cell hepatocytes, and the absence of underlying inflammation or fibrosis. The prognosis is better than HCC associated with cirrhosis.

12. **What types of cirrhosis most commonly are associated with HCC?**
Autopsy studies indicate that 20%–40% of patients dying from cirrhosis harbor HCC. The etiologies of cirrhosis most commonly related to HCC, in order of decreasing risk, are as follows:
1. Alcoholic cirrhosis (alcohol potentiates the carcinogenic risk in nonalcoholic fatty liver disease or viral hepatitis)
2. Nonalcoholic steatohepatitis (1%–3% over 10–15 years)

Box 23.1 Criteria for the diagnosis of HCC

Imaging characteristics of HCC on contrast-enhanced CT or MRI that are diagnostic for HCC and biopsy of the lesion is not needed to establish the diagnosis.

For lesions >1 cm and <2 cm	• Increased contrast enhancement on late arterial phase AND • Washout during portal venous phase AND • Peripheral rim enhancement on delayed phases OR • Increased contrast enhancement on late arterial phase and 50% growth in diameter within 6 months
For lesions ≥2 cm	• Increased contrast enhancement on late arterial phase and washout on delay/portal venous phase or late capsule enhancement OR • Increased contrast enhancement on late arterial phase and 50% growth in diameter within 6 months

CT, Computed tomography; *HCC,* hepatocellular carcinoma; *MRI,* magnetic resonance imaging.

---

3. Chronic hepatitis C (over 5 years, 7% of patients with hepatitis C virus cirrhosis develop HCC)
4. Chronic hepatitis B (even in the absence of cirrhosis)
5. Hemochromatosis
6. Alpha-1-antitrypsin deficiency

13. What clinical and laboratory findings should raise suspicion for HCC?

Most patients with HCC are asymptomatic and lesions are detected on screening. If symptoms develop, they are related to abdominal pain from hemorrhage or paraneoplastic syndromes. Clinical findings can include:

1. New abdominal pain or weight loss
2. Hepatomegaly
3. Hepatic bruit
4. Acute hemoperitoneum
5. Blood-tinged ascitic fluid
6. Persistent fever
7. Sudden increase in serum alkaline phosphatase
8. Increasing ratio of aspartate aminotransferase to alanine aminotransferase
9. Polycythemia or persistent leukocytosis
10. Hypoglycemia
11. Hypercalcemia
12. Hypercholesterolemia
     Findings 9–12 are paraneoplastic syndromes associated with HCC.

14. What primary liver tumor occurs in young adults without underlying cirrhosis?

The fibrolamellar variant of HCC is a distinctive, slow-growing subtype of hepatic neoplasm, occurring at a mean age of 26. Patients seldom have a history of prior liver disease. Unlike typical HCC, men and women are equally affected. Fibrolamellar tumors usually present with abdominal pain, due to a large, solitary mass, most often in the left lobe (75%). The AFP level is normal. Patients with fibrolamellar carcinoma typically do not have underlying chronic liver disease.

The term fibrolamellar characterizes the microscopic appearance of this lesion; thin layers of fibrosis separate the neoplastic hepatocytes. A fibrous central scar may be seen in imaging studies. Because patients with this HCC variant do not have cirrhosis, it is important to recognize because nearly one-half of these tumors are resectable at the time of diagnosis.

15. What factors predispose to the development of cholangiocarcinoma?

Cholangiocarcinomas, which account for about 10% of primary liver cancers, arise as adenocarcinomas from bile duct epithelium. Painless jaundice is the most frequent clinical presentation of this tumor. Risk factors for cholangiocarcinoma include:

• PSC
• Liver fluke infestation

- Chronic ulcerative colitis
- Congenital cystic liver diseases, choledochal cysts

    Only about 25% of cholangiocarcinomas occur in the setting of cirrhosis. However, in more than half of the cases, an underlying liver disease is not found in patients with cholangiocarcinoma. Although there are no proven screening tests for serum cholangiocarcinoma, CA 19-9 and MRI abdomen with MRCP are frequently used to screen patients with PSC for cholangiocarcinoma.

16. What is a Klatskin tumor?

Cholangiocarcinomas at the hilar bifurcation of the hepatic ducts are referred to as Klatskin tumors. Peripheral (or intrahepatic) and extrahepatic bile duct cholangiocarcinomas are other subtypes. Delayed tumor enhancement on CT after intravenous contrast is noted in approximately 75% of intrahepatic cholangiocarcinomas. The characteristic desmoplastic reaction accompanying these tumors often makes them poorly visible in imaging studies and difficult to diagnose on biopsy. The diagnosis may require endoscopic retrograde cholangiopancreatography with brushings of a malignant-appearing stricture with cytology or fluorescent in situ hybridization analysis, endoscopic ultrasound (EUS) with biopsy, or both. The newly developed cholangioscopy technology is very useful in making diagnosis by direct visualization and tissue acquisition with forceps biopsy for histology. Resection is the mainstay of treatment, but unfortunately the majority of lesions are unresectable. In some circumstances, liver transplantation may be an option for treatment. Highly selected cases of hilar cholangiocarcinoma that undergo neoadjuvant chemoradiation and staging laparoscopy before transplantation have acceptable posttransplant survival. Unfortunately, most are unresectable when diagnosed and thus require palliative drainage of obstructive jaundice by endoscopic, percutaneous, or surgical methods.

17. When should liver transplantation be considered in patients with HCC?

Patients who meet the Milan criteria should be considered for transplantation. In some regions of the country, locoregional therapy is used to downstage more advanced HCC to meet the Milan criteria and be considered for transplantation. See Table 23.4.

Table 23.4 Liver Transplant Criteria for Hepatocellular Carcinoma.	
MILAN CRITERIA	**UCSF**
Solitary lesion ≤5 cm Or Three or fewer nodules less than 1–3 cm in diameter And No macroscopic vascular invasion or extrahepatic disease	Solitary lesion ≤6.5 cm Or Three or fewer lesions with the largest lesion ≤4.5 cm and cumulative diameter ≤8 cm And No macroscopic vascular invasion or extrahepatic disease

UCSF, University of California San Francisco.

18. When should resection be considered in patients with HCC?

HCC is resectable in only approximately 10% of patients in the United States because underlying cirrhosis with portal hypertension and hepatic synthetic dysfunction precludes resection. Noninvasive methods to determine the presence of portal hypertension include thrombocytopenia, splenomegaly, and vibration-controlled elastography. Five-year survival rates with surgical treatment range between 17% and 40%. Most patients succumb to intrahepatic recurrence of tumors. The multifocal nature of HCC carcinogenesis explains this poor prognosis. Selection criteria for resectability of HCC include:

- Child-Pugh class A cirrhosis
- Solitary lesion <5 cm
- Absence of significant portal hypertension defined as hepatic wedge pressure gradient <10 mm Hg
- Lack of vascular invasion or extrahepatic spread

19. What other therapies are available for the management of HCC?

Both radiofrequency and microwave ablation are direct application of thermal energy by percutaneous or surgical means, which destroys unresectable areas of HCC. Radiofrequency and microwave ablation are superior to percutaneous ethanol injection by decreasing local recurrence rates and enhancing directed tissue necrosis.

    Transarterial chemoembolization (TACE) involves the selective administration of chemotherapy, followed by embolization, into the hepatic artery branch feeding the tumor. TACE confers a survival advantage compared to supportive therapy. It is frequently used to delay tumor progression "bridge therapy" in patients awaiting liver transplantation.

    Another modality used to treat HCC is radioembolization which introduces Yttrium90 through the hepatic artery blood supply. This modality may be used for tumors too large for TACE or in patients with portal vein thrombosis who are not candidates for TACE. In a randomized clinical trial of patients with early or intermediate HCC comparing transarterial radioembolization (TARE) to TACE with drug-eluting beads, the median overall survival rate in the TARE and TACE groups was 30.2 and 15.6 months, respectively, $P = .006$.

Atezolizumab with bevacizumab has largely replaced sorafenib as first-line systemic therapy for HCC. In a randomized trial of patients with unresectable HCC atezolizumab-bevacizumab was associated with a 42% reduction in death compared to sorafenib.

20. **Who should be screened for HCC? Describe a typical screening strategy.**

Patients with cirrhosis, especially those at high risk of HCC, should be screened. Screening is done routinely in people with cirrhosis including viral-induced cirrhosis (hepatitis B and C) and cirrhosis related to metabolic liver disease.

Serial AFP measurements and hepatic ultrasound studies are the most commonly used screening tools. Optimal screening intervals are not established, but AFP levels and ultrasound every 6 months are common practice. Although surveillance may not have a definite impact on mortality rate with only one randomized trial demonstrating a survival advantage (Zhang study), it allows more tumors to be amenable to curative resection. Other newer biomarkers such as AFP-L3% and DCP offer marginal improvement in combination with AFP.

21. **What benign tissue abnormality may simulate a focal liver mass?**

Focal fatty infiltration may appear similar to the focal hepatic lesions described above. Focal fatty liver is often seen in alcoholism, obesity, diabetes mellitus, malnutrition, corticosteroid excess or therapy, and AIDS. MRI may be necessary to fully characterize this entity. An interesting aspect of focal fat is its rapid disappearance once the inciting disease process is corrected. The LI-RADS criteria provide a standardized way for radiologists to report the classification of liver tumors. A LI-RADS-5 liver mass has a greater than 95% probability of being HCC and does not require liver biopsy even if the AFP is normal.

22. **What new imaging techniques are under development to evaluate focal liver masses?**

MRI angiography, which permits the rapid acquisition of arterial and venous sequences, has shown promise in the detection of small HCCs missed by triphasic CT scanning.

Positron emission tomography (PET scan) is currently being studied to improve the difficult detection of cholangiocarcinoma. PET scans are also playing an increasing role in the detection of hepatic metastases from colorectal cancer when liver resection is contemplated. PET scans are not useful for HCC because HCCs are not PET avid.

EUS with fine-needle aspiration (FNA) or biopsy has also been reported to aid in the diagnosis of suspected cholangiocarcinoma when other tissue-sampling methods such as intraductal cytology have failed to provide a diagnosis. EUS can also be utilized to biopsy liver masses, particularly those located in the left lobe of the liver.

23. **Why is fine-needle biopsy of hepatic masses controversial?**

Establishing a diagnosis for a focal liver mass by FNA cytology is more problematic than one would think, owing to subtle histopathologic differences between normal hepatocytes and benign lesions or even well-differentiated hepatomas. The literature reveals a wide range of sensitivity for FNA-based diagnosis of primary hepatic lesions. The most optimistic studies report sensitivities and specificities >90%. Hemangiomas, FNH, and HCC appear to be more difficult to diagnose accurately by FNA; sensitivity ranges between 60% and 70% in many series. Rigorous protocols making use of two or more imaging studies to characterize a benign lesion can have accuracy and sensitivity as high as 80%–90%. When HCC is suspected, the use of MRI, CT, and angiography (in selected cases) can confirm the diagnosis in >95% of patients without the use of FNA. Biopsy of a liver mass is preferred over FNA.

Another controversy about the use of FNA in HCC is the risk of needle-tract seeding and tumor spread into the circulation, a risk that may be as high as 5%. With the increasing use of liver transplantation in the treatment of HCC, this complication can have grave consequences.

FNA plays a dominant role in the setting of suspected metastatic disease to the liver and inoperable primary cancers. When surgical resection of a lesion, based on clinical and imaging findings, is deemed necessary, preoperative biopsy is generally not advocated.

24. **What should be done when small incidental liver lesions are found?**

Lesions <1 cm are common incidental findings on liver imaging. In the vast majority of cases they represent benign entities such as small cysts or hemangiomas. Their small size makes further characterization by other radiographic studies or percutaneous biopsy problematic, and usually impossible. If the lesion is too small to characterize then repeat imaging in 3–6 months can be performed to determine if there is interval growth making the lesion amenable to biopsy if warranted.

Simple, thin-walled hepatic cysts, regardless of size, need no further follow-up when definitively documented by ultrasound. Otherwise, clinical follow-up by repeating the imaging study in 6 months is recommended. This provides verification that the lesion has not grown in size. Interval growth of such lesions should prompt further workup.

25. Outline a logical approach to the evaluation of a focal hepatic mass.
The workup of a focal liver mass must occur in the context of a carefully considered differential diagnosis. Associated symptoms, the presence of underlying liver disease or extrahepatic malignancy, drug and occupational exposures, and laboratory abnormalities must be assessed before proceeding with further radiographic studies. Symptomatic lesions and lesions noted incidentally are likely to have different etiologies. The patient's age and sex are important clues. Cirrhosis requires a modified approach because of the increased likelihood of HCC. See Chapter 69 for a comprehensive discussion and examples of imaging options for the evaluation of liver lesions. See Box 23.2.

Box 23.2 Evaluation of Liver Lesions

INCIDENTAL LESIONS	CIRRHOSIS OR RISK FACTORS FOR CHOLANGIOCARCINOMA
Small lesions <1 cm → repeat study in 6 months Simple cysts → verify with ultrasound Hemangiomas → triphasic CT with contrast → 99Tc-labeled red blood cell scan (for lesions >2 cm) or gadolinium-enhanced MRI FNH → triphasic CT with contrast → gadolinium-enhanced MRI → ? biopsy Hepatic adenoma → history of OCPs → rule out hemangioma and FNH → resection (outlined above)	HCC → AFP → triphasic CT → MRI with contrast or MRI angiography Cholangiocarcinoma → CA 19-9 → triphasic with delayed-phase CT → MRCP, ERCP with cholangioscopy for cytology, FISH and biopsy, and PET scan
Symptomatic lesions	**History of malignancy**
Hepatic adenoma → history of OCPs → rule out hemangioma/FNH → resection Liver abscess → sepsis → ultrasound → triphasic CT (rim enhancement)	Metastases → triphasic CT with contrast → if resection is considered → PET scan (to rule out multiple metastasis)

AFP, Alpha-fetoprotein; *CT,* computed tomography; *ERCP,* endoscopic retrograde cholangiopancreatography; *FISH,* fluorescent in situ hybridization; *FNH,* focal nodular hyperplasia; *HCC,* hepatocellular carcinoma; *MRCP,* magnetic resonance cholangiopancreatography; *MRI,* magnetic resonance imaging; *OCPs,* oral contraceptive pills; *PET,* positron emission tomography.

BIBLIOGRAPHY

Available Online

WEBSITES

Available Online

CHAPTER 24

DRUG-INDUCED LIVER DISEASE

Anand V. Kulkarni, MD, DM and K. Rajender Reddy, MD, FACP, FACG, FRCP, FAASLD

 Additional content available online

1. **What is drug-induced liver injury (DILI)?**
   DILI is a diagnosis of exclusion that can be either dose-dependent or idiosyncratic and can present with a wide spectrum of liver injury ranging from cholestatic and hepatocellular to mixed pattern and can either be acute or chronic and is also known as a leading cause of acute liver failure (ALF).

2. **How many drugs are there with known DILI potential?**
   There are approximately 1100 drugs implicated in causing DILI.

3. **How common is drug-induced liver disease? Is there any regional variation of DILI across the world?**
   The annual incidence of DILI is 14–19 per 100,000 population in the United States. The incidence of DILI is higher in the Asia-Pacific region, especially in China, where the reported annual incidence is 24 per 100,000 population. This is because of the higher incidence of tuberculosis (TB) and thus the need for anti-TB treatment, and the widespread and unregulated use of complementary and alternative medicines in the Asia-Pacific region.

4. **What class of drugs are commonly implicated in DILI?**
   Antimicrobials followed by herbal and dietary supplements (HDSs).

5. **What are the most common drugs causing liver injury?**
   Amoxicillin-clavulanate, isoniazid, and acetaminophen are common causes of DILI. Amoxicillin-clavulanate is the most common antibiotic prescribed (6 million prescriptions/year in the United States), and liver injury develops in 1 in 2500 prescriptions.

6. **What are the types of DILI, and how to identify them?**
   There are four main types of liver injury: (1) hepatocellular, (2) cholestatic, (3) mixed, and (4) steatotic.
   The identification of the first three types of DILI is based on the R score (Fig. 24.1). R is the ratio of serum alanine transaminase (ALT)/upper limit of normal (ULN) of ALT divided by serum alkaline phosphatase (ALP)/ULN of ALP, with ALT and ALP concentrations in units per liter. Steatotic pattern is identified based on histology.

7. **Are there any clinical features (on history) to identify the type of injury?**
   Patients commonly present with symptoms of hepatitis: nausea, vomiting, abdominal pain, or can be asymptomatic in hepatocellular injury. Jaundice and pruritus are features often found in those with cholestasis which can be disabling. Mixed injury may be associated with both features. The more important aspects to recognize DILI are the history of exposure to drug, the signature of the drug in causing liver injury, the latency, and the absence of other causes for liver injury. Even a single dose of an implicated drug can cause liver injury.

8. **Why is it important to identify the type of injury?**
   The type of injury determines the management and helps in predicting the outcome. Idiosyncratic hypersensitivity injury may respond to corticosteroids. Severe acute liver injury may evolve into ALF and in some cases may

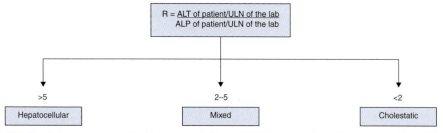

Fig. 24.1 Classification of drug-induced liver injury based on the R score. *ALP,* Alkaline phosphatase; *ALT,* alanine transaminase; *ULN,* upper limit of normal.

necessitate consideration of liver transplantation. The responsible drug can often be identified based on the type of injury. Drugs causing hepatocellular, cholestatic, mixed, and steatotic patterns of injury are described in Table 24.1.

9. **Can serum bilirubin levels help in identifying the type of injury?**
Serum bilirubin is variable in DILI and cannot aid much in diagnosis. However, in patients with cholestatic pattern or mixed type, bilirubin is elevated >2 the ULN (with elevated conjugated levels). The degree of bilirubin elevation in hepatocellular jaundice has more prognostic value (discussed further under Hy's law).

10. **Is there any role of liver biopsy in DILI?**
Liver biopsy may help identify or support the clinical pattern of liver injury. Occasionally, unique features such as bile duct paucity and microvesicular steatosis may suggest specific considerations and aid in prognostication. Often the diagnosis of DILI is based on clinical considerations.

11. **What is the gold-standard test for DILI?**
As such, there is no gold standard. The causality assessment methods help diagnose DILI and are largely used as research tools. The diagnosis of DILI is mostly made on clinical grounds and dependent on the signature of the implicated drug, latency for DILI, and the exclusion of other causes of liver injury. Tools to assess causality include the following:
1. Roussel-Uclaf Causality Assessment Method (RUCAM);
2. Maria and Victorino clinical diagnostic scale; and
3. Digestive Disease Week Japan.

Table 24.1 Medications Commonly Associated With Various Drug-Induced Liver Injury (DILI) Patterns.

HEPATOCELLULAR	CHOLESTATIC	MIXED	STEATOTIC: MICROVESICULAR MIXED MICRO- AND MACROVESICULAR
Acetaminophen Amiodarone Allopurinol	Amoxicillin-clavulanate Amiodarone Azathioprine Anabolic steroids/andro-gens/estrogens/OCPs	Azathioprine Allopurinol Amiodarone Amoxicillin Amitriptyline Ampicillin	Aflatoxin β1; amiodarone
Isoniazid Inhaled anesthetics	Chlorpromazine Captopril	Flutamide Flavocoxib	L-Asparaginase methotrexate
Fluoroquinolones	Fluoroquinolones	Fluoroquinolones	Coumadin; halothane tetra-/trichloroethylene
Macrolides Minocycline	Trimethoprim-sulfamethoxazole Sulfasalazine	Sulfasalazine	Aspirin; minocycline
NSAIDs Nitrofurantoin		Cimetidine	Cocaine; tamoxifen
Carbamazepine Phenytoin Valproate	Carbamazepine Phenytoin	Carbamazepine Phenytoin	Valproic acid
Statins Sulfonamides		Imipramine	Deferoxamine; tetracyclines
HAART (nevirapine, abacavir, and maraviroc carry black box warning)			Didanosine

HAART, Highly active antiretroviral therapy; *NSAIDs,* nonsteroidal anti-inflammatory drugs; *OCPs,* oral contraceptive pills.

Table 24.2 Roussel-Uclaf Causality Assessment Method.

ENZYME PATTERN EXPOSURE	HEPATOCELLULAR			CHOLESTATIC OR MIXED		
Timing from	Initial exposure	Subsequent exposure	Pts	Initial exposure	Subsequent exposure	Pts
Drug start	5–90 days	1–15 days	+2	5–90 days	1–90 days	+2
	<5 or >90 days	>15 days	+1	<5 or >90 days	>90 days	+1
Drug stop	≤15 days	≤15 days	+1	≤30 days	≤30 days	+1
Course	Difference between peak ALT and ULN value			Difference between peak Alk P (or bili) and ULN		
	Decrease ≥50% in 8 days		+3	Decrease ≥50% in 180 days		+2
After stopping the drug	Decrease ≥50% in 30 days		+2	Decrease <50% in 180 days		+1
	Decrease ≥50% in >30 days		0	Persistence or increase or no information		0
	Decrease <50% in >30 days		−2			
Risk factor	Ethanol: yes		+1	Ethanol or pregnancy: yes		+1
	Ethanol: no		0	Ethanol or pregnancy: no		0
Age	≥50 years		+1	≥50 years		+1
	<50 years		0	<50 years		0
Other drugs	None or no information		0	None or no information		0
	Drug with suggestive timing known hepatotoxin with suggestive timing		−1	Drug with suggestive timing known hepatotoxin with suggestive timing		−1
	Drug with other evidence for a role (e.g., + rechallenge)		−2	Drug with other evidence for a role (e.g., + rechallenge)		−2
Competing causes	All groups I[a] and II[b] ruled out		+2	All groups I and II ruled out		+2
	All of the group I ruled out		+1	All of the group I ruled out		+1
	4–5 of the group I ruled out		0	4–5 of the group I ruled out		0
	<4 of group I ruled out		−2	<4 of group I ruled out		−2
	Nondrug causes highly probable		−3	Nondrug causes highly probable		−3
Previous information	Reaction in product label		+2	Reaction in product label		+2
	Reaction published; no label		+1	Reaction published; no label		+1
	Reaction unknown		0	Reaction unknown		0
Rechallenge	Positive		+3	Positive		+3
	Compatible		+1	Compatible		+1
	Negative		−2	Negative		−2
	Not performed or not interpretable		0	Not performed or not interpretable		0

Alk P, Alkaline phosphatase; *ALT,* alanine transaminase; *bili,* bilirubin; *Pts,* points; *ULN,* upper limit of normal.
[a]Group I includes hepatitis A, B, C, and E, biliary obstruction, alcohol misuse, and hypotension/shock.
[b]Group II includes cytomegalovirus, Epstein-Barr virus, and herpes infection.

RUCAM is a widely used tool to assess causality. RUCAM scores can range between −9 and +14 (Table 24.2).

However, rechallenge is rarely performed, and the score ranges between −7 and +11. A score of ≤0: DILI excluded; 1–2: DILI unlikely; 3–5: DILI possible; 6–8: DILI probable; and ≥9: DILI highly probable. Even the best-known drugs fall into the category of probable DILI range, and rarely are drugs categorized in the highly probable range. RUCAM gives a fair idea about causality and the possible course of DILI.

12. What are the drawbacks of the RUCAM scoring system?

RUCAM has very limited intra- and interrater reliability (~0.5). It is 86% sensitive and 90% specific to reflect causality probability. RUCAM cannot aid in the diagnosis of chronic DILI, HDS-induced liver injury, or DILI in preexisting liver disease.

13. Can DILI be chronic, and how common is it?

Persistence of abnormal laboratory, imaging, or histopathologic features of the liver injury for ≥6 months after the onset of DILI is termed chronic DILI. DILI progresses to chronicity in 10%–15% of patients.

14. What are the types of chronic DILI, and how to manage them?

There are four types of chronic DILI (Table 24.3).

15. Can medications cause ALF?

Yes. Some of the examples apart from acetaminophen include antibiotics (amoxicillin, nitrofurantoin, sulfonamides, ciprofloxacin, and ofloxacin), antifungals (terbinafine, itraconazole, ketoconazole, and terbinafine), anti-TB drugs (isoniazid, rifampin, and dapsone), and antiepileptics (phenytoin and valproate).

16. What are the main modulators of DILI?

- The drug (dose, duration, and class)
- The host (age, sex, body mass index, and genetic and immunologic factors)
- The environment (diet, other toxins, antioxidants, and probiotics)

17. Are there any differential diagnoses of DILI?

Yes, DILI is mostly a diagnosis of exclusion. A detailed history, complete physical examination, and review of laboratory and imaging studies are extremely important. The diagnosis of DILI requires exclusion of other etiologic possibilities such as viral, autoimmune, and cardiovascular diseases; exposure to other toxins (alcohol, industrial toxins, etc.); inheritable disorders; gallstones; primary biliary cholangitis; primary sclerosing cholangitis; and malignant causes. Withdrawal of the offending agent and close observation often provide adequate circumstantial evidence for the diagnosis. In short, heightened clinical awareness for a drug causing injury, the phenotype, along with latency for the injury, in a case satisfying a RUCAM score ≥6 can reliably help in the diagnosis of DILI. Liver biopsy should be considered when discontinuation of the medication is not followed by prompt improvement.

18. What variables influence susceptibility to DILI?

Several factors influence the susceptibility to DILI. Some are discussed in Table 24.4.

19. Does the genetics of the individual play any role in DILI?

Amoxicillin-clavulanic acid is the most studied drug in terms of genetic association. Certain human leukocyte antigen (HLA) haplotypes such as DRB1*1501, DRB1*15, and DRB1*0602 have been identified as influencing the risk of DILI caused by amoxicillin-clavulanate. The most significant association has been observed for haplotype HLA DRB1*15:01 (increased risk of autoimmune-like DILI). Other medications with significant HLA associations include abacavir, flucloxacillin (DRB*57:01), isoniazid (HLA DAB*0201 and DQA*0103), lapatinib, lumiracoxib, ticlopidine, and ximelagatran. Furthermore, *CYP2E1* mutations and *N*-acetyltransferase 2 slow acetylators are the non-HLA genes associated with an increased risk of DILI due to isoniazid.

20. Does the presence of preexisting liver disease increase the risk of DILI?

Chronic hepatitis B and C are associated with an increased risk of liver injury with highly active antiretroviral therapy, azithromycin, and isoniazid. Otherwise, generally, preexisting chronic liver disease (CLD) is not a risk factor for DILI. However, patients who develop DILI in the background of CLD have increased mortality (threefold) compared to those who do not have underlying CLD.

21. How is acetaminophen toxic to the liver?

Acetaminophen is the most common cause of drug-induced ALF and the second most common cause of death from poisoning in the United States. Acetaminophen-related injury can have two phenotypes: (1) as an intentional overdose and (2) as a therapeutic misadventure when even lower doses of acetaminophen in a chronic alcohol user/abuser cause liver injury. The mechanism of liver injury is explained in Fig. 24.2.

Table 24.3 Types, Diagnosis, and Management of Chronic Drug-Induced Liver Injury (DILI).

TYPE	SYMPTOMS AND SIGNS	DIAGNOSIS	EXAMPLES	MANAGEMENT	PROGNOSIS
Autoimmune-like DILI	AIH-like features	Serology and liver biopsy features of AIH with a history of drug exposure. Positive DILI risk alleles for AIH.	Nitrofurantoin, minocycline, alpha-methyldopa, hydralazine	Withdrawal of the drug. Immunosuppressants (steroids ± azathioprine) till hepatic biochemical tests normalize.	Excellent drug-induced AIH rarely relapses.
VBDS	Pruritus, fatigue and jaundice, hypercholesterolemia, and skin xanthomata	Elevation in ALP and serum bilirubin >6 months with the paucity of bile ducts in >50% of portal tracts on histology (performed within a month of onset) in the absence of other causes of bile duct injury (PBC, PSC, obstruction, etc.).	Amoxicillin-clavulanate, fluoroquinolones, azithromycin, carbamazepine, lamotrigine, allopurinol, ibuprofen, temozolomide, and nevirapine.	Antihistamines and bile acid resins for pruritus. Plasma exchange for severe itching. Vitamins A, D, E, and K replacement ?Ursodeoxycholic acid/?Steroids/calcineurin inhibitors.	8%–10% progress to requiring liver transplant. 20% liver-related mortality.
DISH	Elevation in hepatic biochemical tests; right upper quadrant abdominal pain	Biopsy features of NASH.	Amiodarone, methotrexate, tamoxifen, valproate, nucleoside reverse transcriptase inhibitors, 5-fluorouracil, and irinotecan.	Withdrawal of drug.	1 in 4 methotrexate-induced steatohepatitis may progress to cirrhosis.
NRH SOS	Asymptomatic to features of portal hypertension	Regenerative nodules but without fibrosis. SOS: nonthrombotic fibrosis of hepatic sinusoids and small intrahepatic veins.	Azathioprine: 0.5% at 5 years and 1.5% at 10 years develop NRH Oxaliplatin (SOS > NRH). Other chemotherapeutic agents: 6-thioguanine, busulfan, bleomycin, cyclophosphamide, chlorambucil, cytosine arabinoside, carmustine, and doxorubicin.	Withdrawal of drug. Management of portal hypertension in advanced disease. Consider defibrotide.	Good.

AIH, Autoimmune hepatitis; *ALP*, alkaline phosphatase; *DISH*, drug-induced steatohepatitis; *NASH*, nonalcoholic steatohepatitis; *NRH*, nodular regenerative hyperplasia; *PBC*, primary biliary cholangitis; *PSC*, primary sclerosing cholangitis; *SOS*, sinusoidal obstruction syndrome; *VBDS*, vanishing bile duct syndrome.

Table 24.4 Variables Influencing the Susceptibility to Drug-Induced Liver Injury (DILI).

Age	Aspirin and valproic acid more frequently cause Reyes syndrome in younger individuals. Acetaminophen, isoniazid, and halothane affect older individuals more frequently.
Sex	Females are more prone to DILI and drug-induced acute liver failure.
Nutrition	Malnutrition increases the risk of acetaminophen toxicity due to lower glutathione stores, while obesity is associated with an increased risk of liver injury fibrosis/cirrhosis due to halothane, tamoxifen, and methotrexate.
Enzyme inducers	Substances (phenobarbital, phenytoin, ethanol, cigarette smoke, and grapefruit juice) that induce the hepatic cytochrome P450 system can alter drug metabolism and potentiate hepatotoxicity.
Drug-drug interactions	Valproic acid increases chlorpromazine-induced cholestasis. Rifampin potentiates isoniazid hepatotoxicity. Chronic alcohol ingestion enhances acetaminophen and isoniazid hepatotoxicity.
Excess alcohol intake	Increased risk of liver injury with acetaminophen, isoniazid, and methotrexate.
Diabetes, psoriasis, and renal failure	Increased risk of hepatic fibrosis with methotrexate.

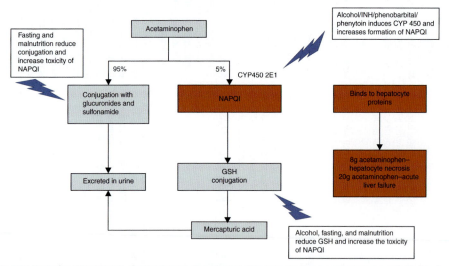

Fig. 24.2 Mechanism of hepatotoxicity of acetaminophen. Normally, most of the acetaminophen is conjugated and excreted in the urine. Glutathione also detoxifies NAPQI (*N*-acetyl-*p*-benzoquinone-imine). Accumulation of the toxic metabolite NAPQI is responsible for liver injury and results in severe hepatocyte centrilobular necrosis. *GSH*, glutathione; *INH*, isoniazid.

22. How is acetaminophen toxicity treated?

The Rumack-Matthew nomogram helps predict the likelihood of liver injury from acetaminophen and directs the therapy. The antidote for acetaminophen overdose is *NN*-acetylcysteine (NAC) which should be administered at 140 mg/kg orally, followed by 17 maintenance doses of 70 mg/kg every 4 hours. However, most patients with ALF cannot tolerate oral NAC. For such patients, intravenous NAC diluted in 5% dextrose at a loading dose (150 mg/kg) is given slowly over 15 minutes, followed by a 4-hour infusion (50 mg/kg) and a 100 mg/kg infusion over 16 hours is the Food and Drug Administration-recommended treatment of choice. Ipecac is given if the time of ingestion is less than 4 hours. Activated charcoal is typically not administered because it can interfere with the absorption of orally administered NAC.

23. **What is the difference between intrinsic and idiosyncratic liver injury?**
    - Intrinsic (predictable) liver injury: All individuals generally develop liver injury at high doses, and injury typically occurs within a week of exposure. This type of injury is reproducible, dose-dependent, and is typically an acute hepatocellular injury. For example, acetaminophen, cyclophosphamide, and busulfan.
    - Idiosyncratic (unpredictable) liver injury: Idiosyncratic reactions occur when a drug causes nondose-related (unpredictable) DILI, and injury occurs variably after exposure. This type of injury may not be reproducible, is dose-independent, and can be hepatocellular, cholestatic, or mixed pattern. Idiosyncratic injury may or may not be associated with immunoallergic phenomenon. The latency for nonimmunoallergic idiosyncratic DILI is longer (90 days to a year). For example, isoniazid, chlorpromazine, amoxicillin-clavulanate, nitrofurantoin, minocycline, diclofenac, and phenytoin. Idiosyncratic reactions may or may not be accompanied by immunoallergic manifestations such as fever, peripheral eosinophilia, skin rash, and arthralgias. Latency is usually shorter (occurring within 3–90 days) in idiosyncratic immunoallergic injury. For example, phenytoin, trimethoprim-sulfamethoxazole, fluoroquinolones, and macrolides.

24. **Describe Mallory-Denk bodies, peliosis hepatis, and phospholipidosis.**
    - Mallory-Denk bodies are cytoplasmic hyaline inclusions in hepatocytes and may develop as a result of alcoholic or nonalcoholic steatohepatitis.
    - Peliosis hepatis is the presence of cystic, blood-filled cavities (vascular lesions) distributed randomly throughout the liver parenchyma.
    - Phospholipidosis is the excessive accumulation of phospholipids in cells, which can be seen as foamy macrophages or cytoplasmic vacuoles on light microscopy, or lamellar inclusions or myeloid bodies in electron microscopy. The causes of these are tabulated in Table 24.5.

25. **What are the common drug-induced hepatic neoplasms?**
    - Hepatocellular carcinoma: Androgenic steroids, estrogenic steroids, thorium oxide (Thorotrast), and vinyl chloride
    - Angiosarcoma: Thorium oxide (Thorotrast), vinyl chloride, arsenic, and androgenic steroids
    - Hepatic adenoma: Estrogenic steroids and androgenic steroids

26. **What drugs are known to cause hepatic granulomas?**
    The drugs causing granulomas can be memorized by this mnemonic (Mackenna's Gold).
    MACKENNa'S: M—Mineral oil; A—Allopurinol; C—Chlorpromazine; K—Quinidine, Quinine; E—pEnicillin; N—Nitrofurantoin; N—INH; S—Sulfonamides.
    GOLD: G—Gold; O—OCP, Oxacillin; L—phenyLbutazone; D—Diazepam, Diltiazem.

27. **How should patients receiving long-term methotrexate be monitored for chronic hepatitis and cirrhosis?**
    Methotrexate is an antifolate and antimetabolite agent that is used widely for psoriasis and rheumatoid arthritis.

Table 24.5 Drugs and Chemicals Associated With Mallory-Denk Bodies, Peliosis Hepatis, and Phospholipidosis.

MALLORY-DENK BODIES	PELIOSIS HEPATIS	PHOSPHOLIPIDOSIS
Amiodarone	Anabolic steroids, arsenic, glucocorticoids, danazol, medroxyprogesterone, and OCPs	Amantadine, amiodarone, amitryptilline, and propranolol
Diethylstilbestrol, glucocorticoids, and ethanol	Azathioprine; tamoxifen	Chloroquine, chlorpheniramine, and chlorpromazine
Griseofulvin	Thioguanine and Thorotrast	Desipramine, imipramine, and trimipramine
Nifedipine and tamoxifen	Vinyl chloride and vitamin A excess	Amikacin, gentamicin, trimethoprim-sulfamethoxazole, chloramphenicol, and ketoconazole

OCP, Oral contraceptive pill.

- Methotrexate is thought to cause liver injury by direct toxicity by inhibiting RNA and DNA synthesis in the liver and causing cellular arrest.
- Risk factors for methotrexate-induced fibrosis include advanced age (>60 years), uncontrolled diabetes mellitus, obesity, chronic alcohol use, daily dosing of methotrexate, psoriasis, and nonsupplementation of folic acid, apart from the cumulative dose (1.5 g) and duration of therapy (>2 years).

28. How to monitor patients who receive methotrexate?

Patients with preexisting liver disease should be monitored with hepatic biochemical tests every month for 6 months, then every 3 months.

Patients with psoriasis should be monitored approximately every 8–12 weeks with hepatic biochemical tests, and if they are altered, that is, ≥3-fold the ULN, the treatment should be held, and consideration to reinitiation can be given after they normalize. Traditionally, liver biopsy has been done after achieving a cumulative dose threshold of 1.5 g in those at risk and then followed with periodic liver biopsies after again further cumulative dose of 1.5–2.0 g. However, with the advent of noninvasive modalities of assessing hepatic fibrosis, such as transient elastography, liver biopsy is being done less frequently. Patients with rheumatoid arthritis need not be monitored regularly unless the patient has other risk factors for drug-induced fibrosis (as discussed above).

29. How is methotrexate-induced liver injury classified, and what are the recommendations for changing methotrexate therapy based on liver biopsy findings?

Roenigk histopathologic classification of methotrexate toxicity includes (1) fatty infiltration, (2) nuclear variability, (3) portal inflammation and necrosis, and (4) fibrosis as components. There is no fibrosis in grades I and II, IIIa has mild fibrous septa, IIIb has bridging (moderate) fibrosis, and IV is cirrhosis.

For grades I and II, it is recommended to continue therapy and repeat biopsy after 1.5–2 g of cumulative dose.

For grade IIIa the drug can be continued, and a repeat biopsy is suggested in 6 months.

For grades IIIb and IV the drug needs to be discontinued.

30. What is the mechanism of liver injury in immune checkpoint inhibitor (ICI) therapy?

Immune checkpoints are normally present in liver tissue to prevent self-reactivity of T cells and promote tolerance. This mechanism is exploited by tumor cells for proliferation. ICIs prevent the inactivation of T cells and augment T cell activation against tumor cells. This immune activation may lead to inflammatory side effects termed as immune-related adverse events (irAEs). irAE can affect the skin, gastrointestinal tract, liver, lung, and heart. The incidence of liver injury due to ICI ranges between 1% and 16%.

31. What are the common ICIs known to cause DILI, and how to manage them?

Ipilimumab (CTLA 4 inhibitor): incidence reported in up to 16%
Ipilimumab + nivolumab (PD1 inhibitor): incidence reported in up to 13%
Durvalumab (PDL1 inhibitor): incidence reported in up to 12%
Atezolizumab (PDL1 inhibitor): incidence reported in up to 9%

DILI occurs after 1–3 doses/months of ICI therapy and is a mixed picture in the initial phase, followed by the hepatocellular type of injury later. Low-titer ANA may be positive in approximately 50% of patients. Diagnosis is based on RUCAM scoring and clinical considerations. Majority of DILI due to ICI resolve spontaneously within 5–9 weeks. Corticosteroids (1 mg/kg) with or without mycophenolate mofetil is the treatment of choice for grade 3 (transaminases >5–20 times the ULN, bilirubin >3–10 times) and grade 4 (transaminases >20 times and bilirubin >10 times) toxicity. Hepatitis B virus reactivation must be ruled out before initiating steroids in ICI-induced DILI.

32. What are the commonly noticed drugs in clinical practice to cause liver injury, and how to manage them?

The commonly noticed drugs in clinical practice to cause liver injury are discussed in Table 24.6.

33. What commonly used recreational drugs are associated with hepatotoxicity?

- Cocaine: Patients with cocaine hepatotoxicity may present with jaundice or fatigue and generalized malaise. Cocaine toxicity also may cause coagulopathy, rhabdomyolysis, and disseminated intravascular coagulation (DIC). The mechanism of hepatotoxicity is thought to be due to an intermediate toxic metabolite. The clinical phenotype is usually acute hepatic necrosis. Liver biopsy typically shows zone III necrosis and fatty change, suggesting related ischemia. It is usually self-limited, but fatalities have been reported mainly resulting from its major systemic effects. Liver injury may be multifactorial and include coexistent viral liver disease (hepatitis B, C, and delta) and acetaminophen or alcohol use.
- 3,4-Methylenedioxymethamphetamine (MDMA, ecstasy): MDMA is a dangerous synthetic amphetamine commonly used for abuse. It is a potent central nervous system stimulant that causes euphoria and increases cognitive abilities. Amphetamines undergo extensive metabolism by the hepatic P450 system, and injury is thought to be secondary to the generation of toxic metabolites. Liver injury is usually hepatocellular type and

Table 24.6 Drugs Commonly Causing Drug-Induced Liver Injury (DILI) in Clinical Practice.

COMMON DRUGS CAUSING DILI	TYPE AND MECHANISM OF INJURY	KEY POINTS
Amoxicillin-clavulanate	Hepatoceullar/cholestatic/mixed Can occur up to 6 weeks after the last intake of drug.	Majority recover with symptomatic management.
INH	Mechanism: INH→ acetylisoniazid→ hydrolyzed to monoacetylhydrazine→ then activated to toxic metabolites. Advanced age, female sex, alcohol, Asian race, and slow acetylator increase injury risk. Rifampicin and pyrazinamide increase the risk of INH toxicity.	Second commonest drug to cause ALF. Stop INH if ALT is more than three times the ULN with symptoms or more than five times the ULN without symptoms.
Nitrofurantoin	Immune-mediated hepatocellular injury may have fever and rash.	Some reports of HLA association (HLA-DR6 and 2). Injury resolves after drug withdrawal. Corticosteroids may be beneficial.
Azithromycin	Cholestatic>>hepatoceullar Can lead to bile duct loss (vanishing bile duct). Can occur up to 3 weeks after stopping of drug.	Liver injury is more frequent in patients with preexisting liver disease. May be associated with severe skin reactions.
Minocycline	Hepatocellular injury with autoimmune features. Occurs after long latency.	Doxycycline, another tetracycline, causes cholestatic injury after short latency.
TMP-SMZ	Injury due to SMZ cholestatic/mixed > hepatocellular. Idiosyncratic liver injury. TMP rare, no immunoallergic features.	More frequent in HIV-infected individuals. Can cause DRESS.
Amiodarone	Can cause any type of injury. 25% have asymptomatic elevations in AST, and ALT often resolve spontaneously despite the continuation of the drug Amiodarone and its metabolite N-desethylamiodarone accumulate in lysosomes of the liver, causing phospholipidosis; if the drug accumulates in the mitochondria, it causes lipid peroxidation and steatohepatitis.	Liver biopsy: Mallory bodies with steatosis, neutrophilic infiltrates, and perivenular fibrosis/micronodular cirrhosis: akin to alcohol injury (called pseudoalcoholic cirrhosis). Monitor ALT levels regularly if dose >400 mg/day. Decrease the dose or stop if ALT >3× ULN. Perform a liver biopsy if elevations persist.
Statins	Severe DILI is rare. Safe to use even in patients with chronic liver disease. Act as haptens on cellular targets in susceptible hosts.	Contraindicated in decompensated cirrhosis.
Anabolic steroids Methyltestosterone, methandrosteno-lone, oxymetholone, danazol, fluoxyme-sterone, stanazol, norethandrolone, and oxandrolone	Cause cholestasis or canalicular liver injury. Oral anabolic steroids, alkylation of the C-17 position of testosterone. Induce androgen-stimulated genes and promote cell growth and development.	Increased off-label use to improve athletic performance. Androgenic steroids must be discontinued if liver injury develops. Liver injury is usually reversible, but fatalities have been reported.

Table 24.6 Drugs Commonly Causing Drug-Induced Liver Injury (DILI) in Clinical Practice.

COMMON DRUGS CAUSING DILI	TYPE AND MECHANISM OF INJURY	KEY POINTS
OCPs Tamoxifen	Estrogens and OCPs inhibit bilirubin and bile acid secretion through estrogen's effects on receptors that modulate bile metabolism. It can cause liver injury, fatty liver, steatohepatitis, and cirrhosis. Liver injury is due to an idiosyncratic reaction to tamoxifen metabolites. Presents as cholestatic, mixed, or hepatocellular injury.	
PTU Methimazole	PTU typically results in hepatocellular liver injury. Methimazole liver injury is typically cholestatic.	PTU hepatotoxicity can lead to ALF. Methimazole causes self-limited injury.
Phenytoin	Phenytoin can cause various types of liver injury, including allergic hepatitis, cholestasis, granulomatous liver disease, and fulminant hepatic failure. Formation of the reactive arene oxide metabolite followed by the formation of the o-quinone leads to haptens and immune activation. Systemic symptoms include fever, malaise, lymphadenopathy, splenomegaly, and rash.	Hepatic biochemical tests can be elevated 2- to 100-fold (ALT > AST) and ALP levels 2- to 8-fold. It can cause leukocytosis and atypical lymphocytes suggesting mononucleosis and eosinophilia, but lupus-like syndrome and pseudolymphoma are rare. Cessation of the drug leads to the resolution of toxicity in most cases. Corticosteroids may help. However, if liver failure develops, the case–fatality ratio can go up to 40%. Because of cross-reactivity, carbamazepine, oxcarbazepine, and fosphenytoin should be avoided.

ALF, Acute liver failure; *ALT*, alanine transaminase; *AST*, aspartate transaminase; *ALP*, alkaline phosphatase; *DRESS*, drug rash eosinophilia and systemic symptoms; *HLA*, human leukocyte antigen; *INH*, isoniazid; *OCPs*, oral contraceptive pills; *PTU*, propylthiouracil; *TMP-SMZ*, trimethoprim-sulfamethoxazole; *ULN*, upper limit of normal.

can be severe enough to cause ALF and death. Ecstasy can cause various systemic effects, including cardiac arrhythmias, DIC, acute renal failure, and hyperthermia.

34. Can herbal therapies cause liver injury?

The composition of herbal remedies is variable and unregulated. Some have the potential to cause liver injury. Patients with preexisting liver disease should be extremely cautious and consult their physicians. Some noted herbs include: *Larrea tridentate* (chaparral used in Mexico and the United States), kava (*Piper methysticum* used as a recreational drug in Hawaii), *Jin Bu Huan* (*Lypocodium serratum* used in the United States as an analgesic and sedative), Dai-saiko-to (Chines herb used in Japan for liver disease), *Teucrium chamaedrys* (blossoms of germander found in Europe and the Middle East), *Tinospora crispa* (used for diabetes mellitus), *Psoralea corylifolia* (for vitiligo), *Centella asiatica* (for leprosy), Liv.52 (contains capers, wild chicory, arjuna, black nightshade, and yarrow), *Atractylis gummifera* (in the Mediterranean regions—antipyretic, antiemetic, abortifacient, and a diuretic), and *Callilepsis laureola* (used in Africa).

35. How to assess the prognosis of patients with DILI?

Most patients recover within 6 months. Factors associated with poor prognosis are:
1. Model for End-Stage Liver Disease (MELD) score >19.
2. Modified Hy's law: Mortality is 10% if the bilirubin is >2× the ULN and AST or ALT >3× the ULN in the absence of other causes of bilirubin elevation (Gilbert syndrome; hemolysis or drug-induced indirect hyperbilirubinemia) or liver failure.

Table 24.7 Grading of Drug-Induced Liver Injury (DILI) Severity.

GRADE	INTERNATIONAL DILI GROUP	GRADE	US DILIN
1 (mild)	ALT ≥5 or ALP ≥2 and bilirubin <2 the ULN	1 (mild)	Increased ALT and/or ALP with bilirubin <2.5 mg/dL and INR <1.5
2 (moderate)	ALT ≥5 or ALP ≥2 and bilirubin ≥2 the ULN	2 (moderate)	Increased ALT and/or ALP with bilirubin ≥2.5 mg/dL or INR ≥1.5
		3 (moderate–severe)	Grade 2 + need for hospitalization
3 (severe)	Grade 2 or symptomatic hepatitis and one of the following: 1. INR ≥1.5 2. Ascites and/or encephalopathy in <26 weeks and absence of underlying cirrhosis 3. Other organ failures due to DILI	4 (severe)	Increased ALT and/or ALP and bilirubin ≥2.5 mg/dL with one of the following: 1. Liver failure (INR >1.5, ascites or encephalopathy) 2. Other organ failures due to DILI
4 (fatal)	Death or transplantation due to DILI	5 (fatal)	Same as the International Working Group

ALP, Alkaline phosphatase; *ALT*, alanine transaminase; *DILI*, drug-induced liver injury; *INR*, international normalized ratio; *ULN*, upper limit of normal; *US DILIN*, US Drug-Induced Liver Injury Network.

3. Ghabril DILI calculator: An online calculator can predict 6-month mortality. MELD score, albumin, and Charlson Comorbidity Index are the components of the score (DILI CAM-GIHEP) (http://gihep.com/calculators/hepatology/dili-cam/).

36. **Are there biomarkers to predict mortality in DILI?**
Cytokeratin 18, osteopontin, and macrophage colony-stimulating factor receptor 1 are some of the markers assessed to predict mortality and transplant need.

37. **How to assess the severity of DILI?**
There are two severity classifications: the US Drug-Induced Liver Injury Network (US DILIN) and International DILI Expert Working Group (Table 24.7). US DILIN has five grades and includes hospitalization (grade 3), while the International group has four grades and does not include hospitalization criteria.

ACKNOWLEDGMENT

We thank the previous authors of the chapter for *Gastrointestinal and Liver Secrets*: Dr. Cemal Yazici MD, Dr. Mark W. Russo MD, MPH, FACG, and Dr. Herbert L. Bonkovsky MD.

CLINICAL VIGNETTE

Available Online

BIBLIOGRAPHY

Available Online

WEBSITES

Available Online

ALCOHOLIC LIVER DISEASE, ALCOHOLISM, AND ALCOHOL WITHDRAWAL

Pranav Penninti, DO, Landon Brown, MD and Ashwani K. Singal, MD, MS, FACG, FAASLD, AGAF

 Additional content available online.

1. What are the criteria for the diagnosis of alcohol-associated liver disease (ALD)?
ALD in an individual with liver disease is diagnosed in the setting of harmful alcohol use (>2 drinks per day in females and >3 drinks per day in males during the last 12 months or longer) and exclusion of other causes of liver disease (Table 25.1).

Table 25.1 Criteria for Diagnosis of Alcohol-Associated Liver Disease.

CRITERIA FOR DIAGNOSIS OF ALCOHOL-ASSOCIATED LIVER DISEASE
Evidence of liver disease with (1) elevated transaminases and/or steatosis on imaging or (2) clinical, biochemical, or imaging features of cirrhosis
Harmful alcohol use (>2 drinks per day in females and >3 in males) during the last 12 months or more
Exclusion of other etiologies of liver disease: viral hepatitis, autoimmune hepatitis, PBC, Wilson disease, hereditary hemochromatosis, and A1AT deficiency

A1AT, Alpha-1 antitrypsin; *PBC*, primary biliary cholangitis.

2. What are the epidemiologic factors of alcohol use and alcoholism?
Per the 2019 National Survey on Drug and Health on alcohol use over the prior month, 54.9% of adults consumed alcohol, 25.8% reported binge drinking (>4 drinks in females and >5 in males over 2 hours' period), and 6.3% endorsed harmful drinking. Alcohol use disorder (AUD) afflicts 5.6% of the US adult population, with over 2 million people diagnosed with alcohol-associated cirrhosis in the United States in 2017. Alcohol contributes to about 27% of cirrhosis-related deaths worldwide and in the United States. Increasing disease burden with related morbidity and mortality has been increasing worldwide, especially among young individuals, <40 years of age, who are at the prime of their productive life. Further, due to industrialization and several other factors, the burden is increasing in developing countries such as India and China. In the last 2 years since the coronavirus disease pandemic in March 2020, alcohol consumption has substantially increased, resulting in an increase in new cases of ALD as well as a worsening of those with preexisting disease. A modeling study predicted an additional 18,700 cases of decompensated cirrhosis and 8000 additional ALD-related deaths from 2020 to 2040.

3. What is the definition of a standard alcoholic drink?
One of the unmet needs in the field is harmonizing the definition of an alcoholic drink across the world. Currently, a standard drink is defined differently across the world based on the amount of pure alcohol as 8 g in the United Kingdom, 10 g in France and Southeast Asia, 12 g in Germany and Italy, 14 g in Canada and the United States, and 20 g in Austria. The percentage of pure alcohol (weight by volume) is 5% in beer, 9% in wine, and 45% in hard liquor. Hence, 12 oz of beer, 5 oz of wine, and 1.5 oz of hard liquor constitute a standard alcoholic drink in the United States.

4. What are the disease modifiers for the development of advanced liver disease in patients with AUD?
Duration and amount of alcohol use are the most important factors in predisposing an individual to develop ALD. However, not all individuals with harmful alcohol use develop ALD, suggesting the role of other factors related to host or to environment. Host factors include sex and ethnicity with females, Hispanics, and Native Americans, who are at a higher risk of developing ALD. Genetic polymorphisms of patatin-like phospholipase domain protein

3 (*PNPLA3*), membrane-bound *O*-acyltransferase domain 7 (*MBOAT7*), and transmembrane 6 superfamily member 2 (*TM6SF2*) also predispose to ALD and its severity. Environmental factors like obesity and concomitant hepatitis B or C infections are synergistic in mediating a higher risk for advanced ALD. Patterns of alcohol use like binge drinking and drinking outside meals increase the predisposition to develop ALD. In contrast, coffee consumption is associated with a reduced risk of ALD.

5. How does the liver metabolize alcohol?

About 90% of alcohol metabolism is via the enzyme alcohol dehydrogenase (ADH) in hepatocytes. Alcohol oxidation via cytochrome P450 2E1 (CYP2E1) in the smooth endoplasmic reticulum is another major pathway. While the catalytic efficiency of CYP2E1 is much lower than ADH, it has a 10-fold higher binding affinity for ethanol. The final route of ethanol metabolism is via catalase, using hydrogen and ethanol as substrates. All three pathways produce acetaldehyde, a highly toxic substrate to hepatocytes. Acetaldehyde is oxidized to acetate in the mitochondria by acetaldehyde dehydrogenase resulting in disequilibrium in the NADH+/NAD ratio with the generation of multiple reactive oxidative species, leading to oxidative stress.

6. What is the pathogenesis of ALD?

The pathogenesis of ALD is complex with the involvement of several pathways (Fig. 25.1). Altered redox potential from alcohol metabolism enhances lipogenesis, decreases fatty acid oxidation, and impairs very-low-density lipoprotein secretion. Alcohol induces increased gut permeability leading to bacterial endotoxemia and an inflammatory signaling cascade. Liver injury and cytokine-mediated activated hepatic stellate and vascular endothelial cells result in the laying down of collagen, fibrosis, and portal hypertension. Hepatocyte regeneration, an adaptive response to hepatocyte injury, is impaired by alcohol-induced inhibition of DNA synthesis and microRNA signaling leading to progressive hepatocyte injury and liver failure.

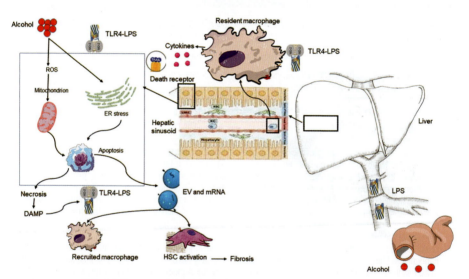

Fig. 25.1 Pathogenesis of alcohol-associated liver disease. Alcohol leads to hepatotoxicity via direct and indirect mechanisms. Direct injury occurs via reactive oxygen species (ROS) which cause oxidative stress and endoplasmic reticulum (ER) stress leading to hepatocyte apoptosis. Indirect effect occurs through the gut-liver axis. Alcohol leads to increased intestinal permeability and bacterial translocation with bacterial lipopolysaccharides (LPS) binding to Toll-like receptor 4 (TLR4) on hepatic macrophages triggering an inflammatory cascade with cytokines leading to apoptosis and necrosis of hepatocytes, subsequently releasing damage-associated molecular patterns (DAMPs) which perpetuate inflammation. Cell death leads to the extrusion of extracellular vesicles (EV) and messenger ribonucleic acid (mRNA) which recruit neutrophils to activate hepatic stellate cells (HSC) which lie down collagen, thereby leading to fibrosis.

7. What is the spectrum of ALD?

ALD is characterized by steatosis, steatohepatitis, steatofibrosis, and cirrhosis (Fig. 25.2).

Hepatic steatosis, defined with large fat droplets (macrosteatosis) in >5% of hepatocytes, extends from zone three outwards with increasing severity. Alcohol foamy degeneration is a rare variant with small fat droplets (microvesicular steatosis) and is associated with mitochondrial dysfunction and usually occurs without steatohepatitis or fibrosis. Steatohepatitis with features of inflammation (hepatocyte ballooning and cytoskeleton

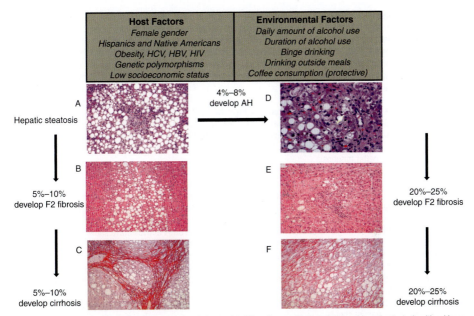

Fig. 25.2 Disease modifiers for the development of alcohol-associated liver disease. (A) Alcohol-induced hepatic steatosis with evidence of fat droplets within the hepatocytes. (B) 5%–10% of patients with hepatic steatosis progress to F2 fibrosis which is typified by fibrous expansion of the portal areas. (C) Cirrhosis is seen on a trichrome stain with bridging fibrosis. (D) Alcohol-associated hepatitis (AH) is characterized histologically by hepatocyte ballooning, neutrophilic infiltration, Mallory-Denk bodies, and cholestasis. (E) 20%–25% of patients with alcohol-associated hepatitis develop F2 fibrosis. (F) 20%–25% of those with F2 fibrosis go on to develop cirrhosis. *HBV*, Hepatitis B virus; *HCV*, hepatitis C virus; *HIV*, human immunodeficiency virus.

disruption with the formation of Mallory-Denk bodies) is a severe form with accelerated progression to cirrhosis. Steatofibrosis begins with perivenular fibrosis extending outward along the sinusoids in a chicken-wire pattern. Cirrhosis develops as a micronodular form and is a risk factor for hepatocellular carcinoma (HCC).

8. **What is the risk of developing HCC in a patient with alcohol-associated cirrhosis?**
The risk of HCC in ALD cirrhosis is 1%–3% annually. It is recommended to perform biannual screening for HCC among patients with ALD and cirrhosis.

9. **Can ALD and non-alcohol-associated fatty liver disease (NAFLD) be differentiated histologically?**
Although it may be difficult to differentiate ALD from NAFLD based on histology, there are subtle differences. For example, foamy degeneration, neutrophilic lobular inflammation, sclerosing hyaline necrosis, and canalicular cholestasis are more often observed in ALD.

10. **What is the clinical presentation of ALD?**
Based on the degree of fibrosis, ALD can be stratified into early ALD and advanced ALD. Individuals with early ALD (fibrosis stage 0–2) are asymptomatic and may present with incidental detection of fatty liver on imaging and/or elevated liver enzymes.
   Individuals with advanced ALD (fibrosis stage 3–4) may be asymptomatic (compensated cirrhosis) or present with decompensation events (ascites, jaundice, gastrointestinal bleeding, hepatic encephalopathy, or HCC). Laboratory findings may show abnormal liver synthetic function with elevated serum bilirubin, prothrombin time, and decrease in serum albumin levels. Findings of portal hypertension may be seen like splenomegaly, abdominal veins (caput medusa), and portal venous enlargement on liver Doppler ultrasound.

11. **What are the clinical criteria for the diagnosis of alcohol-associated hepatitis (AH)?**
Although liver biopsy is the gold standard for definitive AH diagnosis, invasiveness, cost, and a turnaround time of 2–4 days limit its widespread use. Hence, criteria for clinical diagnosis of AH were proposed by the National Institute of Alcohol Abuse and Alcoholism based on the consensus of experts: (1) serum bilirubin >3 mg/dL, (2) aspartate aminotransferase (AST) >50 and <400, AST/alanine aminotransferase (ALT) ratio >1.5, (3) chronic

heavy alcohol use until at least 60 days prior, and (4) exclusion of other causes of liver disease, cholangitis, and HCC. If all these criteria are met (probable AH), the patient can be treated as AH and for inclusion in clinical trials. Transjugular liver biopsy is recommended if ≥1 criteria are not met (possible AH). AH superimposed on ALD is a common precipitant of acute on chronic liver failure (ACLF), a syndrome characterized by multiorgan failure with the potential for high short-term mortality, and should be considered in this clinical setting. AH and infections are the most common precipitants of ACLF and are present either alone or in combination in 97% of patients with ALD and ACLF in one study.

12. What are the characteristic histologic findings of AH?

Typical histologic findings in AH include hepatocyte ballooning, lobular, neutrophil-predominant inflammation, cholestasis (hepatocyte, ductular, or canalicular), steatosis, megamitochondria, and Mallory-Denk bodies. Of these, ballooning and cholestasis are associated with worse patient survival, while megamitochondria and neutrophilic infiltration confer better prognosis.

13. What is the role of noninvasive tests for fibrosis risk assessment in ALD?

Noninvasive serologic and radiologic tests have emerged as valuable tools in fibrosis risk stratification in patients with any liver disease including ALD (Table 25.2). Fibrosis-4 (FIB-4) is an example of a cost-effective screening test to assess the risk of advanced fibrosis in ALD. Obesity, ongoing alcohol use, and inflammation can confound the results. Patented serologic tests such as Enhanced Liver Fibrosis and FibroTest have shown a high degree of sensitivity and specificity. However, these tests are limited by the need for laboratory values other than standard of care workup and cost. Transient elastography (TE) interpretation in patients with ALD should account for active alcohol use and inflammation with AST and bilirubin measurements. Magnetic resonance elastography (MRE) quantifies liver stiffness accurately but is limited by availability, cost, and lack of data in ALD. FIB-4 and TE have excellent sensitivity and negative predictive value. If either or both of these tests are suggestive of advanced fibrosis or cirrhosis, further testing with MRE, patented serum tests, or liver biopsy may be performed based on physician and/or patient choice.

Table 25.2 Noninvasive Tests for the Diagnosis of Advanced Fibrosis (>stage 3) in Alcohol-Associated Liver Disease.

TEST	CUTOFF VALUE	SENSITIVITY AND SPECIFICITY (95% CI)
Serologic Markers		
• FIB-4	≥3.25	58% and 91%
• ELF	≥10.5	79% and 91%
• FibroTest	≥0.58	67% and 89%
Imaging Techniques (LSM)		
• Ultrasound transient elastography	≥15 kPa	86% and 94%
• Magnetic resonance elastography	≥3.31 kPa	96% and 95%

ELF, Enhanced Liver Fibrosis; *FIB-4*, Fibrosis-4; *LSM*, liver stiffness measure; *kPa*, kilopascals.

14. How is AUD defined?

The Diagnostic and Statistical Manual of Mental Disorders, fifth edition diagnosis of AUD requires 2 of 11 criteria over a previous 12-month period. These criteria broadly cover areas of craving, tolerance, withdrawal symptoms, and persistent use despite deleterious personal, social, and professional harms. AUD identification test or AUDIT, with self-reported answers to a 10-item questionnaire (each question reported on 0–4 scale), is another validated accurate tool. AUD is diagnosed at a score >8, with severe AUD at a score >15. AUDIT-C, a shorter version consisting of the first three questions of the AUDIT, is equally accurate and simple to use in clinic.

15. How do you screen for ALD and AUD?

The U.S. Preventive Services Task Force recommends performing screening for AUD in all adults at every medical encounter. Individuals with AUD (AUDIT-C ≥4 in males or ≥3 in females) should be screened for ALD using liver biochemical tests and liver ultrasound. Those identified as having advanced fibrosis or cirrhosis should be referred to hepatologists for further management. AUD should be treated for any spectrum of ALD using brief intervention (counseling on alcohol-related harms) for mild AUD, and referral to an addiction team for patients with severe AUD (Fig. 25.3).

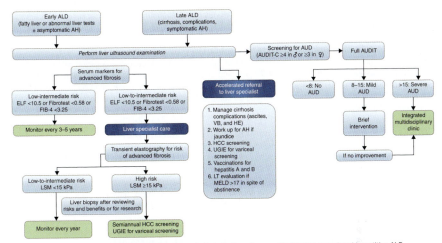

Fig. 25.3 Screening algorithm for alcoholic use disorder and alcoholic liver disease. *AH*, Alcohol-associated hepatitis; *ALD*, alcohol-associated liver disease; *AUD*, alcohol use disorder; *AUDIT*, alcohol use disorders identification test; *AUDIT-C*, alcohol use disorders identification test-consumption; *ELF*, enhanced liver fibrosis test; *HCC*, hepatocellular carcinoma; *HE*, hepatic encephalopathy; *LSM*, liver stiffness measurement; *LT*, liver transplant; *MELD*, Model for End-stage Liver Disease; *UGIE*, upper gastrointestinal endoscopy; *VB*, variceal bleed. (Modified from Singal AK, Mathurin P. Diagnosis and treatment of alcohol-associated liver disease: a review. JAMA. 2021;326(2):165-176.)

16. What are the emerging biomarkers of alcohol use?

As alcohol metabolism follows first-pass metabolism, the blood alcohol concentration can only allow detection of alcohol use for a few hours after consumption. However, alcohol metabolites can detect alcohol use for a longer period. Urine ethyl glucuronide (EtG), a water-soluble alcohol metabolite, detects alcohol use over a 4-day period with 62%–89% sensitivity and 93%–99% specificity. Data are emerging on EtG in hair samples with an ability to detect alcohol use over a few weeks to months. Phosphatidylethanol, a phospholipid metabolite of alcohol, can identify alcohol use over a few days to up to 4 weeks with 90%–99% sensitivity and 100% specificity.

17. What are the behavioral treatment options for the management of AUD?

Brief intervention uses the FRAMES model, which consists of feedback on risk, responsibility for change, advice on options, empathy, and enhancing self-efficacy. Cognitive behavioral therapy helps to understand drinking triggers and to develop coping mechanisms. Motivational interviewing elicits internal change and reasons, which motivate an individual to make positive change. Groups such as Alcoholics Anonymous provide kinship and a long-term support system.

18. What are the pharmacotherapy options for the treatment of AUD in patients with ALD?

Disulfiram, naltrexone, and acamprosate are US Food and Drug Administration (FDA) approved to treat AUD. Disulfiram inhibits aldehyde dehydrogenase increasing acetaldehyde levels, leading to flushing, vomiting, and sweating, thereby dissuading patients from alcohol use. Naltrexone, a nonselective agonist of opioid receptors, acts on the reward-sensing areas of the brain to reduce alcohol craving. Acamprosate modulates glutamate neurotransmission and is approved to prevent relapse in patients who are abstinent at the time of medication initiation. However, none of these have been studied in patients with ALD. Disulfiram is entirely metabolized in the liver and should be avoided in patients with ALD. Acamprosate is entirely metabolized outside the liver and is likely the safest for use in ALD. Of non-FDA approved medications, baclofen, a GABA-B agonist, has a documented efficacy and safety in patients with ALD including AH. Gabapentin and topiramate are other non-FDA approved, safe options.

19. How is alcohol withdrawal managed in a hospitalized patient?

Inpatient management of alcohol withdrawal should be considered in patients with risk factors for several alcohol withdrawal syndrome (AWS) such as a history of sustained drinking, history of alcohol withdrawal, history of delirium tremens, and age >30 years. The inpatient management of AWS is focused on preventing withdrawal seizures and delirium tremens. The Clinical Institute Withdrawal Assessment for Alcohol (CIWA) is a validated tool that helps assess AWS severity and guide further management. Supportive measures including judicious intravenous fluids, thiamine, multivitamins including folate, and antiemetics are instituted. Benzodiazepines reduce the risk of withdrawal seizures, delirium tremens, and mortality, with short-acting agents (lorazepam and oxazepam) used cautiously to avoid precipitation of hepatic encephalopathy. Patients with severe AWS refractory to benzodiazepines need intensive care unit care with the use of propofol, dexmedetomidine, or phenobarbital.

20. What is the role of integrated care management in patients with ALD?

Simultaneous management of AUD along with the management of liver disease is associated with reduced alcohol use and readmission, improvement in liver disease, and patient survival. An integrated approach by hepatologists and an addiction team in a multidisciplinary care model within one location provides a holistic treatment focused on individual patient's needs. Data are emerging on better outcomes of this model compared to the siloed management of AUD and liver disease.

21. What are the barriers to the management of AUD in patients with ALD?

Patients with ALD do not often receive treatment for their second pathology of AUD and the focus remains on managing their liver disease. In a large analysis of veterans with ALD and AUD, only 14% received some form of AUD treatment, with only 0.5% receiving pharmacologic treatment. Barriers to AUD management in patients with ALD can be at the level of patients (stigma of ALD diagnosis, poor insight and understanding of disease, focus on liver care, and fear of repercussions at the personal and professional level), clinicians (lack of time for AUD screening and lack of training for AUD management), and administration (insurance coverage, cost of care, and transportation of sick patients).

22. What are the pharmacotherapy options for patients with severe AH?

Currently, corticosteroids are the only available and recommended pharmacologic therapy to treat severe AH. A meta-analysis of randomized studies (including the largest randomized, placebo-controlled, multicenter STOPAH study) showed the benefit of corticosteroids in reducing 30-day mortality by 46%. There was no survival benefit beyond 1 month. Pentoxifylline was ineffective and is currently not recommended. In a randomized controlled trial, a combination of N-acetylcysteine infusion and oral prednisolone versus prednisolone alone showed improved 1-month survival, but not at 3 or at 6 months.

23. How is eligibility for corticosteroid treatment determined?

Corticosteroids are indicated for patients with severe AH as defined by Maddrey discriminant function >32, Model for End-stage Liver Disease (MELD) >20, or hepatic encephalopathy (Fig. 25.4). Active infection, gastrointestinal bleeding, acute pancreatitis, psychosis, hepatorenal syndrome/renal failure, and poorly controlled diabetes mellitus are relative contraindications for corticosteroids. In a retrospective, international multicenter cohort study, the maximum benefit of corticosteroids was observed in patients with MELD scores between 25 and 39.

24. How are steroids monitored in the management of severe AH?

For eligible patients, oral prednisolone 40 mg/day or intravenous methylprednisolone 32 mg/day for patients unable to take oral medications is initiated. Corticosteroid response is assessed on day 7 using the Lille score, which can be calculated online, with the major component being a change in bilirubin from baseline. With a range of 0–1, a score of ≥0.45 signifies nonresponse to corticosteroids, and it is recommended to discontinue treatment among these patients to avoid the risk of bacterial or fungal infections without further benefit. Among responders (Lille score <0.45), corticosteroids are continued for another 3 weeks. In a recent study, Lille score on day 4 of treatment performed similarly to the day 7 score and can be used for making an earlier decision regarding the continuation of treatment.

25. What are the limitations of corticosteroid therapy for severe AH?

About 30%–40% of patients are ineligible to receive corticosteroids due to contraindications for their use. Among patients treated with corticosteroids, only 50%–60% of patients respond to treatment which can only be determined after 4–7 days of administration of treatment. It must be recognized that these contraindications are not absolute, and corticosteroids can be used after adequate treatment of infection, gastrointestinal bleeding, or hepatorenal syndrome, with similar responses as in patients without these conditions. Furthermore, the durability of the response is only for 1 month. These limitations of corticosteroids result in their heterogeneous use with only 25%–40% of eligible patients receiving corticosteroids.

26. What is the role of nutritional supplementation in patients with ALD and AH?

Malnutrition is frequent in ALD and AH, leading to worse outcomes. A daily protein intake of 1.2–1.5 g/kg and caloric intake of 25–40 kcal/kg is recommended. Patients with poor oral intake (<1200–1500 calories/day) should receive supplementation preferably through enteral route. Vitamins and minerals should be replaced for potential associated deficiencies.

27. What are the emerging therapies for AH?

Given the limitations of corticosteroids, there remains an unmet need for newer effective therapies. Over the last decade, several therapeutic targets have emerged in the management of ALD and AH. Of these, fecal microbiota

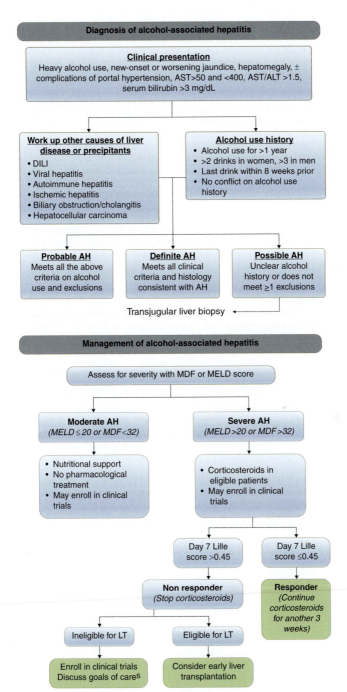

Fig. 25.4 Algorithms for the diagnosis of alcohol-associated hepatitis (AH) (*above panel*) and management of AH (*below panel*). *ALT*, Alanine aminotransferase; *AST*, aspartate aminotransferase; *DILI*, drug-induced liver injury; *LT*, liver transplant; *MDF*, Maddrey discriminant function; *MELD*, Model for End-stage Liver Disease. (Modified from DiMartini AF, Leggio L, Singal AK. Barriers to the management of alcohol use disorder and alcohol-associated liver disease: strategies to implement integrated care models. Lancet Gastroenterol Hepatol 2022;7(2):186-195.)

transplant (FMT), interleukin-22 (IL-22), granulocyte colony–stimulating factor (G-CSF), and DUR-928 have shown promise. Data are also emerging on the benefits of FMT in reducing craving and promoting abstinence. Data on G-CSF are mixed and controversial, with benefits reported from Asia, but not in studies performed in Europe. Currently, phase 2 and 3 studies are ongoing to examine the role of G-CSF, DUR-928, and IL-22 in the management of patients with AH.

28. **What is the role of early liver transplantation (LT) in patients with ALD?**
Early LT, transplant performed prior to a defined period of abstinence, has emerged as a salvage treatment for patients with decompensated alcohol-associated cirrhosis or with severe AH. Several studies have observed that the minimum of 6 months of abstinence from alcohol (6-month rule) is not a strong predictor of relapse to alcohol use after transplantation. In fact, psychosocial status of the candidate, younger age, and previous failed rehabilitation attempts are stronger variables associated with relapse to alcohol use after LT. In a prospective study challenging the 6-month rule, early LT in selected 26 patients with severe AH compared to 26 patients with severe AH not selected for early LT showed a survival benefit at 6 months and at 2 years (77% vs. 23%). Post-transplant alcohol relapse occurred in three patients (heavy in one) at 2 years. The selection criteria for LT were as follows: first episode of decompensation, nonresponse to corticosteroids, excellent psychosocial status with consensus among treating teams, and patient signed contract on maintaining abstinence after LT. Since then several case series, prospective, and retrospective studies have shown similar findings. Currently, most societies recommend of early LT in selected patients with decompensated ALD and AH. However, there remains an unmet clinical need for objective criteria and protocol for patient selection to optimize the management of these patients maintaining rational use of donor organs.

29. **What is the role of alcohol abstinence in determining long-term patient survival among patients with ALD?**
Abstinence is the single most important factor in determining long-term survival in patients with ALD. After an episode of AH, 1-year mortality was 44% and 29% among relapsers to alcohol use and abstainers, respectively. Abstinence is also associated with improvement in fibrosis and portal hypertension which can be significant resulting in delisting from the liver transplant list.

30. **What is the magnitude of alcohol relapse after transplant in patients with pretransplant AUD, and how does this impact outcomes?**
ALD is the leading cause of LT in the United States contributing to 40%–45% of all LT performed in 2018. Liver graft and patient survival at 5 years are over 80%. Furthermore, the alcohol relapse rate is not significantly different, when comparing patients undergoing early LT versus LT after $\geq$6 months of abstinence. The annual incidence of alcohol relapse is approximately 5% for any alcohol use and 3% for heavy drinking. Relapse to heavy drinking impacts long-term patient survival with the risk of recurrent alcoholic cirrhosis, AH, and malignancy (especially of the aerodigestive tract) being the commonest reasons of patient mortality.

31. **What are the federal policies to reduce the risk and progression of liver disease?**
Minimum unit price of alcohol, taxation, and control over advertising and promotion of alcohol are federal policies with documented benefits in reducing per capita alcohol consumption and associated morbidity and mortality from ALD. Studies have shown a direct correlation between the number of alcohol control policies within a country with ALD-related morbidity and mortality in that specific country.

CLINICAL VIGNETTE

Available Online

BIBLIOGRAPHY

Available Online

CHAPTER 26

VASCULAR LIVER DISEASE

Dawn M. Torres, MD and Clemence C. White, DO

 Additional content available online.

BACKGROUND

1. **Which vessels supply blood and are responsible for oxygen delivery to the liver?**
   1. Hepatic artery proper (HAP): supplies 30% of the liver's blood supply and ~60% of its oxygen supply.
      a. Abdominal aorta → celiac trunk → common hepatic artery → HAP
   2. Portal vein (PV): supplies 70% of total liver blood flow. It carries ~40% of oxygen supply. The PV delivers intestinal nutrients, drugs, and inflammatory mediators directly to the liver after intestinal absorption.
      a. Formed most commonly by the union of the splenic and superior mesenteric veins
      b. Additional tributaries: inferior mesenteric, cystic, and left and right gastric veins

2. **Name the vessels that compose the portal vein.**
   Venules drain blood from the intestinal and splenic capillaries and form the superior and inferior mesenteric veins and the splenic vein. These veins join to form the portal vein that subsequently divides into tributaries that eventually branch into fenestrated capillaries (sinusoids) of the liver.

   Splenic vein ⎫
   Inferior mesenteric vein ⎬ Portal vein
   Superior mesenteric vein ⎭

3. **Describe blood flow at the microscopic level in the liver.**
   Blood flows down a pressure gradient from the portal venule and hepatic arteriole (derived from the portal vein and hepatic artery, respectively) through sinusoids. Fenestrated endothelial cells line these sinusoids. They supply sheets of hepatocytes before draining into the central venule.

4. **What is the conventional way to divide the liver into lobes?**
   The liver is traditionally divided into four hepatic lobes based on appearance, not functionality. They are the right, left, caudate, and quadrate. The left lobe is separated from the right by the falciform ligament.

5. **How many functional segments compose the liver and what is unique about them?**
   Using the system according to Couinaud, there are eight segments of the liver. Each segment functions independently with its own vascular inflow, outflow, and biliary drainage (Fig. 26.1).

6. **What is unique about the caudate lobe?**
   The caudate lobe is segment one and uniquely drains directly into the inferior vena cava (IVC).

7. **Describe the three "zones" of the hepatic lobule with respect to blood flow.**
   The hepatocytes can be defined by their proximity to either the portal triad or central venules. Zone 1 includes hepatocytes surrounding the portal tract where they receive the most oxygenated blood but also are the first exposed to any toxins. Zone 2 includes hepatocytes found in the intermediate area between the periportal and perivenular areas. Zone 3 is made up of perivenular hepatocytes that are the most susceptible to hypoxic-mediated injury (Fig. 26.2).

BUDD-CHIARI SYNDROME

8. **What is Budd-Chiari syndrome (BCS) and which blood vessels are involved?**
   BCS is anything that interrupts or decreases blood flood out of the liver. This commonly involves complete or partial thrombosis of one or all major hepatic veins (HVs) (right, middle, and left) or small HVs. In Asia, pure IVC obstruction or combined IVC-HV obstruction is more commonly diagnosed. Primary BCS is defined by an abnormality intrinsic to the vessels, whereas secondary BCS is where the inciting injury is extrinsic to the veins.

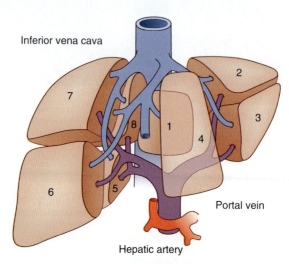

Fig. 26.1 Vascular and surgical anatomy of the liver. According to Couinaud, there are eight functional segments in the liver, which receive blood supply via the portal vein and hepatic artery. Efferent drainage is through the right, middle, and left hepatic veins. The caudate lobe (segment 1) has a separate and direct outflow into the vena cava via the dorsal hepatic veins.

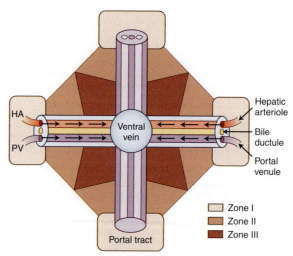

Fig. 26.2 Rappaport hepatic lobule with portal (zone I), sinusoidal (zone II), and pericentral hepatocytes (zone III). *HA,* Hepatic arteriole; *PV,* portal venule.

9. What are the causes of secondary BCS?
The causes of secondary BCS can be seen in Box 26.1.

10. What are the clinical features of BCS?
BCS presentation is variable with acute, chronic, and asymptomatic forms. Right upper quadrant (RUQ) abdominal pain, fever, ascites, liver and spleen enlargement, and unexplained liver dysfunction are important features. Ascites protein greater than 3 g/dL and a serum-ascites albumin concentration gradient of 1.1 g/dL is consistent with BCS, cardiac, or pericardial disease. BCS is diagnosed through Doppler ultrasound (US), magnetic resonance imaging (MRI), or computed tomography (CT) scan.

Box 26.1 Secondary Causes of Budd-Chiari Syndrome

Centrally Located Primary Hepatic Tumors
- Hepatocellular carcinoma
- Large nodules of focal nodular hyperplasia
- Polycystic liver disease
- Primary hepatic hemangiosarcoma
- Epithelioid hemangioendothelioma

Extrahepatic Tumors
- Renal adenocarcinoma
- Adrenal adenocarcinoma
- Sarcoma of the IVC
- Right atrial myxoma

Other Causes
- Kinking of the HV after hepatic resection or transplantation
- Parasitic and nonparasitic cysts

Blunt Abdominal Trauma
- Intra-abdominal hematoma
- IVC thrombosis related to trauma
- Herniation through a ruptured diaphragm

Cardiac Dysfunction
- Right heart failure with severe tricuspid insufficiency
- Constrictive pericarditis

HV, Hepatic vein; *IVC,* inferior vena cava.

11. **What is the Janus kinase 2 (JAK2)?**
JAK2 is a tyrosine kinase found only in hemopoietic progenitor cells. JAK2 V617F mutation is strongly implicated in the pathogenesis of myeloproliferative disorders (MPDs); they are found in approximately 90% of patients with polycythemia vera and 50% of patients with essential thrombocythemia and idiopathic myelofibrosis.

12. **What is the role of JAK2 mutations and other hypercoagulable states in BCS?**
About 41% of patients with BCS have MPDs. On diagnosis of BCS, a stepwise analysis for different underlying mutations is recommended starting with JAK2 V617F, flow cytometry for paroxysmal nocturnal hemoglobinuria, factor V Leiden and prothrombin *G20210A* gene mutations, and analysis for lupus anticoagulant and antiphospholipid antibody.

13. **What is the typical patient with fulminant or acute BCS?**
A pregnant woman or one on oral contraceptives will present with abdominal pain, hepatomegaly, jaundice, and ascites. Serum aminotransferase levels are >1000 U/L with alkaline phosphatase 300–400 IU/L, and serum bilirubin levels <7 mg/dL. Rapid deterioration of hepatic function and resulting encephalopathy and renal failure are seen in fulminant cases. Acute BCS requires immediate intervention for revascularization in an effort to prevent the need for liver transplantation. The clinical presentation depends on the location of the thrombus, its stage, and the rapidity of evolution (Fig. 26.3).

14. **How often are patients with BCS asymptomatic?**
Asymptomatic BCS accounts for up to 20% of cases and can be incidentally diagnosed.

15. **When should a liver biopsy be performed for BCS?**
Liver biopsy is reserved for cases in which Doppler US, MRI, or CT scan has not demonstrated the obstructed hepatic venous outflow tract.

16. **What are the histopathologic features of BCS?**
The predominant hepatic histologic features include centrilobular congestion, hemorrhage, sinusoidal dilatation, and noninflammatory cell necrosis. In delayed diagnoses, fibrosis develops in the centrilobular areas and to a lesser extent in the periportal areas.

17. **Why does BCS result in a massive caudate lobe?**
Caudate lobe hypertrophy is found in 75% of patients with BCS because of the separate venous drainage into the IVC that is not affected by obstruction of the HVs.

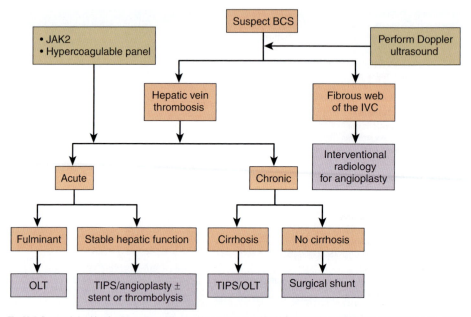

Fig. 26.3 Proposed algorithm for diagnostic and therapeutic management of Budd-Chiari syndrome (BCS). *IVC,* Inferior vena cava; *JAK2,* Janus kinase 2; *OLT,* orthotopic liver transplantation; *TIPS,* transjugular intrahepatic portosystemic shunt.

18. What is the role of hepatic venography in BCS?

Hepatic venography has been the gold standard for the evaluation of HVs, but other noninvasive radiographic modalities are generally adequate for diagnosis. Venography is now reserved for diagnosing difficult cases and for precise delineation of obstructive lesions before planning treatment.

19. What is the radiographic modality of choice if you suspect BCS?

US is considered the initial imaging modality of choice with a sensitivity and specificity of more than 80%. Doppler US provides information on vessel patency and blood flow direction. Absent or reversed hepatic venous flow is considered diagnostic for BCS. Both contrast-enhanced MRI and contrast CT can also diagnose BCS as well as provide indirect evidence such as enlarged caudate lobe or altered perfusion pattern as it relates to the caudate lobe and venous flow obstruction (Fig. 26.4).

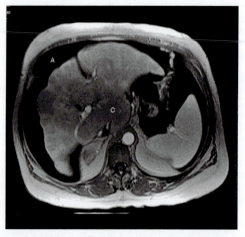

Fig. 26.4 Magnetic resonance image showing features of Budd-Chiari syndrome, including hepatomegaly with caudate lobe hypertrophy, ascites, and splenomegaly. *A,* Ascites; *C,* caudate lobe.

20. What is the role of medical management?

The goal of medical therapy is to prevent the extension of clot and prevent further hepatic necrosis using anticoagulants and to relieve fluid retention using diuretics and a low-sodium diet. Medical therapy is considered successful if ascites is controlled and liver biochemical studies improve, although this approach is successful only in a minority of patients.

21. What is considered medical therapy in BCS?

All patients with BCS should receive therapeutic anticoagulation. Indefinite anticoagulation therapy is considered in patients with an underlying hypercoagulable disorder. Thrombolytic agents can be considered in patients with a strong clinical suspicion for acute or subacute BCS and no contraindications to the use of thrombolytic agents.

22. What is the role of transjugular intrahepatic portosystemic shunt (TIPS)?

The role of TIPS is to decompress congested liver segments by creating an alternative venous outflow tract. TIPS is useful for treating combined hepatic-vein and IVC obstruction and can be effective in patients with fulminant BCS awaiting liver transplantation. In chronic BCS, TIPS is an effective bridge to liver transplant in those with refractory ascites or variceal bleeding.

23. What underlying hypercoagulable states can be cured with a liver transplant?

Liver transplantation will definitively cure an underlying hypercoagulable state caused by protein C, protein S, or antithrombin deficiency. Patients with other underlying hypercoagulable conditions require long-term anticoagulation.

24. What are the long-term outcomes for patients transplanted for BCS?

The prognosis after transplantation for BCS is good with reported 5-year survival rates of 75%–95%, although an increased risk of hepatic artery and portal vein thrombosis (PVT) has been reported. Patients with blood dyscrasias, such as polycythemia rubra vera, require treatment with hydroxyurea and aspirin to reduce long-term complications after transplantation.

PORTAL VEIN THROMBOSIS

25. How is portal vein thrombosis (PVT) classified?

1. Acute: PVT presumed to be present for <6 months
2. Chronic: occurs when an acute PVT does not resolve, and collateral blood vessels develop "cavernous transformation"

26. How do patients present with symptomatic PVT?

The main clinical features include sudden onset of abdominal pain and a systemic inflammatory response, often with fever. Partial thrombus might be associated with fewer symptoms.

27. What is the initial workup in a patient with a newly diagnosed PVT?

1. The initial workup includes searching for local, inflammatory, or general risk factors. In the absence of liver disease, evaluation for a prothrombotic state should be considered as myeloproliferative neoplasms are found in 25% of patients with PVT (Box 26.2).
2. In patients with cirrhosis an extensive evaluation for thrombophilic conditions is not necessary unless family history or routine laboratory testing raises other concerns.
3. Exclusion of malignant venous obstruction with appropriate contrast-enhanced imaging studies is mandatory.

Box 26.2 Risk Factors and Conditions Associated With Portal Vein Thrombosis

Local Risk Factors
- Cirrhosis
- Trauma
- Focal malignant lesions

Inflammatory Lesions
- Crohn disease
- Pancreatitis
- Duodenal ulcers

General Risk Factors
- Myeloproliferative disorder
- Hypercoagulable state

28. **What radiographic findings are associated with PVT?**
Doppler US shows the absence of flow within the portal vein or its branches. CT scan can provide additional information regarding the extent of the thrombus, the presence of related malignancy, or inflammatory lesions.

29. **How often does intestinal infarction occur with recent PVT and how does it present?**
Intestinal infarction has been reported in 2%–28% of patients with recent PVT, with 20%–60% mortality. Intestinal infarction should be suspected in patients with persisting intense pain despite adequate anticoagulation, hematochezia, guarding, ascites, or multiorgan failure with metabolic acidosis.

30. **What is the prevalence of PVT?**
PVT in patients without cirrhosis is a rare disease with less than 0.05% prevalence. In patients with cirrhosis the incidence of PVT rises with severity of liver disease: ~1% in compensated cirrhosis and up to 25% in likely transplant candidates.

31. **What is the efficacy of anticoagulation in PVT?**
Patients with acute PVT should be treated with anticoagulation as data support increased recanalization rates of the portal vein with therapy. Duration is unclear but most advocate at least 6 months of therapy or longer if there is another reason to do so. Long-term therapy for permanent prothrombotic conditions should be considered.

32. **What are other available treatment options for recent PVT?**
Local or systemic thrombolytic therapy should be considered as adjunct therapy in recent PVT in whom intestinal ischemia persists despite anticoagulation. Similarly, surgical thrombectomy is an option for patients who require surgery for an intestinal infarction.

33. **What are the goals of therapy for PVT?**
Prevent thrombus extension to the mesenteric veins; prevent complications of intestinal ischemia and achieve recanalization to prevent the development of portal hypertension and portal cholangiopathy.

34. **What are the outcomes of anticoagulation therapy in patients with recent PVT?**
Spontaneous recanalization occurs infrequently with complete recanalization in 40% and partial in 15%. Anticoagulation does prevent the extension of the clot in the portal system, as well as in intestinal ischemia. Most importantly, complications of anticoagulation appear to be uncommon.

35. **What treatment options are available for chronic PVT?**
Anticoagulation should be considered in patients with permanent prothrombotic conditions, although bleeding risk from esophageal varices should be established. Primary prophylaxis for variceal bleeding should be instituted prior to beginning anticoagulation.

SINUSOIDAL OBSTRUCTION SYNDROME

36. **What is the pathogenesis behind sinusoidal obstruction syndrome (SOS; also known as hepatic veno-occlusive disease [VOD])?**
SOS is caused by circulatory obstruction at the level of the sinusoid secondary to injury to perivenular epithelium leading to sinusoidal congestive obstruction. Occlusion of the central vein occurs more commonly in severe cases.

37. **What are risk factors for developing SOS?**
1. **Hematopoietic stem cell transplantation (HSCT) with an incidence rate of 15%
2. High-dose chemotherapy: cyclophosphamide, oxaliplatin, and gemtuzumab ozogamicin
3. Hepatic irradiation or embolization with yttrium-90-labeled microspheres
4. Thiopurines (azathioprine, 6-thioguanine, and thioguanine), and calcineurin inhibitor (Tacrolimus)
5. Consumption of pyrrolizidine alkaloid–containing plants, typically in herbal teas
6. Preexisting liver disease
7. Lung disease, particularly reduced diffusion capacity <70%

38. **What are the clinical features of SOS?**
Clinical presentation ranges based on the presence of symptoms and timing from the inciting insult. Acute presentations occur 1–3 weeks after exposure with nonspecific symptoms such as weight gain, ascites, RUQ pain, and hepatomegaly; or in severe cases, acute hepatic dysfunction leads to multiorgan failure and death. Subacute SOS occurs months or even years after exposure and presents with symptoms of fatigue, ascites, hepatic encephalopathy, or varices.

39. How is the diagnosis of SOS made?

SOS is considered in the appropriate clinical setting such as after HCT with weight gain, RUQ pain, hepatomegaly, and jaundice in the absence of other causes such as sepsis, renal, or heart failure. A transvenous liver biopsy with an elevated hepatic venous pressure gradient of more than 10 mm Hg in the appropriate clinical setting is highly suggestive of SOS, although the disease may be patchy and the liver biopsy can be falsely negative.

40. What are the preventive measures for SOS?

Ursodeoxycholic acid 12 mg/kg divided into two doses is recommended as prophylactic therapy for SOS in all patients undergoing HSCT. Also, adjusting the chemotherapy regimens before transplantation in patients with cirrhosis and optimizing liver status through avoidance of other hepatotoxic medications like azole antifungals and treating hepatitis C are all recommended.

41. What is the treatment of SOS?

1. Defibrotide infusion is the only the United States Food and Drug Administration–approved treatment for SOS and is recommended for the treatment of moderate-to-severe SOS.
2. Supportive therapy with diuretics to manage fluid retention is the mainstay of treatment. Paracentesis may be used as needed for ascites.
3. TIPS and liver transplantation have yielded mixed results and are not routinely recommended.

HEREDITARY HEMORRHAGIC TELANGIECTASIA

42. What is hereditary hemorrhagic telangiectasia (HHT; Rendu-Osler-Weber syndrome), and which genes are involved?

1. HHT is a rare (1 in 5000–8000 people) autosomal dominant multisystemic vascular disorder that affects the liver 2/3 of the time, particularly with HHT type 2. Vascular malformations result from a mutation in the activin receptor–like kinase type 1 gene that encodes for transmembrane proteins involved in the transforming growth factor–β signaling pathway. Disruption in blood vessel wall integrity from defects in vascular remodeling promotes the formation of a variety of vascular malformations, notably in the liver and gastrointestinal (GI) tract.
2. Three genes are implicated: *ENG* (Endoglin), *ACVLR1* (hepatic arteriovenous malformations [AVMs]), and *SMAD4* (GI tract AVMs).

43. What are the liver manifestations of HHT?

These can range from small telangiectasia to larger AVMs like a connection between the hepatic artery and HV. Presentation ranges from clinically silent to a hyperdynamic circulation with portosystemic shunting leading to ascites and encephalopathy.

44. How do vascular malformations lead to presinusoidal portal hypertension?

Microscopic and macroscopic vascular malformations occur with direct arteriovenous and portovenous shunts that progressively enlarge. Portal hypertension develops from chronic sinusoidal hypertension secondary to increased blood flow and increased fibrous tissue deposition at the portal and periportal levels.

45. Describe the clinical presentations seen in overt HHT liver disease (from most to least common) (Fig. 26.5).

1. High-output heart failure caused by intrahepatic shunting of blood
2. Biliary disease caused by ischemia of the biliary tree, which can lead to severe cholestasis with or without recurrent cholangitis
3. Portal hypertension (ascites more common, variceal hemorrhage)
4. Portosystemic encephalopathy
5. Intestinal ischemia

46. What other structural abnormalities are observed in HHT with liver vascular malformation (LVM)?

The prevalence of focal nodular hyperplasia is greater with LVMs (2.9%) than the general population (Fig. 26.5). This may lead to erroneous diagnosis of cirrhosis with hepatocellular carcinoma, neither of which is directly associated with HHT. Liver biopsy is not recommended for substantial bleeding risk. Cross-sectional imaging may confirm the diagnosis.

47. What is the treatment of LVMs?

Asymptomatic LVMs do not warrant therapy. Symptomatic LVMs consist of standard therapy for specific complications including heart failure, portal hypertension, and biliary ischemia. Bevacizumab and/or liver transplant is warranted in nonresponders to standard therapy.

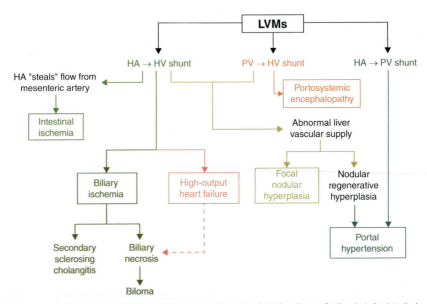

Fig. 26.5 Liver vascular malformations (LVMs) can lead to a variety of hepatic and extrahepatic complications including intestinal ischemia, biliary ischemia, high-output heart failure, focal nodular hyperplasia, portosystemic encephalopathy, and portal hypertension. Which of these secondary downstream manifestations will occur depends upon the type and severity of the shunt: hepatic artery (HA) → hepatic vein (HV), portal vein (PV) → HV or HA → PV.

PELIOSIS HEPATIS

48. **What is peliosis hepatis?**
    Peliosis hepatis is a rare disorder characterized by focal destruction of hepatocytes and sinusoidal endothelial cells, leading to multiple cystic spaces filled with blood within the liver. Patients are usually asymptomatic, but fatal intra-abdominal hemorrhage or hepatic failure may rarely occur.

49. **What factors have been linked to the pathogenesis of peliosis hepatis?**
    1. Infection with *Bartonella* species—bacillary peliosis hepatitis
    2. Other infections including tuberculosis, human immunodeficiency virus, and syphilis
    3. Immune disorders including hematologic malignancies or when taking immune suppression after transplantation
    4. Drugs including steroids, oral contraceptives, azathioprine, and other immune-suppressive medications

HEPATIC ARTERY ANEURYSMS

50. **What are the causes of hepatic artery aneurysms (HAAs)?**
    The primary causes are atherosclerosis, medio-intimal arterial wall degeneration, trauma, and infection. Vasculitis and connective tissue disorders are less commonly implicated.

51. **What are the clinical presentation of HAAs?**
    Most HAAs are asymptomatic and found incidentally in imaging. Ruptured HAAs into the biliary tract will present as hemobilia with jaundice, pain, and GI bleeding (Quincke triad). They are rarely present as mycotic (infected) aneurysm or can rupture into retroperitoneal or peritoneal space.

52. **What is the general management in HAAs?**
    Monitoring with serial imaging is typical HAA <2 cm and has no symptoms. The American College of Gastroenterology recommends endovascular or surgical intervention for all HAA >2 cm.

ISCHEMIC HEPATITIS

53. What are the hallmark findings of ischemic hepatitis (shock liver)?
There is a massive increase in aspartate aminotransferase, alanine aminotransferase, bilirubin, prothrombin time, and lactate dehydrogenase levels after an episode of systemic hypotension or decreased cardiac output. Once hemodynamic instability has been corrected, values return to normal within 7–10 days.

54. What are the long-term outcomes of ischemic hepatitis?
Patients tend to be older and acutely ill in the intensive care setting. Most deaths are attributed to septic shock, cardiogenic shock, or cardiac arrest. Fulminant hepatic failure is rare and seems to be restricted to patients with long-standing congestive heart failure and cardiac cirrhosis.

CONGESTIVE HEPATOPATHY

55. What is congestive hepatopathy?
Congestive hepatopathy is a chronic liver injury attributed to a spectrum of cardiovascular conditions with right-sided heart failure, leading to increased central venous pressure.

56. What are the histopathologic characteristics that correlate to the finding of "nutmeg liver"?
Hepatic venous hypertension leads to central vein hemorrhage, sinusoidal engorgement, and fibrosis of the terminal hepatic venules. The nutmeg appearance reflects the alternating patterns of hemorrhage and zone 3 necrosis.

MISCELLANEOUS

57. How does polyarteritis nodosa (PAN) vasculitis manifest as a liver disease?
PAN is a systemic necrotizing vasculitis with immune complex deposition in small- and medium-sized arteries resulting in hepatic infarction, abscess, and cholecystitis in severe cases. Diagnosis is confirmed when a tissue biopsy reveals necrotizing arteritis.

58. What is the most common vascular tumor of the liver?
Hepatic hemangioma (also referred to as cavernous hemangiomas) are benign tumors with a 2%–20% general prevalence found more commonly in women. Lesions smaller than 5 cm are usually asymptomatic, lesions larger than 5 cm may cause abdominal pain, and those larger than 10 cm are at risk for rupture with bleeding or can lead to disseminated intravascular coagulation (Kasabach-Merritt syndrome). MRI is the diagnostic modality of choice. Treatment with surgical resection or liver transplantation is reserved for large tumors.

ACKNOWLEDGMENT
The authors would like to acknowledge the contributions of Drs Marcello Kugelmas and Angleo Paredes, who were coauthors of this chapter in previous editions.

BIBLIOGRAPHY
Available Online

METABOLIC-ASSOCIATED FATTY LIVER DISEASE (MAFLD): NONALCOHOLIC FATTY LIVER DISEASE/METABOLIC DYSFUNCTION–ASSOCIATED STEATOTIC LIVER DISEASE (NAFLD/MASLD) AND METABOLIC DYSFUNCTION–ASSOCIATED STEATOHEPATITIS (MASH)

Dawn M. Torres, MD and Stephen A. Harrison, MD

 Additional content available online.

1. **Compare metabolic dysfunction–associated steatotic liver disease (MASLD) and metabolic-associated liver disease (MAFLD).**
   MASLD is defined by the accumulation of intrahepatic fat (steatosis) in the absence of significant alcohol use (~2–3 drinks per day for a male or ~1–2 drinks per day for a female) and the exclusion of other chronic liver diseases. MAFLD was proposed as a new nomenclature to reflect the pathogenesis of metabolic syndrome and make the diagnosis more one of inclusion rather than exclusion. However, this has not been widely adopted as of yet. MAFLD requires the presence of hepatic steatosis plus one of the following three conditions:
   • overweight or obesity
   • presence of type 2 diabetes
   • evidence of metabolic dysregulation

2. **What is the difference between MASLD, metabolic dysfunction–associated steatohepatitis (MASH), and nonalcoholic fatty liver (NAFL)?**
   MASH is a subset of MASLD, which in addition to hepatic steatosis, has histologic evidence of hepatocyte injury to include lobular inflammation, ballooning degeneration, with or without Mallory hyaline, and variable fibrosis. NAFL are those with metabolic fatty liver that do not have MASH. New nomenclature was recently adopted to replace NAFLD with MASLD.

3. **What is the natural history of patients with NAFL and MASH?**
   Patients with NAFL have a more favorable prognosis with one-fourth progressing to MASH and a much lower risk for progression to cirrhosis than their MASH counterparts. The clinical course of patients with MASH is variable. Natural history studies of patients with MASH suggest up to 20% progress to cirrhosis. The time course of progression is also highly variable, and while progression to cirrhosis typically takes a decade or more, it can occur rapidly over a few years.

4. **How is the mortality of a patient with MASLD compared to the general population?**
   All-cause mortality, liver-related mortality, cancer incidence (mostly hepatocellular carcinoma [HCC]), cardiovascular disease, and type 2 diabetes mellitus are higher in patients with MASLD.

5. **How do patients with MASLD present?**
   Patients with MASLD are often noted to have mildly elevated serum aminotransferases on routine blood work or hepatic steatosis on imaging. The majority of patients are asymptomatic, although a small but clinically notable fraction of patients complain of right upper quadrant discomfort. This symptom, which can range in presentation from a dull ache to sharp, severe pain, has been attributed to capsular swelling in the setting of hepatomegaly, although it is not always associated with liver enlargement and does not correlate with disease severity.

6. **What does the serologic workup for patients with MASLD show?**
Serologic workup is typically negative, although antinuclear antibody and anti–smooth muscle antibody may be positive in up to one-third of cases, in titers of up to 1:640. As a marker of inflammation, serum ferritin may be elevated. Ferritin levels more than 1.5 times the upper limit of normal predict more advanced MASLD histologic findings, and further study to assess the genetic markers of hereditary hemochromatosis or hepatic iron overload (via liver biopsy) should be considered in this scenario.

7. **Describe the typical patient with MASLD.**
Most patients are overweight, middle-aged adults, although the disease can present in childhood with a rising incidence secondary to the increasing numbers of obese children. There is an even distribution between males and females.

8. **What is the prevalence of MASLD and MASH?**
The exact prevalence of MASLD is unknown and it is easily the most common chronic liver disease in the developed world. Global prevalence is estimated at 25%. A higher prevalence of up to 75% is seen in patients with type 2 diabetes with MASLD.
Given the lack of histologic data in most prevalence studies, the rates of MASH within the larger MASLD population are uncertain, although autopsy data suggest an overall MASH prevalence of 3% to 6%. Two prospective prevalence studies in more than 1000 middle-aged Texans collectively, presenting for colon cancer screening, demonstrated a higher MASH prevalence of 12%–14%, and among morbidly obese patients undergoing bariatric surgery, prevalence rates of 91% for MASLD and 35% for MASH have been demonstrated.

9. **Are certain ethnic populations at greater risk of MASLD or MASH?**
Evidence suggests increased MASLD prevalence in Hispanic populations and a lower prevalence in African American individuals despite similar rates of comorbid conditions. Asian populations have also been shown to have more advanced diseases at a lower body mass index than their White counterparts.

10. **Are any genes associated with MASLD?**
Homozygosity for the patatin-like phospholipase domain-containing protein 3 rs738409 has been associated with increased rates of MASLD, often with increased inflammation and fibrosis. This gene family is involved in lipid metabolism and intrahepatic fat storage. Numerous other genes, including the glucokinase regulatory proteins (*GCKR* genes), have also been associated with prevalence and risk of disease progression such as HSD17B13 and TM6SF2.

11. **How can you distinguish between MASLD and MASH?**
The short answer to this is liver biopsy—it remains the gold standard and is the only test that can provide clear-cut evidence of steatohepatitis. Imaging studies, such as ultrasound (US), computed tomography, and magnetic resonance imaging, are very good at diagnosing steatosis with upward of 95% sensitivity and 80% specificity. Elastography, typically US-based, is able to estimate hepatic fibrosis and is used routinely to risk stratify patients.

12. **What noninvasive markers are available for either the diagnosis of MASH or fibrosis?**
As shown in Box 27.1, noninvasive scoring systems are useful to initially risk stratify those at greatest risk for MASH with advanced fibrosis. The MASLD fibrosis score and the fibrosis index based on four factors are the most commonly used. If these suggest a patient is intermediate to high risk, further evaluation with transient elastography is indicated. Liver stiffness measures >8 kPa predict at least intermediate risk and liver biopsy may be considered consistent with the established American Gastroenterological Association clinical care pathway (Fig. 27.1).

13. **How is the severity of the disease determined in patients with MASH?**
Hepatic histologic characteristics are the ultimate indicator of the degree of hepatic injury. The Brunt classification system is the predominant system used to assess hepatic histologic findings in which grade is defined by the degree of steatosis and inflammation and stage is based on the degree of fibrosis (Box 27.2).

14. **Are there other causes of fatty liver besides insulin resistance, obesity, and metabolic syndrome?**
Alcohol-induced steatohepatitis is indistinguishable from MASH on liver biopsy, but a lifetime adult drinking history of more than 20 g/day in males or more than 10 g/day in females supports alcohol as the primary cause of the patient's liver disease. A combination of lower alcohol intake, even as low as 40 g/week, with coexisting insulin resistance, may also lead to steatohepatitis. Other comparatively rare causes of hepatic steatosis with or without steatohepatitis are outlined in Table 27.1. Although these conditions compose less than 5% of cases of hepatic steatosis or steatohepatitis, they are important to recognize given their specific and unique treatments.

Box 27.1 Noninvasive Markers to Diagnose Metabolic Dysfunction–Associated Steatohepatitis (MASH) or Advanced Fibrosis

Laboratory Tests
- APRI $\geq$1.5 (significant fibrosis)
- AST/ALT ratio $\geq$0.8
- Proprietary tests: FibroTest, FibroMeter, HepaScore, and ELF

Scoring Systems
- BARD score
- FIB-4 score
- MASLD fibrosis score

Radiologic Studies
- Conventional imaging (for steatosis, not MASH or fibrosis)
- US
- CT
- MRI
- Fibrosis assessment:
  - Transient elastography
  - MR elastography
  - ARFI
  - 2D-SWE

ALT, Alanine aminotransferase; *APRI*, AST-to-platelet ratio index; *ARFI*, acoustic radiation force impulse imaging; *AST*, aspartate aminotransferase; *BARD*, BMI, AST/ALT ratio, presence of diabetes; *BMI*, body mass index; *CT*, computed tomography; *ELF*, enhanced liver fibrosis; *FIB-4*, fibrosis index based on four factors—age, AST, ALT, and platelets; *MR*, magnetic resonance; *MRI*, magnetic resonance imaging; *MASLD*, metabolic dysfunction–associated steatotic liver disease; *MASH*, metabolic dysfunction–associated steatohepatitis; *PPV*, positive predictive value; *SWE*, shear wave elastography; *US*, ultrasound.

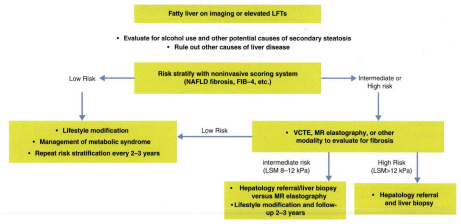

Fig. 27.1 Metabolic dysfunction–associated steatotic liver disease (MASLD) algorithm. *ALT*, Alanine aminotransferase; *AST*, aspartate aminotransferase; *DM*, diabetes mellitus; *HTN*, hypertension; *IFL*, isolated fatty liver; *LFT*, liver function test; *MUFA*, monounsaturated fatty acid; *MASH*, metabolic dysfunction–associated steatohepatitis; *pts*, patients; *PUFA*, polyunsaturated fatty acid; *SFA*, saturated fatty acid; *TZD*, thiazolidinediones. (From Kanwal F, Shubrook JH, Adams LA, Pfotenhauer K, Wong VW-S, Wright E, et al. Clinical care pathway for the risk stratification and management of patients with nonalcoholic fatty liver disease. Gastroenterology. 2021;161(5):1657-1669.)

15. What is the cause (pathogenesis) of MASLD, in particular MASH?

Insulin resistance is thought to be the common denominator in an intricate pathway that includes the accumulation of triglycerides in hepatocytes and ends with the activation of stellate cells that promote collagen deposition and fibrosis development. The intervening steps are thought to involve oxidative stress with increased levels of proinflammatory cytokines, decreased levels of cytoprotective cytokines, mitochondrial dysfunction, endoplasmic reticulum stress, altered gut microbiota, cellular autodigestion, and molecular endotoxins leading to apoptosis, as well as genetic factors that promote hepatic steatosis, necroinflammation, and fibrogenesis.

Box 27.2 Brunt Classification	
Grade 1	Up to 66% steatosis, minimal ballooning hepatocytes predominantly in zone 3, scattered PMNs, possibly intra-acinar lymphocytes with no or mild portal inflammation
Grade 2	Steatosis of 33%–66%, more prominent PMNs, obvious ballooning hepatocytes; mild-to-moderate portal and intra-acinar chronic inflammation also present
Grade 3	Marked steatosis, marked ballooning, intra-acinar inflammation with PMNs associated with ballooned hepatocytes, mild-to-moderate portal chronic inflammation
Stage 1	Zone 3 perisinusoidal/pericellular fibrosis to a mild-to-moderate degree
Stage 2	Zone 3 perisinusoidal/pericellular fibrosis with focal or extensive periportal fibrosis
Stage 3	Zone 3 perisinusoidal/pericellular fibrosis and early bridging portal fibrosis
Stage 4	Cirrhosis

PMN, Polymorphonuclear neutrophil.

Table 27.1 Causes of Hepatic Steatosis or Steatohepatitis.

CAUSE	COMMENT
Drugs	
Associated with Steatohepatitis	Steatosis (more frequently) and rarely steatohepatitis
Tamoxifen (and other estrogen	Can occur with normal serum aminotransferases
agonists)	Three months into treatment up to 4 years after stopping
Amiodarone	1%–3% of patients
Calcium channel blockers	Usually reverses on discontinuation of drug
Glucocorticoids	Rare cases of cirrhosis or acute liver failure
Methotrexate	Controversial association
Irinotecan	Mediated by ↑ serum triglycerides and glucose
Oxaliplatin	Pseudoalcoholic steatohepatitis
	Chemotherapy-associated steatohepatitis
Associated with steatosis	
Valproic acid	
Ibuprofen	
Aspirin	
Tetracycline	
Zidovudine/didanosine/stavudine	
Surgery	
Jejunal-ileal bypass	
Biliopancreatic diversion	
Extensive small bowel resection	
Miscellaneous	
Total parenteral nutrition	Jejunal diverticulosis
Bacterial overgrowth	
Abetalipoproteinemia	
Hepatitis C virus	

16. How do you treat patients with MASLD?

Lifestyle changes and management of their metabolic syndrome are the mainstay of therapy. A moderate reduction in caloric intake of approximately 500 calories per day, along with exercise designed to expend 400 kcal four times per week, is thought to be adequate to produce biochemical and histologic improvement, although large, well-designed studies are lacking. Modification of cardiovascular risk factors is essential as patients with MASLD are at an increased risk for cardiovascular events. In particular, statins can be used safely to manage hyperlipidemia.

17. What is the optimal treatment for patients with biopsy-proved MASH?

No single treatment has been shown to be universally efficacious and applicable to all patients in the treatment of MASH. Treatments are typically grouped into lifestyle interventions, pharmacologic therapies, or surgical interventions. Currently, there are no US Food and Drug Administration (FDA)–approved therapies for MASH, although this remains an area of intense investigation and it is thought that within the next few years, some therapy will be available to augment lifestyle guidance.

18. Describe the optimal lifestyle modification approach for patients with MASH.

Lifestyle interventions include caloric reduction and increased activity levels similar to what is recommended for isolated patients with fatty liver. There is also evidence to support diet composition modification such as low glycemic index diets with reduced fructose and saturated fatty acid intake. Increased intake of omega-3 fatty acids may also be of benefit.

The optimal physical training regimen has not been established and both resistance and cardiovascular training appear beneficial. Exercise of either aerobic or resistance training three to four times per week for 30–45 minutes of at least moderate intensity seems a reasonable recommendation. Although these interventions are safe and efficacious, they are difficult to sustain over long periods and are difficult to apply to clinical practice. While exercise can improve intrahepatic triglyceride independent of weight loss, the most robust data suggest 10% weight loss (from either diet, exercise, or both) is an effective treatment for MASH.

19. What is the role of coffee and MASLD?

Caffeinated coffee is composed of several bioactive compounds with favorable effects on chronic liver diseases such as hepatitis C virus (HCV), in which studies have linked its consumption with decreased hepatic fibrosis in patients. A recent cross-sectional study found an inverse relationship between the amount of caffeinated coffee consumed and hepatic fibrosis in patients with MASH. Moderate daily regular caffeinated drip coffee may be considered a reasonable adjunct to a multidisciplinary treatment plan for patients with MASLD (Hold the cream and sugar!).

20. What FDA-approved medical therapies exist for MASH?

There are no FDA-approved medical therapies. Numerous agents, including antioxidants, cytoprotective agents, lipid-lowering medications, weight-loss agents, and diabetic medications, have all been evaluated with mixed results. Vitamin E and thiazolidinediones (pioglitazone) have been the most studied with beneficial effects on MASH histologic findings. Pioglitazone use is limited due to its side effect profile, which includes weight gain (~2–5 kg after 1 year of therapy, peripheral edema, congestive heart failure exacerbation, and osteoporosis. Histologic benefits do not appear to be sustained with cessation of medication.

21. What is the role of vitamin E in the treatment of MASH?

The antioxidant vitamin E has been studied in adult MASH with generally beneficial results. A dose of 800 IU once daily demonstrated significant improvements in hepatic steatosis and inflammation but not fibrosis, although another smaller trial suggested fibrosis improvement with treatment. Once considered a completely benign therapy, vitamin E has been reported to increase cardiovascular risk, all-cause mortality, hemorrhagic stroke, and prostate cancer rates. It may be considered a second-line therapy in nondiabetic patients with biopsy-proven MASH that fail lifestyle intervention.

22. What are potential future therapies for MASH?

The newer diabetic medications, including the incretin mimetics/glucagon-like peptide–1 agonists such as liraglutide, semaglutide, and exenatide, have shown initial promise and studies are ongoing. The nuclear hormone receptor agonist obeticholic acid has shown efficacy in several large trials but has been limited by side effects, including pruritus and lipid abnormalities, and is not FDA-approved for MASH. Thyroid-hormone receptor-β agonists, peroxisome proliferator–activated receptor agonists, fibroblast growth factor–21 agonists, and inhibitors of lipogenic key enzymes including fatty acid synthase are other classes of medications being studied.

23. What is the role of bariatric surgery as a treatment for MASH?

Studies in patients undergoing bariatric surgery for morbid obesity demonstrate that surgical weight loss improves MASH histologic findings. Early studies in patients undergoing biliopancreatic diversion showed some concern over the worsening of hepatic fibrosis, but the vast majority of studies using either Roux-en-Y gastric bypass or gastric sleeve have shown significant improvement in hepatic histologic findings, with even total resolution of steatohepatitis reported. These studies offer compelling evidence that bariatric surgery in morbidly obese patients improves steatohepatitis. These invasive procedures may be considered for those with comorbid conditions that would justify the risks of an invasive surgical procedure. Endoscopic weight loss procedures are also being studied for this indication.

24. **Where does MASH cirrhosis rank for liver transplant indication?**
    Decompensated cirrhosis or HCC caused by MASH is currently the second most common indication for liver transplantation in the United States.

25. **What is the role of hepatic steatosis in liver transplant donors?**
    Up to 30% of all livers evaluated for transplant show some steatosis. Donor livers with 30% steatosis are considered acceptable, donor livers with 30%–60% steatosis are considered with caution, and donor livers with more than 60% steatosis are considered unsuitable by many transplant centers. Macrovesicular steatosis appears to be an independent risk factor for graft survival with >30% macrosteatosis demonstrating a 71% adjusted risk of 1-year graft failure ($P = .007$).

26. **What are the outcomes of a liver transplant for MASH cirrhosis?**
    Data are mixed with older studies reporting similar 1- and 5-year survival but a more recent study showed decreased 1-year survival compared to HCV or alcohol-related liver disease with death from cardiovascular or cerebrovascular disease. Post-transplant MASLD is common occurring in >50% of patients with a subset of these demonstrating MASH histology. Recurrent MASH cirrhosis in the first five years at rates ranging from 1% to 14%.

CLINICAL VIGNETTE

Available Online.

BIBLIOGRAPHY

Available Online.

CHAPTER 28

OVERVIEW OF LIVER TRANSPLANTATION

Karen Chang, DO, Rebecca Salvo, DO and Zeid Kayali, MD, MBA

 Additional content available online

1. **List the diseases for which liver transplantation is performed.**
   Acute liver failure (ALF) or complications of cirrhosis:
   - Autoimmune hepatitis
   - Chronic gastrointestinal blood loss due to portal hypertensive gastropathy
   - Chronic viral hepatitis
   - Hepatocellular carcinoma (HCC)
   - Nonalcoholic steatohepatitis (NASH)
   - Primary biliary cirrhosis
   - Primary sclerosing cholangitis

   Liver-based metabolic conditions with systemic manifestations:
   - α1-Antitrypsin deficiency
   - Familial amyloidosis
   - Glycogen storage disease
   - Hemochromatosis
   - Primary oxaluria
   - Wilson disease

   Systemic complications of chronic liver disease:
   - Hepatopulmonary syndrome
   - Portopulmonary hypertension
   - Hepatopulomnary syndrome
   - Esophageal varices
   - Ascites
   - Hepatic encephalopathy
   - HCC

   Evaluation for liver transplantation should be considered once a patient with cirrhosis has experienced complications such as ascites, hepatic encephalopathy, variceal hemorrhage, or hepatocellular dysfunction that results in a Model for End-stage Liver Disease (MELD) score of ≥15 or refractory to medical therapy. Furthermore, potential liver transplant (LT) candidates with worsening renal dysfunction or other evidence of rapid hepatic decompensation should have a prompt evaluation for an LT.

2. **What is the current basis for prioritizing patients for cadaveric transplantation?**
   The MELD score was first established in 2000 to assess mortality following transhepatic intrajugular portosystemic shunt (TIPS) placement in patients with cirrhosis. It was subsequently shown to be a good predictor of 90-day mortality following liver transplantation and was adopted by the United Network for Organ Sharing (UNOS) for the purposes of prioritization of cadaveric liver transplantation in 2002. The MELD score was an improvement over the previous use of the Child-Turcotte-Pugh (CTP) score in which it used objective data and emphasized a "sickest first" allocation of donor livers. An online MELD calculator can be found here: https://optn.transplant.hrsa.gov/data/allocation-calculators/meld-calculator.

   The MELD score incorporates the serum measurements of creatinine, total bilirubin, and international normalized ratio (INR) in the following formula:

   MELD score = 9.6 × ln (creatinine mg/dL) + 3.8 × ln (bilirubin mg/dL) + 11.20 × ln (INR) + 6.4

   Since the adoption of the MELD score, the rate of waiting list mortality significantly dropped from 30% in 2001 to 15% in 2005. However, some conditions place patients at higher risk of mortality such as HCC, hepatopulmonary syndrome, cystic fibrosis with progressive pulmonary compromise, portopulmonary syndrome, and cholangiocarcinoma. MELD "exception points" are added to move these individuals higher on the transplant list. Recent studies have shown that the MELD score also has its disadvantages. Some discrepancies can be accounted for by different laboratory limits in serum measurements. For example, creatinine is only a rough estimation of glomerular filtration rate and is influenced by extrarenal factors such as total muscle mass, ethnicity, and gender. The MELD-Na, which includes serum sodium in the calculation, provides better statistical performance for the risk of death among LT candidates: 7% of waiting list deaths could be averted using the

MELD-Na score. Serum sodium measurement is also subject to laboratory variation just as INR and creatinine and can be altered by therapeutic interventions (e.g., vaptans and diuretics).

3. For patients with chronic liver disease, when is the appropriate time to refer for liver transplantation?

Evaluation for LT should not be deferred even if a reversible component is identified, as the course of chronic liver disease remains unpredictable. In many cases, liver transplantation referrals begin when the MELD score exceeds 15 while on optimized medical therapy.

4. Which patients with HCC are considered and prioritized for transplantation?

HCC is the most common primary hepatic malignancy in adults and is currently the leading indication for LT in the United States. HCC typically occurs in the setting of cirrhosis, though in chronic HBV infection, HCC can arise in the absence of cirrhosis. LT remains the definitive treatment of choice for HCC in patients with cirrhosis.

The Milan criteria, introduced by Mazzaferro in 1996, restrict LT in adults with HCC as follows: (1) single tumor diameter ≤ 5 cm; (2) not more than three foci of tumor, each ≤ 3 cm; (3) no angioinvasion; and (4) no extrahepatic involvement. Patients who meet the Milan criteria have a posttransplant survival rate of 75% at 4 years. In the most recent modification of the MELD score, patients with a solitary HCC measuring ≤ 2 cm do not receive additional MELD points. If patients otherwise meet Milan criteria, they are placed on the transplant list with their biologic MELD score and automatically receive 28 points, and continue to accrue 10% increments every 3 months until the score of 34. Strategies to expand criteria for LT and HCC include downgrading the tumor by the use of locoregional therapy, such as transarterial chemoembolization (TACE) so that the Milan criteria are met.

5. What is the risk of HCC in patients with hepatitis C, and how has this influenced trends in liver transplantation?

Approximately 71 million people in the world today are chronically infected with the hepatitis C virus (HCV) and are at a greatly increased risk for the development of HCC. Patients with HCV-induced HCC are generally older than those with HBV-related tumors, as HCC can occur at any point during HBV infection, in contrast to HCV, when it is more likely in cirrhosis. Long-term follow-up of a large group of patients with chronic hepatitis C and cirrhosis found a cumulative 5-year frequency of HCC of just over 5%. The rate was higher among those with cirrhosis, at 7%. Treatment of hepatitis C with direct-acting antiviral agents (DAAs) results in a cure rate of over 90%; it also results in the regression of hepatic fibrosis and a lower-than-expected rate of HCC in those with the sustained biologic response. However, HCC may still occur in a patient with cirrhosis after DAAs have eliminated HCV.

Successful treatment of HCV with DAAs has dramatically decreased the number of these patients with decompensated cirrhosis listed for LT in the United States. Now, HCC arising in HCV patients with cirrhosis is an ever-increasing indication for LT. In these patients with compensated cirrhosis, TACE or transarterial radioembolization (TARE) therapy prior to liver transplantation is widely accepted, either as a bridge between treatments while the patient is on the waiting list or to downstage Milan criteria. Other possible locoregional treatments include ablation with radiofrequency ablation or cryoablation. TARE shows similar complication and survival rates compared to TACE, while producing a higher quality of life. For tumors <3 cm in size, it results in a 5-year survival that is comparable to transplantation and surgical resection. Similarly, ablation also produces survival outcomes similar to surgical resection in tumors <3 cm. Combination therapy with TACE and ablation provides the best outcomes for large tumors 3–5 cm in size.

6. Given the high waiting list mortality, is living donor liver transplantation (LDLT) an option and how much of the donor's liver is necessary for a viable transplant?

Experience with LDLT in Asian countries has suggested that a standard liver volume (SLV) threshold (a graft >40% of the recipient's SLV) is required to prevent small-for-size syndrome (SFSS). The SFSS refers to functional impairment of the partial liver graft during the first postoperative week (coagulopathy, cholestasis, encephalopathy, and ascites). Most adult-to-adult LDLTs in the United States use the right hepatic lobe for donation. Up to 38% of donors experience complications related to hepatic donation in the first 2 years following surgery. LDLT recipients may also have more biliary complications than recipients of cadaveric organs.

7. Who are potential recipients of LDLT?

The Adult-to-Adult Living Donor Liver Transplantation Cohort Study funded by the NIH demonstrated comparable survival rates and many survival benefits of LDLT over traditional deceased donor liver transplant (DDLT).

- LDLT allows patients to be transplanted at a much earlier stage with less severe disease and associated comorbidities. The survival benefit is even seen in patients with MELD scores <15. A significant number of these patients have decompensated cirrhosis with severe symptoms, and they are at a high risk of mortality despite a lower MELD score. It is these lower MELD but symptomatically ill patients who probably are the best candidates to consider for LDLT.
- Patients with HCC are another group that may gain significant benefits from LDLT. These transplants can significantly shorten waitlist time and eliminate the 20%–30% dropout from the waitlist due to tumor

progression. For patients with HCC exceeding the Milan criteria and unable to obtain exception points, LDLT may be a possible option as they may be excluded from DDLT by many transplant centers.

- The protocol for evaluation of the donor includes a complete history and physical examination, liver biochemical tests and serologic testing for viral infection, various imaging studies, and liver biopsy in addition to a psychosocial evaluation to ensure that there is no coercion, and an advocate is appointed to safeguard the donor's interests. In addition to testing and imaging studies, the donor liver will need to be at least 40% of the recipient's SLV or ≥0.8% of the graft-recipient weight ratio.
- SFSS is characterized by hyperbilirubinemia, ascites, coagulopathy, and encephalopathy. Pathophysiology appears to be driven by hepatic hyper-perfusion and congestion. To prevent SFSS, it is crucial to maintain large hepatic venous drainage for adequate outflow. Recipient conditions such as poor nutrition and sarcopenia can increase the risk of SFSS, as can a donor age ≥60 years, and fatty donor livers.

8. What is the definition of ALF (fulminant hepatic failure)?

In the United States the original definition of ALF is the development of encephalopathy and coagulopathy within 8 weeks of the illness onset without preexisting liver disease, which distinguishes ALF from decompensated cirrhosis or acute-on-chronic liver failure.

The King's College criteria is a prognostic tool used to identify patients who would most benefit from urgent liver transplantation. It predicts mortality risk based on acetaminophen versus non-acetaminophen ALF.

The following criteria identify *acetaminophen-associated ALF* with a poor prognosis and are unlikely to recover spontaneously:
- pH <7.30 more than 24 hours after ingestion, or

All of the following:
- Prothrombin time (PT) >100 seconds or INR >6.5
- Serum creatinine >3.4 mg/dL or anuria
- Grade 3 or 4 encephalopathy

The following criteria identify *non-acetaminophen-associated ALF* with a poor prognosis and unlikely to recover spontaneously:
- Prothrombin time >100 seconds or INR >6.5 or

Any three of the following:
- Age <10 years or >40 years
- Unfavorable etiology such as non-A, non-B hepatitis, and drug reaction
- Duration of jaundice before onset of encephalopathy more than 7 days
- PT more than 50 seconds (INR >3.5)
- Serum bilirubin more than 17.5 mg/dL

ALF escalates medical priority regardless of MELD score. These patients are placed into Status 1A or Status 1B priority. Status 1A patients have acute (sudden and severe onset) liver failure and are not likely to live more than a few days without a transplant. Status 1B is reserved for very sick, chronically ill patients younger than 18 years old.

9. A 21-year-old female is admitted following an overdose of acetaminophen. How is it determined whether she should be referred for liver transplantation?

The most common cause of ALF is acetaminophen toxicity. Acute ingestion of acetaminophen may cause severe hepatic injury via the formation of the toxic metabolite *N*-acetyl-*p*-benzoquinone imine via the cytochrome P450 system. Chronic alcohol ingestion may result in the induction of the cytochrome P450 system, which decreases the amount of acetaminophen required to cause hepatotoxicity. *N*-Acetylcysteine (NAC), a glutathione precursor, should be given in all cases of suspected acetaminophen overdose regardless of the dose or timing of acetaminophen ingestion. Early administration of NAC is recommended not only in patients with acetaminophen hepatotoxicity but should also be given in cases of non-acetaminophen ALF with grade 1 or 2 encephalopathy, in which it is associated with a significant survival benefit.

Donor organ allocation system prioritizes patients with ALF so that most patients receive transplants within 48–72 hours of waitlisting. Mortality on the waitlist is the highest for acetaminophen-related ALF. Studies have identified 5 clinical factors that correlate with poor outcomes: body mass index (BMI) ≥ 30 kg/m², serum creatinine level ≥2 mg/dL, recipient age ≥50 years, the need for inotropic support, and the use of life support.

In a US study the survival rate was 81% when none of these factors were present, and 42% when four were present. Objective evidence of brain stem injury should preclude LT, as well as confirmed systemic fungal infection. The overall 1-year patient survival rate following LT for ALF in the United States was 78.6%.

10. Is human immunodeficiency virus (HIV) infection a contraindication to liver transplantation?

In 2013 the HIV Organ Policy Equity (HOPE) Act was passed in the United States. HOPE reversed the previous federal ban on the use of organs "infected with the etiologic agent for AIDS." The intention was to increase the number of organs available to HIV-positive recipients. The use of highly active antiretroviral therapy (HAART) has changed the selection process for patients who are HIV-positive. From 2008 to 2018, persons with HIV accounted for 0.6% of liver transplantation in the United States. It increased steadily over that time, from 22 transplants in 2008 to 63 transplants in 2018. Solid-organ manifestations of HIV can be divided into the pathologic effects: (1) HIV infection of the organ, (2) opportunistic pathogens infecting the organ, and (3) consequences of HAART.

The selection criteria for patients with HIV are evolving but require:
- Patient on HAART treatment
- CD4 count 200 mm^3 or higher
- Absence of HIV-related infections or malignancies

In HIV-infected candidates who meet these criteria, survival following liver transplantation is comparable to patients without HIV; however, individuals coinfected with HCV and HIV have significantly lower posttransplant survival rates. Currently, there is active research in assessing the safety of HIV-living donors with HIV-positive recipients as well as HIV-negative recipients. Careful recipient and donor selection are important in optimizing outcomes in this population.

11. Is liver transplantation an effective management option for cholangiocarcinoma?

In most cases, cholangiocarcinoma remains a relative contraindication for liver transplantation; however, some transplant centers have reported acceptable outcomes in highly-selected individuals. LTs are more commonly performed in unresectable cases of early-stage (stages I and II) perihilar cholangiocarcinoma (tumor size <3 cm, without nodal involvement) in which protocols involving neoadjuvant chemotherapy followed by liver transplantation are associated with recurrence-free survival rates of 65% in the following 5 years. In cases of intrahepatic cholangiocarcinoma, liver transplantation is generally not performed because of very high recurrence rates. Overall, transplantation for cholangiocarcinoma is done under a research protocol and each must be reviewed and approved by the regional UNOS.

12. What conditions are considered absolute contraindications to liver transplantation?

Absolute contraindications include the following:
- Extrahepatic malignancy (excluding squamous cell carcinoma of the skin)
- Active uncontrolled sepsis or infection
- Active alcohol or illicit drug use
- Psychosocial factors precluding recovery after transplantation
- Uncontrolled cardiopulmonary disease (coronary artery disease, congestive heart failure, valvular disease, pulmonary hypertension, restrictive lung disease, and severe chronic obstructive pulmonary disease)

Relative contraindications include the following:
- Advanced age (65 years old)
- Obesity (BMI >35–40 kg/m^2)
- Portal vein or mesenteric vein thrombosis
- Cholangiocarcinoma (see earlier discussion)
- Psychiatric illness
- Poor social support
- HIV infection (see earlier discussion)

In 2019 the American Association for the Study of Liver Diseases (AASLD) Practice Guidance on alcoholic liver disease recommended that "[liver transplant] can be considered in carefully selected patients with favorable psychosocial profiles with severe alcoholic hepatitis not responding to medical therapy" and did *not* include the requirement of ≥6 months of sobriety.

13. An LT candidate develops worsening renal failure. At what point should a simultaneous liver and kidney transplantation (SLKT) be considered?

Consideration for SLKT requires at least one of the following criteria: (1) the presence of chronic kidney disease (CKD), (2) sustained kidney injury, or (3) metabolic disease. The number of SLKTs has increased over the last several years, particularly with the option of a "safety net." The "safety net" option is for LT recipients who fail to recover renal function or develop advanced kidney dysfunction within 60–365 days after receiving LT alone.

14. Do LT candidates with hepatorenal syndrome (HRS) require kidney transplantation?

HRS occurs in patients with cirrhosis and ascites due to hypovolemia and renal hypoperfusion in the setting of hyperdynamic circulation, reduction in cardiac output, and severe renal vasoconstriction. Two types of HRS are defined as follows:
1. **AKI-HRS** (acute kidney injury-HRS; formerly known as HRS type 1): a rise of creatinine at least twofold above baseline/admission creatinine, or a serum creatinine level of 4 mg/dL with an acute increase of ≥0.3 mg/dL or initiation of renal replacement therapy (RRT).
2. **CKD-HRS** (formerly known as HRS type 2): a more gradual increase in creatinine, usually at least a 50% increase in the last 7 days or a rise in creatinine of ≥0.3 mg/dL in the <48 hours.

Additional diagnostic criteria include the following:
- No improvement or partial improvement in creatinine after 48 hours of diuretic withdrawal and volume expansion with intravenous albumin.

- No shock, exposure to nephrotoxic medications, or evidence of parenchymal kidney disease (proteinuria >500 mg/day, hematuria >50 red blood cells per high-power field, or abnormal kidney imaging).

If the patient meets the definition for HRS, then the patient should receive prompt pharmacologic therapy: vasoconstrictor therapy with albumin supplementation. Patients who do not recover and who are deemed ineligible for LT may undergo TIPS as it can improve portal hypertension. However, TIPS increases the risk of transient ischemia to the liver and hepatic encephalopathy. RRT is not a treatment for AKI-HRS and is considered a bridge for LT. Patients who are not deemed to be transplant candidates are not considered candidates for RRT.

Although AKI-HRS is associated with progressive renal failure, requirement for RRT, and a very high mortality risk, the associated renal dysfunction is potentially reversible following LT. Data suggest that most individuals who undergo LT within 4–6 weeks of the onset of AKI-HRS will recover renal function and may not require a kidney transplant. The "safety net" kidney transplant is a possible option for those whose HRS does not resolve or worsens post-LT.

15. Is acute alcoholic hepatitis considered for LT? Which features of a patient's psychosocial profile connote a good prognosis for continued abstinence from alcohol prior to liver transplantation?

Alcohol-associated hepatitis (AH) is associated with a mortality rate of >70% and is refractory to medical treatment in many cases. The National Institute of Health (NIH) AH diagnostic criteria: onset of jaundice within 60 days in the setting of heavy alcohol consumption in the last 6 months with laboratory evidence of hepatitis demonstrating total bilirubin of >3 mg/dL, an aspartate aminotransferase level more than 1.5 times the alanine aminotransferase level and exclusion of all other known etiology of liver disease. Patients with AH with a Maddrey discriminant function of >32 or MELD >20 are classified as severe AH. If medical therapy is not effective, then LT remains the only life-saving option. Several studies have confirmed similar posttransplant survival rates in those with AH compared to those with alcoholic cirrhosis and other indications for liver transplantation.

Three- and five-year survival rates ranged from 84% to 87%. The selection of patients with AH for liver transplantation can be especially challenging as it is important to identify patients who have a poor prognosis without transplantation but are likely to maintain abstinence. Because the ability to predict both is difficult, selection practices vary widely across transplant centers. Patients presenting with AH should not have a previous decompensating event. Those who have already had decompensated liver disease and have recurrent alcohol use portends poor insight. There is a trend of emerging literature that suggests that the 6-month period of alcohol abstinence requirement before LT is an inadequate measurement of the risk of relapse, though some insurance plans will not assist with costs unless this criterion has been met.

This may penalize patients with recent drinking and a low risk of relapse as they may not survive waiting the full 6-month period. Recent guidelines recommend that transplant centers focus on psychosocial evaluation to select patients who are less likely to relapse. Several scores have been developed in an attempt to select lower-risk patients. These scores have some commonalities among them: they favor the presence of social integration indicators (e.g., presence of supportive family, spouse or partner, stable home and work, insight into alcohol use disorder) and negatively rate a history of failed rehabilitation attempts or preexisting psychiatric disorders. However, it remains clear that there is no single measure that reliably predicts relapse of alcohol use after LT.

16. Which factors measured in the recipient prior to transplant correlate with reduced postoperative survival?

Reports have suggested that pretransplant clinical factors such as Child-Pugh class and MELD score are not good predictors of survival after transplantation. Though early posttransplant outcomes have improved in the last 30 years, long-term survival rates have remained stable. Before the introduction of direct antiviral agents against HCV, hepatitis C recurrence in the graft was almost universal and made more progressive due to posttransplant immunosuppression. Patients with advanced cirrhosis related to metabolic syndrome and who have poor nutritional status pretransplant are at risk of developing NASH after LT. There is a strong association between metabolic syndrome and negative cardiovascular outcomes, which account for >10% of mortality late after transplantation. There is a 15%–30% increase in the prevalence of diabetes after LT. Tobacco use after transplantation represents an important modifiable risk factor. Recurrence of primary sclerosing cholangitis (PSC) may occur in 10%–30% of patients and is relatively insensitive to changes in immunosuppression and no specific intervention has been found to slow progression. Recurrence of autoimmune hepatitis (AIH) is observed in about 10% of patients with an average time posttransplant of 2 years. In contrast to PSC, AIH does respond to intensification of immunosuppression and reintroduction of steroids. Advanced age is also an independent prognostic factor in posttransplant survivability. In the United States, the proportion of patients listed for LT over the age of 60 years increased from 19% in 2002 to 41% in 2014, likely due to an increasing percentage of NASH and/or HCC as the indication for transplant.

17. Which immunosuppressants are used in liver transplantation? What are their mechanisms of action and side effects?

Immunosuppressants' mechanisms of action and side effects can be seen in Table 28.1.

Table 28.1 Mechanism of Action and Side Effects of Immunosuppressants.

DRUG	MECHANISM OF ACTION	SIDE EFFECTS
Tacrolimus Cyclosporine	Calcineurin inhibitors: block T cell proliferation through inhibition of key signaling phosphatase calcineurin -cyclosporine→cyclophilin -tacrolimus→FK-binding protein -pimecrolimus→macrophilin-12 suppresses IL-2-dependent proliferation of T cells	Nephrotoxicity, hepatotoxicity, lymphomas, infections (viral, bacterial, fungal), hypertension, hyperlipidemia, hyperkalemia, hypomagnesemia, glucose intolerance, gum hyperplasia, tremor, and hirsutism
Sirolimus Everolimus	*mTOR* inhibits IL-2 mediated signal transduction cell cycle arrest in the G1 phase prevents cell cycle progression and proliferation	Infections, lymphocele, thrombocytopenia and leukopenia, rash, bone marrow suppression, proteinuria, impaired wound healing, hepatotoxicity, interstitial lung disease, hyperlipidemia, *risk of hepatic artery thrombosis*, and teratogenicity
Mycophenolate	Inhibits de novo purine (guanosine nucleotide) synthesis to selectively inhibit T and B lymphocyte proliferation suppressing the cell-mediated immune response and antibody formation	Infections, leukopenia, anemia, pure red cell aplasia, nausea, vomiting, diarrhea, and teratogenicity
Azathioprine	Purine analog that converts to its active metabolites, 6-MP, and 6-TGN by the action of HPRT and TPMT enzymes inhibits purine synthesis, decreased circulating B and T lymphocytes, decreased immunoglobulin synthesis, and IL-2 secretion	Bone marrow suppression, leukopenia, hepatotoxicity, infections, pancreatitis, hypersensitivity syndrome (rash myalgias, malaise, elevated liver enzymes, hypotension), nausea, vomiting, and diarrhea
Corticosteroids	Sequester CD4+ lymphocytes in reticuloendothelial system. Inhibition transcription of cytokines (IL-1, IL-2, IL-6, TNF, and IFN-y)	Infections, sodium and fluid retention, hypertension, Cushingoid features, psychosis, growth retardation myopathy, muscle weakness, skin thinning, leukocytosis, carbohydrate intolerance and diabetes mellitus, osteoporosis and increased fracture risk, aseptic necrosis of femoral head, cataracts, and glaucoma
Daclizumab Basiliximab	Humanized and chimeric CD 25 *monoclonal antibody* blocks IL-2 receptor and selectively inhibits T cell activation	Hypersensitivity reaction
Antithymocyte Globulin	Antibody against multiple T cell surface antigens causing polyclonal depletion of lymphocytes	Cytokine release, lymphopenia, opportunistic infections, posttransplant lymphoproliferative disease, malignancy

6-MP, Mercaptopurine; *6-TGN*, thioguanine; *HPRT*, hypoxanthine-guanine phosphoribosyltransferase; *IFN*, interferon; *IL*, interleukin; *mTOR*, mammalian target of rapamycin; *TNF*, tumor necrosis factor; *TPMT*, thiopurine methyltransferase.

18. What is the typical immunosuppressive regimen used with LT?

Immunosuppression regimens after LT vary by individual and transplant center. With the advent of new immunosuppressive agents, the rates of rejection have decreased. Regimens should be individualized for efficacy and safety with care taken to understand those who may be predisposed to certain adverse effects. In general, a reasonable approach is to include various agents with diverse side effect profiles and de-escalate drugs when feasible. Corticosteroids are utilized in the early postoperative period. Calcineurin inhibitors (CNIs) remain the backbone of early and late-phase immunosuppressive regimens despite side effects. Antimetabolites (mycophenylate and azathioprine) are frequent choices for steroid and/or CNI-sparing strategies. Combination regimens are now favored to synergize benefits and reduce toxicities.

Table 28.2 Common Drug Interactions.

DRUGS THAT INCREASE IMMUNOSUPPRESSANT SERUM CONCENTRATION	DRUGS THAT DECREASE IMMUNOSUPPRESSANT SERUM CONCENTRATION
Amiodarone	Antiseizure medications, enzyme-inducing (carbamazepine, fosphenytoin, phenobarbital, phenytoin, and primidone)
Azole antifungals	
Cimetidine	
Ethinyl estradiol	
HART boosting agents (ritonavir, cobicistat)	Enzalutamide
Macrolide antibiotics (erythromycin, clarithromycin, azithromycin, fidaxomicin)	Nafcillin
Non-dihydropyridine calcium channel blockers (diltiazem, nicardipine, nifedipine, and verapamil)	Rifamycins (rifampin, rifabutin, and rifapentine)
Prokinetic agents (metoclopramide and cisapride)	Terbinafine
Protease inhibitors (atazanavir, nelfinavir, and saquinavir)	

HAART, Highly active antiretroviral therapy

19. What are the major drug interactions to avoid in an LT?

Both CNIs, tacrolimus and cyclosporine, use p-glycoprotein and are metabolized mostly in the liver by cytochrome enzymes/P450-3A4 system. Therefore, they have significant drug interactions. Drugs that inhibit liver microsomal enzyme function can impair the metabolism of CNI, leading to increased CNI blood concentrations and toxicity. Alternatively, enzyme-inducing drugs increase the metabolism of CNI and may result in lowered cyclosporine blood levels and an increased risk of transplant rejection (Table 28.2). If these medications are necessary, dose adjustments and drug monitoring are required.

20. How do you differentiate between acute and chronic rejection (CR)?

Acute cellular rejection (ACR) should be suspected after the elevation of liver enzymes in the early postoperative period, usually within the first month. However, labs alone are not specific enough to differentiate from other causes of graft dysfunction or even CR. A liver biopsy is required for definitive diagnosis. The diagnosis of ACR is based on the Banff criteria. ACR is divided into three categories based on histologic findings: portal inflammation, bile duct inflammation, and subendothelial inflammation of portal veins or terminal hepatic venules with each scored on a scale from 1 to 3 based on degree of damage. By definition, chronic or ductopenic rejection occurs months to years after LT, however, may occur only after a few months posttransplant and lead to graft failure in the first year. Generally, these patients present with progressive cholestatic graft dysfunction. These patients may be asymptomatic or may present with cholestatic pattern elevation in alkaline phosphatase and bilirubin. CR is characterized by destruction of the portal bile ducts or biliary epithelial atrophy also known as "vanishing bile duct syndrome." It can also demonstrate a decreased number of hepatic arterioles in the portal tract or obliterative arteriopathy. Other findings can include interstitial inflammation and fibrosis, atrophy of parenchymal cells, and disruption of lymphatics.

21. Describe the other posttransplant complications manifested by elevated liver enzymes

Posttransplant complications include primary graft injury (both immune-related and nonimmune), vascular complication, biliary, or infections (Table 28.3).

Immune-mediated graft dysfunction is frequently a result of rejection. Rejection can present with any biochemical pattern abnormality and some degree of cholestasis will be seen in both acute and CR.

Hepatic artery thrombosis (HAT) is the most serious vascular complication in the posttransplant period occurring in 2%–6% of cases. HAT can present with any biochemical profile of liver test abnormality but is more likely to present with significant hepatocellular pattern early postoperation. Doppler ultrasound is the first diagnostic test of choice if there is suspicion with angiogram or surgical exploration to follow if suspicion is high.

Biliary complications are the most common technical complication following an LT. Bile leaks commonly occur within the first month of transplant and can affect 2%–25% of transplant patients. Biliary strictures occur in 5%–15% of patients and tend to occur in the later postoperative period at 5–8 months. These both can present as elevation in liver tests, usually cholestatic in nature, abdominal pain, jaundice, and pruritus. Nonanastomotic strictures are caused by ischemic damage from hypoperfusion, mainly HAT, immunochemical reaction from ABO-incompatible grafts, AIH, PSC, and chronic ductopenic rejection.

Lastly, infections should be considered in the differential for all degrees and patterns of liver biochemistry abnormalities.

Table 28.3 Complications With Elevated Liver Enzymes.

PRIMARY GRAFT DYSFUNCTION	
NONIMMUNE	**IMMUNE**
Preservation injury Primary infection Recurrent Infection Recurrent primary liver disease (i.e., NASH and alcohol) Drug-induced (immunosuppression and antibiotics)	Rejection (acute, chronic, and antibody-mediated) Recurrence of autoimmune hepatitis, PBC, and PSC
Vascular Hepatic artery stenosis Hepatic artery thrombosis Portal vein thrombosis	
Biliary Bile leak Biliary structure	
Infection Viral Bacterial Fungal	

NASH, Nonalcoholic steatohepatitis; *PBC*, primary biliary cholangitis; *PSC*, primary sclerosing cholangitis.

22. **How often is it necessary to perform a second LT, and for what reasons are re-transplantations performed?**

    About 10% of all LT procedures are re-transplants. Improvements in immunosuppression, operative technique, and organ procurement have enhanced the probability of long-term graft survival. However, despite this, some LTs fail. The primary indications for re-transplant in the early postoperative time period have been early graft failure from venous thrombosis, HAT, ischemic-type biliary lesions, and acute rejection. Late re-transplant is usually due to the recurrence of the initial disease. Most commonly autoimmune hepatitis (36%–68%), primary biliary cirrhosis (21%–37%), and primary sclerosing cholangitis (20%–25%). The introduction of DAAs has significantly decreased the need for transplantation for hepatitis C and has improved outcomes following re-transplant. Similarly, the evolution of antiviral drugs and hepatitis B immunoglobulin (HBIg) has also dramatically improved outcomes in recurrent hepatitis B. Previously, recurrent HBV was considered a futile indication for re-transplant with a 2-year survival of less than 50%. Now with nucleoside and nucleotide analogs and HBIg, recurrent hepatitis B has declined to less than 10%. Most transplant centers have switched to HBIg-free protocol utilizing lifelong tenofovir or entecavir to reduce viral relapse after transplant.

23. **Describe the long-term metabolic complications that occur in the LT recipient.**

    Metabolic syndrome, which includes hypertension, hyperglycemia, dyslipidemia, and obesity, is one of the most common complications following an LT. Prevalence ranges from 44% to 58%. Metabolic syndrome when combined with immunosuppression is the main risk factor for the development of cardiovascular disease.

    Hypertension is usually caused by immunosuppressive drugs as a result of their effect on the renal system and the systemic changes they induce. CNIs, more commonly cyclosporine, create hypertension by vasoconstriction of the afferent arteriole causing resorption of sodium and water and therefore, volume expansion. Steroids can also cause hypertension due to their mineralocorticoid effect. Dyslipidemia can occur in up to 70% of posttransplant patients. This is in part due to alteration in hepatic synthesis as well as medication effects. Both CNIs and steroids may be implicated. The majority of patients after transplant will also develop CKD. The etiology remains multifactorial with the most common causes including chronic CNI use, hypertension, diabetes, obesity, dyslipidemia, pretransplant kidney disease, and perioperative AKI. The incidence of new-onset diabetes after transplant (NODALT) ranges from 14% to 44%. Risk factors for the development of NODALT include prediabetes, previous steatosis or steatohepatitis, and receiving a graft with steatosis, or graft from donors after circulatory death. Steroids and CNI increase insulin resistance and reduce beta cell secretion. NODALT is associated with a high risk of developing cardiovascular disease and posttransplant mortality.

24. **Are LT recipients at increased risk of developing cancer?**

    Patients undergoing liver transplantation are at increased risk of developing de novo malignancies (DNMs). Previous studies have shown that patients undergoing orthotopic liver transplantation (OLT) have a two- to four-fold increased risk of developing DNM compared to age and sex-matched controls. Skin cancers are the most common DNM in adult LT recipients accounting for almost 40% of malignancies in these patients. Nonmelanoma skin cancers (such as squamous cell carcinoma, basal cell carcinoma, and Kaposi sarcoma) account for most of these and occur at a 20- to 70-fold higher rate than the general population. The relative risk for Kaposi sarcoma is up to 500-fold higher accounting for 0.2%–3.5% of all DNMs. Posttransplant lymphoproliferative disorder (PTLD) is the second most common DNM occurring after OLT representing about 35% of nonskin malignancies. Most PTLDs are caused by Epstein-Barr virus. The overall incidence ranges from 1% to 3% in adults and most commonly occurs in the first year after transplant, presumably due to higher doses of immunosuppression.

Colorectal cancer is often diagnosed between years 1 and 4 with the highest risk at year 5 in patients with PSC. The risk of colorectal cancer in the PSC population is increased to 5.6%. Additionally, patients undergoing OLT are at a two- to three-fold higher risk of developing lung cancer compared to the general population. Head and neck cancers are less common but are the most serious DNMs. Tobacco is a risk factor in the development of tongue and pharyngeal cancer. Equally, alcohol and alcoholic liver diseases have been associated with the development of oropharyngeal, squamous cell carcinoma of esophagus, skin, lung, colorectal cancer, PTLD, and HCC in patients undergoing OLT.

25. **What factors contribute to metabolic bone disease after transplantation?**
Bone disease is an important cause of morbidity after liver transplantation. The majority of patients undergoing LT already have some degree of bone disease prior to LT. Abnormal bone metabolism and osteoblast dysfunction seen in chronic liver disease is further aggravated by excess alcohol use, hyperbilirubinemia, hypogonadism, and decreased insulin-like growth factor. After an LT, almost all liver recipients will have accelerated bone loss in the first 4 months postoperatively. This is mostly attributed to medication effects of corticosteroids, possibly CNI's as well as reduced mobility in postoperative patients. After the first 4 postoperative months, there is a gain in bone mass and a gradual decrease in fracture risk. Corticosteroids can also cause osteonecrosis, usually affecting the femoral head.

CLINICAL VIGNETTE

Available Online.

BIBLIOGRAPHY

Available Online.

CHAPTER 29

ASCITES

Nathalie A. Pena Polanco, MD and Kalyan Ram Bhamidimarri, MD, MPH, FACG, FAASLD

⊕ **Additional content available online**

1. **What is the clinical significance of the development of ascites in patients with cirrhosis?**

   Ascites is the accumulation of fluid within the peritoneal cavity, typically the first event that results from clinical decompensation of patients with cirrhosis, associated with a significant reduction in 5-year survival rates. It is important to note that cirrhosis is not the only cause of ascites, and other systemic conditions, such as heart failure, peritoneal carcinomatosis, alcoholic hepatitis, and fulminant liver failure can account for its development. The differential diagnosis of ascites can be categorized according to their pathophysiology (Table 29.1).

2. **What are the most commonly used clinical tools in the diagnosis of ascites?**

   Ascites is diagnosed when large amounts of fluid are present in the peritoneal cavity.

   Initial evaluation should include a thorough clinical history and physical examination, with ultrasonography-guided abdominal paracentesis (when feasible) for the characterization of peritoneal fluid. Analysis of the peritoneal fluid, by measuring the albumin and protein content, provides information about the etiology of cirrhosis, whereas analysis of the cell count, Gram stain, and/or bacterial cultures, is paramount in the diagnosis of spontaneous bacterial peritonitis (SBP).

   Diagnostic paracentesis should always be performed upon identification of first episode of ascites, either in the inpatient or outpatient setting, at the time of hospitalization of patients with cirrhosis and ascites, and if SBP or secondary bacterial peritonitis is suspected.

3. **How should a diagnostic paracentesis be performed?**

   Paracentesis is a safe procedure associated with low rate of complications, even in patients with a certain degree of coagulopathy (international normalized ratio >1.5 and platelet count <50,000/mL), without the need for fresh frozen plasma or platelet infusion, although it should be avoided in cases of disseminated intravascular coagulation. Employing sterile technique, paracentesis needle should be inserted in an area that is dull to

Table 29.1 Differential Diagnosis of Ascites Categorized According to Pathophysiology.

MECHANISM	DIFFERENTIAL DIAGNOSIS
Portal hypertension	Cirrhosis Alcoholic hepatitis Acute liver failure Hepatic vein occlusion (Budd-Chiari syndrome) Heart failure Constrictive pericarditis Dialysis ascites
Hypoalbuminemia	Nephrotic syndrome Malnutrition Protein-losing enteropathy
Peritoneal disease	Malignant ascites Tuberculous peritonitis Fungal peritonitis Peritoneal dialysis Eosinophilic gastroenteritis Starch granulomatous peritonitis
Miscellaneous	Chylous ascites Pancreatic ascites Myxedema Hemoperitoneum

percussion. A site in the *left lower quadrant* two finger-breadths cephalad from the anterior superior iliac spine and two finger-breadths medial to this landmark appears to be the best site for needle insertion. Because the panniculus is less thick in this area, the needle traverses less tissue. Therapeutic taps in the lower quadrants drain more fluid than midline taps. Scars should be avoided, as they are often sites of collateral vessels and adherent bowel. Between 30 and 50 mL of ascitic fluid should be withdrawn for analysis.

4. **Which tests are frequently obtained in the analysis of ascitic fluid, and what is their clinical indication?**
Analysis of the ascitic fluid should be guided by the clinical course and setting of each patient. At the time of initial diagnosis of ascites, both ascitic fluid albumin and protein levels should be obtained, since calculation of the serum-ascites albumin gradient (SAAG) allows to classify the etiology of ascites based on the presence of portal hypertension. An SAAG >1.1 g/dL is indicative of portal hypertension with an accuracy of 97%, while lower gradients are associated with other causes of ascites (Table 29.2). In patients with portal hypertension, ascitic fluid protein levels >2.5 g/dL suggest the presence of cardiac ascites rather than cirrhosis, which usually presents with a protein level <2.5 g/dL. Protein concentration should be obtained during recurrent episodes of ascites only if primary prophylaxis of SBP is indicated or if secondary bacterial peritonitis is suspected in hospitalized patients; in the latter group, tests such as glucose concentration and lactate dehydrogenase levels can also be helpful when secondary bacterial peritonitis is suspected. Cell count with differential should always be obtained regardless of the clinical setting. An absolute polymorphonuclear (PMN) leukocyte count of $\geq$250 cells/mm^3 (PMN = total white blood cell [WBC] count $\times$ % PMN cells) provides presumptive evidence of bacterial infection of ascitic fluid. Culture of the ascitic fluid should be considered in all hospitalized patients; bedside inoculation of the ascitic sample into blood culture bottles increases the sensitivity of the culture to >90% in the diagnosis of SBP. An elevated WBC count with a predominance of lymphocytes suggests peritoneal carcinomatosis or tuberculous peritonitis. The diagnosis of abdominal tuberculosis has been historically challenging, with bacteriologic tests (smear and/or culture) showing poor sensitivities, but the use of nucleic acid amplification tests is very helpful. When pancreatic and neoplastic etiologies are suspected ascitic cytology and amylase levels should be obtained.

5. **How should the results of the SAAG be interpreted?**
The SAAG is calculated by:

$$SAAG = \frac{(\text{albumin concentration in serum}) - (\text{albumin concentration in ascites})}{(\text{serum and ascites samples are obtained simultaneously})}$$

This gradient is physiologically based on oncotic-hydrostatic balance and is related directly to portal pressure. In cases of *portal hypertension*, the SAAG will be high ($\geq$1.1 g/dL), with cirrhosis being the cause in more than 80% of cases. Other conditions that result in ascites due to portal hypertension include heart failure, alcoholic hepatitis, acute liver failure, massive hepatic metastases, hepatic vein occlusion (Budd-Chiari syndrome), constrictive pericarditis, portal vein thrombosis, myxedema, fatty liver of pregnancy and even mixed ascites (presence of multiple concurrent causes, including at least one that causes portal hypertension). Low-gradient ascites is found in the *absence of portal hypertension* and are usually due to peritoneal disease (Table 29.2).

Table 29.2 Classification of Ascites Based on Serum-Ascites Albumin Gradient (SAAG) and Ascitic Fluid Protein Content.

SAAG	DIFFERENTIAL DIAGNOSIS
High (SAAG $\geq$1.1 g/dL) confirms the presence of portal hypertension	Ascitic fluid protein <2.5 g/dL: cirrhosis
	Ascitic fluid protein >2.5 g/dL: post-sinusoidal (i.e., heart failure/constrictive pericarditis, hepatic vein occlusion)
Low (SAAG <1.1 g/dL) excludes portal hypertension	Peritoneal carcinomatosis Tuberculous peritonitis Pancreatitis Biliary ascites Nephrotic syndrome Serositis Bowel obstruction or infarction

6. **What is the current classification for ascites, and what is it based on?**
Ascites can be classified based on the amount of fluid accumulated in the abdomen and the response to treatment:
- **Grade 1** (only detected by ultrasound) or responsive ascites: fully mobilized with diuretic therapy ± moderate dietary sodium restriction
- **Grade 2** (moderate symmetric distention of abdomen) or recurrent ascites: recurs on at least three occasions within a 12-month period despite dietary sodium restriction and adequate diuretic therapy.
- **Grade 3** (marked distension of the abdomen) or refractory ascites: cannot be mobilized or early recurrence cannot be prevented by medical therapy.

7. **Describe the initial management of ascites in patients with cirrhosis.**
Moderate dietary sodium restriction and diuretic therapy are the mainstays of treatment in patients with cirrhosis and ascites, with more invasive interventions required in cases of refractory ascites.
- Dietary sodium restriction (2 g/day) is recommended to achieve net fluid loss; reducing dietary sodium intake and increasing urinary sodium excretion mobilize ascitic fluid by creating a net negative balance of sodium. Nonetheless, care should be taken to prevent malnutrition and sarcopenia. Fluid restriction is only recommended in the presence of moderate or severe hyponatremia (serum sodium ≤125 mmol/L).
- Diuretic therapy is required in most patients, even if adherent to dietary sodium restriction. Monitoring body weight is recommended to assess the efficacy of diuretics, with weight loss of up to 1 kg/day tolerated in patients with edema. Aldosterone antagonists (such as spironolactone) alone can provide adequate response in the initial episode of ascites, whereas combination with loop diuretics (furosemide, bumetanide) is usually required in the long term. The recommended starting dose of spironolactone is 100 mg/day, and for furosemide, it is 40 mg/day. If response to initial doses is not optimal, assessment of sodium excretion can further guide management; in patients with ascites, a 24-hour sodium excretion of <80 mmol/day usually indicates an insufficient diuretic dose, whereas higher excretion rates are associated with noncompliance with dietary restriction. Doses can be progressively increased every 72 hours to 400 and 160 mg/day, respectively, according to response and tolerability. Once ascites is controlled, minimal effective doses of diuretics should be maintained to minimize the risk of adverse reactions.
- In patients with tense ascites (grade 3), large-volume paracentesis (LVP) with concomitant human albumin infusion is the treatment of choice with diuretic therapy instituted after the reduction of intra-abdominal pressure to minimize the need for LVP in the future. This strategy is recommended in cases of hyponatremia as well. Management of refractory ascites (RA) is discussed separately.

8. **What is the definition of RA?**
RA develops in about 11% of patients after an initial episode of ascites, associated with 1-year survival barely above 30%; it is defined as ascites that cannot be mobilized or that recurs after LVP despite dietary sodium restriction and diuretic therapy. Based on the response to diuretics, it can be further classified as follows:
- Diuretic-resistant ascites: lack of response to sodium restriction at maximum doses of diuretics (400 mg of spironolactone and 160 mg of furosemide daily).
- Diuretic-refractory ascites: use of maximal doses of diuretics is precluded due to associated side effects, such as hyponatremia, electrolyte abnormalities, acute kidney injury (AKI), and gynecomastia (aldosterone antagonist), among others.

  Dietary sodium restriction is still recommended, while diuretics are usually discontinued, given that they are either not effective or have already caused complications that preclude their use. Long-term albumin treatment can be effective and safe, associated with decreased need for LVP, fewer complications and liver-related hospitalizations, improvement in circulatory function, and even improved survival in some cases; however, more randomized controlled trials are required before recommending long-term use of outpatient albumin infusions. Given that medical therapy provides limited benefit, the first-line treatment of RA is recurrent LVP and albumin infusion. Repeated LVP is more effective in controlling ascites than conventional diuretic treatment, is associated with a lower incidence of complications, and patients show similar survival compared to those who use diuretic use alone. In eligible patients, placement of a transjugular intrahepatic portosystemic shunt (TIPS) can provide better ascites control than LVP, albeit an increased risk of hepatic encephalopathy (HE). Despite initial conflicting data, most recent studies show that the use of TIPS is associated with increased survival when compared to LVP for the management of RA. Patients with RA should be referred for transplant evaluation. For patients who are neither TIPS nor transplant eligible, a referral to palliative care is reasonable; the use of abdominal drains can be an alternative to serial LVP for patients whose goals are comfort-focused; however, more data are needed prior to their routine recommendation and widespread use.

9. **Which intervention has proven to decrease the risk of post–paracentesis circulatory dysfunction (PPCD)?**
Studies have shown that total paracentesis (removing all the ascitic fluid present) is as effective and safe as repeated partial paracentesis. Several physiologic changes take place during the paracentesis; an acute increase

in cardiac output occurs while the systemic vascular resistance decreases, resulting in a slight reduction of blood pressure. Right atrial pressure falls acutely due to the reduction of intrathoracic pressure, and pulmonary capillary wedge pressure decreases after 6 hours. PPCD (defined by an increase in plasma renin activity or aldosterone concentrations) can occur hours or days after the procedure, and volume expansion, done more effectively with albumin when compared to other synthetic plasma expanders, should start as the paracentesis is completed. Albumin is used as plasma expander because it maintains the initial improvement in circulatory function seen after paracentesis and prevents the subsequent activation of vasoconstrictor systems and impairment in renal function. PPCD, which can lead to renal dysfunction, is associated with a shorter time to first readmission, re-accumulation of ascites, and survival. Therefore for those in whom greater than 5 L ascites is removed, it is recommended that albumin be administered at a dose of 6–8 g/L of ascites removed. Using the 2015 International Ascites Club definition for AKI in patients with cirrhosis, a recent study found that up to 23% of patients with cirrhosis can develop PPCD-associated AKI. Development of PPCD is an independent predictor of early mortality, estimated at 73% in this group, and an advanced Model for End-stage Liver Disease-sodium (MELD-Na) score was the only identified risk factor for AKI development after paracentesis.

10. Which patients with cirrhosis and ascites should be considered for TIPS?

TIPS is a side-to-side portocaval shunt created inside the liver by connecting a main portal branch with a large hepatic vein, with the purpose of reducing ascites formation by decreasing portal pressure, increasing (transiently) the effective arterial blood volume and decompressing both the portal venous system and the hepatic microcirculation. When compared to LVP, it is more effective in preventing recurrence of ascites, and when using covered stents that improve primary shunt patency, higher survival rates at 1-year are also noted (93% vs. 52%). Other than transplantation, it is the only intervention that acts directly on the pathogenesis of ascites, and in general, is considered second-line therapy for the treatment of refractory ascites. Alternatively, TIPS is strongly recommended in patients not fulfilling a strict definition of RA but requiring at least three LVP for tense ascites in a year despite optimal medical therapy, as well as in carefully selected patients with cirrhosis and RA. Contraindications to TIPS placement, independent of clinical setting, include very advanced disease (Child-Pugh >13 points), episodes of recurrent overt HE (without an identifiable precipitating factor), heart failure, and pulmonary hypertension.

11. Is there currently any indication for the use of permanent abdominal drains or other types of shunts in the management of ascites?

A recent meta-analysis described the current evidence available on the use of permanent indwelling peritoneal catheters (PIPC), used as an alternative for patients with RA who are ineligible for LT or TIPS, and for whom LVP is difficult. A total of 18 studies were included, with a total of 176 patients. Successful insertion rate was 100%, the use of prophylactic antibiotics was variable, and two-thirds of the studies recommended their use as a palliative measure. Rates of bacterial peritonitis varied from 0% to 42% across individual studies with an overall combined rate of 17%, and cellulitis at catheter insertion site was reported in 9 of 147 (6%) patients. Other non-infectious complications included transient hyponatremia (11%), rise in creatinine (8%), leakage of ascites at exit sites (8%), catheter occlusion (6%), and accidental catheter displacement (1%). Median survival ranged between 6 weeks and 5 months. The authors acknowledged that the studies were heterogeneous, of poor quality with small sample sizes, using a variety of different indwelling catheters, hence making direct comparison impossible; therefore these results should be interpreted with care. A recent American Association for the Study of Liver Diseases guidance on palliative care and symptom-based management states that PIPCs may be an alternative to serial LVP for patients with RA who are transplant and TIPS ineligible and whose goals are comfort-focused.

The automated low-flow ascites pump (alfapump®) is an implantable device that drains ascites directly into the urinary bladder, associated with high rates of infectious complications and need for recurrent LVP, and its use is not routinely recommended in the United States.

12. What is the pathogenesis of spontaneous infections in patients with cirrhosis?

The development of spontaneous infections is significantly increased in patients with cirrhosis compared to the general population; infectious complications are recognized in up to a third of hospitalized patients with cirrhosis, with SBP and urinary tract infection the most common sources. Multiple factors are at play in the pathogenesis of these, including alterations in the microbiome (characterized by intestinal bacterial overgrowth and dysbiosis); the combination of increased intestinal permeability caused by alterations in tight-junction processes and transcytosis of bacteria; genetic predisposition—certain genetic mutations of Toll-like and Nod-like receptors that recognize extracellular bacteria have been found in patients with cirrhosis and increased risk of SBP; and importantly, the presence of cirrhosis-associated immune dysfunction, defined by the simultaneous occurrence of immunodeficiency and persistent activation of immune system cells with their associated production of inflammatory cytokines. Bacteria can translocate to mesenteric lymph nodes and eventually to the systemic circulation; when ascites is present and seeded by bacteria, both SBP and bacterascites can develop, on occasion with positive blood cultures or spontaneous bacteremia (SB). Bacterial infection should be suspected when a patient with cirrhosis deteriorates, even if typical symptoms of infection are not present. In the United States, infections remain an important cause of mortality in patients with cirrhosis: a study of hospitalized patients with cirrhosis published in 2015 revealed that the risk of dying from sepsis has been progressively increasing over time, despite a decrease in mortality from gastrointestinal bleeding, hepatorenal syndrome (HRS), or hepatocellular carcinoma during the same time frame. Worldwide, the rate of acute on chronic liver failure (ACLF) development in hospitalized patients with cirrhosis who either present with a bacterial infection or develop one during their hospital stay reaches a staggering 48%, with SBP and pneumonia being the most frequent inciting events.

13. Explain how SBP develops in patients with cirrhosis.

Increased bacterial translocation has been associated with the development of SBP. Patients with intestinal bacterial overgrowth are more frequently affected by SBP than those without, and it has been noted that decreasing the bacterial burden reduces the severity of liver disease and infectious complications in patients with liver disease. Thus bacterial overgrowth, coupled with failure of the intestinal barrier, in the state of immune deficiency found in cirrhosis provides a favorable milieu for the development of SBP. Bacterial translocation does not occur in prehepatic portal hypertension where liver function is normal and immune dysregulation is absent.

14. What are the variants of ascitic fluid infection?

Ascitic fluid infection can be spontaneous or secondary to an intra-abdominal, surgically treatable source of infection; in patients with cirrhosis, the vast majority is spontaneous. SBP is diagnosed by the presence of a fluid PMN $\geq 250/mm^3$ in the absence of a secondary intra-abdominal source of infection or inflammation; isolation of the microorganism, if possible, is important for guiding antibiotic therapy. Bacterascites, on the other hand, is defined by a positive bacteriologic culture of the ascitic fluid in the setting of a PMN $<250/mm^3$ and can be monobacterial or polybacterial (usually caused by contamination).

15. What is the clinical significance of differentiating spontaneous from secondary peritonitis?

Bacterial peritonitis can arise from perforation or acute inflammation of the intra-abdominal organs, abdominal wall infections, or previous surgical procedures, and in these situations is referred to as secondary bacterial peritonitis. This condition often requires surgical intervention for resolution, a stark difference when compared to SBP, in which pharmacologic therapy is the mainstay of treatment. Given the difference in the management of these two conditions, prompt differentiation is essential. It should be noted that although surgical intervention is the treatment of choice for most cases of secondary bacterial peritonitis, it can, in turn, precipitate significant clinical deterioration in the patient with cirrhosis.

The following criteria, although highly sensitive in the detection of secondary bacterial peritonitis, have low sensitivity but are employed in clinical practice to differentiate the etiology of ascitic fluid infections in selected cases:

1. Lack of response to antibiotic therapy is defined as absence of a significant decrease (or even an increase) in ascitic fluid PMN cell count in follow-up paracenteses.
2. Presence of polybacteria in ascites fluid culture, especially if anaerobic bacteria or fungi are observed.
3. At least two of the following findings in the ascitic fluid: glucose levels $<50\,mg/dL$, protein concentration $>10\,g/L$, or lactic dehydrogenase concentration $>$ normal serum levels.

A recent retrospective, multicenter observational study identified two factors independently associated with secondary peritonitis in patients with cirrhosis admitted to the intensive care unit (ICU): an ascitic leukocyte count $>10,000/mm^3$ and absence of laboratory signs of decompensated cirrhosis. Most positive cultures were polymicrobial, and the associated 1-year mortality rate was 80%; none of the patients who did not receive surgical intervention survived the hospitalization.

16. Which patients are at higher risk of developing SBP?

Patients with an *ascitic total protein level $<1.5\,g/dL$* with *advanced liver disease* (defined by Child-Turcotte-Pugh score ≥ 9 points with serum bilirubin $\geq 3\,mg/dL$) or *renal impairment* (characterized by serum creatinine $\geq 1.2\,mg/dL$, urea nitrogen $\geq 25\,mg/dL$, or sodium $\leq 130\,mmol/L$) have a 1-year probability of developing SBP estimated to be higher than 60%. Patients with *prior history of SBP* also have a probability close to 70% of SBP recurrence at 1-year, which decreases to less than a third of that if antibiotic prophylaxis is used.

17. Is a positive culture required to establish the diagnosis of SBP?

If SBP is suspected clinically, empiric antibiotic therapy should be started immediately after diagnostic paracentesis. In hospitalized patients with ascites, a diagnostic paracentesis should always be pursued, and delay ($>12\,hours$ after presentation) has been associated with a 2.7-fold increase in mortality from SBP. SBP is diagnosed based on analysis of the ascitic fluid *PMN $\geq 250\,cells/mm^3$*. Despite using sensitive methods, culture of ascitic fluid is negative in as many as 60% of patients suspected of having SBP with an increased neutrophil count, and therefore a positive culture is not required to make the diagnosis, although it remains essential to guide antibiotic therapy. Patients with an ascitic fluid *PMN $\geq 250\,cells/mm^3$ and negative culture* have *culture-negative SBP*.

18. **What is the treatment of choice for suspected SBP?**

Response to initial antibiotic therapy has been declining over time due to the emergence of multidrug-resistant organisms (MDROs), bacteria with acquired nonsusceptibility to at least one agent in three or more antimicrobial categories, and this has been reflected in current guidelines. Whereas third-generation cephalosporins traditionally achieved a high success rate and were thus recommended to all patients with SBP, present guidelines propose their use based on local bacterial prevalence, namely *in settings where MDROs are not common.* Antibiotic choice should be broader in patients with increased risk of MDRO infections, such as those with prior health care exposure and use of antibiotics in the 3 months prior to hospitalization. Recent data show that in critically ill patients and those with nosocomial infections, initial use of carbapenems may lead to higher resolution rates and lower mortality than the use of third-generation cephalosporins. Overall, patients with risk factors for MDRO should receive piperacillin/tazobactam with vancomycin added if they have had a prior infection or a positive surveillance swab for methicillin-resistant *Staphylococcus aureus*; daptomycin should be chosen instead if the organism was a vancomycin-resistant enterococcus. Patients with recent exposure to piperacillin/tazobactam should receive meropenem. Length of treatment should be 5–7 days.

For patients with cirrhosis and SBP, renal dysfunction is the main prognostic factor, associated with high mortality rates. Dual therapy of antibiotics plus albumin (at a dose of 1.5 g/kg of body weight at the time of diagnosis, followed by 1 g/kg on day 3) has shown a reduction in the incidence of renal impairment and associated mortality in comparison with antibiotic monotherapy, and its use is recommended by current guidelines.

19. **What is the clinical significance of MDRO infection?**

Globally, the prevalence of infections caused by MDROs in patients with cirrhosis is close to 34%, roughly double than that in the United States. Infections caused by multidrug resistance (MDR) bacteria are associated with lower rates of resolution, higher incidence of septic shock and new organ failures (need for mechanical ventilation or renal replacement therapy [RRT]), as well as higher in-hospital mortality than those caused by non-MDR bacteria. Considering this, adequate empirical antibiotic treatment is fundamental to improve in-hospital and 28-day survival.

20. **Should diagnostic paracentesis be repeated during the treatment of SBP?**

Traditionally, treatment with cefotaxime (2 g intravenous [IV] every 12 hours for 5 days) achieved a rapid decrease of PMN cell count in patients with SBP, with response rates (bacteriologic clearance) slightly higher than 90%, and therefore repeat paracentesis was not necessary if the patient had the expected response to treatment (Fig. 29.1). Considering progressively increasing rates of treatment failure (decrease in PMN count <25% from baseline) attributed to MDROs, a diagnostic paracentesis should be repeated 48 hours after initiation of treatment to assess response, particularly if patients are not improving clinically, if an organism has not been isolated, or on the other hand, if cultures show polymicrobial growth, raising suspicion for secondary peritonitis. A negative response should lead to broadening antibiotic therapy and pursuing further testing to rule out a secondary source of peritonitis, which may require surgical intervention.

21. **Does bacterascites represent a real peritoneal infection? Should it be treated?**

Bacterascites (ascitic fluid PMN count <250 cells/mm^3 with a positive culture) can result from secondary bacterial colonization of ascites from an extraperitoneal source, which usually presents with systemic symptoms and signs of infection, and warrants treatment. In other cases, bacterascites ensues from the spontaneous colonization of ascitic fluid and can either be clinically asymptomatic or lead to symptoms, in which case treatment should also be offered. On the other hand, in asymptomatic patients, bacterascites can represent only a transient and self-resolving colonization or the first step in the development of SBP. In these situations, treatment with antibiotics should not be offered, as bacteria often clear spontaneously, but paracentesis should be repeated to rule out progression to SBP.

22. **What does the presence of bacterial DNA in blood and ascitic fluid represent in patients with cirrhosis?**

Although the presence of bacterial DNA in plasma and/or ascites is associated with bacterial translocation, its prevalence in patients with proven SBP and bloodstream infections is similar to that in patients with sterile ACLF (~70%), and it does not indicate increased mortality in patients with cirrhosis with suspected infection. Using multiplex polymerase chain reaction for risk stratification is therefore not recommended.

23. **Which patients with liver disease should receive prophylaxis against bacterial infection?**

Antibiotic prophylaxis can be either primary, for patients with ascites without a history of SBP, or secondary, for those with a prior episode.

- Primary prophylaxis: Prior data showed that in patients with ascitic fluid protein < 1.5 g/dL and advanced liver disease or renal dysfunction, the use of norfloxacin decreased rate of SBP development from 61% to 7%, while significantly increasing the probability of survival at 3 months and 1 year (48%–60%). Despite this significant benefit, a recent study has failed to replicate increased survival from norfloxacin prophylaxis. In the setting of

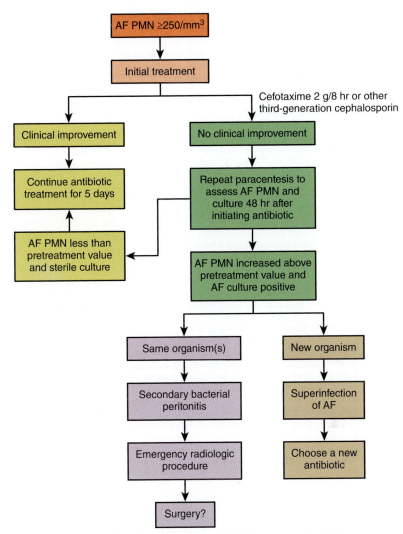

Fig. 29.1 Management of spontaneous bacterial peritonitis. *AF*, ascitic fluid; *PMN*, polymorphonuclear (cells).

decreased efficacy and lack of effect on mortality, as well as potential for other complications, and insufficient evidence to support it, routine use of primary prophylaxis for patients with low serum protein levels is no longer routinely recommended on current guidelines, and rather tailored based on risk-benefit ration of the individual patient. On the contrary, there are sufficient data supporting the use of antibiotics for primary prophylaxis in patients with cirrhosis and acute gastrointestinal hemorrhage, who are at high risk of SBP development. IV ceftriaxone is considered to be the agent of choice rather than norfloxacin, given the emergence of quinolone-resistant organisms.

- Secondary prophylaxis: Patients with a prior episode of SBP are at high risk of recurrence, generally because the risk factors that lead to the initial infection are still present. It has been proven that daily norfloxacin use decreases the rate of recurrence significantly, and it was routinely used until it was discontinued in the United States in 2014, with a reasonable alternative at this time being daily oral ciprofloxacin.

24. **Are there alternative prophylactic treatments to quinolones for preventing bacterial infections in cirrhosis?**
    The recurrence of SBP in patients receiving secondary antibiotic prophylaxis was originally reported at a rate of 20%–26% over 20 years ago. Despite the increased prevalence of quinolone-resistant (~70%) and MDR (~10%)

bacteria on the first episode of SBP, recent studies found that the recurrence rate for patients on secondary prophylaxis with norfloxacin remains superior to placebo, although the efficacy to prevent SBP, not death, decreased over time. In patients with known MDRO colonization, fluoroquinolone-based prophylaxis for SBP seems to be less efficient, and alternative antibiotics might need to be considered.

Other agents have been used when quinolones are not a viable option, however, there are no sufficient high-quality data to support the routine use of sulfamethoxazole/trimethoprim or rifaximin for secondary prophylaxis, but their use for this purpose has been documented.

25. Should a diagnostic thoracentesis be performed in patients with cirrhosis and pleural hydrothorax?

Hepatic hydrothorax (HH), a transudative pleural effusion secondary to portal hypertension, is present in 4%–12% of patients with cirrhosis, usually unilaterally and in more than 75% of cases confined to the right side. It is important to exclude other causes of effusion, in particular infection, malignancy, and/or cardiopulmonary processes, and therefore a diagnostic thoracentesis for fluid analysis is essential. In a small percentage of patients with cirrhosis and HH, ascites may not be evident; however, a serum to pleural fluid albumin gradient >1.1 g/dL is suggestive of HH. Furthermore, spontaneous bacterial empyema (SBE), although rare, can be present in about 10% of patients with HH, even in the absence of SBP. Prompt diagnosis of SBE is imperative to provide appropriate therapy, given its high mortality. A recent retrospective study showed that patients with SBE who underwent thoracentesis after 24 hours after presentation had higher rates of inpatient mortality (41% vs. 7%) and ICU admission compared to patients who received early thoracentesis.

26. What is the treatment of hepatic hydrothorax?

The initial treatment of hepatic hydrothorax is the same as that of ascites: salt restriction, diuretics, and large-volume paracentesis with albumin supplementation, if ascites is present. Despite these interventions, therapeutic thoracentesis is eventually required, and since fluid reaccumulates rapidly, in many cases repeat thoracentesis is needed to manage symptoms. Bleeding and pneumothorax are the main complications of thoracentesis, although it can be performed without the transfusion of platelets or plasma. Ultimately, patients with refractory hydrothorax might need TIPS and should be referred for transplant evaluation. The use of chest tubes should be avoided, as it has been linked to increased mortality stemming from clinical decompensation. Lower rates of infection (~5%) have been recently reported with the use of indwelling tunneled pleural catheters, and although there are no sufficient data to recommend routine use, they can be considered in select patients who need recurrent thoracentesis.

27. What are the diagnostic criteria for SBE?

It can be diagnosed by the presence of a transudative effusion, in the absence of underlying pneumonia, with either of the following:

- $\geq 250/mm^3$ of PMN cells in addition to positive pleural fluid culture, or
- $\geq 500/mm^3$ PMN cells with negative pleural fluid cultures (culture-negative SBE)

28. What is the treatment of SBE?

SBE develops when a preexisting hydrothorax becomes infected, which has been reported in >10% of patients with cirrhosis and has been associated with increased mortality. Because of the high risk for complications, the choice of adequate antibiotic therapy is important, and current guidelines recommend a similar approach as that utilized in the management of paracentesis (refer to Question 16). As previously discussed, the spread of resistant bacteria in the health care environment during the last two decades has led to a significant increase in infections caused by MDROs, which in turn are associated with increased rates of therapy failure and poor outcomes, including increased mortality. Therefore the setting and local prevalence of MDRO should be considered when choosing antibiotic therapy for SBE. For community-acquired SBE, a third-generation cephalosporin can still be used with good results; the same applies for cases of health care–associated SBE in areas with low MDRO prevalence; however, in those where the prevalence is high, SBE should be treated in the same manner as nosocomial cases, using carbapenems alone or with daptomycin, vancomycin, or linezolid if there is a high prevalence of MDR Gram-positive bacteria or evidence of sepsis. Repeat thoracentesis and fluid analysis should be performed 48 hours after initiating antibiotic therapy, particularly if infection with an MDRO organism is suspected or if the clinical condition of the patient continues to deteriorate. As in cases of HH, chest tube insertion should be avoided.

29. Should umbilical hernias be repaired in patients with cirrhosis and ascites?

In patients with cirrhosis and ascites, the incidence of umbilical wall hernias ranges from 20% to 40%, much higher than the 2%–4% prevalence seen in the general population. Cirrhosis-induced sarcopenia, together with secondary fascial weakness and enlargement of preexistent umbilical fascial defects from increased intra-abdominal pressure, are at the root of this higher incidence. Complications such as spontaneous leakage of ascites, peritonitis, and even evisceration can occur, resulting from necrosis of the overlying skin, caused by large-volume ascites. In cases where ascites is not optimally controlled in the perioperative period, rates of postoperative recurrence (up to 75%), wound infection, peritonitis, and leakage increase significantly. The MELD score has been identified as an independent risk factor for both morbidity and mortality, as well as the Child-Pugh classification, with a score >7 or CP-C classification found to be independent factors for morbidity and 90-day mortality. Based on this, it is accepted that patients with CP class A or MELD <10 can be considered for elective surgery due to lower risk of complications, whereas for patients with CP class B/C or MELD >10, medical therapy should be optimized prior to attempting intervention, either with optimization of diuretic therapy or with recurrent paracentesis or TIPS placement for patients with refractory ascites. It is worth noting that immediately after these procedures the portal pressure decreases, thus decompressing the abdominal wall defect, and a small risk of hernia incarceration ensues. For patients with MELD scores >15 or CP class C, the perioperative morbidity and mortality is exceptionally high and thus should only undergo hernia repair at the time of liver transplants if they qualify for it. Many studies have concluded that, when possible, hernia repair should be performed in the elective rather than emergency setting, to prevent the development of complications and inferior outcomes postoperatively. For patients with complicated hernias that require emergent surgical intervention, perioperative management of ascites should be aggressively pursued, and in some cases, even TIPS placement has been considered for better control.

30. What is the impact of hyponatremia in patients with cirrhosis?

Hyponatremia (serum sodium concentration <130 mmol/L) is a common complication of cirrhosis, found more frequently in later stages of the disease, with a prevalence ranging between 20% and 60% and associated with poor outcomes, including increased instances of HE, refractory ascites, and hepatorenal syndrome, as well as decreased quality of life and increased health care burden, and therefore not surprisingly associated with increased mortality (even after transplant). Considering the accuracy of hyponatremia to predict waitlist mortality when added to the MELD score, it was eventually incorporated in 2016 to determine transplant priority.

Dilutional hyponatremia develops as portal hypertension and splanchnic arterial vasodilation cause a decrease in the mean arterial pressure, translating to a lower effective blood volume that causes decreased renal perfusion, activation of the sympathetic nervous system and arginine vasopressin release, culminating in activation of the renin-angiotensin-aldosterone system and resulting sodium and water retention. Urine osmolality is usually UOsm ≥100 mOsm/kg due to urine not being maximally diluted.

31. How is dilutional hyponatremia managed?

Patients with cirrhosis and hyponatremia are frequently asymptomatic, and treatment is considered only if symptoms develop (nausea, lethargy, confusion, and seizures) or if the degree of electrolyte abnormality becomes moderate to severe, usually at a level <125 mEq/L. Management should be guided by the duration of hyponatremia and the severity of symptoms; in severe, symptomatic hyponatremia, correction by 4–6 mEq/L within the first hour (usually with hypertonic saline) is recommended, whereas a goal of 4 mmol/L/day is more appropriate for patients with chronic hyponatremia. Treatment relies on discontinuation of diuretics, correction of hypokalemia (improves cellular Na-K exchange), and creation of a negative free water balance with fluid restriction to 1–1.5 L/day, although patient adherence and efficacy are limited. Albumin administration is recommended for severe hyponatremia (<120 mEq/L). Vasopressin antagonists cause only a transient increase in serum sodium levels and have been found to cause hepatocellular injury at high doses; thus their use is limited to situations when clinical benefit outweighs the risks, such as in patients planning to undergo liver transplantation.

32. What is the role of antihypertensive medications in the management of patients with cirrhosis and ascites?

The use of beta-blockers has been proven to reduce the incidence of ascites, thus increasing decompensation-free survival in patients with compensated cirrhosis; they are also routinely used for primary and secondary prophylaxis of variceal hemorrhage in patients with cirrhosis, as their effect on portal hypertension decreases the risk of bleeding. Despite these benefits, a *window hypothesiswindow hypothesis* proposes that the beneficial effects of these medications are lost in the last stages of cirrhosis, leading to increased mortality, and recommending their discontinuation in that setting. Current guidelines recommend caution regarding the use of beta-blockers in patients with RA, hypotension (as indicated by systolic blood pressure <90 mm Hg), hyponatremia, or renal dysfunction (serum creatinine [sCr] >1.5 mg/dL).

In patients with cirrhosis and ascites, mean arterial pressure is an independent predictor of survival, thus hypotension should be prevented. Maintaining adequate arterial pressure in this population depends on the activation of endogenous vasoconstrictor systems, and therefore antihypertensive medications such as angiotensin-converting enzyme inhibitors, angiotensin II receptor antagonists, and α-1 adrenergic blockers should not be used.

33. What is the definition of HRS?

Originally, HRS was described as a "functional" category of renal failure in patients with cirrhosis, caused by reduced renal perfusion secondary to the reduction of the effective circulating volume (as a result of splanchnic and systemic arterial vasodilation and inadequate cardiac output), as well as overactivity of vasoactive systems. Since 2007 it was classified as HRS-1 and HRS-2; however, new definitions and diagnostic criteria have been adopted: HRS-1 has been renamed HRS-AKI, whereas HRS-2 is now HRS-NAKI (non-AKI). Furthermore, it is now thought that systemic inflammation, oxidative stress, and other factors (such as direct tubular damage from bile salts) play a role in the development of HRS, and that rather than a purely "functional" entity, an actual underlying structural component may be involved (increased levels of tubular injury biomarkers have been found in HRS-AKI, thus explaining the lack of response to therapy seen in patients with HRS and progressive increase in inflammation (Fig. 29.2). Taking these points into account, a recent position paper by the International Club of Ascites provided an update on the definition, classification, diagnosis, pathophysiology, and treatment of HRS and is worth noting the following changes in recent years:

- AKI is now defined as an *absolute increase in sCr of ≥0.3 mg/dL from baseline* (previously a set value of ≥1.5 mg/dL was used) *or an increase of ≥50% from baseline.* The main etiologies of AKI in cirrhosis are *prerenal AKI* (main causes are hypovolemia and HRS-AKI) and acute tubular necrosis, which in turn, can be difficult to differentiate from HRS-AKI.
- It is recognized that systemic inflammation plays a role in the development of organ failure and acute decompensation in patients with cirrhosis.
- With the increase of nonalcoholic steatohepatitis (and associated metabolic derangements, such as diabetes and hypertension) as a cause of cirrhosis, more patients with cirrhosis now have underlying structural chronic kidney disease (CKD).
- Lastly, HRS has been proposed to be a possible phenotype of renal dysfunction that occurs in patients with cirrhosis, and both the nomenclature and definitions of HRS-1 and HRS-2 have been reclassified:
  - HRS-AKI (previously HRS-1): Increase in sCr ≥0.3 mg/dL within 48 hours or ≥50% from baseline, among other criteria (Box 29.1). Originally, HRS-1 was defined as a rapid and progressive reduction of renal function defined by a doubling of the initial serum creatinine to a level greater than 2.5 mg/dL or a 50% reduction in the initial 24-hour creatinine clearance to a level less than 20 mL/min in less than 2 weeks).
  - HRS-NAKI (previously HRS-2): While previous definitions of HRS-2 only assumed a more chronic development of renal dysfunction without a definitive timely, HRS-NAKI has been further classified either in the context of CKD or acute kidney disease (AKD):
    - HRS-AKD: eGFR <60 mL/min per 1.73 m^2 for <3 months or increase in sCr <50% from baseline
    - HRS-CKD: Glomerular filtration rate <60 mL/min per 1.73 m^2 for >3 months

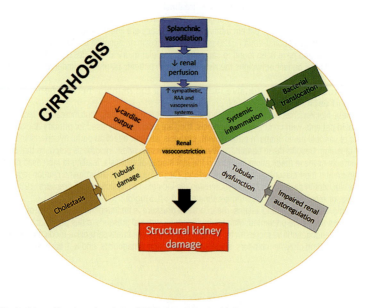

Fig. 29.2 Pathophysiology of hepatorenal syndrome. *RAA,* Renin-angiotensin-aldosterone.

34. **What is the clinical significance of the change in HRS-AKI definition?**

By changing the sCr cutoff in the previous HRS-1 definition, clinicians can initiate treatment at a lower sCr level, even with small changes in absolute value, rather than having to wait for a later stage of AKI, where the efficacy of vasoconstrictor therapy is limited. ACLF, present in up to a third of hospitalized patients with cirrhosis and associated with a high mortality rate, is characterized by the development of multiorgan dysfunction and systemic inflammation as a distinct entity, rather than decompensation from cirrhosis, and usually results from an identifiable trigger. In this setting, renal dysfunction has been associated with significantly high short-term mortality and, if coexisting with another organ failure, defines the presence of ACLF, which can be graded based on the severity of renal dysfunction. Patients with ACLF should be referred for liver transplant consideration, given poor prognosis, and therefore an early diagnosis if essential.

35. **What are the criteria for diagnosis of HRS-AKI?**

The criteria can be seen in Box 29.1.

Box 29.1 Diagnosis of HRS-AKI

- Cirrhosis with ascites.
- Diagnosis of AKI based on increase in serum creatinine greater than 0.3 mg/dL from baseline within 48 hours or a percent increase in serum creatinine of $\geq$50% which is known or presumed to have occurred within the preceding 15 days and/or urinary output $\leq$0.5 mL/kg of body weight $\geq$6 hours.
- No full or partial response after at least 2 days of diuretic withdrawal and volume expansion with albumin. The recommended dosage of albumin is 1 g/kg of body weight per day up to a maximum of 100 g/day.
- Absence of shock.
- No current or recent treatment with nephrotoxic drugs.
- Absence of parenchymal kidney disease as indicated by proteinuria greater than 500 mg/day, microhematuria (greater than 50 red blood cells per high-power field), urinary injury biomarkers (if available), and/or abnormal renal ultrasonogram.

---

36. **Describe the treatment of patients with HRS.**

Treatment should be instituted as soon as AKI is suspected, with general measures including:

- Discontinuation of diuretics and/or beta-blockers, as well as any nephrotoxic drugs (vasodilators, nonsteroidal anti-inflammatory drugs)
- Volume replacement

HRS-AKI is the underlying cause of AKI in 15%–43% of cases, characterized by a poor prognosis with a median survival of $\leq$3 months, highlighting the importance of prompt treatment. Pharmacologic therapy rests on volume expansion with albumin in combination with vasoconstrictors, with an average response rate close to 50% in patients with HRS-AKI when terlipressin or norepinephrine are used. If no response is noted over 4 days of treatment with maximal tolerated doses of vasoconstrictors, therapy can be discontinued, whereas treatment can be continued for up to 14 days if improvement is observed. A recently published trial (CONFIRM) compared the use of terlipressin (currently not available in the United States) to placebo in combination with albumin, in a large cohort of North American patients with HRS-AKI, finding that reversal of HRS was achieved in 32% of patients on terlipressin therapy, compared to only 17% in the placebo arm. Albumin is thought to contribute to the management of HRS by maintaining or increasing the cardiac output, which can sometimes be further reduced by terlipressin when administered alone, and thus explaining the higher effectiveness of this combination which is administered at a dose of 20–40 g/day. Terlipressin can be administered either as a bolus or a continuous IV infusion, which has been related to a lower incidence of side effects. Norepinephrine is given as a continuous infusion starting at 0.5 mg/hr, with the goal of achieving an increase in either mean arterial pressure of 10 mm Hg or in urine output to >200 mL/4 hr. Midodrine, α-1 adrenergic agonist with effect on the splanchnic circulation, is an oral vasoconstrictor usually administered in combination with subcutaneous or IV octreotide and albumin when other vasoconstrictors are not available, however, the rate of renal function recovery with this regimen is significantly lower than that achieved by terlipressin therapy.

Other interventions have been considered in the management of HRS-AKI: TIPS is not recommended due to the lack of data to support its use in this setting, whereas RRT has typically been started only as a bridge to transplantation in patients who are candidates, given high mortality associated with RRT in HRS.

37. **How can AKI be prevented in patients with cirrhosis?**

AKI can be prevented by avoiding precipitating factors, such as gastrointestinal bleeding and bacterial infections; for example, AKI can frequently complicate the course of SBP and contribute to increased mortality rates, but the use of IV albumin in combination with antibiotics for the management of SBP has been proven to decrease this complication. Along the same lines, prevention of PPCD with albumin replacement after LVP is associated with decreased incidence of renal injury.

38. **Which patients with cirrhosis and ascites should be evaluated for liver transplantation?**
    This information can be seen in Box 29.2.

Box 29.2 Referral Criteria for Transplant Evaluation in Patients With Cirrhosis and Ascites

- Patients with grade 2 or 3 ascites
- Patients with persistent ascites 12 months after TIPS placement (once patency confirmed)
- Patients with refractory ascites and liver dysfunction that precludes TIPS placement
- Patients with hepatic hydrothorax[a]
- Patients with cirrhosis who develop HRS (both HRS-AKI and HRS-NAKI)

[a]Additional criteria, if met, can be used to request MELD exception points in patients with recurrent hepatic hydrothorax.

AKI, Acute kidney injury; *HRS*, hepatorenal syndrome; *MELD*, Model for End-stage Liver Disease; *NAKI*, non-AKI; *TIPS*, transjugular intrahepatic portosystemic shunt.

CLINICAL VIGNETTE

Available Online

BIBLIOGRAPHY

Available Online

CHAPTER 30

LIVER ABSCESS

Jorge L. Herrera, MD

 Additional content available online

1. **What are the two major categories of liver abscess?**
   There are two types of liver abscess: pyogenic and amebic. Pyogenic abscesses are the most common, comprising 80% of all abscesses in Western countries. Pyogenic liver abscess originate from infections involving either aerobic/anaerobic Gram-negative or Gram-positive bacteria, or fungal infections. Amebic abscesses are more common in India, sub-Saharan Africa, Mexico, Central, and South America, resulting from infection with *Entamoeba histolytica*. Differentiation between the two types of abscesses is important because management differs.

2. **Describe the clinical features of pyogenic liver abscess.**
   Pyogenic liver abscesses (PLA) are most common among older male patients, approximately 2.5 males are affected for every 1 female. The prevalence has been increasing due to more instrumentation of the biliary tract and higher number of patients with diabetes, immunosuppression, liver resection, transplantation, and malignancy, all of which are risk factors. The clinical findings are nonspecific consisting of fever, malaise, anorexia, weight loss, and right upper quadrant pain. Fever can be absent in up to 20% of cases. Only 37% present with the classic findings of fever and right upper quadrant tenderness, reinforcing the nonspecific nature of signs and symptoms. Diaphragmatic irritation can result in referred pain to the right shoulder, cough, or hiccups. Due to the subacute presentation, the mean duration of symptoms before hospital admission is around 26 days.

3. **What are the clinical features of amebic liver abscess?**
   Amebic abscess are 10 times more common in males than in females. Within the United States, this predominantly affects young Hispanic male migrants from affected areas or travelers to developing countries. Amebic abscess usually appears 8–20 weeks (median 12 weeks) after the patient has left an endemic area, but may develop years after exposure. Concurrent hepatic abscess and amebic dysentery are unusual. Among the population at risk, there is a close relationship between excessive alcohol intake and the development of amebic abscess. Amebic abscess may develop without prior symptomatic amebic enteritis, or follow a bout of enteritis 4 days to 20 weeks later. Compared to PLA, patients with amebic abscess are often more acutely ill. Fever is present 85% of the time. Abdominal pain is typically well localized to the right upper quadrant. If there is involvement of the diaphragmatic surface of the liver, this may lead to right-sided pleural pain, referred shoulder pain, cough, or hiccups. Gastrointestinal symptoms occur in 10%–30% of patients which includes nausea, vomiting, abdominal cramping, distention, diarrhea, and constipation.

4. **What laboratory features are distinctive in patients with liver abscess?**
   Results of routine laboratory tests are not diagnostic for pyogenic or amebic liver abscess. Leukocytosis, normocytic anemia, and elevated C-reactive protein and erythrocyte sedimentation rate are common. Eosinophilia is characteristically absent in both pyogenic and amebic abscesses. More than 90% of patients have a higher elevation in alkaline phosphatase (AP) compared to aspartate aminotransferase (AST) and alanine aminotransferase (ALT). Hyperbilirubinemia is seen with biliary involvement and is less common in those with cryptogenic abscess. The presence of jaundice in cases of amebic liver abscess, while uncommon (10%), is a sign of severe disease. Hypoalbuminemia is common and a level less than 2 g/dL carries a poor prognosis. Blood cultures are positive in less than 50% of patients with pyogenic abscess and 75%–90% of aspirates from the abscesses are positive for bacteria on Gram stain. A positive blood culture in cases of PLA is associated with increased mortality. Aspiration of amebic abscess is not diagnostic as trophozoites are located only in the wall of the abscess.

5. **What are the most common sources of pyogenic liver abscess?**
   Biliary tract disease is the most common known source of PLA accounting for 35% of cases. Initially, gallstone disease was the predominant cause, more recently, malignant biliary strictures have become the most common cause of biliary-related pyogenic abscesses. Abscesses have also been shown to arise as a late complication of endoscopic sphincterotomy or surgical biliary-intestinal anastomosis. Malignant tumors of the pancreas, common bile duct, and ampulla account for 10%–20% of hepatic abscesses originating in the biliary tree. Parasitic invasion of the biliary tree by roundworms or flukes can also lead to biliary infection and hepatic abscess. Abscesses occurring from a biliary source tend to be multiple and small in size involving both lobes of the liver.

Less commonly pyogenic abscess can occur as a complication of bacteremia from bacterial seeding through the portal vein from underlying abdominal disease. Abdominal diseases associated with this are diverticulitis, appendicitis, gastrointestinal malignancy, and inflammatory bowel disease. Up to 40% of cases of PLA have no obvious source of infection and are defined as cryptogenic. Diabetes is particularly common among patients with cryptogenic liver abscess. Pyogenic infection may be carried to the liver in hepatic arterial blood flow from distant localized infections, such as endocarditis or severe dental disease.

6. List the organisms that commonly cause pyogenic liver abscess.

Numerous bacteria have been found to cause liver abscesses. Currently, the most common are Gram-negative organisms occurring 50%–70% of the time. *Escherichia coli*, which was once the most common aerobic Gram-negative bacteria cultured, is gradually being overtaken by *Klebsiella pneumoniae*, particularly in Asia. *Klebsiella* is most common in those with underlying diabetes or malignant disease (Table 30.1). A particularly virulent strain of *K. pneumoniae*, genotype K1, has been described which can cause catastrophic septic ocular or central nervous system complications from PLA, even in otherwise healthy hosts. Aerobic Gram-positive organisms account for about 25% of infections. Anaerobic infection is often present but its prevalence is difficult to quantitate given the difficulties in culturing anaerobic organisms. Anaerobic coverage is usually included in the empiric therapy of PLA. Fungal abscess has also been found in immunocompromised individuals and those with hematologic malignancies.

Table 30.1 Bacteriology of Pyogenic Liver Abscess.

GRAM-NEGATIVE AEROBES (50%–70%)	GRAM-POSITIVE AEROBES (25%)	ANAEROBES (40%–50%)
Escherichia coli	Streptococcus faecalis	Fusobacterium nucleatum
Klebsiella sp.	β Streptococci	Bacteroides sp.
Proteus sp.	α Streptococci	Bacteroides fragilis
Enterobacter sp.	Staphylococci	Peptostreptococcus sp.
Serratia sp.	Streptococcus milleri	Actinomyces sp.
Morganella sp.	Clostridium sp.	
Actinobacter sp.		
Pseudomonas sp.		

7. Do negative cultures from an abscess aspirate indicate a nonpyogenic abscess?

Although cultures from abscess contents are usually positive, a negative culture can occur with improper handling, prior antibiotic therapy, or anaerobic infection. Proper collection and culture techniques are important for growing anaerobic organisms. Culture material should be transported to the lab immediately in the same syringe used for aspiration to avoid exposure to the air. Never submit swabs for the culture of liver abscess. Anaerobic organisms may require at least several days and up to 1 week or more for sufficient growth to establish a diagnosis. For this reason, a Gram stain of the aspirate is of paramount importance. If the Gram stain shows organisms and no growth is seen on the culture within 2 or 3 days, this is suggestive of anaerobic organisms. All aspirated material should be cultured for aerobic, anaerobic, and microaerophilic organisms. In patients with no prior antibiotic therapy, a Gram-negative stain should raise suspicion for an amebic liver abscess.

8. What is the pathogenesis of amebic abscess?

Ingestion of the *E. histolytica* cysts from fecal-contaminated food or water initiates infection. Excystation then occurs in the intestinal lumen producing trophozoites that use galactose and *N*-acetyl-DD-galactosamine (Gal/GalNAc) specific lectin to adhere to the colonic mucin layer leading to invasion of the colon and colonization. About 90% of the time trophozoites aggregate in the intestinal mucin layer and form new cysts resulting in a self-limited asymptomatic infection. However, 10% of the time Gal/GalNAc-specific lectin causes lysis of the colonic epithelium and invasion of the colon by trophozoites. Colitis is then worsened by activation of the host immune system leading to upregulation of nuclear factor-kB, lymphokines, and neutrophils. Once intestinal epithelium invasion occurs <1% of the time, this can lead to hematogenous dissemination and eventual liver and/or brain abscess.

9. **What abnormalities can be detected in standard radiologic studies of patients with liver abscess?**
A chest radiograph may be abnormal in 50%–80% of patients with liver abscess. Right-lower lobe atelectasis, right pleural effusion, and an elevated right hemidiaphragm may be clues to the presence of a liver abscess. Perforation of a pyogenic liver abscess into the thoracic cavity may result in empyema. In plain abdominal films, air can be seen in the abscess cavities in 10%–20% of cases. Gastric displacement due to enlargement of the liver also may be seen. These features are not sensitive to the diagnosis of liver abscess.

10. **Which imaging studies should be obtained in evaluating a suspected liver abscess?**
Imaging results are similar for pyogenic and amebic abscesses with ultrasonography and computerized tomography (CT) being the most common initial imaging modalities used. Ultrasonography is noninvasive, readily available, and highly accurate, with a sensitivity of 80%–90%. It is the preferred modality to distinguish cystic from solid lesions and in most patients is more accurate than CT scanning for visualizing the biliary tree. Ultrasonography, however, is operator dependent and its accuracy may be affected by the patient's habitus or overlying gas. CT is also very sensitive and abscesses are usually described as hypodense. A rim of contrast enhancement can be seen in less than 20% of cases. CT is also able to detect gas in the abscess and the location of the abscess related to adjacent structures. It also provides an assessment not only of the liver but also of the entire peritoneal cavity, which may provide information about the primary lesions causing the liver abscess. Magnetic resonance imaging does not add much to the sensitivity of CT scanning. Abscesses have low signal intensity on T1-weighted images and high signal intensity on T2-weighted images with enhancement using gadolinium.

11. **What areas of the liver are usually affected by hepatic abscess?**

Right lobe only	60% of patients
Both lobes	20%–30% of patients
Left lobe only	5%–20% of patients

12. **How can the location, size, and number of liver abscesses help determine the source?**
PLA arising from a biliary source tend to be multiple and of small size involving both lobes of the liver. Septic emboli from the portal vein may be solitary and tend to be more common in the right lobe of the liver because most of the portal vein flow goes to the right lobe. Abscesses arising from a contiguous source tend to be solitary and localized to one lobe only.
Amebic liver abscesses tend to be solitary and large. Most commonly, they are located in the right lobe of the liver. The right lobe receives a major part of the venous drainage from the cecum and ascending colon, which are the parts of the bowel most commonly affected by amebiasis. Abscesses located in the dome of the liver or complicated by a bronchopleural fistula are typically amebic in origin.

13. **When should a hepatic abscess be aspirated?**
Hepatic abscesses should be aspirated if they are thought to be pyogenic and not amebic. Patients with multiple abscesses, diabetes, coexistent biliary disease, or an intra-abdominal inflammatory or malignant process are more likely to have pyogenic abscess. In such patients, aspiration under ultrasound (US) guidance with Gram stain and culture helps to guide antibiotic selection. In a recent US series, antimicrobial resistance was found in 40% of isolates. Aspiration of amebic abscess will not be diagnostic but should be considered under the following circumstances:
- When pyogenic abscess or secondary infection of an amebic abscess cannot be excluded
- When the patient does not respond after 5–7 days of adequate therapy for amebic liver abscess
- When the abscess is very large, usually greater than 5 cm, particularly in the left lobe, which increases risk of rupture
- When a large abscess is causing severe pain

14. **In what situation should an amebic liver abscess be treated by surgical drainage?**
When the amebic abscess is located in the left lobe of the liver, inaccessible to needle drainage, or if there is no dramatic response to therapy within the first 24–48 hours surgical drainage should be performed. Complications of left-lobe amebic abscess, such as cardiac tamponade, are associated with high mortality and require prompt intervention to prevent their occurrence. Laparoscopic drainage is the preferred approach because this has been shown to have shorter surgery time, less blood loss, faster recovery times, and shorter hospital stays when compared to open drainage.

15. **Does aspiration of an amebic hepatic abscess yield diagnostic material in most patients?**
    No. Trophozoites are found in less than 20% of aspirates, as trophozoites are mainly located in the cyst wall and not in the abscess cavity. Although classically the contents of amebic abscess are described as anchovy paste in appearance, in practice, most aspirated material does not conform to this description. The contents of an amebic abscess are typically odorless. Foul-smelling aspirates or a positive Gram stain should suggest a pyogenic abscess or secondarily infected amebic abscess.

16. **How often is the biliary tree involved in patients with amebic liver abscess?**
    Bile is lethal to amoebas thus infection of the gallbladder and bile ducts does not occur. In patients with a large amebic or pyogenic abscess, compression of the biliary system may result in jaundice, but cholangitis occurs only with a secondary bacterial infection.

17. **How can the diagnosis of an amebic abscess be confirmed?**
    Amebic abscesses are best differentiated from pyogenic abscesses by the following serologic tests:

Hemagglutination	Gel diffusion precipitin
Indirect immunofluorescence	Complement fixation
Counterimmunoelectrophoresis	Latex agglutination
Immunoelectrophoresis	Enzyme-linked immunosorbent assay

Serologic tests are positive only in patients with invasive amebiasis, such as hepatic abscess or amebic colitis. They are negative in asymptomatic carriers. With the exception of complement fixation, these tests are highly sensitive (95%–99%). Hemagglutination (IHA) is extremely sensitive and a negative test excludes the diagnosis; a titer greater than 1:512 is present in almost all patients with invasive disease. IHA, however, remains positive for many years, and a positive result may indicate prior infection. Gel diffusion precipitin (GDP) titer usually becomes negative 6 months after the infection and this is the test of choice for patients from endemic areas with prior exposure to amebiasis. A high GDP titer in a patient with hepatic abscess suggests an amebic abscess, even if the patient has a prior history of invasive amebiasis. A commercially available serum antigen test (TechLab *E. histolytica* II kit, Virginia, United States) detecting circulating Gal/GalNAc antigen has been found to be a sensitive test for diagnosis of hepatic amebic abscess even in patients previously exposed to amoeba. This test, however, is not widely available in the United States. In general, the choice of serologic tests depends on availability and epidemiologic considerations.

18. **Describe the treatment for pyogenic liver abscess.**
    A combination of systemic antibiotics and percutaneous drainage has become the treatment of choice for the management of PLA (Fig. 30.1). Treatment is based on the size of the abscess. Abscesses that are smaller

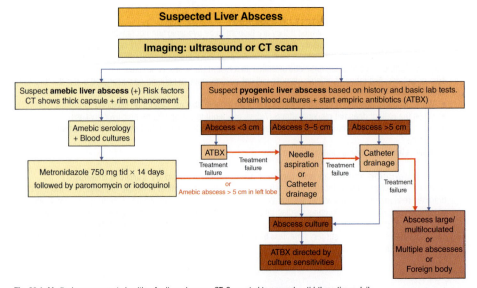

Fig. 30.1 Medical management algorithm for liver abscess. *CT*, Computed tomography; *tid*, three times daily.

Table 30.2 Empiric Treatment of Pyogenic Liver Abscess.

DRUG	ADULT DOSAGE/COMMENTS
Cefotaxime and metronidazole	2 g IV q 8 hr 500 mg IV q 8 hr
Piperacillin/tazobactam	3.375 g IV q 6 hr
Ertapenem, imipenem, meropenem, or doripenem	If suspected or documented antibiotic-resistant Gram-negative organisms
Beta-lactam + aminoglycoside	Preferred for septicemic, seriously ill patients
Vancomycin + aminoglycoside + metronidazole	Suitable for penicillin-allergic individuals

IV, Intravenous.

than 3 cm in diameter can be treated with antibiotics alone and close follow-up to assess for response. Empiric antibiotic coverage needs to cover against anaerobes, Gram-negative and Gram-positive aerobes, and enterococci. Most pathogens found in PLA are now resistant to ampicillin and many to fluoroquinolones. Taking this into consideration, third- and fourth-generation cephalosporins, piperacillin/tazobactam, aminoglycosides, and carbapenems remain effective empiric treatment options. Initial empiric antibiotic therapy should consist of either a third-generation cephalosporin and metronidazole or piperacillin/tazobactam. The latter regimen is preferred when enterococcal infection is suspected. Combination therapy with beta-lactam and an aminoglycoside is preferred for septicemic infections in seriously ill patients. Vancomycin is a good choice for enterococcus coverage or in cases of penicillin allergy. Vancomycin should be combined with gentamycin and metronidazole for Gram-negative and anaerobic coverage. Recently, beta-lactamase-producing Enterobacteriaceae have been reported in Asia as an increasing cause of pyogenic abscess, necessitating broader antimicrobial coverage. Table 30.2 lists recommended antibiotic regimens for the empiric therapy of PLA.

Intravenous (IV) antibiotics should be continued for 2–3 weeks and then orally for up to 6 weeks. If the abscess is greater than 3 cm or the patient is not responding to antibiotics alone, percutaneous drainage should be done. Although controversial, some studies have shown that intermittent percutaneous image-guided drainage is equally effective as continuous catheter drainage. Most experts prefer continuous catheter drainage for larger (≥5 cm) abscess. Surgical drainage should be considered in any patient with no clinical response after 4–7 days of drainage, multiple large or loculated abscess, ruptured abscess, or intra-abdominal disease. The combination of percutaneous drainage with IV antibiotics results in a 76% cure rate, compared with 65% for antibiotic alone and 61% for surgery alone. Concurrent endoscopic therapy to relieve biliary obstruction is mandatory for the resolution of the abscess. Recurrence is more common in those with underlying biliary disease compared to those who have a cryptogenic cause.

19. **Describe the treatment for amebic liver abscess.**
Oral or IV metronidazole has been shown to be effective for extraintestinal amebiasis (Fig. 30.1). The duration of treatment is usually 7–10 days. Response to treatment occurs within 96 hours and cure rates exceed 85%. Parasites persist in the intestine 40%–60% of the time in those receiving metronidazole. For that reason, following treatment with metronidazole patients should be given an oral luminal amebicide to prevent recurrence (Table 30.3). Metronidazole and paromomycin should not be given together because diarrhea is a common side effect of paromomycin making it difficult to assess the patient's response to therapy. Percutaneous drainage of

Table 30.3 Treatment of Amebic Liver Abscess.

DRUG	ADULT DOSAGE
Initial therapy—Amebicidal agent: Metronidazole	750 mg tid for 7–10 days
Followed by a Luminal agent: Paromomycin	25–35 mg/kg/day tid for 7 days
or Iodoquinol	650 mg tid for 20 days
or Diloxanide furoate	500 mg tid for 10 days

tid, Three times daily.

the abscess should be considered in patients who have no clinical response to drug therapy within 3–5 days of initiation, those with a large cavity size in which rupture is believed to be imminent, and abscesses in the left lobe at risk for rupturing into the pericardium. Surgical drainage is done only when the abscess is inaccessible to needle drainage. Abscess fluid should be sent for Gram stain and cultures to exclude bacterial superinfection.

20. List the potential complications of pyogenic liver abscess.
Untreated, PLA has a mortality rate of 100%. Potential complications include rupture into the peritoneal cavity leading to subphrenic, perihepatic, or subhepatic abscess or peritonitis. Rupture can also occur into the pleural space leading to empyema while rupture into the pericardium can lead to pericarditis and tamponade. In 5%–10% of patients with *K. pneumoniae,* pyogenic abscess septic emboli can occur involving the lungs, brain, and eyes.

21. List the potential complications of amebic liver abscess.
Complications of amebic liver abscess are similar to those of PLA. Because of the close proximity to the diaphragm, rupture into the pleural space can occur which can lead to empyema. This can then spread further producing lung abscess or bronchopleural fistula. Since abscesses are mostly seen in the right lobe, pericardial extension is only seen in 1%–2% and is associated with patients who have left lobe involvement. A serious pericardial effusion may indicate impending rupture. Constrictive pericarditis occasionally follows suppurative amebic pericarditis. Brain abscess from hematogenous spread has also been reported.

22. What is the prognosis for patients with liver abscess?
The prognosis depends on the rapidity of diagnosis and the underlying illness. Patients with amebic liver abscess generally do well with appropriate treatment, morbidity, and mortality rates are low at 1%–3%. Response to treatment is prompt and dramatic. Healing of the abscess may lead to residual scar tissue associated with subcapsular retraction. Occasionally, in patients with large abscess, a residual cavity surrounded by fibroconnective tissue may persist.

The mortality rate associated with pyogenic liver abscess has been reduced to 5%–10% with prompt recognition, adequate drainage, and antibiotic therapy. Mortality is highly dependent on the underlying disease process. Morbidity remains high at 50%, primarily because of the complexity of therapy and the need for prolonged drainage.

CLINICAL VIGNETTE

Available Online

BIBLIOGRAPHY

Available Online

WEBSITES

Available Online

CHAPTER 31

INHERITABLE FORMS OF LIVER DISEASE

Mohammed Eyad Alsabbagh, MD and Bruce Raymond Bacon, MD

 Additional content available online

HEMOCHROMATOSIS

1. **How do we classify the various iron-loading disorders in humans?**
   The usual way to classify iron-overload syndromes is to distinguish between hereditary hemochromatosis (HH), secondary iron overload, and parenteral iron overload.
   - *HH* results in increased iron absorption from the gut, with preferential deposition of iron in the parenchymal cells of the liver, heart, pancreas, and other endocrine glands. Most HH (approximately 85%–90%) is found in patients who are homozygous for the C282Y mutation found in *HFE*, the gene for hemochromatosis. Over the past several years, however, mutations in other genes have been found that can lead to iron overload. These include mutations in transferrin receptor-2 (TfR2), ferroportin, hemojuvelin, and hepcidin.
   - In secondary iron overload, some other stimulus causes the gastrointestinal tract to absorb increased amounts of iron. Here, the increased absorption of iron is caused by an underlying disorder rather than by an inherited defect in the regulation of iron absorption. Examples include various anemias caused by ineffective erythropoiesis (e.g., thalassemia, aplastic anemia, red cell aplasia, and some patients with sickle cell anemia), chronic liver disease, and, rarely, excessive intake of medicinal iron.
   - In parenteral iron overload, patients have received excessive amounts of iron as either red blood cell transfusions or iron-dextran given parenterally. In patients with severe hypoplastic anemias, red blood cell transfusion may be necessary. Over time, patients become significantly iron-loaded. Unfortunately, some physicians give iron-dextran injections to patients with anemia that is not due to iron deficiency; such patients can become iron-loaded. Parenteral iron overload is always iatrogenic and should be avoided or minimized. In patients who truly need repeated red blood cell transfusions (in the absence of blood loss), a chelation agent should be initiated to prevent toxic accumulation of excessive iron.

2. **What are neonatal iron overload and African iron overload?**
   - Neonatal iron overload is a rare condition that is probably related to an immune-mediated intrauterine hepatic defect. Infants are born with modest increases in hepatic iron and many patients do very poorly; liver transplantation can be lifesaving.
   - African iron overload, previously called Bantu hemosiderosis, was thought to be a disorder in which excessive amounts of iron were ingested from alcoholic beverages brewed in iron drums. Recent studies have suggested that this disorder does have a genetic component and some patients have mutations in ferroportin. Thus Black patients may be at risk for developing iron overload from an inherited disease.

3. **How much iron is usually absorbed per day?**
   A typical Western diet contains approximately 10–20 mg of iron, which usually is found in heme-containing compounds. Normal daily iron absorption is approximately 1–2 mg, representing approximately a 10% efficiency of absorption. Patients with iron deficiency, HH, or ineffective erythropoiesis absorb increased amounts of iron (up to 3–6 mg/day).

4. **Where is iron normally found in the body?**
   The normal adult male contains approximately 4 g of total body iron, which is roughly divided between the 2.5 g of iron in the hemoglobin of circulating red blood cells, 1 g of iron in storage sites in the reticuloendothelial system of the spleen and bone marrow and the parenchymal and reticuloendothelial system of the liver, and 200–400 mg in the myoglobin of skeletal muscle.

   Iron is bound to transferrin in both the intravascular and extravascular compartments. Storage iron within cells is found in ferritin and, as this amount increases, in hemosiderin. Serum ferritin is proportional to total body iron stores in patients with iron deficiency or uncomplicated HH and is biochemically different from tissue ferritin.

5. **Discuss the genetic defect in patients with HH.**
   In 1996 the gene responsible for hemochromatosis was identified and named *HFE. HFE* codes for a major histocompatibility complex (MHC) type 1–like protein. A single missense mutation results in the loss of a cysteine at amino acid position 282 with replacement by a tyrosine (C282Y). As a result, *HFE* fails to interact with β_2-microglobulin (β_2M), which is necessary for the function of MHC class 1 proteins.

Later on, it was demonstrated that the *HFE*/β_2M complex binds to TfR and is necessary for TfR-mediated iron uptake into cells. C282Y homozygosity is found in approximately 85%–90% of patients with hemochromatosis. A second mutation, whereby a histidine at amino acid position 63 is replaced by an aspartate (H63D), is common but less important in cellular iron homeostasis. A third mutation has been characterized whereby serine is replaced by cysteine at amino acid position 65 (S65C). Like H63D, S65C has little effect on iron loading unless it is present as a compound heterozygote with the C282Y mutation.

It is important to note the role of hepcidin, a 25-amino acid peptide produced in the liver, as the principal regulator of iron absorption. Hepcidin in normal amounts interferes with the activity of ferroportin at the basolateral surface of the enterocyte, preventing iron absorption. Thus, when there is hepcidin deficiency, there is an increase in iron absorption despite the fact that individuals are in fact iron-loaded. Hepcidin is found to be deficient in patients with HFE, TfR2, hemojuvelin, and hepcidin gene mutation, thus explaining the iron overload in these patients.

6. What are the most common symptoms and physical findings in patients with HH?

Most patients are asymptomatic and identified by abnormal iron studies or elevated liver enzymes on routine screening chemistry panels or by screening family members of a known patient. Nonetheless, it is useful to be aware of the symptoms that patients with more established HH can exhibit. Typically, they are nonspecific and include fatigue, malaise, and lethargy. Other more organ-specific symptoms include cirrhosis, hepatocellular carcinoma, new-onset diabetes secondary to pancreatic iron deposits, skin hyperpigmentation and porphyria cutanea tarda, and congestive heart failure.

7. How is the diagnosis of hemochromatosis established?

Patients with abnormal iron studies on screening blood work, elevated liver enzymes, positive family history of hemochromatosis, or any of the symptoms and physical findings mentioned above should have iron studies either repeated or performed for the first time. These studies include serum iron, total iron-binding capacity (TIBC) or transferrin, and serum ferritin. The transferrin saturation (TS) should be calculated from the ratio of iron to TIBC or transferrin. If the TS is greater than 45% or if the serum ferritin is elevated, hemochromatosis should be strongly considered, and mutation analysis of *HFE* should be performed. If patients are homozygous for the C282Y mutation or compound heterozygotes (C282Y/H63D) and younger than the age of 40 years or in those with normal liver enzymes (alanine aminotransferase and aspartate aminotransferase) and a ferritin level less than 1000 ng/mL, no further evaluation is necessary.

8. Is there a place for liver biopsy in the diagnosis of hemochromatosis?

Liver biopsy is not needed to confirm diagnosis after genetic testing, however, in those patients with abnormal liver enzymes or markedly elevated ferritin (greater than 1000 ng/mL), a percutaneous liver biopsy *should* be performed! The main purpose for performing the biopsy in these individuals is to determine the degree of fibrosis because markedly elevated ferritin levels and elevated liver enzymes were found to be major risk factors for advanced fibrosis. At the same time, the biopsy enables us to do routine histologic examination, including Perls Prussian blue staining for storage iron and biochemical determination of hepatic iron concentration (HIC). The hepatic iron index (HII) can be calculated. Calculation of the HII was more important in the past than it is now because we have genetic testing.

9. Are genetic tests available for determining non-HFE-linked causes of HH?

Yes, diagnostic DNA laboratories have developed assays for hemojuvelin, hepcidin, ferroportin, and TfR2 in addition to HFE mutation analysis.

10. How commonly do abnormal iron studies occur in other types of liver diseases?

In various studies, approximately 30%–50% of patients with chronic viral hepatitis, alcoholic liver disease, and nonalcoholic steatohepatitis have abnormal serum iron studies. Abnormalities in serum iron studies in the absence of HH are more commonly seen in hepatocellular than in cholestatic liver diseases. The serum ferritin can be markedly elevated in patients with alcoholic and nonalcoholic fatty liver disease (NAFLD). In general, an elevation in TS is much more specific for HH. Thus, if the serum ferritin is elevated and the TS is normal, another form of liver disease may be responsible. In contrast, if the serum ferritin is normal and the TS is elevated, the likely diagnosis is hemochromatosis, particularly in young patients. Differentiation of HH in the presence of other liver diseases can be done with the use of genetic testing (*HFE* mutation analysis for C282Y and H63D).

11. Is magnetic resonance imaging (MRI) useful in diagnosing hemochromatosis?

In massively iron-loaded patients, MRI shows the liver to be black, consistent with the kinds of changes associated with increased iron deposition. In more subtle and earlier cases, overlap is tremendous, and imaging studies are not useful. With the new advancements in radiology, HIC can be assessed to a good degree using a new software in T2-weighted images. However, as mentioned earlier, diagnosis relies on genetic testing, but if

HIC is to be assessed in patients with non-C282Y homozygote, then MRI can be used instead of a liver biopsy to assess HIC.

12. On liver biopsy, what is the typical cellular and lobular distribution of iron in HH?
In patients with hemochromatosis, iron is found in the cytoplasm and the periportal hepatocytes (zone 1). In heavier iron loading in older patients, iron is still predominantly hepatocellular, but some iron may be found in Kupffer cells and bile ductular cells. The periportal-to-pericentral (zones 1–3) gradient is maintained but may be less distinct in more heavily loaded patients. When patients develop cirrhosis, the pattern is typically micronodular, and regenerative nodules may show less intense iron staining. In patients with secondary iron overload, the accumulation is mainly in Kupffer cells as compared to the hepatocytes.

13. How useful is HIC?
Since genetic testing has become readily available, liver biopsy and determinations of HIC and HII are less important. Nonetheless, whenever a liver biopsy is performed on a patient with suspected HH, the quantitative HIC should be obtained. In symptomatic patients, HIC is typically greater than 10,000 mcg/g. The iron concentration threshold for the development of fibrosis is approximately 22,000 mcg/g. Lower iron concentrations can be found in cirrhotic HH with a coexistent toxin, such as alcohol or hepatitis C or B virus. Young people with early HH may have only moderate increases in HIC.

14. How is the HII used in diagnosing HH?
The HII, introduced in 1986, is based on the observation that HIC increases progressively with age in patients with homozygous HH. In contrast, in patients with secondary iron overload or in heterozygotes, there is no progressive increase in iron over time. Therefore the HII was thought to distinguish patients with homozygous HH from patients with secondary iron overload and heterozygotes. The HII is calculated by dividing the HIC (in micromoles per gram) by the patient's age (in years). A value greater than 1.9 was thought to be consistent with homozygous HH. With the advent of genetic testing, we have learned that many C282Y homozygotes do not have phenotypic expression to the degree that would cause an elevated HII, and they will not have increased iron stores. Thus the HII is no longer the gold standard for the diagnosis of HH. The HII is not useful in patients with parenteral iron overload.

15. How do you treat a patient with HH?
Treatment of HH is relatively straightforward and includes weekly or twice-weekly phlebotomy of 1 unit of whole blood. Each unit of blood contains approximately 200–250 mg of iron, depending on the hemoglobin. Therefore a patient who presents with symptomatic HH and who has up to 20 g of excessive storage iron requires the removal of more than 80 units of blood, which takes close to 2 years at a rate of 1 unit of blood per week. Patients need to be aware that this treatment can be tedious and prolonged. Some patients cannot tolerate the removal of 1 unit of blood per week, and occasionally, schedules are adjusted to remove only a unit every other week. In contrast, in young patients who are only mildly iron-loaded, iron stores may be depleted quickly with only 10–20 phlebotomies. The goal of initial phlebotomy treatment is to reduce tissue iron stores, not to create iron deficiency. Important to note the marker to monitor the treatment response is ferritin and not TS which takes a longer time to drop. Once the ferritin is less than 50 ng/mL, the majority of excessive iron stores has been successfully depleted, and most patients can go into a maintenance phlebotomy regimen (1 unit of blood removed every 2–3 months). At this point, usually, TS has reached 50% and the goal of maintenance treatment is to keep ferritin 50–100 ng/mL and TS ~50%.

We do not routinely restrict iron in the diet, but it is important to avoid iron supplements and vitamin C and also advise patients to read the labels of their supplements which frequently contain iron.

16. What kind of a response to treatment can you expect?
Many patients feel better after phlebotomy therapy has begun, even if they were asymptomatic before treatment. Energy level may improve, with less fatigue and less abdominal pain. Liver enzymes typically improve once iron stores have been depleted. Increased hepatic size diminishes. Cardiac function may improve, and approximately 50% of patients with glucose intolerance are more easily managed. Unfortunately, advanced cirrhosis, arthropathy, and hypogonadism do not improve with phlebotomy.

17. What is the prognosis for a patient with hemochromatosis?
Patients who are diagnosed and treated before the development of cirrhosis can expect a normal life span. The most common causes of death in hemochromatosis are complications of chronic liver disease and hepatocellular cancer. Patients who are diagnosed and treated early should not experience any of these complications.

18. **Because hemochromatosis is an inherited disorder, what is the practitioner's responsibility to family members once a patient has been identified?**

    Once a patient has been fully identified, all first-degree relatives should be offered screening with genetic testing (*HFE* mutation analysis for C282Y) and tests for TS and ferritin. If genetic testing shows that the relative is a C282Y homozygote or a compound heterozygote (C282Y/H63D) and has abnormal iron studies, HH is confirmed.

α_1-ANTITRYPSIN DEFICIENCY

19. **What is the function of α_1-antitrypsin (α_1-AT) in healthy people?**

    α_1-AT is a protease inhibitor synthesized in the liver. It is responsible for inhibiting trypsin, collagenase, elastase, and proteases of polymorphonuclear neutrophils. In patients deficient in α_1-AT the function of these proteases is unopposed. In the lung, this can lead to a progressive decrease in elastin and the development of premature emphysema. The liver fails to secrete α_1-AT and aggregates of the defective protein are found, leading by unclear means to the development of cirrhosis. More than 75 different protease inhibitor (Pi) alleles have been identified. Pi MM is normal, and Pi ZZ results in the lowest levels of α_1-AT.

20. **How common is α_1-AT deficiency?**

    α_1-AT deficiency occurs in approximately 1 in 2000 people.

21. **Where is the abnormal gene located?**

    The gene is located on chromosome 14 and results in a single amino acid substitution (replacement of glutamic acid by lysine at the 342 position), which causes a deficiency in sialic acid and a tendency to aggregation.

22. **What is the nature of the defect that causes α_1-AT deficiency?**

    α_1-AT deficiency is a protein-secretory defect. Normally, this protein is translocated into the lumen of the endoplasmic reticulum, interacts with chaperone proteins, folds properly, is transported to the Golgi complex, and then is exported out of the cell. In patients with α_1-AT deficiency, the protein structure is abnormal because of the deficiency of sialic acid, and the proper folding in the endoplasmic reticulum occurs for only 10%–20% of the molecules, with resultant failure to export via the Golgi complex and accumulation within the hepatocyte.

    Environmental factors play a major role in patients who develop clinical manifestations, smoking, for example, significantly increases the risk of developing chronic obstructive pulmonary disease (COPD) in Pi ZZ patients, similarly having fatty liver or alcohol consumption can lead to earlier cirrhosis in these patients.

23. **Describe the common symptoms and physical findings of α_1-AT deficiency.**

    Adults with liver involvement may have no symptoms until they develop signs and symptoms of chronic liver disease. Similarly, children may have no specific problems until they develop complications from chronic liver disease. In adults with lung disease, typical findings include premature emphysema with the classical type being basal panacinar emphysema.

24. **How is the diagnosis of α_1-AT deficiency established?**

    It is useful to order α_1-AT levels and phenotype in all patients evaluated for chronic liver disease and in patients with COPD because no clinical presentation suggests the diagnosis (apart from premature emphysema). Certain heterozygous states can result in chronic liver disease; for example, SZ, as well as ZZ patients, can develop cirrhosis. MZ heterozygotes usually do not develop disease unless they have some other liver condition, such as alcoholic liver disease or chronic viral hepatitis. When these genotypes are identified, the diagnosis is confirmed.

25. **What histopathologic stain is used to diagnose α_1-AT deficiency?**

    Periodic acid-Schiff (PAS)-diastase. PAS stains both glycogen and α_1-AT globules a dark, reddish-purple, and diastase digests the glycogen. Thus, when a PAS-diastase stain is used, the glycogen has been removed by the diastase, and the only positively staining globules are those resulting from α_1-AT. In cirrhosis, these globules characteristically occur at the periphery of the nodules and can be seen in multiple sizes within the hepatocyte. Immunohistochemical staining also can be used to detect α_1-AT globules, and electron microscopy can show characteristic globules trapped in the Golgi apparatus. So, the typical read of the biopsy of a patients with α_1-AT liver disease would be PAS-positive, diastase-resistant globules.

26. **How is α_1-AT deficiency treated?**

    The main intervention relies on early diagnosis and counseling individuals with the genetic variants of α_1-AT to avoid active and passive smoking, avoid alcohol and risk factors for NAFLD, and treat any coexisting viral hepatitis.

    For patients with α_1-AT-related decompensated liver disease, we manage the complications of liver disease and offer liver transplantation for the patients who are good candidates. With liver transplantation, the phenotype becomes that of the transplanted liver.

In certain patients with severe lung disease, who are nonsmokers and failed symptomatic and supportive therapy, pooled human IV α_1-AT can be given weekly with some benefit. Lung transplant can also be an option for patients with advanced emphysema.

27. **What is the prognosis for patients with α_1-AT deficiency? Should family screening be performed?**
The prognosis depends entirely on the severity of the underlying lung or liver disease. Typically, patients who have lung disease do not have liver disease, and those who have liver disease do not have lung disease, although in some patients both organs are severely involved. In patients with decompensated cirrhosis, the prognosis relates largely to the availability of organs for liver transplantation. Patients with transplants typically do fine. Family screening should be performed with α_1-AT levels and phenotype. This screening is largely for prognostic information and to provide counseling to avoid risk factors for lung and liver disease.

WILSON DISEASE

28. **How common is Wilson disease?**
Wilson disease has an estimated prevalence of 1 in 30,000 people.

29. **Where is the Wilson disease gene located?**
The abnormal gene responsible for Wilson disease, an autosomal recessive disorder, is located on chromosome 13. The gene has homology for the Menkes disease gene, which also results in a disorder of copper metabolism. The Wilson disease gene (called *ATP7B*) codes for a P-type adenosine triphosphatase, which is a membrane-spanning copper–transport protein that causes a defect in the transfer of hepatocellular lysosomal copper into bile. This defect results in the gradual accumulation of tissue copper with subsequent hepatotoxicity.

30. **What is the usual age of onset of Wilson disease?**
Wilson disease is characteristically a disease of adolescents and young adults. Clinical manifestations have not been seen before the age of 5 years. By 15 years of age, almost one-half of the patients have some clinical manifestations of the disease. Rare cases of Wilson disease have been identified in patients in their 40s or 50s and even up into their 80s.

31. **Which organ systems are involved in Wilson disease?**
The liver is uniformly involved. All patients with neurologic abnormalities caused by Wilson disease have liver involvement. Wilson disease also can affect the eyes, kidneys, joints, and red blood cells. Thus patients can have cirrhosis, neurologic deficits with tremor and choreic movements, ophthalmologic manifestations such as Kayser-Fleischer rings, psychiatric problems, nephrolithiasis, arthropathy, and hemolytic anemia.

32. **What are the different types of hepatic manifestations in Wilson disease?**
The typical patient who presents with symptoms from Wilson disease already has cirrhosis. However, patients can present with chronic hepatitis, and in all young people with chronic hepatitis, a serum ceruloplasmin level should be performed as a screening test for Wilson disease. Rarely, patients can present with fulminant hepatic failure, which is uniformly fatal without successful liver transplantation. Finally, patients can present early in the disease with hepatic steatosis. As with chronic hepatitis, young patients with fatty liver should be screened for Wilson disease.

33. **How is the diagnosis of Wilson disease established?**
Wilson disease evaluation should be considered in young patients with acute liver failure, chronically elevated liver enzymes, and unexplained neurologic or psychiatric symptoms. Initial evaluation should include measurement of serum ceruloplasmin and, if abnormal, a slit-lamp examination to evaluate for Kayser-Fleischer rings *and* a 24-hour urinary copper level. Approximately 85%–90% of patients have depressed serum ceruloplasmin levels, but a normal level does not rule out the disorder. The presence of all three: low ceruloplasmin, high 24-hour urinary copper, and a KF ring confirms the diagnosis. If there is any clinical suspicion and the ceruloplasmin is decreased or the 24-hour urinary copper level is elevated, more testing should be done.
Liver biopsy should be performed for histologic interpretation and quantitative copper determination. Histologic changes include hepatic steatosis, chronic hepatitis, or cirrhosis. Histochemical staining for copper with rhodamine is not particularly sensitive. Usually, in established Wilson disease, hepatic copper concentrations are greater than 250 mcg/g (dry weight). Although elevated hepatic copper concentrations can occur in other cholestatic liver diseases, the clinical presentation allows an easy differentiation between Wilson disease and primary biliary cirrhosis, extrahepatic biliary obstruction, and intrahepatic cholestasis of childhood.
Genetic testing is now more easily accessible and gaining an important role in the diagnosis of Wilson disease. In patients with high suspicion, especially if liver biopsy is not possible, genetic testing can help with

making the diagnosis. Given the presence of over 500 different mutations in the *ATP7B* gene, genetic testing should not be performed as a first test.

34. What forms of treatment are available for patients with Wilson disease?

The mainstay of treatment has been the use of a copper-chelating agent: D-penicillamine or trientine. Because D-penicillamine is frequently associated with side effects, trientine is now used more frequently. Maintenance therapy with dietary zinc supplementation also has been used. Twenty-four-hour urinary copper should be checked regularly every 6–12 months with a target range of 200–500 mcg. If urine copper levels are low and treatment adherence is confirmed, the dose of the medication should be increased. Neurologic disorders can improve with therapy. Patients who present with complications of chronic liver disease or with fulminant hepatic failure should be quickly considered for orthotopic liver transplantation. Wilson disease is cured by liver transplant with no recurrence post-transplant.

35. Is it necessary to perform family screening for Wilson disease?

Wilson disease is an autosomal recessive disorder, and all first-degree relatives of the patient should be screened. If the ceruloplasmin level is reduced, a 24-hour urinary copper level should be obtained, followed by a liver biopsy for histologic examination and quantitative copper determination. Genetic testing can be valuable for family screening if genotyping has been done on the proband and is available to family members.

36. Compare Wilson disease and HH.

Both disorders involve abnormal metal metabolism and are inherited as autosomal recessive disorders. The mechanism of tissue damage is probably related to metal-induced oxidant stress for both disorders. In HH the gene is on chromosome 6, whereas in Wilson disease the abnormal gene is on chromosome 13. HH occurs in approximately 1 in 250 people, but Wilson disease occurs in only approximately 1 in 30,000. The inherited defect in HH causes increased absorption of iron by the intestine, with the liver a passive recipient of the excessive iron; in contrast, the inherited defect in Wilson disease is in the liver, resulting in decreased hepatic excretion of copper with excessive deposition and subsequent toxicity. Although the liver is affected in both Wilson disease and HH, the other affected organs are variable. In hemochromatosis, the heart, pancreas, joints, skin, and endocrine organs are affected; in Wilson disease, the brain, eyes, red blood cells, kidneys, and bone are affected. Both disorders are fully treatable if the diagnosis is made promptly before the development of end-stage complications.

The reader is referred to Chapter 32, where histologic examples of most of the inheritable forms of liver disease discussed in this chapter can be reviewed.

CLINICAL VIGNETTE

Available Online

BIBLIOGRAPHY

Available Online

WEBSITES

Available Online

LIVER HISTOPATHOLOGY

Jacqueline Birkness-Gartman, MD and Kiyoko Oshima, MD, PhD

 Additional content available online

LIVER BIOPSY

1. **Explain the role of liver biopsy.**
   - Diagnosis: Biopsy can determine the cause of liver injury in patients with atypical clinical features or coexisting disorders such as steatosis and hepatitis C.
   - Prognosis: Assessing fibrosis is of particular importance in determining the risk of complications, including hepatocellular carcinoma (HCC).
   - Treatment: Histologic analysis can inform treatment plans. For example, the amount of ongoing inflammation can guide therapy in patients with autoimmune hepatitis.

2. **What laboratory testing and medication management is necessary before liver biopsy?**
   - Measurement of complete blood count including platelet count and prothrombin time/international normalized ratio is recommended.
   - Antiplatelet medication should be discontinued 7–10 days prior to biopsy.
   - Warfarin should be discontinued at least 5 days prior to biopsy.

3. **What are the contraindications for liver biopsy?**
   - Absolute: Uncooperative patient, severe coagulopathy, infection of hepatic bed, and extrahepatic biliary obstruction.
   - Relative: Ascites, morbid obesity, possible vascular lesion, amyloidosis, and hydatid disease.

4. **What are the criteria for an adequate liver biopsy?**
   - Ideally, at least 11 portal tracts should be present. The minimum requirement is five portal tracts.
   - Grading and staging accuracy are reduced in biopsies less than 2.0 cm in length. A short specimen may result in a failure to recognize cirrhosis in up to 20% of cases.

HISTOLOGIC AND BASIC PATHOLOGIC FINDINGS

5. **Describe the normal histology of the liver.**
   - The liver consists of portal tracts (containing portal vein branches, hepatic artery branches, and bile ducts) and lobules (hepatocytes and central veins).
   - The liver is organized into zones 1–3 (Fig. 32.1). Blood flows from zone 1 (periportal) to zone 3 (centrilobular), while bile flows in the opposite direction. Zone 3 is the least oxygenated.

6. **What inflammatory cells can be seen on liver biopsy, and what are the associated disease processes?**
   - Neutrophils: Steatohepatitis, drug toxicity, and surgical hepatitis (margination of neutrophils during surgery)
   - Lymphocytes: Viral hepatitis and drug toxicity
   - Plasma cells: Autoimmune hepatitis and drug toxicity
   - Eosinophils: Drug toxicity, parasitic infection, and autoimmune hepatitis

7. **What is steatosis, and how much is seen in a normal liver biopsy?**
   - Steatosis is the accumulation of fat, predominantly triglycerides, in hepatocytes.
   - Normal livers have less than 5% steatosis.

8. **What is the difference between macrovesicular and microvesicular steatosis?**
   - Macrovesicular steatosis can easily be seen on hematoxylin and eosin (H&E) stain as large or small droplets (Fig. 32.2A). It can be caused by alcohol, metabolic syndrome, or medications.
   - Microvesicular steatosis is not easily seen on H&E stain, although the cytoplasm may appear foamy (Fig. 32.2B). It can be seen with acute fatty liver during pregnancy, medications, and metabolic diseases.

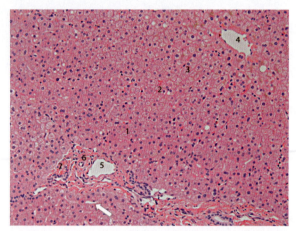

Fig. 32.1 Normal liver (hematoxylin and eosin stain) showing the zones (1–3), central vein (4), portal vein (5), hepatic artery (6), bile duct (7), and hepatic sinusoid (*arrow*).

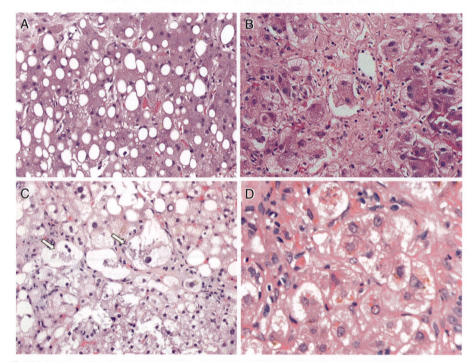

Fig. 32.2 Steatosis and hepatocyte injury (hematoxylin and eosin stains). (A) Macrovesicular large and small droplet steatosis. (B) Microvesicular steatosis. (C) Balloon cell degeneration with Mallory-Denk bodies (*arrows*). (D) Feathery degeneration with bile pigment in hepatocytes.

9. What histologic changes can be seen with hepatocyte injury?

- Balloon cell degeneration: Swollen hepatocytes with wisps of cytoplasmic material. This change occurs when intermediate filaments which form the support network of hepatocytes become damaged. Causes include steatohepatitis, acute hepatitis, and ischemia (Fig. 32.2C).

- Mallory-Denk bodies (Mallory hyaline): Aggregates of intermediate filaments form eosinophilic (pink) rope-like inclusions. Causes include steatohepatitis, drugs (amiodarone), and Wilson disease (Fig. 32.2C).
- Feathery degeneration: Cholestasis results in swollen hepatocytes with wispy cytoplasmic threads (Fig. 32.2D). Feathery degeneration and balloon cell degeneration and sometimes indistinguishable.

10. **What patterns of liver cell necrosis can be seen?**
   - Single-cell necrosis (acidophil/Councilman body): Single hepatocytes show acidophilic (bright pink) cytoplasm and pyknotic nuclei. Causes include viral hepatitis, steatohepatitis, and drugs/toxins (Fig. 32.3A).
   - Interface activity: Necrosis of individual hepatocytes at the limiting plate (between the portal tract and lobule). Causes include viral hepatitis, autoimmune hepatitis, and drugs (Fig. 32.3B).
   - Zonal necrosis: Certain types of injury affect specific zones. Zone 3 necrosis is seen with ischemia or acetaminophen toxicity (Fig. 32.3C). Zone 1 necrosis occurs with certain drugs, toxins, or eclampsia (Fig. 32.3D).
   - Bridging necrosis: Necrosis extending between portal tracts or central veins. Causes include severe autoimmune hepatitis, ischemia, viruses, and drugs.

11. **What types of pigment can be seen in the liver?**
   - Hemosiderin: Golden brown pigment seen in zone 1, due to red cell degeneration.
   - Lipofuscin: Brown granules are seen in zone 3. This is considered a wear-and-tear pigment, seen in older adults.
   - Bile: Green-yellow pigment seen in zone 3. This is an abnormal finding.

12. **What are the causes of cytoplasmic and nuclear inclusions in hepatocytes?**
   - Hepatitis B (HBV): Ground glass hepatocytes with pale pink material in the cytoplasm can be seen with chronic infection (Fig. 32.4A).
   - Cytomegalovirus: Large "cytomegalic" cells with nuclear "owl's eye" inclusions and cytoplasmic inclusions (Fig. 32.4B).

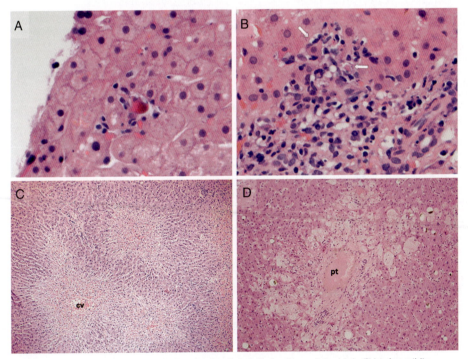

Fig. 32.3 Hepatocyte necrosis patterns (hematoxylin and eosin stains). (A) Single-cell necrosis in a lobule. (B) Interface activity, characterized by necrosis of individual hepatocytes at the limiting plate (*arrows*). (C) Zone 3 necrosis surrounding central veins (cv). (D) Zone 1 necrosis around a portal tract (pt).

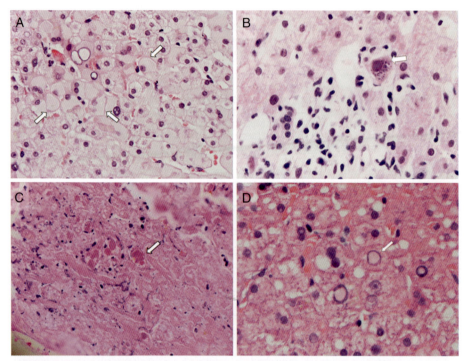

Fig. 32.4 Hepatocyte inclusions (hematoxylin and eosin stains). (A) Ground glass hepatocytes (*arrows*) in chronic hepatitis B infection. (B) Cytomegalovirus nuclear and cytoplasmic inclusions (*arrow*). (C) Herpes simplex virus viral cytopathic effect showing multinucleation (*arrow*). (D) Glycogenated hepatocyte nuclei (*arrow*).

- Herpes simplex virus: Viral cytopathic with the 3 M's: multinucleation, margination of chromatin, and molding (Fig. 32.4C).
- Adenovirus: Smudgy nuclear inclusions.
- Glycogenated nuclei: Nuclei with central clearing, seen with steatohepatitis, diabetes, and Wilson disease (Fig. 32.4D).

13. **What kinds of special stains are used for liver biopsies?**
- Masson trichrome: Highlights fibrosis (Fig. 32.5A).
- Reticulin: Outlines hepatic plates and is used to evaluate architecture, for example, thickening of hepatic plates in HCC (Fig. 32.5B) or collapse in hepatocyte necrosis.
- PAS (periodic acid-Schiff): Highlights glycogen and α1-antitrypsin globules.
- PAS-D (periodic acid-Schiff with diastase): Variant of the PAS stain that uses diastase to remove glycogen. α1-antitrypsin globules can be seen in zone 1 (Fig. 32.5C).
- Perls Prussian blue: Shows the distribution and amount of iron deposition (Fig. 32.5D).
- Rhodamine: Detects copper accumulation.
- Congo red: Detects amyloid.
- Oil red O: Confirms microvesicular steatosis. Requires fresh tissue.

STEATOSIS AND STEATOHEPATITIS

14. **What is the difference between steatosis and steatohepatitis?**
- Steatosis is the accumulation of lipids in hepatocytes (Fig. 32.2A and B).
- Steatohepatitis refers to a combination of steatosis, inflammation, and hepatocyte injury (balloon cell degeneration, Fig. 32.2C). Mallory-Denk bodies can be seen but are not required.

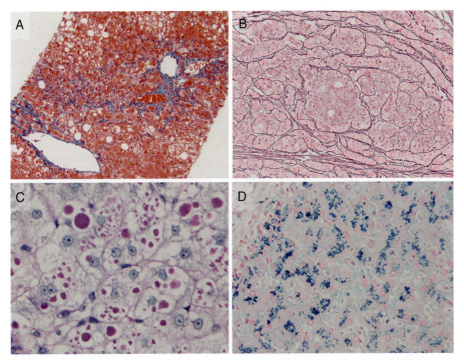

Fig. 32.5 Liver special stains. (A) Trichrome stain showing "chicken wire" pericellular fibrosis in steatohepatitis. (B) Reticulin stain showing expansion of the hepatic plates in hepatocellular carcinoma. (C) Periodic acid-Schiff with diastase–positive globules in α1-antitrypsin deficiency. (D) Perl Prussian blue stain showing iron deposition in hepatocytes.

15. **Can histologic examination distinguish between alcoholic hepatitis and nonalcoholic hepatitis?**

    Not really. Alcoholic hepatitis shows more neutrophils and Mallory hyaline. While it is possible to favor one etiology over the other, clinical correlation is needed.

16. **How does scarring progress with steatohepatitis?**

    Fibrosis starts around the central vein with "chicken wire" fibrosis extending along the sinusoids (Fig. 32.5A). In contrast, fibrosis in viral hepatitis starts from the portal tracts.

17. **How is nonalcoholic steatohepatitis (NASH) graded and staged?**

    - The Brunt system, the clinical research network scoring system (CNR), and Steatosis-Activity-Fibrosis (SAF) scoring system can be used for NASH.
    - Grade is based on the degree of steatosis, hepatocellular ballooning, and lobular inflammation, while stage is based on the progression of fibrosis.

CHRONIC HEPATITIS

18. **What histologic features are typical of chronic hepatitis?**

    Chronic hepatitis is a necroinflammatory process in which hepatocytes are injured. Inflammation is predominantly in the portal tracts with evidence of interface activity.

19. **What is the differential diagnosis of chronic hepatitis pattern?**

    Viral hepatitis, autoimmune hepatitis, drug toxicity, and Wilson disease.

20. **What histologic features are seen in chronic hepatitis B?**

    Ground glass hepatocytes may be seen due to the accumulation of hepatitis B surface antigen in hepatocytes (Fig. 32.4A).

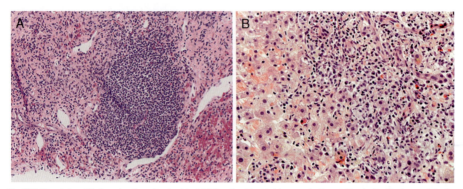

Fig. 32.6 Chronic hepatitis (hematoxylin and eosin stains). (A) Prominent lymphoid aggregates in portal tracts should raise suspicion for hepatitis C. (B) Plasma cell–rich interface activity in autoimmune hepatitis.

21. **What histologic features are seen in chronic hepatitis C?**
    Lymphoid aggregates and mild-to-moderate interface activity are present (Fig. 32.6A). The lobular activity is typically mild with sparse inflammation and acidophil bodies.

22. **What histologic features are seen in autoimmune hepatitis?**
    Classic features include portal and lobular chronic inflammation with interface activity and prominent plasma cells (Fig. 32.6B). Hepatic rosette formation and bridging necrosis may be seen.

23. **What are the grading and staging systems for chronic hepatitis and what is their purpose?**
    - The goal of grading and staging systems is to provide specific histologic criteria for assessing inflammation and fibrosis.
    - Various systems (Knodell, Ishak, Scheuer, Metavir, and Batts-Ludwig) are available, but all are based on portal chronic inflammation, interface activity, lobular necroinflammatory lesions, and fibrosis.

24. **How is chronic hepatitis graded and staged according to the Batts-Ludwig system?**
    The grading and staging of chronic hepatitis can be seen in Table 32.1.

Table 32.1 Grading and Staging of Chronic Hepatitis (Batts and Ludwig).

Grading of Inflammatory Activity	
Grade 1 (minimal)	Mild portal inflammation with scant interface activity
No lobular necrosis	
Grade 2 (mild)	Mild portal inflammation with interface activity
Scant lobular necrosis	
Grade 3 (moderate)	Moderate portal inflammation with interface activity
Spotty Lobular Necrosis	
Grade 4 (severe)	Marked portal inflammation with brisk interface activity Considerable spotty necrosis and areas of confluent necrosis
Staging of Fibrosis	
Stage 1 (portal)	Fibrous portal expansion
Stage 2 (periportal)	Periportal or rare portal-portal septa
Stage 3 (bridging)	Fibrous septa with architectural distortion
Stage 4 (cirrhosis)	Well-defined cirrhotic nodules

BILE DUCT DISEASE

25. What are the histologic features of biliary obstruction?

Centrilobular cholestasis, proliferation of bile ductules associated with neutrophils, and portal tract edema are seen (Fig. 32.7A). Neutrophils around the bile ducts are related to interleukin-8 expressed by ductular cells and do not indicate infection.

26. What are the histologic features of primary biliary cholangitis (PBC)?

PBC affects small bile ducts. Florid bile duct lesions are diagnostic and are characterized by biliary epithelial damage, basement membrane destruction, and a lymphoplasmacytic infiltrate (Fig. 32.7B). Non-necrotizing granulomas are seen in up to 25% of cases.

27. What are the histologic features of primary sclerosing cholangitis (PSC)?

PSC predominantly affects medium to large bile ducts. Onion skin fibrosis with a reduced number of bile ducts is diagnostic, although this finding is present in fewer than 40% of liver biopsies (Fig. 32.7C and D). The most common findings on biopsy are nonspecific fibrosis, portal inflammation, and paucity of normal bile ducts or the same histologic findings as extrahepatic bile duct obstruction. Imaging studies confirm the diagnosis of PSC.

28. What is small duct PSC?

This subset of PSC affects only small bile ducts. Cholangiography is normal and only liver biopsy can confirm the diagnosis.

29. What is overlap syndrome?

The clinical and histologic features of more than one autoimmune process are seen in a patient. The most common overlap is autoimmune hepatitis with PBC or PSC.

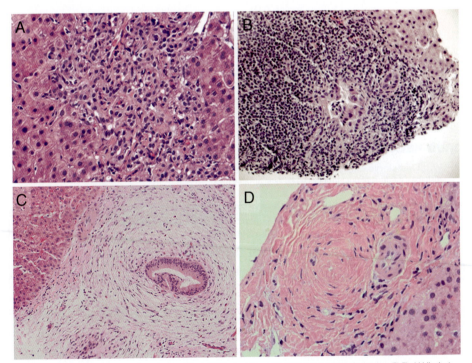

Fig. 32.7 Bile duct disease (hematoxylin and eosin stains). (A) Bile ductular proliferation due to biliary obstruction. (B) Florid bile duct lesion in primary biliary cholangitis. (C) Periductal fibrosis and (D) obliterated bile duct in primary sclerosing cholangitis.

GRANULOMATOUS INFLAMMATION

30. What is a granuloma?

   An aggregate of epithelioid histiocytes (Fig. 32.8).

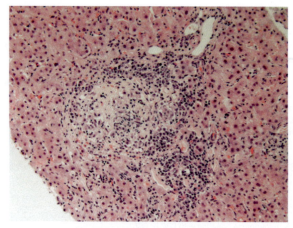

Fig. 32.8 Granuloma in a portal tract (hematoxylin and eosin stain).

31. What are the causes of granulomas in the liver?
   - Infection: mycobacteria, schistosomiasis, and fungal infection
   - Drug toxicity
   - PBC
   - Foreign material
   - Extrahepatic granulomatous diseases: sarcoidosis, chronic granulomatous disease, and inflammatory bowel disease
   - Neoplasms: Hodgkin lymphoma

DRUG-RELATED LIVER INJURY

32. What histologic patterns are seen in drug-related liver injury?

   Histologic patterns of drug toxicity can be seen in Table 32.2.

Table 32.2 Histologic Patterns of Drug Toxicity.	
Histologic Findings	Associated Agents
Massive necrosis	Isoniazid and phenytoin
Zone 3 necrosis	Acetaminophen
Zone 1 necrosis	Halothane
Macrovesicular steatosis	Methotrexate, corticosteroids, total parenteral nutrition, and ethanol
Microvesicular steatosis	Tetracyclines and aspirin (Reye syndrome)
Steatohepatitis and Mallory-Denk bodies	Amiodarone and ethanol
Cholestasis without inflammation	Oral contraceptives and anabolic steroids
Cholestasis with inflammation	Numerous antibiotics
Granulomas	Allopurinol, penicillins, phenothiazines, and phenylbutazone

INHERITED LIVER DISEASE

33. Does the pattern of iron accumulation help to determine the cause?

Yes. Accumulation of iron in hepatocytes can be seen with hereditary hemochromatosis, alcoholic liver disease, and porphyria cutanea tarda. Iron in Kupffer cells indicates multiple transfusions or hemolytic anemia.

34. Describe the histologic features of Wilson disease.

Various histologic patterns can be seen, including portal inflammation, steatosis, Mallory-Denk bodies, and periportal glycogenated nuclei. Quantitative copper testing of liver tissue is useful to confirm the diagnosis.

35. Is Wilson disease the only cause of copper accumulation in the liver?

No. Copper accumulation in the liver is seen with chronic cholestasis because copper is excreted via the biliary system.

36. What are the features of α1-antitrypsin deficiency on liver biopsy?

PAS-positive, diastase-resistant globules are seen in periportal hepatocytes (Fig. 32.5C). Clinical correlation with laboratory testing is required.

VASCULAR DISEASE

37. Do patients with portal hypertension always have cirrhosis?

No. Patients with nodular regenerative hyperplasia, hepatoportal sclerosis, and idiopathic portal hypertension have portal hypertension without cirrhosis.

TRANSPLANTATION

38. What is the role of liver biopsy in the first year after transplantation?

Common causes of abnormal liver enzymes after transplantation include rejection, steatohepatitis, recurrent viral hepatitis, and other recurrent liver diseases (PBC, PSC, and autoimmune hepatitis). Liver biopsy is helpful to differentiate between these possibilities.

39. What are the histologic features of acute cellular rejection (ACR), and how are they graded by the Banff system?

- Portal inflammation, bile duct injury, and endotheliitis (venous endothelial inflammation) are the three main histologic features of ACR (Fig. 32.9).
- The Banff system includes two components. The first is a global assessment of the overall rejection grade (indeterminate, mild, moderate, and severe). The second component involves scoring the three main features on a scale of 0–3 and adding the scores to produce an overall rejection activity index (maximum score of 9).

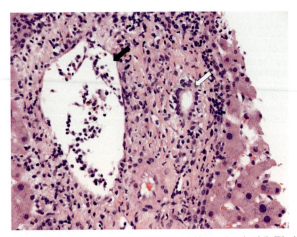

Fig. 32.9 Acute cellular rejection showing portal inflammation, bile duct injury (*white arrow*), and endotheliitis characterized by inflammatory cells lifting up the endothelial cells in a portal venule (*black arrow*) (hematoxylin and eosin stain).

40. **What are the histologic findings of chronic rejection?**

Loss of small bile ducts and obliterative vasculopathy affecting large and medium arteries can be seen, although the latter may require the examination of an explant. Ductopenia is characterized by bile duct loss in more than 50% of portal tracts.

41. **What are the histologic findings of acute graft-versus-host disease (GVHD) involving the liver?**

Acute GVHD can occur in patients who have undergone bone marrow or peripheral blood stem cell transplant and is characterized by bile duct lesions with mononuclear inflammation. Cholestasis may be seen.

NEOPLASMS

42. **What neoplasms can be seen in the liver?**
    - Hepatocellular adenoma (HCA): HCA consists of an abnormal proliferation of hepatocytes and lacks portal tracts. The hepatic plates maintain a normal thickness.
    - Hepatocellular carcinoma: HCC is a malignant proliferation of hepatocytes that shows loss of portal tracts and abnormal architecture. Some tumors show pseudoglandular architecture (Fig. 32.10A). A reticulin stain can be used to highlight expanded hepatic plates (Fig. 32.5B).
    - Cholangiocarcinoma: This malignant neoplasm of the bile ducts typically forms glands with an associated desmoplastic (fibrotic) reaction (Fig. 32.10B).

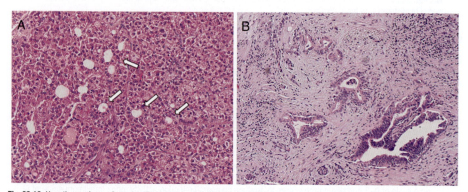

Fig. 32.10 Hepatic neoplasms (hematoxylin and eosin stains). (A) Hepatocellular carcinoma showing pseudoglandular architecture (*arrows*). (B) Cholangiocarcinoma consists of atypical glands with desmoplasia (fibrosis).

43. **Discuss the role of liver biopsy in diagnosing HCC.**

HCC can be diagnosed by imaging studies alone if certain criteria are met. When imaging studies are inconclusive, liver biopsy is required for diagnosis.

44. **Discuss the role of liver biopsy in diagnosing metastatic neoplasms.**

Biopsies can confirm metastasis from a known primary tumor. Some biopsies show a tumor that is probably metastatic but for which no primary tumor is known. In such cases, immunohistochemical stains may guide further workup.

CLINICAL VIGNETTE

Available Online

BIBLIOGRAPHY

Available Online

CHAPTER 33

HEPATOBILIARY CYSTIC DISEASE

Savio John, MD and Ganesh Aswath, MD

 Additional content available online

1. **What are the common types of cysts and cystic diseases seen in the liver?**
   - Cystic diseases of the liver include both liver and bile duct cystic lesions which can overlap. The common cystic diseases include simple cysts (which do not communicate with the biliary tree), echinococcal cysts, polycystic liver disease (PLD; including liver cysts in autosomal dominant polycystic kidney disease [ADPKD] and autosomal dominant PLD [ADPLD]), noninvasive mucinous cystic neoplasm, previously referred to as cystadenomas, cystadenocarcinoma, and biliary cysts. The classification of biliary cysts is discussed separately below.
   - Rarely, liver metastases can appear as cystic lesions due to central necrosis. Certain extrahepatic cysts from the kidneys or adrenal glands can also present as liver cysts.

2. **Provide a differential diagnosis for a cystic hepatic lesion.**
   - It is important to differentiate a simple cyst from a complex cyst. Simple hepatic cysts are benign fluid collections usually surrounded by a thin columnar epithelium and frequently require no treatment, whereas complex-appearing cysts are more concerning for infection or malignancy.
   - Cysts typically cause no symptoms. When patients have fever or severe pain along with single or multiple liver cysts on imaging, the diagnosis is likely to be amebic or bacterial abscess rather than a benign or malignant cyst. A cyst can also present rarely as a palpable mass in the right upper quadrant, cause dull pain in the right upper quadrant, cause obstruction and jaundice if it is located adjacent to main bile ducts, or rarely cause early satiety and vomiting if it is large enough to compress the stomach or the small bowel. Neoplastic cysts are almost always solitary. When there are multiple cysts or if they involve several organs, they are often benign cysts.
   - Differential diagnosis of cystic hepatic lesions is as follows:
     - Simple liver cyst
     - Infectious (abscess, pyogenic, amebic, and *Echinococcal* cyst)
     - PLD
     - Neoplasm (biliary cystadenoma, hamartoma, hepatocellular carcinoma, and cavernous hemangioma)
     - Pseudocyst
     - Hematoma
     - Biloma

3. **What is the significance of a simple hepatic cyst?**
   - Many simple hepatic cysts are solitary, asymptomatic and are frequently found incidentally on imaging. They are not associated with cystic disease in other organs. No treatment is necessary for a simple hepatic cyst.
   - Cyst-related symptoms include abdominal pain, increasing abdominal girth, and obstructive jaundice. If symptoms develop, laparoscopic surgical unroofing of the simple cyst is the first line of definitive therapy. Percutaneous drainage is not recommended as the fluid will reaccumulate, but it will help determine if the patient's symptoms are attributable to the enlarging cyst. A temporary drain is also not recommended because of the risk of infection.

4. **Describe the ultrasonographic, computed tomography (CT), and magnetic resonance imaging (MRI) characteristics of a simple hepatic cyst.**
   - On ultrasound (US), a simple hepatic cyst has a smooth margin with the surrounding parenchyma without an appreciable wall or internal echoes. Failure to meet any of these criteria increases the likelihood of a complex cyst, cyst infection, hydatid cyst, or biliary cyst disease. Ultrasonography is the first, and often the most useful test, which helps confirm that the content of the cyst is fluid and anechoic and that the cyst wall is smooth as in the case of a benign cyst. Benign cysts have a smooth wall without any irregularity and clear contents without septa or debris.
   - On CT, a simple hepatic cyst appears as a thin-walled lesion that does not enhance with iodinated intravenous contrast agents. The density of the lesion is that of water. CT scan helps determine the viscosity of the fluid and location of the cyst within the liver in relation to the bile ducts and other structures. When a complex cyst is

seen in US, a CT scan should be performed to localize the lesion and evaluate for imaging findings that suggest a malignancy.
- On T1-weighted MRI scans, cysts appear as a homogeneous, very-low-intensity lesion. On T2-weighted scans, they can appear as a discrete high-intensity lesion. MRI helps to distinguish hemorrhage into the cyst from complex irregularities and the extension into or involvement of the bile ducts.

5. What are the forms of PLD?
There are two forms of PLD: ADPLD, where cysts are isolated to the liver, and ADPKD, in which patients have cysts in both the liver and the kidney which accounts for 80%–90% of all PLD. More than 75% of all patients with ADPKD also have PLD. Half of PLD cases involve solitary cysts.

6. Describe the clinical manifestations of complicated PLD.
In many patients, liver lesions are diagnosed incidentally during imaging for other reasons. The common complications of PLD are related to the mass effect. Compression of adjacent structures by large cysts may cause chronic pain, anorexia, nausea, occasional vomiting, dyspnea, or obstructive jaundice. Acute pain may be due to cyst rupture or hemorrhage into a cyst. A definitive diagnosis of cyst infection usually requires percutaneous CT- or US-guided fine-needle aspiration.

7. How does the presence of liver cysts affect hepatic function?
Hepatic function usually is not affected by liver cysts. In the absence of complications the serum aminotransferase, bilirubin, and alkaline phosphatase levels typically are within normal range or only slightly elevated.

8. What are the treatment options for patients with symptomatic PLD?
- Typically, cysts with a diameter of more than 5 cm can be treated. Symptomatic liver cysts may be treated either percutaneously or surgically. Simple US- or CT-guided percutaneous aspiration results in rapid reaccumulation of the cyst fluid. The rate of cyst recurrence is greatly reduced by instilling a sclerosing agent, such as ethanol, at the time of aspiration. Percutaneous sclerosis of a liver cyst is contraindicated when the cyst communicates with either the biliary system or the peritoneal cavity. Surgical options include laparoscopic or open cyst fenestration.
- Infected cysts do not resolve with systemic antibiotic therapy alone. Administration of antibiotics should be combined with either percutaneous or surgical drainage.
- Patients with intractable symptoms who have failed other therapies may be candidates for either isolated orthotopic liver transplant or combined liver and kidney transplant if they are dialysis dependent.

9. What disease commonly is associated with PLD?
The majority of PLD occurs as part of ADPKD. There are strong associations between ADPKD and intracranial saccular aneurysms (berry aneurysms, 5%–7%), mitral valve prolapse, and colonic diverticula. Patients with ADPLD have no kidney disease but may have an increased risk for intracranial aneurysms. Some authors recommend that patients with PLD of either type should be screened for intracranial aneurysms by either magnetic resonance or CT angiography. In ADPKD the kidney involvement is extensive with 50% developing end-stage renal disease (ESRD) by the age of 50 years. In the US, ADPKD-ESRD is the indication for 12%–14% of all renal transplants, while it is rare to require liver transplantation.

10. What is hepatic cystic echinococcosis?
Echinococcosis is a parasitic infection caused by the tapeworm *Echinococcus*, with *E. granulosus* being the most common worldwide. *E. multilocularis is* usually known to cause alveolar echinococcosis. Humans are usually infected as intermediate hosts when eggs are ingested through contaminated food or water (Fig. 33.1). The eggs hatch in the duodenum, and the larvae penetrate the intestinal mucosa and are then carried by the circulatory system to the capillary beds of distant organs. The intermediate host creates the hydatid cyst by producing surrounding fibrosis. New scolices bud from the inner wall of the cyst. Over time, daughter cysts may form within the original cyst. More than one-half of all human infections involve the liver and other common sites are the lungs, spleen, kidney, heart, bones, and brain.

11. Describe the typical clinical presentation of hepatic cystic echinococcosis.
Patients may harbor the infection for years until they present with a palpable abdominal mass or other symptoms. The hydatid cyst diameter usually increases by 1–5 cm per year. The symptoms of hepatic cystic echinococcosis are related primarily to the mass effect of the enlarging cyst: abdominal pain from the stretching hepatic capsule, jaundice from compression of the bile duct, or portal hypertension from portal vein obstruction. Approximately 20% of patients have cysts that rupture into the biliary tree and may have symptoms like those of choledocholithiasis or cholangitis. Rupture of a cyst into the peritoneal cavity may cause an intense antigenic response, resulting in eosinophilia, bronchial spasm, or anaphylactic shock.

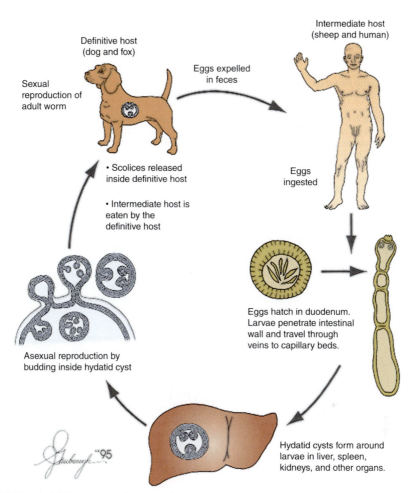

Fig. 33.1 Life cycle of *Echinococcus granulosus.*

Definitive host
(dog and fox)

Intermediate host
(sheep and human)

Sexual
reproduction of
adult worm

Eggs expelled
in feces

• Scolices released
inside definitive host

• Intermediate host is
eaten by the
definitive host

Eggs
ingested

Eggs hatch in duodenum.
Larvae penetrate intestinal
wall and travel through
veins to capillary beds.

Asexual reproduction by
budding inside hydatid cyst

Hydatid cysts form around
larvae in liver, spleen,
kidneys, and other organs.

12. How is cystic echinococcosis diagnosed?

Confirming a diagnosis of cystic echinococcosis involves diagnostic imaging and serologic tests. CT scans may show the hydatid cyst as a sharply defined, low-density lesion with spikelike septations. The presence of a calcified rim of daughter cysts greatly enhances the specificity of the CT findings. When imaged by US, the hydatid cyst appears as a complex mass with multiple internal echoes from debris and septations. Enzyme-linked immunosorbent assay or indirect hemagglutinin serologic assays for echinococcal antibodies are positive in approximately 85%–90% of patients. Recovery of scolices from a suspected hydatid cyst by percutaneous needle aspiration is diagnostic, but this technique must be used with caution because of the risk of fulminant peritonitis from spilling scolices into the peritoneal cavity.

13. What are the treatment options for hepatic cystic echinococcosis?

• The optimal treatment of hepatic cystic echinococcosis depends on the local expertise and the characteristics of the individual patient. Cysts with a single compartment that are <5 cm in size may be treated with albendazole alone. Surgical cyst resection generally is the preferred method of therapy for large or infected cysts. Percutaneous cyst drainage and irrigation with a scolicidal agent (puncture, aspiration, injection, and reaspiration) and adjunctive albendazole is a safe and effective alternative therapy for those with uncomplicated cysts >5 cm or for patients who are not surgical candidates. Albendazole therapy reduces the recurrence rate of both techniques.

- Pretreatment magnetic resonance cholangiopancreatography (MRCP)/endoscopic retrograde cholangiopancreatography (ERCP) helps to rule out cyst communication with the biliary or pancreatic duct systems. Persistent postoperative biliary fistulas may be diagnosed and treated by ERCP with endoscopic sphincterotomy.

14. Describe the five major classes and subtypes of congenital bile duct cysts.
    The classification of bile duct cysts can be seen in Fig. 33.2 and Table 33.1.

15. Compare the main features of Caroli disease and Caroli syndrome.
    - Caroli disease is a rare condition characterized by congenital cystic dilation of the larger intrahepatic bile ducts, which may be segmental, in the absence of an obstructive cause. It is associated with bile stasis, which can cause recurrent intrahepatic calculi and cholangitis. Typically it does not affect liver parenchyma. Hepatic fibrosis and its sequelae are not present in Caroli disease.
    - Caroli syndrome is an autosomal recessive condition that is more common than Caroli disease. Cystic dilation of large and small intrahepatic ducts can occur. Hepatic fibrosis is always present, which can lead to portal hypertension. Histologic examination generally reveals ductal plate malformation.
    - Caroli syndrome exists on a spectrum with congenital hepatic fibrosis and autosomal recessive polycystic kidney disease (ARPKD). All three are associated with mutations in the gene *PKHD1* (Table 33.2). The clinical spectrum of ARPKD is widely variable. There is a mortality rate of 30%–50% in the neonatal period, generally resulting from severe kidney disease. However, many survive into adulthood.
    - Treatment of Caroli disease and syndrome. Treatment is patient specific depending on disease pattern. Ursodeoxycholic acid helps to prevent choledocholithiasis, and antibiotics are used to treat cholangitis. Many patients may undergo ERCP for stone removal and duct stenting. Partial hepatic resection may be performed if the disease is isolated to one lobe of the liver. Liver transplantation can be considered in select cases.
    - Both Caroli disease and syndrome have an increased risk for cholangiocarcinoma.

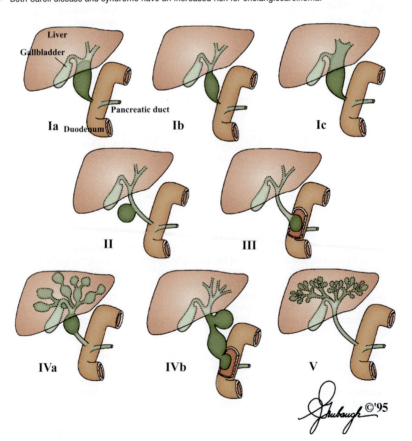

Fig. 33.2 Classification of bile duct cysts.

Table 33.1 Genes Associated With Bile Duct Cysts.

LIVER DISEASE	GENE	PROTEIN	ASSOCIATED RENAL DISEASE
Congenital hepatic fibrosis Caroli syndrome	*PKHD1*	Fibrocystin/polyductin	ARPKD
Autosomal PLD	*PKD1/2*	Polycystin-1 and -2	ADPKD
Isolated PLD	*SEC63/PRKCSH*	SEC63/hepatocystin	None
PLD	*NPHP1-8*	Nephrocystins	Medullary cystic kidney disease

ADPKD, Autosomal dominant polycystic kidney disease; *ARPKD*, autosomal recessive polycystic kidney disease; *PLD*, polycystic liver disease.

Table 33.2 Todani Classification of Biliary Cysts With Treatment Options.

TODANI CLASSIFICATION OF BILE DUCT CYSTS	TYPE	INTRA-HEPATIC	EXTRA-HEPATIC	MALIG-NANT POTENTIAL	TREATMENT
Type Ia: cystic extrahepatic bile duct dilation[a]	1a		✓	High	*RYHJ*, Roux-en-Y hepaticojejunostomy.
Type Ib: segmental extrahepatic bile duct dilation[a]	1b		✓		
Type Ic: fusiform, diffuse, or cylindrical bile duct dilation[a]	1c		✓		
Type II: extrahepatic duct diverticula	2		✓	Low	Cyst excision (often laparoscopic)
Type III: choledochocele	3		✓	Low	Sphincterotomy or endoscopic cyst excision
Type IVa: multiple intrahepatic and extrahepatic duct cysts[b]	4a	✓	✓		RYHJ and cholecystectomy ± partial hepatectomy
Type IVb: multiple extrahepatic duct cysts	4b		✓	High	
Type V: intrahepatic duct cysts, also associated with Caroli disease	5	✓		High	Largely supportive. Occasionally surgery/ transplant

[a]Type I is the most common occurring type (80%–90%).
[b]Usually associated with an anomalous pancreaticobiliary junction.

16. **Describe the typical clinical presentation of a bile duct cyst.**

Presentation can vary widely based on the type of cyst. Many of these are asymptomatic and can be picked up incidentally on imaging. The classic clinical presentation of a bile duct cyst is the triad of abdominal pain, jaundice, and abdominal mass. It occurs more commonly in infants and children than adults. Other presenting symptoms include cholangitis or pancreatitis. Due to the overlap with cystic kidney disease, patients may have manifestations of ARPKD.

17. **What hepatobiliary cystic neoplasm with malignant potential can be mistaken for a simple cyst, PLD, or hydatid cyst?**
Hepatobiliary cystadenoma is a rare neoplasm that has thick irregular walls and internal septations, distinguishing it from a simple cyst. Abdominal pain is the most common symptom. These cysts are lined with biliary epithelium and have a high potential for transformation to cystadenocarcinoma. The treatment of choice is surgical resection of the entire neoplasm.

18. **What is the incidence of malignancy within a congenital bile duct cyst?**
    - It is difficult to precisely estimate the risk of carcinogenesis in choledochal malformations. The reported incidence of malignancy within a congenital bile duct cyst ranges from 10% to 30%. This may be an overestimation because the true incidence of bile duct cyst disease is unknown. Malignancy has been reported in all types of bile duct cysts and the probability of malignancy increases with the age of the patient at presentation. It is thought that pancreaticobiliary reflux causes inflammation and eventually dysplasia in patients with congenital bile ducts.
    - Cholangiocarcinoma is the most serious complication of congenital bile duct disease. Early detection is the best preventive measure. Primary sclerosing cholangitis (PSC) accounts for 30% of cholangiocarcinoma. When PSC is the underlying diagnosis, an US and serum CA 19-9 are obtained yearly in patients with noncirrhosis and every 6 months in patients with cirrhosis.

19. **Describe the preferred treatment for patients with bile duct cyst disease.**
The preferred treatment for patients with bile duct cyst disease can be seen in Table 33.1.
Treatment is largely supportive. For choledochal cysts, the preferred treatment is complete surgical excision with hepatoenterostomy. Complete excision significantly reduces but does not eliminate the risks of developing bile duct malignancy, strictures, and cholangitis. Patients with symptomatic intrahepatic bile duct cyst disease may require segmental resection or liver transplantation.

20. **What is the role of cholangiopancreatography in patients with bile duct cyst disease?**
    - MRCP allows for visualization of the biliary tree. Patients with extrahepatic bile duct cysts have an increased incidence of anomalous pancreaticobiliary junction.
    - Direct cholangiopancreatography—percutaneously, endoscopically, or intraoperatively—allows definitive identification of the pancreatic duct insertion, which may be important in surgical planning if MRCP is not feasible. In addition, cholangiography can distinguish multiple intrahepatic bile duct cysts from multiple hepatic cysts, which can appear similar on CT.
    - ERCP should be performed with caution in patients with suspected Caroli disease or Caroli syndrome because of the increased risk of recurrent cholangitis and sepsis. ERCP, however, remains a useful tool for the management of acute cholangitis caused by bile duct stones.

21. **What are von Meyenberg complexes?**
These are usually asymptomatic, diagnosed incidentally, or at autopsy. Rarely, they may be associated with portal hypertension. Kidneys may show medullary sponge change. Microhamartomas can be associated with polycystic disease. Histologically, microhamartomas consist of groups of rounded biliary channels, lined by cuboidal epithelium and often containing inspissated bile. These biliary structures are embedded in a mature collagenous stroma. They are usually located in, or near, portal tracts. The appearances suggest congenital hepatic fibrosis but in a localized form. During hepatic arteriogram, multiple microhamartomas lead to stretching of the arteries and blushing in the venous phase.

CLINICAL VIGNETTE

Available Online

BIBLIOGRAPHY

Available Online

CHAPTER 34

GALLBLADDER DISEASE: CAUSES, COMPLICATIONS, AND THERAPIES

Kevin D. Platt, MD and Michael D. Rice, MD

 Additional content available online

1. **What is the prevalence of gallstones in Western populations?**
   The prevalence of gallstone disease is estimated to be between 10% and 20% of adults in Western countries and can greatly vary by race and region.

2. **What are the different types of gallstones?**
   Gallstones are classified as cholesterol, pigmented, or mixed stones based on their chemical composition. Approximately 90% of gallstones are cholesterol (>50% cholesterol), or mixed (30%–50% cholesterol). The remaining 10% are brown and black pigmented stones.
   - Cholesterol stones: usually form in individuals with a genetic or environmental predisposition to bile that is supersaturated with cholesterol. Most stones have a mixed composition with small amounts of calcium palmitate and bilirubinate salts.
   - Brown pigment stones: soft, clay-like consistency found in bile ducts, but not the gallbladder, often is associated with infection or prior manipulation of the biliary system.
   - Black pigment stones: form in the gallbladder from bilirubin precipitation; result from hemolysis and consist primarily of calcium bilirubinate.

3. **What are the risk factors for cholesterol gallstones?**
   Unalterable risk factors for gallstone disease include female sex, advanced age, ethnicity, and pregnancy. Potentially modifiable risk factors include diet (e.g., high in carbohydrates), obesity, metabolic syndrome, physical activity, rapid weight loss, and use of certain medications (e.g., oral contraceptives and estrogen replacement therapy).

4. **Name physiologic factors associated with cholesterol gallstone formation.**
   - Cholesterol supersaturation of bile: The amount of cholesterol secreted by the liver into bile exceeds the solubilizing capacity of bile acids and phospholipids in bile.
   - Biliary stasis: Stasis of bile in the gallbladder concentrates bile, accelerating crystal nucleation and impairing emptying of crystals into the duodenum.
   - Nucleation: Cholesterol crystals precipitate from supersaturated bile, which usually occurs in the gallbladder.

5. **What is the significance of biliary sludge?**
   Biliary sludge is composed of microscopic precipitates of cholesterol or calcium bilirubinate, which represents the earliest stages of gallstone formation. Over time, these crystal precipitates can expand and develop into gallstones. Biliary sludge can cause symptoms indistinguishable from those of gallstones.

6. **Describe the characteristics of uncomplicated biliary colic.**
   Biliary colic is characterized by severe, episodic pain in the epigastrium or right upper quadrant that is a consequence of a temporary obstruction of the biliary tree. This pain can occur postprandially, often has no inciting triggers, and typically resolves on its own. The pain may radiate to the right shoulder and be associated with nausea or vomiting. Protracted and progressive pain lasting more than 6 hours should prompt consideration of gallstone complications.

7. **What are the complications of gallstone-related disease?**
   - Acute cholecystitis: Infection of the gallbladder, most commonly caused by gallstone disease (calculous) leading to cystic duct obstruction (>90%), with the minority of cases being related to bile stasis and hypoperfusion (acalculous). Presents with right upper quadrant pain, fever, and leukocytosis associated with gallbladder inflammation.
   - Choledocholithiasis: Bile duct stones, generally result from the migration of gallstones from the gallbladder into the biliary tree.

- Cholangitis: Infection in the bile duct occurs when biliary obstruction results in cholestasis and infection. This is most often secondary to a bile duct stone but can also occur in the setting of malignancy, prior biliary instrumentation, biliary strictures secondary to surgery or chronic pancreatitis, or other infectious or autoimmune cholangiopathies.
- Gallstone pancreatitis: Passage of gallstones through the biliary tract can trigger acute pancreatitis either by obstruction of the flow from the pancreatic duct or by obstructing the ampulla.

8. **What is the treatment of choice for patients with symptomatic stones?**
Laparoscopic cholecystectomy is the treatment of choice for symptomatic cholelithiasis to prevent complications of gallstone disease (Fig. 34.1). Patients with common bile duct stones (choledocholithiasis) are at increased risk for complications and should undergo stone extraction and cholecystectomy.

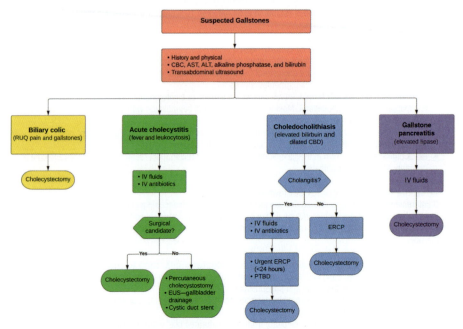

Fig. 34.1 Algorithm for diagnosis and management of gallstones and their complications. Note: These conditions are not mutually exclusive. For example, patients with cholecystitis may also have common bile duct (CBD) stones or cholangitis. *ALT,* Alanine aminotransferase; *AST,* aspartate aminotransferase; *CBC,* complete blood count; *ERCP,* endoscopic retrograde cholangiopancreatography; *EUS,* endoscopic ultrasound; *IV,* intravenous; *PTBD,* percutaneous transhepatic biliary drainage; *RUQ,* right upper quadrant.

9. **What is the best imaging test for detecting gallbladder stones and acute cholecystitis?**
Transabdominal ultrasonography can diagnose gallstones with a sensitivity and specificity of more than 90%. On ultrasound, gallstones appear as high-amplitude echoes with post-acoustic shadowing (Fig. 34.2A). While computed tomography (CT) and magnetic resonance imaging can detect gallbladder stones, ultrasound is preferred as it is safe, widely available, and cheap. Ultrasound findings suggestive of acute cholecystitis include gallbladder wall thickening >3 mm, pericholecystic fluid, and a positive sonographic Murphy sign (Fig. 34.2B). The diagnosis of cholecystitis is *not* made based on ultrasound findings alone. Diagnosis is determined based on the clinical findings above, in combination with consistent ultrasound findings.

10. **Should patients with asymptomatic stones undergo cholecystectomy?**
The risk of developing gallstone-related symptoms is estimated to be 2%–4% per year. In patients with gallbladder stones, complications usually occur after the development of uncomplicated biliary colic, so prophylactic cholecystectomy is not indicated. Approximately 20% of initially asymptomatic patients will eventually develop symptoms, therefore, it is recommended that they be educated about the symptoms of gallstone disease so they can seek treatment before complications arise. Patients without true biliary-type pain who are diagnosed with cholelithiasis should not undergo surgery.

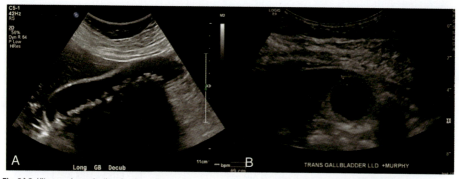

Fig. 34.2 Ultrasound examination showing gallstones (A) which appear as high-amplitude echoes within the gallbladder with post-acoustic shadowing. (B) Imaging findings suggestive of acute cholecystitis with gallbladder distention, gallbladder wall thickness, pericholecystic fluid, and sonographic Murphy sign.

11. How should patients with acute cholecystitis be managed?

Patients with acute cholecystitis should be hospitalized for supportive care and given antibiotics with coverage of Gram-negative organisms and anaerobes. Early cholecystectomy (within 7 days of presentation) is associated with shorter hospital stays compared with delayed treatment (1–2 months). Early cholecystectomy can usually be completed laparoscopically but has higher rates of conversion to open procedures compared to patients with uncomplicated gallstones. Delayed cholecystectomy is associated with an increased risk for recurrent biliary complications.

12. What treatment options are available for patients who are not surgical candidates?

While cholecystectomy remains the standard of care in the management of acute cholecystitis, in patients deemed unfit for surgery due to acute illness and/or significant medical comorbidities, there are a variety of nonoperative approaches, which may serve as a bridge to future cholecystectomy or may be used as destination therapy.

- Percutaneous cholecystostomy: A drainage catheter is placed into the gallbladder percutaneously.
- Transpapillary cystic duct stent: Endoscopic retrograde cholangiopancreatography (ERCP) is performed, the cystic duct is cannulated, and a transpapillary stent is deployed with one pigtail in the gallbladder and the other in the duodenum.
- Endoscopic ultrasonography (EUS)-guided gallbladder drainage: A lumen-apposing metal stent is placed endoscopically from the gastric or duodenal lumen into the gallbladder.

13. What are common complications of cholecystectomy?

The most common complication of cholecystectomy is bile duct injury, with an incidence of 0.5%. This can range in severity from minor bile leaks to complete bile duct transection. While the majority can be treated with endoscopic interventions, some require surgical repair. The risk of major bowel or blood vessel injury is approximately 0.02%. Peritonitis, postoperative bleeding, and intra-abdominal abscesses all occur in fewer than 0.5% of cases. Overall perioperative mortality varies between 0% and 0.3%.

14. Are there medical therapies for gallstone-related diseases?

Oral bile acid dissolution therapy using ursodeoxycholic acid (Ursodiol) can help reduce the cholesterol saturation of bile and can lead to the gradual dissolution of cholesterol-rich gallstones. However, studies have shown a lack of effectiveness in preventing symptoms and complications of gallstone disease, with a recurrence rate over 50% at 5 years, and up to 80% at 10 years. It may be considered in nonsurgical candidates (particularly with small, <1 cm, noncalcified cholesterol-rich stones) or in some cases as primary prophylaxis.

15. What modalities are useful to diagnose common bile duct stones?

The evaluation and management strategy of patients with suspected bile duct stones differs depending on the pretest probability (Fig. 34.3). Patients at high risk for choledocholithiasis should undergo ERCP prior to cholecystectomy, while patients at low risk should proceed directly to cholecystectomy. Patients at intermediate risk should be referred for either EUS, magnetic resonance cholangiopancreatography, or intraoperative cholangiography. All three of these modalities have high sensitivity (>90%) and specificity for choledocholithiasis and can identify patients in need of endoscopic therapy, with the choice between them often based on local expertise and availability of resources (Fig. 34.4).

Probability	Predictors of Choledocholithiasis	Recommended Management
High	1. CBD stone visualized on ultrasound or cross-sectional imaging or 2. Total bilirubin >4 mg/dL *and* dilated CBD (>6 mm, or >8 mm in patients who have undergone cholecystectomy) or 3. Ascending cholangitis	ERCP
Intermediate	1. Abnormal liver biochemical tests or 2) Age >55 or 3) Dilated CBD	EUS vs. MRCP
Low	None of the above	Cholecystectomy

Fig. 34.3 American Society for Gastrointestinal Endoscopy risk stratification and proposed management strategy for choledocholithiasis. *CBD*, Common bile duct; *ERCP*, endoscopic retrograde cholangiopancreatography; *EUS*, endoscopic ultrasound. (Modified from ASGE Standards of Practice Committee, Buxbaum JL, Abbas Fehmi SM, Sultan S, Fishman DS, Qumseya BJ, et al. ASGE guideline on the role of endoscopy in the evaluation and management of choledocholithiasis. Gastrointest Endosc. 2019;89(6):1075-1105.)

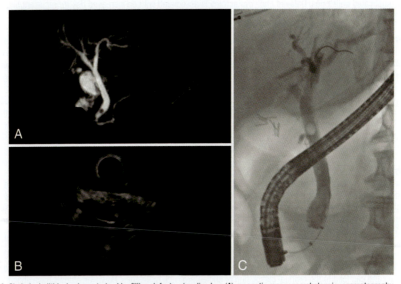

Fig. 34.4 Choledocholithiasis characterized by filling defects, visualized on (A) magnetic resonance cholangiopancreatography, (B) endoscopic ultrasound, and (C) endoscopic retrograde cholangiopancreatography.

16. ## What is acute cholangitis and what are the key points in its management?

Acute cholangitis is clinically characterized by fever, jaundice, and biliary pain (Charcot triad) as a result of bile duct obstruction and subsequent infection. Delays in diagnosis and therapy can give rise to septic shock.
- Intravenous fluids.
- Antibiotics aimed at Gram-negative organisms and *Enterococcus* species.
- Biliary decompression within 24 hours of clinical presentation. ERCP is the preferred method. Percutaneous biliary drainage is an alternative drainage method if endoscopic drainage is not available or not technically feasible.

17. **How should pregnant females with symptomatic or complicated gallstones be managed?**
    Laparoscopic cholecystectomy can be performed during pregnancy if the indication is urgent, regardless of trimester, however, the second trimester is the safest. Symptomatic bile duct stones should be treated with ERCP, which should be performed by an experienced endoscopist with care to minimize radiation exposure. Patients with gallbladder and bile duct stones who are asymptomatic after bile duct clearance should undergo cholecystectomy postpartum.

18. **What is Mirizzi syndrome?**
    Mirizzi syndrome occurs when a stone becomes impacted in the neck of the gallbladder or cystic duct, causing extrinsic compression of the common bile duct or common hepatic duct. Mirizzi syndrome usually presents with symptoms of cholecystitis with the addition of jaundice. Because of the jaundice, the presentation may be confused with acute cholangitis.

19. **What is a porcelain gallbladder?**
    Porcelain gallbladder is characterized by intramural calcification of the gallbladder wall. The diagnosis can be made by plain abdominal radiography, ultrasonography, or abdominal CT. Prophylactic cholecystectomy is recommended to prevent the development of carcinoma, which may occur in more than 30% of cases.

CLINICAL VIGNETTE

Available Online

BIBLIOGRAPHY

Available Online

ENDOSCOPIC RETROGRADE CHOLANGIOPANCREATOGRAPHY PLUS SPHINCTER OF ODDI DYSFUNCTION

Samuel Han, MD and Raj J. Shah, MD, MASGE, AGAF, FACG

 Additional content available online

1. What are the signs and symptoms of acute cholangitis?
- Charcot triad includes fever and/or chills, right upper quadrant abdominal pain, and jaundice.
- Reynolds pentad includes Charcot triad as well as altered mental status and hypotension, both of which are suggestive of sepsis.

   Cholangitis represents a biliary infection in association with a partial or complete biliary obstruction with elevation in intraductal pressure resulting in cholangiovenous or cholangiolymphatic reflux. Severity of cholangitis can be measured using the Tokyo criterion: (1) mild cholangitis defined as acute cholangitis responding to initial medical treatment, (2) moderate cholangitis defined as acute cholangitis that does not respond to initial medical treatment and is not accompanied by organ dysfunction, and (3) severe cholangitis defined as the presence of organ dysfunction. Acute cholangitis remains the only clear indication for emergent endoscopic retrograde cholangiopancreatography (ERCP).

2. What is the role of early ERCP in gallstone pancreatitis?
ERCP is indicated in cases of gallstone pancreatitis only when cholangitis and/or biliary obstruction are present. Early ERCP does not reduce the risk of mortality (relative risk: 0.74, 95% confidence interval [CI]: 0.18–3.03) or the risk of local or systemic adverse events in cases without cholangitis.

3. In patients with large bile duct stones, is endoscopic papillary dilation after sphincterotomy favored over sphincterotomy alone?
In cases of large (>1 cm) bile duct stones, endoscopic sphincterotomy followed by endoscopic papillary large balloon dilation (EPLBD) is favored over sphincterotomy alone. Papillary dilation is associated with a higher rate of complete clearance of large stones (pooled odds ratio: 2.8, 95% CI: 1.4–5.7) compared to sphincterotomy alone. Furthermore, there is a decreased requirement for mechanical lithotripsy when papillary dilation is performed and there is no increase in adverse event rate with the addition of papillary dilation to sphincterotomy.

4. What is the role of ERCP in Mirizzi syndrome?
Mirizzi syndrome is defined as common hepatic duct obstruction caused by extrinsic compression from an impacted stone in the cystic duct or infundibulum of the gallbladder with symptoms that often include jaundice, fever, and right upper quadrant pain. ERCP or magnetic resonance cholangiopancreatography allows for diagnosing Mirizzi syndrome and ERCP with stent placement above the level of obstruction can bridge the patient until definitive surgical management (cholecystectomy). While standard ERCP techniques are limited in treating cystic duct stones, transpapillary cholangioscopy enables direct visualization and treatment of cystic duct stones clearing a path to subsequent laparoscopic cholecystectomy in medically appropriate patients. Advances in cholangioscopy-guided lithotripsy including laser and electrohydraulic lithotripsy have increased success rates in treating cystic duct stones. If endoscopic expertise is not available to treat the stones, open cholecystectomy may be required for these cases.

5. What is the role of biliary stents in the management of choledocholithiasis?
In cases of difficult choledocholithiasis (e.g., bile duct stones larger than the downstream bile duct diameter) and an inability to clear the bile duct at index ERCP, plastic or metal stent placement provides temporary decompression and may facilitate stone removal at subsequent ERCP. In retrospective and small series, stent placement has been associated with a significant decrease in stone burden and number, which is thought to be secondary to fragmenting the stones by direct mechanical friction and dilating the papilla. It is important to ensure that a follow-up procedure, or referral to a tertiary center, with an anticipation for the requirement of advanced endoscopic techniques, such as cholangioscopy, be planned for ductal clearance.

6. **What role does ERCP play in the biliary drainage strategy for patients with malignant hilar strictures?**

Hilar strictures are those within 2 cm of the hepatic bifurcation. In patients with malignant hilar strictures, biliary drainage is performed via either ERCP or percutaneous transhepatic biliary drainage. However, due to lower morbidity and lower risk of seeding metastasis, first-line biliary drainage should be attempted via ERCP with stent placement dependent on the nature of the malignancy, symptoms, and the patient's goals of care. A review of predrainage imaging studies is critical to assess target intrahepatic ducts. Stent placement is attempted to drain all segments where contrast has been injected with the goal of draining >50% of the viable liver to prevent jaundice and recurrent cholangitis. Two or three stents, when necessary, are recommended over the placement of a single stent, and metal stents can be considered in patients with a short life expectancy. Since hilar metal stent placement is permanent, caution is warranted given the risk of potentially blocking (jailing) adjacent segments of the liver.

7. **What is the role of ERCP in primary sclerosing cholangitis?**

ERCP can be helpful in making the diagnosis of primary sclerosing cholangitis, but its main application is in tissue sampling and treatment of symptomatic dominant strictures. Defined as a narrowing measuring <1.5 mm in diameter in the common hepatic duct and <1 mm in the intrahepatics, dominant strictures are typically suggested by noninvasive imaging and diagnosed by cholangiography. Clinical presentation includes rising cholestatic liver enzymes, pruritus, jaundice, or cholangitis. Endoscopic evaluation typically entails sampling of the dominant stricture by brush cytology, intraductal biopsies, and fluorescence in situ hybridization to rule out malignancy. Treatment of the stricture will typically consist of dilation with or without stenting although a randomized trial found no difference in stricture recurrence rates in comparing dilation/stenting with dilation alone.

8. **How is the type of stent chosen in the management of extrahepatic benign biliary strictures?**

Extrahepatic benign biliary strictures, including chronic pancreatitis-related biliary strictures, post–liver transplant anastomotic strictures, and post–cholecystectomy strictures, can be treated endoscopically via placement of a plastic or fully covered (and removable) metal stent. A landmark randomized controlled trial compared multiple plastic stents with a single fully covered metal stent in patients with benign biliary strictures and found no difference in stricture resolution rates (85.4% plastic stents vs. 92.6% metal stent), but importantly, metal stenting was associated with significantly fewer procedures. A recent randomized trial also demonstrated that metal stents can be left in place for a year in patients with chronic pancreatitis-related strictures. Whether metal or plastic stenting is chosen, incremental upsizing of the total stent diameter is necessary for stricture resolution.

9. **What are methods for biliary cannulation when unsuccessful with standard techniques?**

A number of advanced maneuvers have been developed to facilitate biliary cannulation in challenging cases. If a guidewire is able to be inserted into the pancreatic duct, a number of options are available. The double-guidewire technique may be employed, during which biliary cannulation is performed keeping the wire in the pancreatic duct to potentially straighten the common channel which contains the intramural aspect of the bile duct and enhances the ability to access the bile duct. Alternatively, a transpancreatic septotomy can be performed over the guidewire in the pancreatic duct during which the septum between the pancreatic duct and the bile duct is cut to attempt to expose the bile duct lumen. In both techniques, guidewire access of the pancreatic duct enables pancreatic duct stent placement to help prevent post-ERCP pancreatitis. A randomized trial comparing both techniques found a significantly higher rate of biliary cannulation (84.6% vs. 69.7%) with transpancreatic septotomy with no difference in adverse event rates. A needle knife can also be used in two techniques to perform a precut to enable biliary cannulation. In a conventional precut sphincterotomy, the needle knife is used to cut starting at the papillary/common channel orifice in an upwards direction. A needle knife fistulotomy, on the other hand, involves making a cut in the papillary roof above the papillary orifice in a downward motion without ever directly contacting the orifice. A randomized study found a 0% post-ERCP pancreatitis rate (compared to 9.2%) when using the needle knife fistulotomy technique along with a high cannulation rate (97.9%).

10. **What are the risk factors for post-ERCP pancreatitis?**

Post-ERCP pancreatitis is believed to occur in nearly 10% of ERCPs, with the majority of cases being mild in severity. It is the most common adverse event of ERCP and risk factors for post-ERCP pancreatitis can be patient related and procedure related. Patient-related risk factors include female sex, age <50 years old, prior history of post-ERCP pancreatitis, and suspected sphincter of Oddi dysfunction. Procedure-related risk factors include multiple cannulation attempts (challenging cannulation) and contrast injection into the pancreatic duct.

11. **How can we reduce the risk of post-ERCP pancreatitis?**

A landmark randomized trial found that in patients at high risk for post-ERCP pancreatitis, the administration of rectal indomethacin was associated with a lower risk of pancreatitis (9.2% indomethacin vs. 16.9% placebo). While aggressive peri-procedural fluid hydration has generally been recommended, a multicenter randomized trial comparing aggressive hydration in combination with rectal nonsteroidal anti-inflammatory drugs alone found no difference in post-ERCP pancreatitis rates between the two treatments. Currently, a large randomized study (ClinicalTrials.gov NCT02476279) is evaluating whether the placement of a pancreatic duct stent in combination with rectal indomethacin can further reduce the risk of post-ERCP pancreatitis compared to rectal indomethacin alone.

12. **What are the indications for ERCP during pregnancy? When can ERCP be safely performed during pregnancy?**
ERCP should only be performed during pregnancy for therapeutic indications, primarily choledocholithiasis and/or cholangitis. When possible, all endoscopies should be deferred to the second trimester, however, given the risk of fetal loss with choledocholithiasis and cholangitis, ERCP should be pursued for these indications regardless of the stage of pregnancy. While ERCP appears to be generally safe during pregnancy, all attempts should be made to reduce fluoroscopy use to decrease fetal radiation exposure.

13. **What are ways to reduce fluoroscopy use during ERCP?**
Judicious use of fluoroscopy remains the guiding principle in minimizing the risk of radiation associated with ERCP. In this light, using doses as low as reasonably achievable helps prevent overexposure to patients, endoscopists, and staff. Continued education in optimizing fluoroscopy settings (image frame rate, magnification, and collimation) has been found to decrease ERCP-related radiation. Artificial intelligence can also aid in reducing fluoroscopy by automatically focusing on areas of interest and limiting radiation exposure to that region alone. Lastly, proper shielding in the form of appropriate lead aprons, thyroid shields, eye shields, and structural shields can protect staff from scatter radiation.

14. **What are the quality indicators for ERCP?**
Quality indicators represent ideals or benchmarks by which the performance of individuals or groups of individuals can be compared to. There are a number of quality indicators proposed by the major societies that pertain to ERCP. Of these, several have been designated as priority indicators, denoting their particular importance to the practice of ERCP. Within the intraprocedural quality indicators, priority indicators include achieving a >90% native papilla cannulation rate in patients without surgically altered anatomy, ≥90% success rate in removing common bile duct stones <1 cm, and ≥90% success rate in stent placement for biliary obstruction below the bifurcation. The lone postprocedural prior indicator includes documentation and tracking of the rate of post-ERCP pancreatitis.

15. **What are the different levels of complexity for ERCP?**
The American Society for Gastrointestinal Endoscopy has created a grading system for the complexity level of ERCPs, which range from level 1 (easiest) to level 4 (most difficult). Level 1 tasks include deep cannulation of the duct of interest, biliary stent exchange, and brush cytology. Level 2 tasks include extracting bile duct stones <10 mm, stenting for extrahepatic tumors, placing prophylactic pancreatic duct stents, and treatment of subhilar benign biliary strictures. Level 3 tasks entail extraction of bile duct stones >10 mm, extraction of internally migrated biliary stents, management of pancreatic duct strictures, treating benign biliary strictures above the hilum, and stenting hilar lesions. The most difficult (level 4) tasks involve the removal of pancreatic duct stones, intraductal-guided therapy, papillectomy, and performing ERCP in a post-Whipple or post-bariatric surgery anatomy.

16. **What are indications for cholangioscopy?**
Cholangioscopy allows for direct visualization within the biliary system and potential diagnostic/therapeutic options under visualization. Its most common application is the treatment of difficult bile duct stones, where a randomized trial found a 93% success rate with cholangioscopy-guided lithotripsy in treating stones >1 cm in diameter. In our practice, we generally reserve cholangioscopy for stones that are refractory to EPLBD or if mechanical lithotripsy appears to be too challenging. Another common indication for cholangioscopy includes tissue sampling in indeterminate strictures. Areas of concern (tumor vessels, papillary projections, and intraductal nodules) can be biopsied under direct visualization with increased diagnostic accuracy compared to standard tissue sampling techniques.

17. **What are indications for pancreatoscopy?**
Similar to cholangioscopy, pancreatoscopy has both diagnostic and therapeutic indications. In regard to diagnostic purposes, pancreatoscopy can characterize the presence, location, and extent of intraductal papillary mucinous neoplasms (IPMNs). In main-duct IPMNs, pancreatoscopy can confirm the diagnosis in equivocal cases and can provide presurgical mapping to help delineate surgical borders. In terms of therapeutic purposes, pancreatoscopy-guided lithotripsy can greatly facilitate the treatment of pancreatic duct stones with success rates approaching 90%. Furthermore, pancreatoscopy can also facilitate laser dissection of pancreatic duct strictures in cases of strictures refractory to standard treatments.

18. **Should we perform ERCP for patients with functional biliary sphincter of Oddi dysfunction?**
    The Rome IV Criteria have clarified what was previously known as sphincter of Oddi dysfunction by defining functional biliary sphincter of Oddi disorder as containing all of the following: biliary pain; twice normal elevation in aspartate aminotransferase or alkaline phosphatase or common bile duct >12 mm (but not both); and the absence of the bile duct stones or other structural abnormalities. The landmark Evaluating Predictors and Interventions in Sphincter of Oddi Dysfunction study randomized patients with abdominal pain after cholecystectomy without elevated liver enzymes or a dilated bile duct to ERCP with sphincterotomy or sham treatment. There was no difference in pain improvement between the two treatments, for which reason, ERCP and sphincterotomy are no longer offered to patients not meeting the Rome IV criteria (i.e., without objective data).

19. **Can ERCP be performed in patients with Roux-en-Y gastric bypass?**
    While challenging, ERCP can be performed in patients who have previously received a Roux-en-Y gastric bypass. Enteroscopy-assisted ERCP involves the use of a single-balloon enteroscopy or double-balloon enteroscopy to reach the afferent limb and cannulate the bile duct. Alternatively, a laparoscopy-assisted ERCP entails the placement of a port into the excluded stomach under laparoscopic guidance, through which a duodenoscope can then be used to enter the excluded stomach and access the major papilla. A comparative study found equivalent success rates with both enteroscopy-assisted ERCP (72.5%) and laparoscopy-assisted ERCP (87.2%). The more recent development of the endoscopic ultrasound–directed transgastric ERCP procedure involves the creation of a gastrogastric fistula through the placement of a lumen-apposing metal stent between the excluded stomach and the remnant stomach. This facilitates performing an ERCP through the lumen of the metal stent and has been shown to have a high success rate (98%).

20. **What is the role of ERCP in the treatment of pancreatic duct strictures?**
    ERCP with therapeutic pancreatic duct stenting remains the treatment of choice for patients with painful pancreatic duct strictures and associated upstream ductal dilatation secondary to chronic pancreatitis. While European guidelines recommend treatment with a single 10 Fr stent, additional tandem stents can be placed to match the diameter of the dilated upstream duct. There are limited data regarding the placement of fully covered metal stents for the treatment of refractory pancreatic duct strictures, but generally this is not advised.

21. **What is the role of the use of disposable duodenoscopes?**
    In response to the outbreak of carbapenem-resistant Enterobacteriaceae infections in patients who had received ERCP, significant effort has been made in developing disposable duodenoscopes and disposable tips to reduce the risk of duodenoscope-related infections. With the Food and Drug Administration recommending transition to fully disposable duodenoscope or those with disposable components, identifying select patient populations for these duodenoscopes remains important. Populations such as posttransplant patients and other immunocompromised patients may represent appropriate patient groups for the use of disposable duodenoscopes but the environmental and cost implications of fully disposable duodenoscopes require further investigation.

BIBLIOGRAPHY

Available Online

ACUTE PANCREATITIS

Bradford Jin Chong, MD and Gregory A. Coté, MD, MS

 Additional content available online

1. How common is acute pancreatitis (AP)?

AP is the most frequent gastroenterology diagnosis for hospital admission and is rising in incidence in the United States, from 9.5 to 12.2 cases per 1000 hospitalizations. Worldwide, the incidence of AP has increased by 3.1% every year over the last 40 years. The average duration of hospitalization is 5 days. The majority of AP cases are mild and categorized as interstitial pancreatitis (80%). When AP is complicated by necrosis or organ failure, the clinical course is more severe with mortality up to 30%–40%.

2. What are the most common causes of AP?

Gallstones and alcohol are the most common causes of AP in the United States and worldwide (Fig. 36.1). The rise in gallstone pancreatitis over the last 10 years has affected males (14%–35% increased risk) and females (12%–25%), likely reflecting the increasing prevalence of diabetes and obesity. Alcohol-induced pancreatitis is more commonly observed in males. This probably correlates with higher rates of alcohol abuse and smoking among males. Historically, idiopathic AP has been the next leading cause. With greater use of genetic testing and high-quality imaging such as magnetic resonance cholangiopancreatography (MRCP) and endoscopic ultrasound (EUS), these idiopathic cases are being reclassified as genetic pancreatitis or biliary secondary to microlithiasis, respectively. Drug-induced pancreatitis comprises less than 5% of all AP cases.

Etiologies of Acute Pancreatitis

Other (drugs and trauma) 3%

Idiopathic 10%

Autoimmune 4%

ERCP 5%

Genetic 5%

Hypertriglyceridemia 3%

Gallstone 40%

Alcohol 30%

Fig. 36.1 Etiologies of acute pancreatitis in the United States. *ERCP*, Endoscopic retrograde cholangiopancreatography.

3. What is a helpful pneumonic to remember the many causes of AP?

"**TIGAR-O**."

Toxic-metabolic: Alcohol, tobacco use, hypertriglyceridemia, hypercalcemia, organophosphates, and medications (valproic acid, didanosine, mesalamine, sulfa, furosemide, estrogen, and cannabis)

Idiopathic

Genetic (mutations in genes including *PRSS1*, *SPINK1*, *CFTR*, and *CTRC*)

Autoimmune (autoimmune pancreatitis, immunoglobulin G4–related disease, celiac disease, and vasculitis)

Recurrent AP (excluding other etiologies: trauma, post-endoscopic retrograde cholangiopancreatography [ERCP], ischemic, infection(s)—viruses including human immunodeficiency virus [HIV], coxsackie, cytomegalovirus, and hepatitis B; *Mycoplasma pneumonia*; and *Ascaris lumbricoides*)

Obstructive (gallstones, pancreatic duct stones, a tumor obstructing the pancreatic duct, and ampullary stenosis)

4. Which drugs have been reported to cause AP?

Drug-induced pancreatitis is the cause of up to 2% of patients with AP and can occur immediately upon initiation of the drug, or it can be delayed by months; it must be considered as a potential etiologic factor of AP in all patients. The World Health Organization (WHO) database lists 525 different drugs suspected to cause AP as a side effect.

The causality for many of these drugs remains elusive. Studies have classified the drugs depending on their published weight of evidence, presence of rechallenge and/or consistent drug latency among cases, and exclusion of other causes. The WHO classification is as follows:

- Class 1: drugs with positive rechallenge (1A: excluding other causes for pancreatitis; 1B: not excluding other causes of AP, e.g., alcohol)
- Class 2: drugs with more than four cases reported in the literature with consistent latency
- Class 3: drugs with at least two cases reported with no consistent latency among cases and no rechallenge
- Class 4: no consistent data to relate the drug to AP

Notable Class 1A drugs include mesalamine, trimethoprim/sulfamethoxazole, furosemide, anabolic steroids, estrogen, and tetracycline. Drugs often implicated in AP, such as azathioprine, 6-mercaptopurine, and valproic acid, were classified as Class 1B.

Dipeptidyl peptidase-4 inhibitors have not been shown to cause pancreatitis. Eluxadoline has been associated with increased pancreatitis in postmarketing cases, especially in those with prior cholecystectomy. This is also a reminder that opioids may cause sphincter of Oddi spasm or stenosis, which may trigger AP (this is believed to be the same mechanism for eluxadoline, which is a mu-opioid receptor agonist).

5. How is pregnancy impacted by AP?

AP in pregnancy is a rare condition, with an incidence ranging from 1 per 1000 to 1 per 10,000 pregnancies. Cholelithiasis or microlithiasis is present in 50%–90% of AP associated with pregnancy. Other causes include hyperlipidemia or alcohol use. Most episodes occur during the third trimester or early postpartum. Historically, maternal mortality rates up to 20% and fetal loss up to 50% were seen in AP during pregnancy. However, with advances in neonatal care, the mortality rate for pregnant females with AP is now comparable to that of the general population with AP. Pooled fetal mortality rate in AP has improved over the years as well (12%), with the highest risk during the first trimester (21%).

AP is diagnosed in pregnant females using the same diagnostic criteria (as for the general population) of symptoms, pancreatic chemistries, and/or imaging. Abdominal ultrasound is the imaging modality of choice in pregnant females, although magnetic resonance imaging without gadolinium can be used at any stage of pregnancy. Computed tomography (CT) is not recommended as the initial test of choice due to the risk of fetal exposure to ionizing radiation. Treatment for AP in pregnancy is generally similar to treatment in the general population: fluids, early feeding, pain control, and addressing the underlying etiology. For AP secondary to gallstones, contrary to prior recommendations, cholecystectomy is safe to perform during any stage of pregnancy. In general, cholecystectomy is still advised after the first trimester, when organogenesis is completed and the size of the uterus has not yet obscured potential surgical views. Endoscopists should use x-ray shielding in pregnant patients.

6. Which infectious agents have been implicated in causing AP?

Although an association is debated because of a lack of solid evidence, a vast number of case reports suggest a possible interrelation between infectious agents and pancreatitis. These include the following:

- Viruses: HIV, mumps, coxsackievirus, cytomegalovirus, varicella-zoster, herpes simplex, Epstein-Barr, hepatitis A, hepatitis B, hepatitis E, and influenza A and B
- Bacteria: *Mycoplasma*, *Legionella*, *Leptospira*, *Salmonella*, *Mycobacterium tuberculosis*, and *Brucella*
- Fungi: *Aspergillus* and *Candida albicans*
- Parasites: *A. lumbricoides*, *Toxoplasma*, *Cryptosporidium*, *Clonorchis sinensis*, *Fasciola hepatica*, and taeniasis

7. Is there an association between severe acute respiratory syndrome coronavirus 2 (SARS-CoV-2) infection and AP?

Pancreatic tissue expresses angiotensin-converting enzyme 2, which mediates the entrance of the SARS-CoV-2 virus into gastrointestinal epithelial cells. So, injury of the pancreas could be seen in patients with SARS-CoV-2, and patients with AP and coexistent SARS-CoV-2 are at increased risk for severe AP and increased mortality. However, there is no clear causative relationship between AP and SARS-CoV-2. Moreover, patients hospitalized with SARS-CoV-2 may have increased pancreatic enzymes that reflect other disease processes than AP, including shock, renal failure, severe systemic inflammation, and increased gut permeability.

8. **How do parasitic infections caused by** *C. sinensis* **and** *A. lumbricoides* **cause AP?**
   These parasitic infections cause biliary-pancreatic obstruction. The parasites migrate into the pancreatobiliary tract and can cause AP by blocking the main pancreatic duct and obstructing the drainage of pancreatic secretions.

9. **Is there an increased incidence of AP in patients with HIV and acquired immune deficiency syndrome (AIDS)?**
   Yes. Up to 10% of patients with HIV infection or AIDS develop AP. The cause is usually multifactorial, with drugs and infections being the most common. The likely drugs include didanosine, trimethoprim and sulfamethoxazole, and pentamidine. The most likely HIV-associated infections causing AP are cytomegalovirus, *Cryptosporidium*, and *Toxoplasma*.
   Abnormalities of lipid metabolism have been described in patients with HIV infection receiving a protease inhibitor, including hypertriglyceridemia and hypercholesterolemia, which may lead to AP.

10. **Does blunt trauma to the pancreas cause AP?**
    Penetrating trauma (e.g., gunshot or stab wounds) may cause damage to the pancreas parenchyma and may disrupt its ductal system, resulting in AP.
    However, the most common cause of trauma that results in pancreatitis is blunt trauma, caused by compression of the pancreas against the spine. This is commonly caused by motor vehicle accidents with compression of the pancreas by the steering wheel or seat belt and is usually seen in adults. Bicycle handlebar injury to the abdomen can cause pancreatic trauma in children and adults.
    Trauma-causing AP can range from mild to severe injury, and the latter may include transection of the gland. Nonrupture of the pancreatic duct causes AP, whereas acute rupture of the pancreatic duct may result in pancreatic ascites. Injury may cause pancreatic duct strictures with resulting chronic pancreatitis.

11. **What is pancreas divisum? Is it associated with an increased incidence of recurrent AP?**
    Pancreas divisum is a common congenital anomaly of the pancreatic ducts seen in Caucasians (7%), but less common among other ethnicities. It occurs when the dorsal and ventral pancreatic ducts fail to fuse completely into one pancreatic duct during organogenesis. This results in dorsal duct dominant drainage through the minor papilla; when there is a complete failure of these ducts to fuse, the ventral duct draining into the major papilla (alongside the common bile duct [CBD]) does not communicate with the dorsal pancreatic duct at all (also known as complete pancreas divisum). In patients with pancreas divisum, the majority of the exocrine pancreas drains through an accessory pancreatic duct and through an often smaller and hypoplastic accessory papilla; theoretically, this may lead to more frequent, transient intraductal pressure as the same volume of pancreatic juice is obligated to pass through the minor papilla. Patients with pancreas divisum are more likely to have mutations in genes associated with a higher risk of pancreatitis, including *PRSS1* and *CFTR*. The interaction between the divisum anatomy, other lifestyle behaviors associated with pancreatitis such as smoking, and genetics remains unclear. While millions of Americans have pancreas divisum, only a small number will develop AP. It is not clear if pancreas divisum significantly increases the risk of AP alone or only in association with other etiologic factors.

12. **What is the relationship between hypertriglyceridemia and AP?**
    Hypertriglyceridemia can cause AP in up to 3% of patients. It is a more common cause of AP than hypercalcemia. Serum triglyceride levels greater than 800 mg/dL are classically believed to be causative of AP; however, even modest (>200 mg/dL) elevation is associated with a higher risk of AP.
    Alcohol binge drinking and estrogen therapy can acutely drive moderate hypertriglyceridemia into the 800- to 1000-mg/dL range. These levels need to be determined when patients are on their usual medications and eating a regular diet (not when they are fasting, which results in decreased levels). Short-term treatment of hypertriglyceridemia includes insulin administration and fasting. The role of plasmapheresis in the acute and chronic settings is unclear. Longer-term interventions include dietary fat restriction and lipid-lowering agents (fenofibrates) to reduce the recurrence of AP. Familial chylomicronemia should be ruled out in patients with acute recurrent pancreatitis and refractory hypertriglyceridemia. It remains controversial whether or not hypertriglyceride-induced pancreatitis has a more severe phenotype compared to other etiologies of pancreatitis. Another confounder is that AP may cause transient hypertriglyceridemia as a part of the acute inflammatory syndrome. Retrospective cohort data have, however, demonstrated a positive correlation between the degree of hypertriglyceridemia and outcomes such as organ failure, pancreatic necrosis, and acute collections. If hypertriglyceridemia is suspected, patients should have their levels checked outside of an AP flare; in this context, it is best to check triglyceride levels when fasting and postprandially.

13. What is the relationship between hypercalcemia and AP?

Hypercalcemia from any cause (hyperparathyroidism or paraneoplastic) can increase the risk of having an episode of AP. There is a 10-fold increased risk of AP in patients with primary hyperparathyroidism compared with the normal population. Possible mechanisms are calcium-mediated activation of trypsinogen to trypsin within the pancreas. Malignancies that are associated with hypercalcemia-associated AP include parathyroid carcinoma, multiple myeloma, and adult T cell leukemia/lymphoma. Treatments for hypercalcemia-induced AP entail isotonic fluid resuscitation and bisphosphonates (to curb excessive bone resorption).

14. How is the diagnosis of AP made?

The diagnosis of AP is based on clinical assessment, biochemical analysis, and radiologic evaluation (Box 36.1). Diagnosis requires the presence of two out of three criteria to be positive.

Abdominal pain: Most patients with AP experience epigastric pain that radiates to the back (40%–70%) with nausea and vomiting. Up to 30%–40% of patients do not present with the classic clinical presentation of pain, or their pain presentation is hidden by other clinical symptoms such as altered mental status or multiorgan system failure.

Laboratory tests: Biochemical diagnosis of AP requires serum amylase or lipase to be greater than three times the upper limit of normal (ULN); levels more than five times the ULN are more specific of a pancreatic origin. Other pancreatic enzymes tested in the serum or the urine can be used for diagnosis; however, these tests are not widely available. These tests include pancreatic isoamylase, phospholipase A2, elastase-1, trypsinogen-1, trypsinogen-2, and trypsinogen-3, procalcitonin, trypsinogen-activated protein, carboxypeptidase B activation peptide, trypsin-2-alpha 1 antitrypsin complex, and circulating DNA. These do not appear to be more sensitive than amylase or lipase.

Radiologic imaging: Contrast-enhanced CT is the single best and most readily available test to evaluate the pancreas. It is best used when the diagnosis or cause of AP is uncertain or when AP is severe or complicated by infection. CT is safest after effective hydration and most accurate in estimating the degree of pancreatic necrosis after 48–72 hours. Ultrasound is an excellent imaging test for gallbladder stones but is limited in the examination of the pancreas and CBD because of obesity or gas artifact from the ileus often seen with AP. MRCP is accurate in estimating the severity of pancreatitis, evaluating pancreatic ductal anatomy, and ruling out the presence of CBD or gallbladder stones; however, it is often impractical in patients with severe pancreatitis because image acquisition may take 30–45 minutes and requires frequent, prolonged breath holds. EUS can assess for suspected microlithiasis, CBD, and gallstones. It can also be used therapeutically to sample or drain walled-off necrosis or other fluid collections.

Box 36.1 Acute Pancreatitis Diagnostic Criteria (Revised Atlanta Consensus 2012)

Clinical diagnosis of AP requires two of three criteria:
1. Serum amylase or lipase $\geq 3\times$ the ULN
2. Abdominal pain strongly suggestive of AP (epigastric and radiating to back)
3. Characteristic findings of AP on imaging, with CT the best and most universally available imaging modality

AP, Acute pancreatitis; *BUN*, blood urea nitrogen; *CT*, computed tomography; *ULN*, upper limit of normal.
Data from Banks PA, Acute Pancreatitis Classification Working Group: Classification of acute pancreatitis, 2012: revision of the Atlanta classification and definitions by international consensus, Gut 63:102-111, 2012.

---

15. How does serum amylase compare with serum lipase in the diagnosis of AP?

Serum amylase typically increases within 6–12 hours of AP onset and gradually declines over the first week. Conversely, serum lipase increases within 24 hours of AP onset and remains elevated in the serum for a longer period than serum amylase, thereby making its sensitivity higher compared with serum amylase. Serum amylase levels may be falsely elevated in several nonpancreatic conditions (see Question 16). Total serum amylase is 40% from pancreatic origin and 60% from extrapancreatic sources. Therefore some studies have shown superior specificity of serum lipase compared with serum amylase in the diagnosis of AP; the combination of enzymes does not improve diagnostic accuracy. Fractionation of elevated serum amylase into pancreatic-type isoamylase and salivary-type isoamylase may help in the diagnosis of AP and exclude a pancreatic source. However, most centers have adopted the practice of checking serum lipase alone and reserving amylase for particularly challenging diagnostic dilemmas.

16. What are the causes of hyperamylasemia and hyperlipasemia?

Elevated serum levels of amylase and lipase without pancreatitis can be due to nonpancreatic sources, including salivary gland disorders, hepatobiliary disorders, decreased renal clearance and/or hepatic metabolism, ectopic pregnancy, and increased small bowel permeability, as well as other systemic diseases (Fig. 36.2).

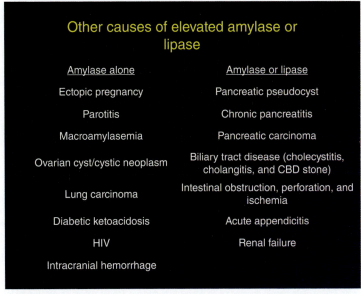

Other causes of elevated amylase or lipase

Amylase alone	Amylase or lipase
Ectopic pregnancy	Pancreatic pseudocyst
Parotitis	Chronic pancreatitis
Macroamylasemia	Pancreatic carcinoma
Ovarian cyst/cystic neoplasm	Biliary tract disease (cholecystitis, cholangitis, and CBD stone)
Lung carcinoma	Intestinal obstruction, perforation, and ischemia
Diabetic ketoacidosis	Acute appendicitis
HIV	Renal failure
Intracranial hemorrhage	

Fig. 36.2 Other causes of elevated amylase or lipase. *CBD,* Common bile duct; *HIV,* human immunodeficiency virus.

17. **Does the magnitude of hyperamylasemia or hyperlipasemia correlate with the severity of AP?**
    No. The levels of amylase and lipase do not correlate with the severity of AP or its prognosis. Serial measurements in patients with AP are not useful to predict prognosis or for altering management; if elevated initially, there is no need to follow levels.

18. **What is the most reliable serum marker for diagnosing gallstone AP?**
    The positive predictive value of alanine aminotransferase three times the upper normal value is 95%, though it has poor negative predictive value. Other biochemical labs such as alkaline phosphatase, bilirubin, lipase, and amylase have failed to reliably distinguish gallstone pancreatitis from other etiologies.

19. **How is AP classified?**
    The revised Atlanta classification (2012) divides AP into mild, moderate, and severe diseases:
    - Mild AP: No organ failure and no local or systemic complications; is associated with a self-limited course.
    - Moderate AP: Organ failure resolves within 48 hours, or local or systemic complications without persistent organ failure.
    - Severe AP: Consists of persistent single or multiorgan failure for more than 48 hours. These patients usually have one or more local complications and are at an increased risk of death.
    - Organ failure can be defined per the Modified Marshall Scoring system:
      - Cardiovascular: Shock (systolic blood pressure less than 90 mm Hg)
      - Respiratory: Pulmonary insufficiency (PaO_2/FiO_2 less than 400)
      - Renal: Renal failure (serum creatinine greater than 1.4 mg/dL)

20. **What prognostic scoring systems are used to assess the severity of AP?**
    Many clinical scoring systems have been developed to predict AP-related complications and hospital outcomes, ranging from Ranson criteria, Glasgow pancreatitis score, Acute Physiology and Chronic Health Evaluation II (APACHE II), Balthazar (CT) severity index, Bedside Index of Severity in AP (BISAP), and Pancreatitis Activity Scoring System. These scoring systems are complex and can be unwieldy in practice, though BISAP uses fewer clinical criteria that can be easily obtained (Table 36.1). Moreover, a BISAP score ≥3 is associated with an increased likelihood of severe AP (odds ratio [OR] 7.3), pancreatic necrosis (OR 4.8), and mortality (OR 9.5). Clinical gestalt based on the patient's risk factors (i.e., presence of organ failure, local complications of pancreatitis, and underlying comorbidities) and biochemical labs (presence of systemic inflammatory response, blood urea nitrogen [BUN], hematocrit, and C-reactive protein) can often guide triage and clinical decision-making in AP.

Table 36.1 Bedside Index of Severity in Acute Pancreatitis (BISAP) Score.

CRITERIA	POINTS
BUN >25 mg/dL	1
Impaired mental status	1
Presence of SIRS (≥2 criteria)	1
Age >60 years	1
Presence of a pleural effusion	1

BUN, Blood urea nitrogen; *SIRS*, systemic inflammatory response system.

21. What is the role of serum markers in assessing the severity of AP?

Several serum markers can in theory be used for prognosis and enable us to distinguish between mild and severe pancreatitis; however, studies have not identified a biochemical panel that can reliably predict a more severe course. Potential markers include trypsinogen activation peptide, polymorphonuclear leukocyte elastase, interleukin (IL)-6, IL-10, IL-8, tumor necrosis factor, platelet activation factor, procalcitonin, antithrombin III, substance P, C-reactive protein, and hematocrit. Only three are clinically useful: C-reactive protein, hematocrit, and BUN.

1. C-reactive protein has been used with good levels of accuracy in predicting severe pancreatitis 48 hours after admission.
2. Hematocrit levels ≥44% at admission and a rise in BUN at 24 hours may be predictive of necrotizing AP and organ failure. Both should decrease with adequate hydration; if these values do not despite intravenous volume, the likelihood of developing pancreatic necrosis is higher.

22. What are the other prognostic indicators in AP?

Mortality during the first week of AP results from systemic inflammatory response syndrome (SIRS). Alcohol-induced AP has been associated with an increased risk of necrotizing pancreatitis and a necessity for artificial ventilation. An interval between the onset of symptoms and hospital admission of less than 24 hours, as well as rebound tenderness or guarding on presentation, is associated with increased severity of AP. An additional prognostic factor is elevated body mass index. Obese individuals tend to have severe AP with increased morbidity and mortality compared with nonobese patients. The presence of visceral adiposity and increased waist circumference are poor prognostic factors.

23. What are the major systemic complications of AP?

- Respiratory failure: Acute respiratory distress syndrome is found in 20% of patients with acute severe pancreatitis. Exudative pleural effusion (with left more frequent than right) may occur, with the diagnosis made via elevated pleural fluid amylase compared to serum amylase.
- Renal failure: Renal hypoperfusion leads to acute tubular necrosis.
- Shock: Shock is caused by third spacing of fluids, peripheral vasodilatation, and/or depressed left ventricular function.
- Hyperglycemia: Insulin deficiency caused by islet cell necrosis or hyperglucagonemia results in hyperglycemia.
- Disseminated intravascular coagulation: Antithrombin III value of 69% at admission was the best cutoff value to predict fatal outcome, having a sensitivity of 81% and specificity of 86%.
- Fat necrosis: Tender red nodules on the skin (subcutaneous tissue) suggest fat necrosis. This is caused by elevated circulating lipase, which can also affect peritoneum, mediastinum, bone, pericardium, pleura, and joints; the latter can mimic acute arthritis.
- Retinopathy (Purtscher disease): Retinopathy is a very rare complication caused by occlusion of the posterior retinal artery with aggregated granulocytes.
- Encephalopathy: Encephalopathy is manifested in several stages ranging from agitation and disorientation to hallucinations and coma.

24. When is infection of pancreatic necrosis (PNec) suspected?

Infection of PNec usually occurs 5–14 days after the onset of the disease (median time 8 days). The hallmark of infected PNec is failure to improve, fever, tachycardia, hypotension, leukocytosis, and worsening abdominal pain. In this case, CT should be performed to diagnose and localize the area of necrosis, and fine-needle aspiration performed (Gram stain and culture) to determine whether the necrosis is sterile or infected. If infected PNec is found and the patient is stable, antibiotics are initiated according to the organism and sensitivity. The presence of gas bubbles within the pancreas or in the retroperitoneum suggests the presence of pancreatic infection. The differential diagnosis for air within a necrotic cavity also includes autofistulization of the collection to the bowel (most commonly the stomach or duodenum). In these cases, patients are usually not as sick as those with infected necrosis; in fact, when the collection begins to drain itself into the bowel, the patient may report improvement in pain, nausea, or anorexia. It is uncommon to have infected necrosis in a stable patient, however. In most cases, fine-needle aspiration to assess for infection is coupled with a plan to begin draining the fluid or necrotic collection because the patient is declining clinically (e.g., persistent or recurrent SIRS, end-organ injury or failure, and inability to advance diet due to pain, nausea, or anorexia).

25. How should PNec be treated?

In patients with AP and sterile necrosis, there is no role for the use of empiric antibiotics, as they may promote the development of resistant organisms or fungal suprainfection. If PNec becomes infected and debridement is needed, historically the standard approach had been open surgical debridement. However, a step-up approach (percutaneous or endoscopic drainage followed, if necessary, by retroperitoneal necrosectomy) has reduced rates of organ failure, health care resource utilization, total costs, and incisional hernia compared to open necrosectomy. There is also no increased risk for reintervention with the step-up approach. In addition to minimally invasive surgical approaches like videoscopic-assisted retroperitoneal debridement and laparoscopic transgastric debridement, endoscopic transmural drainage and/or percutaneous drainage are regarded as appropriate first-line options. Endoscopic drainage of walled-off pancreatic necrosis is performed ideally after 4 weeks, to allow for the walls of the collection to mature and facilitate debridement. Newer endoscopic techniques such as the use of lumen-apposing stents to create the cystgastrostomy (or duodenostomy) tract are challenging this dogma.

Percutaneous drainage should serve as adjunct therapy, for walled-off necrosis with deep extension into paracolic gutters and pelvis; it may also be considered in patients who are too ill for surgical or endoscopic drainage, including in the acute period of 2 weeks. Some collections that do not abut the gastroduodenal wall cannot be treated with endoscopic drainage or debridement; in these cases, a percutaneous drainage approach is preferred.

Mechanical debridement is usually necessary in addition to transmural drainage, especially if there is a large amount of residual solid debris. Endoscopic necrosectomy has been demonstrated to be safe and effective with a definitive resolution rate of 76%, a mortality rate of 5%, and a morbidity rate of 30% (with a mean number of four endoscopic sessions).

26. What is the most common organism isolated in infected PNec?

Infected PNec is usually caused by a single organism (80%). The infection results from a bacterial translocation of intestinal flora via hematogenous, biliary, and lymphatic spread with colonization of the pancreatic necrotic tissue. The organisms most commonly isolated are *Escherichia coli* (50%), *Enterococcus* spp., *Staphylococcus* spp., *Klebsiella* spp., *Proteus* spp., *Pseudomonas* spp., *Streptococcus faecalis*, and *Bacteroides* spp. (and, rarely, *Candida* spp.).

27. What is the ideal administration of fluids in AP?

In AP, the pancreatic microcirculation can be altered via multiple mechanisms: hypovolemia, increased capillary permeability, and microthrombi formation. Intravenous fluids are therefore a mainstay of AP treatment in restoring the pancreatic microcirculation and delaying progression from ischemia to necrosis of the pancreas. Crystalloid fluids are favored over colloids given colloids' risk for intravascular volume overload, renal failure, and coagulopathy. Normal saline resuscitation has been associated with hyperchloremia and metabolic acidosis, which can increase the risk for kidney injury and inflammatory cytokine release. Ringer lactate solution appears to have more favorable physiologic properties compared to normal saline through unclear mechanisms; comparative effectiveness studies have shown a decrease in hospital length of stay and need for intensive care unit admission, compared to normal saline. However, the type of crystalloid solution has not been shown to decrease SIRS, mortality, or end-organ failure. Expert guidelines recommend early fluid resuscitation within the first 24 hours of admission with close monitoring of biochemical markers (e.g., BUN and hematocrit), volume status, and urine output; caution should be taken to avoid overly aggressive fluid therapy, which can lead to respiratory complications and abdominal compartment syndrome. The optimal volume of fluids, rate of infusion, and endpoints for fluid resuscitation in AP remain unknown.

28. When and via what route should nutritional support be initiated in patients with AP?

Early resumption of enteral nutrition should be the goal in the treatment of AP. It should be started as soon as the patient is able to eat; traditional dogma argued that oral intake may stimulate the inflamed pancreas and prolong or worsen the clinical course of AP. This has not been observed in clinical studies. In mild AP, there is no role for parenteral feeding or nasojejunal enteral feeds, because patients tend to start oral intake within 1 week after onset of the disease. If oral feeding is unlikely for a period of more than 5–7 days, other sources of nutrition should be considered; a randomized trial did not demonstrate benefit from early initiation of enteral feeding in patients with predicted severe AP, so this decision can be deferred for the first few days of hospitalization to determine if the patient will be able to initiate oral nutrition within the first week.

Total parenteral nutrition (TPN) is associated with line infections and increased bowel permeability. There is strong evidence that enteral nutrition is superior to TPN as it preserves bowel function and integrity and reduces bacterial translocation (decreasing pancreatic infection). This can be administered via nasojejunal or nasogastric tube feeds; postpyloric placement of a feeding tube is not necessarily required unless there is a component of gastroparesis or gastric outlet obstruction. In addition, enteral nutrition is less expensive than those of TPN. The delivery of elemental or semielemental formulas into the duodenum has been shown to decrease pancreatic stimuli by 50%. Also, a small randomized study showed no difference in morbidity and mortality between nasogastric delivery of nutrition (low-fat, semielemental formula) versus nasojejunal delivery. If TPN is required because of refractory ileus, enteral feeding intolerance, or other contraindication to enteral feeding, adding intravenous fat emulsions when using TPN is generally safe and well tolerated, as long as baseline triglycerides are less than 400 mg/dL and there is no previous history of hyperlipidemia.

29. When should ERCP be performed in gallstone AP?

The routine use of ERCP for presumed gallstone pancreatitis is not justified. Urgent ERCP (typically defined as the first 72 hours of presentation), compared to conservative management for gallstone pancreatitis without acute cholangitis, does not reduce the composite outcome of mortality or major complications including new-onset persistent organ failure, interval development of acute cholangitis, bacteremia, pneumonia, pancreatic necrosis, or pancreatic insufficiency.

Patients with gallstone pancreatitis, but without clear evidence of choledocholithiasis and normal liver function tests, are still at intermediate risk for choledocholithiasis (since by definition acute gallstone pancreatitis occurs when a gallstone transiently obstructs the pancreatic duct at the level of the sphincter of Oddi). Therefore patients should undergo a sensitive test for retained CBD stones. Options include an intraoperative cholangiogram at the time of laparoscopic cholecystectomy. If a stone is visualized but cannot be removed via laparoscopic CBD exploration, postoperative ERCP is indicated. EUS and MRCP are minimally invasive modalities to rule out choledocholithiasis as well; in any case, ERCP should be performed when:
- There is evidence of acute cholangitis in the setting of acute gallstone pancreatitis.
- There is evidence of a persistent CBD stone.

The best clinical predictor to show a persistent CBD stone is an elevated serum total bilirubin level of greater than 4 on hospital day 2. MRCP can be used to determine the presence of choledocholithiasis, with the advantage that it is noninvasive. EUS is equivalent to MRCP and, in the correct clinical setting, can be converted to an ERCP at the same time if a CBD stone is confirmed.

30. Should patients undergo a cholecystectomy after an episode of gallstone AP?

Yes. There is a 20% risk of recurrent biliary complications such as AP, cholecystitis, or cholangitis that occur within 6–8 weeks of the initial episode of gallstone AP. These recurrent complications are associated with increased readmissions and hospital stay.

31. How soon should a cholecystectomy be performed in patients with gallstone AP?

In patients with mild gallstone pancreatitis, laparoscopic cholecystectomy is considered safe within the first week of the index hospitalization. Studies have shown that discharging the patient home to undergo an elective laparoscopic cholecystectomy results in 20% of those patients experiencing adverse events that require readmission before the scheduled surgery, which is usually planned 6 weeks after the initial episode of AP.

In the case of gallstone AP, laparoscopic cholecystectomy should be delayed until 1 week after the initial episode, allowing the patient to recover from the acute episode.

In patients with comorbid diseases who are unable to undergo cholecystectomy, an endoscopic sphincterotomy may be a good choice to prevent further episodes of gallstone AP.

32. What are acute pancreatic fluid collections?

Acute fluid collections are accumulations of fluid resulting from pancreatic inflammation. They occur in up to 57% of patients with severe AP. They do not have communication with any pancreatic duct and lack a clear wall of confinement. Their pancreatic enzyme content level is low, and most of them improve spontaneously within 6 weeks with conservative management. A minority of these fluid collections can develop a true nonepithelialized capsule progressing to a pseudocyst formation (Box 36.2).

33. What are pancreatic pseudocysts?

Pseudocysts are pancreatic fluid collections that have high pancreatic enzyme content, associated with pancreatic duct disruption and initial communication with the pancreatic duct. They usually coalesce between 4 and 6 weeks from the onset of AP. Their capsule lacks an epithelial lining (hence their name). They may occur in any part of the pancreas or peripancreatic area, but they most commonly are located at the body-tail of the pancreas.

34. When should a pseudocyst be suspected?

A pseudocyst should be suspected in a patient after an episode of AP who exhibits:
- No improvement in AP
- Persistent elevation in amylase and lipase levels
- Development of an epigastric mass
- Persistent abdominal pain, nausea, or anorexia after clinical improvement of the acute episode

Box 36.2 Diagnostic Approach to Pancreatic Fluid Collections

	PRESENCE OF FLUID	PRESENCE OF NECROSIS
Four weeks or less from the onset of pancreatitis	Acute peripancreatic fluid collection	Acute necrotic collection
More than 4 weeks from the onset of pancreatitis	Pseudocyst	Walled-off pancreatic necrosis

Adapted from Baron TH, DiMaio CJ, Wang AY, Morgan KA. American Gastroenterological Association Clinical Practice Update: management of pancreatic necrosis. Gastroenterology. 2020;158(1):67-75.e1.

35. What are the indications for pseudocyst drainage?

Pseudocysts should be drained when the patient has persistent or recurrent symptoms; in addition, when a complication such as hemorrhage has occurred, drainage is advised along with a careful evaluation for vascular complications such as the development of a pseudoaneurysm.

36. How are pancreatic pseudocysts drained?

Pseudocysts that meet the criteria for drainage may be treated radiologically, endoscopically, or surgically, depending on their location, size, and relationship with the pancreatic ducts as well as the experience of the physician performing the procedure.
- Asymptomatic pseudocysts are treated conservatively and followed clinically.
- Radiologic drainage is performed via CT-guided percutaneous catheter drainage. This procedure is mostly reserved for high-risk patients who cannot undergo endoscopic drainage since there is a higher risk of developing a cutaneous fistula from a persistent pancreatic duct leak.
- Endoscopic drainage can be performed with the guidance of EUS when the pseudocyst is adherent to the stomach or the duodenum. This has become the preferred modality for draining pseudocysts since EUS and stent technology have made this safer and easier, and patients do not have an external drain. Drainage is accomplished by creating a cystgastrostomy or a cystduodenostomy or by insertion of a stent via the ampulla into the pancreatic duct and into the pseudocyst cavity.

37. What are the possible complications of an untreated pancreatic pseudocyst?
- Infection: Diagnosis made by pseudocyst aspiration; may be treated with drainage.
- Pancreatic ascites: Leakage of the pseudocyst contents or pancreatic duct into the abdominal cavity may occur. Aspiration with analysis of ascitic fluid (high amylase and high protein) may be diagnostic, and placement of a stent into the pancreatic duct is a treatment of choice, combined with the use of octreotide. If this fails, a surgical approach should be considered.
- Fistula formation: Usually occurs after external drainage of the pseudocysts.
- Rupture: Secondary to a rupture of the pseudocyst into the abdominal or thoracic cavities. Manifesting as acute abdomen or pleural effusion. Surgical approach is the treatment of choice.
- Bleeding: Bleeding is the most life-threatening complication. It occurs when the pseudocyst erodes into an adjacent vessel, usually that has formed a pseudoaneurysm from the surrounding inflammatory milieu; blood becomes confined in the cyst versus spontaneous drainage into the gut via the pancreatic duct or a fistula formation, so-called hemosuccus pancreaticus. This condition should be suspected in patients with AP and gastrointestinal bleeding or who have an acute, unexplained decrease in the hematocrit with abdominal pain. This can be diagnosed by CT angiography and should be treated with embolization of the vessel.
- Obstruction: Pseudocysts can cause obstruction of the (1) biliary system (especially the CBD when located at the head of the pancreas), (2) vessels (inferior vena cava and portal vein), (3) duodenum, and (4) urinary system.
- Jaundice: May be due to the pseudocyst occluding the CBD.

CLINICAL VIGNETTE

Available Online

BIBLIOGRAPHY

Available Online

CHAPTER 37

CHRONIC PANCREATITIS

Bradford Jin Chong, MD and Gregory A. Coté, MD, MS

🌐 **Additional content available online**

1. What is the definition of chronic pancreatitis (CP)? Is there a link between acute pancreatitis and CP?

CP is a continuous, irreversible inflammatory and fibrotic condition that results in the impairment of exocrine and endocrine pancreatic function. Historic classifications such as Marseilles-Romeo and Cambridge divided CP into groups based on morphologic characteristics and pancreatogram features, respectively. However, it is now well accepted that CP exists along a disease continuum: acute pancreatitis (many times it is presumed that the acute pancreatitis is subclinical, meaning the patient does not have overt symptoms of acute pancreatitis) acts as the sentinel event of inflammation, and in the setting of repeated pancreatic injury, patients can develop CP. Yet, the frequency of transition to CP is only 10%, and so the pathogenesis of CP is also predicated on sex (higher predilection among males), genetics (*PRSS1*, *SPINK1*, and *CFTR*), and environmental factors (smoking and alcohol) (Fig. 37.1).

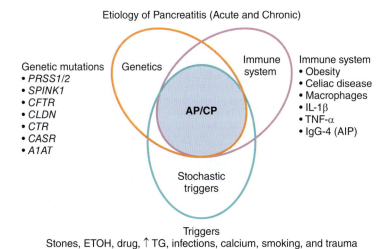

Etiology of Pancreatitis (Acute and Chronic)

Genetic mutations
• *PRSS1/2*
• *SPINK1*
• *CFTR*
• *CLDN*
• *CTR*
• *CASR*
• *A1AT*

Genetics

Immune system

Immune system
• Obesity
• Celiac disease
• Macrophages
• IL-1β
• TNF-α
• IgG-4 (AIP)

AP/CP

Stochastic triggers

Triggers
Stones, ETOH, drug, ↑ TG, infections, calcium, smoking, and trauma

Fig. 37.1 Etiologic factors of acute and chronic pancreatitis. *AIP*, Autoimmune pancreatitis; *AP*, acute pancreatitis; *CP*, chronic pancreatitis; *ETOH*, ethyl alcohol; *IgG*, immunoglobulin G; *IL*, interleukin; *TG*, triglyceride; *TNF*, tumor necrosis factor.

2. How common is CP in adults, and what is the leading cause?

In population studies, incidence of CP has been cited as 4–14 per 100,000 per year and prevalence as 13–52 per 100,000 population. The most common cause of adult-onset CP is alcohol, followed by idiopathic and genetic causes.

An ethyl alcohol (ETOH) consumption threshold of more than five drinks a day for 5–10 years is needed before an associated risk for CP is evident. The North American Pancreatitis Study 2 identified that common genetic variants in *CLDN2* and *PRSS1-PRSS2* loci alter the risk for alcohol-related and sporadic pancreatitis. The *CLDN2* variant was hemizygous and more strongly associated with males, which may explain the increased rates of alcohol-associated CP among males.

3. What are the other causes of CP?

The **TIGAR-O** classification system lists possible causes of CP:

Toxic metabolic: ETOH, tobacco, hypercalcemia, hyperlipidemia, and chronic renal failure

Idiopathic: tropical and cause unknown

Genetic: autosomal dominant, cationic trypsinogen *PRSS1-PRSS2*, autosomal-recessive/modifier genes, *CFTR* mutations, x-linked, claudin (*CLDN2*), *SPINK1* mutations, chymotrypsin-C (*CTRC*), common calcium-sensing receptor (*CASR*), and others

Autoimmune: types 1 and 2

Recurrent and severe acute pancreatitis: postnecrotic (severe acute pancreatitis), vascular diseases or ischemia, and postradiation exposure

Obstructive: pancreas divisum (controversial), sphincter of Oddi dysfunction (controversial), and duct obstruction (tumors and posttraumatic)

4. ## What is autoimmune pancreatitis?

Autoimmune pancreatitis is the most recently described form of CP. It is also known as sclerosing pancreatitis, lymphoplasmacytic pancreatitis, or idiopathic tumefactive CP. The classic (type I) autoimmune pancreatitis often presents as a malignant masquerader: the patient presents with an abdominal mass and jaundice with complaints of abdominal pain. The patient is typically 60–70 years old and more likely to be male (3:1) than female. This type is characterized by the presence of autoantibodies, increased serum immunoglobulin (Ig) levels, and elevated serum Ig4 levels usually at least twofold above the upper limit of normal; the higher the serum IgG4 level, the more specific this marker is in diagnosing the disease. Imaging shows a focal (mass-like) enlargement of the pancreas with pancreatic duct stricture. Pathologic reports show lymphoplasmacytic infiltrate with a predominance of IgG4-positive plasma cells. Cytopathologic confirmation is challenging, although more feasible with iterations in endoscopic ultrasound (EUS) needle technology. This type of CP has been associated with other autoimmune disorders such as primary sclerosing cholangitis, autoimmune hepatitis, primary biliary cirrhosis, Sjögren disease, and scleroderma (Table 37.1). Patients respond well to a short (1–3 months) course of corticosteroids, although there is a high recurrence rate of approximately 41% after discontinuation. For patients with radiographic and/or biochemical relapse, rituximab, azathioprine, or mycophenolate mofetil can effectively maintain disease remission.

HISORt criteria proposed by the Mayo Clinic includes the presence of one or more of the following: (H) histologic examination suggestive of autoimmune pancreatitis; (I) pancreatic imaging suggestive of autoimmune pancreatitis; (S) serologic findings, with an IgG4 more than two times the upper limit of normal; (O) other organ involvement, such as parotid or lacrimal gland involvement, mediastinal lymphadenopathy, or retroperitoneal fibrosis; and (Rt) response to steroid treatment of pancreatic and extrapancreatic manifestations.

On the other hand, type 2 autoimmune pancreatitis presents equally among males and females, typically around 40–50 years old. This type is less associated with IgG4 and extrapancreatic involvement and is more

Table 37.1 Autoimmune Pancreatitis (AIP).

	TYPE 1 AIP (100% JAPAN, 80% UNITED STATES)	TYPE 2 AIP (PREDOMINANT IN EUROPE)
Histologic findings	Lymphoplasmacytic sclerosing pancreatitis	Idiopathic duct-centric pancreatitis
Noninvasive diagnosis	Possible >70% of cases	Definitive diagnosis requires histologic examination
Mean age (years)	70s	50s
Presentation (%)	Obstructive jaundice 75 Acute pancreatitis 15	Obstructive jaundice 50 Acute pancreatitis ≈33
Imaging (%)	Diffuse swelling 40 Focal features 40	Focal features ≈85
IgG4 association	IgG4 ↑↑ serum and positive tissue staining IgG4	Not associated with IgG4
Other organ involvement	Multiple	None
Associated IBD (%)	2–6	16
Responds to steroids	Yes	Yes
Long-term outcome	Frequent relapses	No relapses

IBD, Inflammatory bowel disease; *IgG*, immunoglobulin G.
From Sah RP, Chari ST. Autoimmune pancreatitis: an update on classification, diagnosis, natural history and management. Curr Gastroenterol Rep. 2012;14(2):95-105.

commonly associated with inflammatory bowel disease. Imaging shows more diffuse, as opposed to mass-like, enlargement of the pancreas. Disease relapse is uncommon after steroid treatment.

5. What is tropical or nutritional pancreatitis?

Although its pathophysiology remains unclear, tropical pancreatitis is the most common form of CP affecting persons in areas of India and countries near the equator such as Indonesia, Brazil, and Africa. In India, *SPINK1* mutation is present in 42% of patients with idiopathic CP (compared to 4% of controls), raising the question of whether or not the nomenclature of tropical pancreatitis needs to be revised. Nevertheless, it presents in children and young adults with abdominal pain, severe malnutrition, dilated pancreatic duct with large intraductal calculi, and exocrine–endocrine insufficiency with the development of diabetes mellitus. It may result from protein–calorie malnutrition and it is linked to nutritional antioxidant deficiencies such as zinc, copper, and selenium. Cassava had previously been implicated in tropical pancreatitis, though this association has since been debunked.

6. What is obstructive CP?

Any type of obstruction of the pancreatic duct either malignant or benign may lead to CP or develop as a consequence of CP. It is not clear if the treatment of pancreatic duct obstruction improves the natural history of CP (i.e., reduces the development or worsening of diabetes mellitus or exocrine pancreatic insufficiency). The impact of duct drainage on pain is discussed later in this chapter.

7. What is hereditary pancreatitis?

Hereditary pancreatitis is an autosomal dominant disorder with a high (~80%) penetrance that accounts for <1% of all cases of CP. It affects both sexes equally and presents as episodes of recurrent acute pancreatitis in children aged 10–12 years who then develop CP. Though not as high as originally thought, patients with this condition are predisposed to developing pancreatic cancer with an approximate incidence of 40% by age 70. Autosomal dominant hereditary pancreatitis is caused by a mutation in the cationic trypsinogen gene (*PRSS1*). Autosomal-recessive genetic mutations in pancreatic secretory trypsin inhibitor (*SPINK1*), cystic fibrosis transmembrane conductance regulator (*CFTR*) genes, chymotrypsin-C (*CTRC*), and common calcium-sensing receptor (*CASR*) genes are also associated with a greater risk of CP; the interaction between these genes and environmental risk factors such as smoking remains unclear. For treatment planning and prognostication, genetic testing should be considered for patients with idiopathic CP especially when the onset of disease is <40 years.

8. How is cystic fibrosis (CF) associated with CP?

CF is the most common autosomal-recessive defect in Caucasians. Besides the sinopulmonary disease, CF is also associated with exocrine pancreatic insufficiency. CF is caused by mutations in the *CFTR* gene (more than 1000 different genetic polymorphisms in *CFTR* have been identified, most of which have no clinically significant phenotype). *CFTR* gene mutations cause deranged transport of chloride or other *CFTR*-affected ions, such as sodium and bicarbonate, which leads to thick, viscous pancreatic secretions, resulting in pancreatic duct obstruction and acinar cell destruction. Patients with CF-related pancreatic disease and insufficiency can develop malabsorption symptoms, as well as severe malnutrition. CF should be considered in young patients with pancreatitis, especially who have infertility or pulmonary complications. For these patients, triplet *CFTR* modulator therapy has been effective in improving lung function, though its therapeutic yield for pancreatic function remains to be seen. Atypical *CFTR* mutations often present with little or no sinopulmonary manifestations and become evident in adulthood with the onset of acute recurrent pancreatitis. These individuals have preserved exocrine pancreatic function in youth, allowing for overt parenchymal inflammation (acute pancreatitis) to develop later in life.

9. What is the most common presenting symptom of CP?

Abdominal pain is the most common symptom occurring in up to 80% of the patients. The pain is described as a dull, constant, epigastric discomfort that radiates to the back, worsens 15–30 minutes after meals, improves with sitting or leaning forward, and frequently is associated with nausea and vomiting. Pain patterns vary in CP from none to acute relapsing, to acute relapsing with chronic mild pain, to chronic severe pain with or without acute flares.

10. What are the causes of weight loss in patients with CP?

Causes of weight loss include the following:
- Pancreatic exocrine insufficiency with malabsorption of proteins, carbohydrates, and fat (needs to have more than 90% of nonfunctioning pancreas)
- Uncontrolled diabetes mellitus
- Decreased caloric intake as a result of fear of increasing abdominal pain (sitophobia)
- Early satiety caused by delayed gastric emptying or gastric outlet obstruction—duodenal obstruction

11. Is steatorrhea an early symptom of CP?

No. Steatorrhea occurs when more than 90% of the exocrine function is impaired or insufficient. It signifies advanced disease. It occurs before protein deficiency because lipolysis decreases faster than proteolysis. It manifests as foul-smelling, greasy, loose stools, and liposoluble vitamin deficiency (A, D, E, and K).

Early symptoms of CP are nonspecific and include bloating, abdominal discomfort, pain, and change in bowel habits.

12. What is type 3c or pancreatogenic diabetes?

Pancreatogenic diabetes, or type 3c diabetes, is most often due to CP but can also occur due to pancreatic ductal adenocarcinoma, CF, and prior pancreatic surgery. Whereas type 2 diabetes is primarily driven by impaired insulin sensitivity, the pathophysiology for type 3c diabetes is multifactorial and encompasses deficient insulin production, inflammatory cytokine-induced inhibition of insulin release, hepatic and peripheral insulin resistance, and decreased incretin effect.

Patients with diabetes caused by CP suffer retinopathy and neuropathy at the same levels compared with other types of diabetes. On the other hand, diabetic ketoacidosis and nephropathy are uncommon. Keep in mind that new-onset diabetes with weight loss can be a harbinger of pancreatic ductal adenocarcinoma.

13. Are measurements of serum pancreatic enzymes helpful in the diagnosis of CP?

Pancreatic fibrosis results in the destruction of the acinar cell with subsequent decreased production of amylase and lipase. These enzymes are not helpful in the diagnosis of CP. Levels may be elevated, normal, or decreased despite clinical symptoms of pain. There is no sensitive or specific laboratory test for the diagnosis of CP; however, low levels of trypsinogen or fecal elastase may suggest late-stage CP.

14. What do elevated levels of bilirubin and alkaline phosphatase suggest in a patient with CP?

Elevated levels of bilirubin or alkaline phosphatase in the setting of CP suggest biliary obstruction caused by compression of the intrapancreatic portion of the bile duct secondary to fibrosis, pancreatic mass or carcinoma, and edema of the organ. Also, elevated enzymes may be caused by alcohol intake or other hepatotoxic drugs.

15. What specialized test directly measures pancreatic exocrine function?

Pancreatic exocrine secretions are normally high in bicarbonate (pH = 7.8–8). The *secretin stimulation test*, with or without the administration of cholecystokinin, measures the volume of these pancreatic secretions and the concentration of bicarbonate after the injection of secretin. Historically, this was an invasive test requiring the placement of a duodenal catheter (Dreiling tube) to collect the secretions. Because of its complexity and cumbersome nature, this test has been replaced by endoscopic aspiration of pancreatic secretions and measurements of bicarbonate levels (Table 37.2). Neither are performed in clinical practice frequently given the lack of treatments to delay disease progression, unclear impact on clinical management, and time (30–60 minutes) required to complete the test.

Table 37.2 Secretin Stimulation Test.

BICARBONATE LEVEL (MEQ/L)	RESULTS
<50	Consistent with chronic pancreatitis
50–75	Indeterminate
>75	Normal

16. What conditions may be associated with a false-positive secretin stimulation test?

Primary diabetes mellitus, celiac sprue, cirrhosis, and Billroth II gastrectomy (or other foregut surgery such as gastric bypass) may result in false-positive secretin stimulation tests. Patients in the recovery phase of an episode of acute pancreatitis may also have false-positive results.

17. What indirect tests of pancreatic exocrine function are used?

Indirect tests measure pancreatic enzymes in the serum and stool or any metabolites of the enzymes in serum, urine, or breath after an orally administered compound. Because these studies measure the level of pancreatic maldigestion, the more advanced the disease, the more sensitive will be the measurement. Exocrine function is significantly impaired after 90% of the secretory capacity of the organ is destroyed. Therefore these studies are not sensitive to early-stage pancreatic disease.

Some of the studies are as follows:

- Serum trypsin: very low (20 ng/mL) in patients with advanced CP and steatorrhea
- Fecal chymotrypsin
- Fecal elastase (<100 mcg/g is typically used to define insufficiency): more stable and easier to use than the chymotrypsin stool test
- [14 C]-olein absorption test
- Fecal fat determination: quantitative 72-hour fecal test collected after the patient follows a diet for 3 days that contains 100 g/day of fat
- Breath tests: labeled substrates that are digested by pancreatic enzymes have been proposed for breath tests and are currently under study

18. Are plain abdominal radiographs helpful in the diagnosis of CP?

Yes. The finding of diffuse pancreatic calcifications in plain abdominal radiographs is specific for CP. This is seen in 30%–40% of the patients with CP. Calcifications are not seen in the early stages of the disease, so the utility of abdominal radiographs is mostly in advanced disease and to determine the patient's eligibility for extracorporeal shock wave lithotripsy, which typically requires fluoroscopic guidance to target the calcifications. Calcium deposition is most common with alcohol-related patients in the United States and tropical pancreatitis patients in India.

19. What other imaging modalities are used in the diagnosis of CP?

Ultrasound, computed tomography (CT), and magnetic resonance imaging (MRI) are used to varying degrees to show pancreatic duct dilation, calcifications, pancreatic duct filling defects, and pseudocysts. Ultrasound has a sensitivity of 60%–70% and a specificity of 80%–90%. CT has 10%–20% more sensitivity than ultrasound with similar specificity. MRI shows more detail in the evaluation of the pancreatic duct.

20. What is the role of EUS in the diagnosis of CP?

EUS allows excellent visualization of the pancreatic duct and the parenchyma. CP can be diagnosed based on abnormal ductal findings or abnormal parenchymal findings (see Question 22). A minimum of three criteria are needed to diagnose CP, although the presence of five criteria improves its specificity. As reflected in the Rosemont consensus criteria, the most specific features for CP include the presence of calcifications (shadowing foci) and lobularity with honeycombing.

While none are ready for clinical use, novel imaging techniques such as contrast-enhanced EUS and elastography seem promising for the evaluation of early CP.

21. What are the EUS criteria for the diagnosis of CP?

The EUS criteria for the diagnosis of CP can be seen in Table 37.3.

Table 37.3 Chronic Pancreatitis (Endoscopic Ultrasound Rosemont Criteria).[*]

MAJOR CRITERIA A AND B	MINOR CRITERIA
(A) MPD calculi	Cysts
(B) Hyperechoic foci with acoustic shadowing	Hyperechoic foci without acoustic shadowing
(C) Honeycomb pattern with lobularity	Lobularity without honeycombing
	Stranding
	Irregular MPD contour
	MPD dilation (≥3.5 mm body and 1.5 mm tail)
	Dilated side branches (≥1 mm width)
	Hyperechoic MPD margin

MPD, Main pancreatic duct.
*Suggestive of chronic pancreatitis: 1 major A criteria and <3 minor criteria, OR 1 major B criteria and ≥3 minor criteria, OR ≥5 minor criteria.
*Indeterminate for chronic pancreatitis: 3–4 minor criteria, no major criteria, OR major B criteria alone or with <3 minor criteria.
*Normal: <2 minor criteria, no major criteria.
*Consistent with chronic pancreatitis: 1 major A criteria and ≥3 minor criteria, OR 1 major A criteria and 1 major B criteria, OR two major A criteria.
Adapted from Catalano MF, Sahai A, Levy M, Romagnuolo J, Wiersema M, Brugge W, et al. EUS-based criteria for the diagnosis of chronic pancreatitis: the Rosemont classification. Gastrointest Endosc. 2009;69(7):1251-1261.

22. **What is the role of endoscopic retrograde cholangiopancreatography (ERCP) in the diagnosis of CP?**

ERCP was previously the test of choice to confirm abnormalities in the pancreatic duct in patients with moderate-advanced CP. It was considered the gold standard in evaluating the pancreas with a sensitivity of 90% and a specificity of 100%. However, it is an invasive and risky procedure (complications of 5% and mortality of 0.1%). With the development of new technology, such as magnetic retrograde cholangiopancreatography (MRCP) and EUS, the role of ERCP has been limited to planned interventions (e.g., stone extraction). Findings on ERCP suggestive of CP include the characteristic *chain of lakes* beading of the main pancreatic duct, ecstatic side branches, and intraductal filling defects. ERCP with intraductal brushing of a pancreatic duct stricture is rarely used to distinguish benign from malignant pancreatic duct obstruction, since EUS with fine-needle aspiration provides better diagnostic accuracy with less risk. In autoimmune pancreatitis the main pancreatic duct is narrowed with areas of stenosis (similar to the cholangiogram of a patient with primary sclerosing cholangitis), as opposed to CP with a dilated duct with areas of stenosis.

23. **What is the role of MRCP in the diagnosis of CP?**

MRCP is an excellent initial study for the evaluation of CP, because it is a noninvasive test and evaluates both pancreatic parenchyma and ducts. Studies show good correlation with the ductular findings obtained in MRCP with those obtained in ERCP. MRCP visualizes ductular anatomy, including strictures, and is able to identify cysts not connected with the ductular system. Its limitations are the inability to evaluate areas where the pancreatic duct is small (pancreatic tail or side branches). Secretin-enhanced MRCP can help characterize subtle pancreatic disease by improving imaging of the pancreatic duct anatomy; however, this adds a significant cost to the study.

24. **What is the most common complication of CP?**

The most common complication of CP is the development of pseudocysts, which occurs in 20%–40% of patients. Pseudocysts should be suspected in patients with stable CP who have:
- Persistent abdominal or back pain
- Development of an epigastric mass that may cause obstructive symptoms, such as nausea, vomiting, and jaundice

Pseudocysts can be:
- Acute (resolution within 6 weeks) or
- Chronic (no self-resolution and persisting for longer than 6 weeks)

25. **How are pseudocysts treated?**

Asymptomatic pseudocysts are generally treated conservatively. Symptomatic pseudocysts can be treated via percutaneous, endoscopic, or surgical drainage depending on their location, size, experience of the physician performing the procedure, and relationship with the pancreatic ducts.

Surgery is typically offered to patients when:
- Percutaneous or endoscopic drainage is technically infeasible or unsuccessful (incomplete drainage).
- Additional indications for surgery, such as a symptomatic disconnected pancreatic tail due to complete pancreatic duct obstruction.
- Suspicion for malignancy:
  Percutaneous drainage is preferred for immature fluid collections that require drainage due to known or suspected infection or in individuals who cannot tolerate general anesthesia.

Endoscopic drainage is almost invariably performed with EUS imaging to ensure precise localization of the pseudocyst and avoid intervening structures such as blood vessels. Drainage is typically deferred until the pseudocyst wall has matured (typically at least 4 weeks) and is adherent to the stomach or the duodenum; however, newer stent technology with the use of lumen-apposing stents seems to allow for a shorter time between cyst onset and drainage. The procedure is performed by creating a cystogastrostomy or a cystoduodenostomy, leaving one or more transmural stents to ensure adequate drainage. For smaller cysts that are in communication with the main pancreatic duct, transpapillary drainage can be completed via ERCP.

26. **What are other complications of CP?**

- Distal common bile duct (CBD) obstruction occurs in 5%–10% of patients with CP. Compression of the intrapancreatic portion of the CBD at the head of the pancreas by edema, fibrosis, or pseudocyst causes jaundice, pain, dilated ducts, and potentially cholangitis. If untreated, it may lead to secondary sclerosing cholangitis and biliary cirrhosis.
- Diabetes mellitus is a late complication and occurs in up to one-third of patients with CP. The pathophysiology of pancreatogenic diabetes remains unclear, although volume loss of parenchyma and immunogenic mechanisms play a role.
- Duodenal obstruction occurs in 5% of patients with CP. External compression of the duodenum by the pancreas causes nausea, vomiting, weight loss, gastric outlet obstruction, and postprandial fullness.
- External pancreatic fistulas occur after surgical or percutaneous drainage of a pseudocyst or wall of necrosis.

- Internal pancreatic fistulas occur spontaneously after pancreatic duct rupture or pseudocyst leakage.
- Pseudoaneurysms are a result of a pseudocyst eroding into the splenic vein causing hemosuccus pancreaticus.
- Splenic vein thrombosis is caused by pancreatic inflammation or pseudocyst obstruction in the pancreas with subsequent gastric varices formation (i.e., sinistral portal hypertension).
- Patients with CP have a lifetime risk of developing *pancreatic adenocarcinoma* of 4%.

27. **How is distal CBD obstruction diagnosed and treated?**
Distal CBD stricture should be suspected in the setting of CP, often presenting first with an elevated alkaline phosphatase. Subsequently, jaundice or ascending cholangitis may occur. CBD strictures within the intrapancreatic segment of the bile duct are caused by inflammation, fibrosis, or pseudocyst formation at the head of the pancreas. Imaging studies such as MRCP may demonstrate narrowing of the distal CBD in the form of gradual tapering, bird beak stenosis, or an hourglass stricture.
   Treatment options in the case of no complications (cholangitis and secondary biliary cirrhosis) include observation of the patients for at least 2 months with serial liver function tests (LFTs). If any complication or persistently elevated LFTs are seen, biliary decompression is warranted. Endoscopic biliary stent is often chosen as the first-line treatment for CBD strictures, though it can require frequent stent exchanges because of blockage or migration. Surgical biliary bypass with cholecystojejunostomy or choledochojejunostomy provides more durable long-term outcomes than endoscopic therapy and therefore may be preferred for younger patients or those who relapse after a complete course of endoscopic therapy. If pseudocyst is the cause of the biliary obstruction, decompression of the pseudocyst should be the initial approach.

28. **How is duodenal obstruction diagnosed and treated?**
Duodenal obstruction is suspected in the setting of early satiety and postprandial abdominal bloating or diagnosis of gastric outlet obstruction. It is best diagnosed by upper gastrointestinal series. Treatment includes initial supportive therapy; however, persistent obstruction warrants a surgical approach, usually gastrojejunostomy. If biliary obstruction is also present, biliary bypass or surgical resection of the pancreatic head may be performed.

29. **How are pancreatic fistulas treated?**
Medical treatment of pancreatic fistulas can be attempted through the administration of a somatostatin analog (octreotide 100–250 mcg subcutaneously every 8 hours) to reduce pancreatic secretions. Often this is coupled with pancreatic rest through jejunal feeding or total parenteral nutrition and nothing by mouth. This approach may take several weeks and its efficacy is variable—especially for higher volume fistulae.
   If feasible, ERCP should be offered to localize the site of pancreatic duct leak. The resolution rate with a transpapillary stent placement is very high (>90%) if the leak can be traversed with a transpapillary stent or if observed from the pancreatic tail. The resolution rate is lower when there is complete pancreatic duct disruption or disconnection. Surgical treatment via resection or creation of a pancreaticojejunostomy to the disconnected segment of pancreas is required when medical and endoscopic interventions have failed.

30. **How is pancreatic ascites or pancreatic pleural effusion diagnosed?**
There needs to be a high index of clinical suspicion. The diagnosis is made by examining the fluid obtained from the paracentesis or thoracentesis, which typically has an elevated concentration of amylase (normal amylase level <150 IU/L, but it is usually >1000 IU/L), lipase, and albumin more than 3 g/dL. The serum-albumin ascites gradient is less than 1.1 g/dL. Treatment of the ascites or pleural effusion is palliative (paracentesis or thoracentesis, sometimes with the placement of an indwelling catheter) until control of the pancreatic duct leak can be achieved.

31. **How can CP lead to portal hypertension and gastric varices?**
The splenic vein travels above the body and tail of the pancreas. Chronic inflammation with CP may lead to splenic vein thrombosis in approximately 12% of patients. Splenic vein thrombosis leads to intrasplenic venous hypertension, splenomegaly, and collateral formation of gastric varices through the short gastric veins. Although massive gastrointestinal bleeding can occur from gastric varices caused by CP, it is an uncommon occurrence. Splenectomy is the treatment of choice if bleeding persists, although splenic artery embolization and splenic vein stenting can be attempted in selected cases.

32. **Are signs of fat-soluble vitamin deficiencies highly suggestive of CP?**
No. Although absorption of fat-soluble vitamins (A, D, E, and K) is decreased in CP, clinical manifestations of deficiency of these vitamins are uncommon. However, longstanding CP may be associated with vitamin D deficiency and other fat-soluble vitamin deficiencies. One should also consider the concomitant presence of small intestinal bacterial overgrowth, which can result in vitamin deficiencies.

33. Do patients with CP have increased risk for osteoporosis?

Yes, patients with CP are at increased risk for both osteopenia and osteoporosis. The pathogenesis of bone loss is likely multifactorial and related to the proinflammatory state in pancreatitis, malabsorption (vitamin D deficiency), alcohol and tobacco use, and opioid use. Periodic assessment of bone health is advised in patients with CP, though there is a lack of evidence-based guidelines for monitoring bone health.

34. Can patients with CP develop vitamin B_{12} malabsorption?

Yes. Pancreatic proteases usually destroy cobalamin-binding proteins and allow the B_{12} to bind to the intrinsic factor. In pancreatic insufficiency, vitamin B_{12}, instead of binding to intrinsic factor, competitively binds to the cobalamin-binding protein, which decreases the absorption of the vitamin in the terminal ileum. Vitamin B_{12} malabsorption can occur in 40% of the patients with CP because of the lack of pancreatic proteases. The treatment of choice is pancreatic enzyme supplementation.

35. How is steatorrhea from CP treated?

Steatorrhea occurs when less than 10% of the exocrine pancreas is functional. The main therapeutic modality in the treatment of steatorrhea is pancreatic enzyme replacement.

Pancreatic enzyme replacement consists of lipase to prevent fat malabsorption and other pancreatic enzymes to treat malassimilation. In a standard-size adult the initial starting dose is approximately 36,000 IU of pancrelipase during each meal. It is recommended to take the capsules after 1–2 bites into the meal, in order to ensure adequate mixing with the chyme as it enters the duodenum. Pancreatic enzymes tend to be inactivated by acid. They are available in two forms: nonenteric (easily inactivated by gastric acid, appropriate for achlorhydric and Billroth II patients) and enteric-coated form, which improves effectiveness in the presence of gastric acid. However, lipase is only released from coated spheres once the pH is higher than 5, which occurs in distal segments of the gut in some patients with exocrine pancreatic insufficiency. Therefore proton-pump inhibitors should be given concomitantly. If patients are on adequate dosing for enzyme replacement therapy and still symptomatic, it is important to rule out other nonpancreatic etiologies for diarrhea, including small intestinal bacterial overgrowth.

There are limited data supporting the use of specific diet regimens in the setting of CP. Medium-chain triglycerides, which do not require lipase for absorption, may be given as a supplement. Very-low-fat diets should be avoided since this may result in inadvertent nutritional deficiencies; appropriate use of pancreatic enzyme replacement therapy should allow for at least a modest amount of fat intake.

36. What are nonsurgical modalities for pain control in CP?

Abdominal pain is the most common symptom of CP. It is important to initially consider lifestyle modifications such as alcohol and smoking cessation; small, low-fat meals; and the use of nonopioid analgesics such as amitriptyline and pregabalin. In the case that these measures do not work, a step-up approach is usually needed.

With persistent abdominal pain, the approach can be dichotomized between medical treatment and surgical treatment.

Medical treatment for persistent pain includes the following:
- Pancreatic enzyme replacement therapy has been suggested to decrease abdominal pain by blocking cholecystokinin receptors and diminishing the stimulation of the pancreas. There are no conclusive trial data to support its use for pain relief in CP; however, it may improve abdominal distention and diarrhea associated with malassimilation.
- Antioxidant regimens (combination of beta-carotene, vitamin C, vitamin E, selenium, and methionine) do not have a consistent impact on chronic pain, although selected individuals appear to derive a benefit. Given their low risk, such a regimen could be attempted in selected individuals.
- Neuromodulators, particularly pregabalin, provide pain relief in CP. Potential associations between pain experience and psychiatric disease also give credence to neuromodulators as potential adjunctive therapy in CP.
- Opioid analgesics may be needed in patients with inadequate control with previous measures; however, opioid dependence is a significant risk if pain persists.
- Celiac plexus blockage by alcohol or steroids has limited long-term effectiveness in decreasing pain, lasting 3–6 months. However, it may decrease the need for oral opioids. Short-term side effects include postural hypotension and diarrhea.

37. Does endoscopy have a role in pain control in CP?

Endoscopy is designed to treat pancreatic duct obstruction, under the premise that pancreatic duct hypertension is causing pain. Therefore ERCP is typically offered to patients with CP who have a main pancreatic duct stone or stricture, typically defined by a dilated (≥ 6 mm) pancreatic duct upstream. No randomized study with adequate statistical power has confirmed the effectiveness of endoscopic management of CP pain. Some small studies have shown that endoscopic sphincterotomy with pancreatic stricture dilation and pancreatic duct stent placement relieves recurrent pain associated with CP, although response rates are typically 30%–50% and with limited durability for many. Other studies have shown pain improvement after the removal of pancreatic stones with the combination of pancreatic duct sphincterotomy, extracorporeal lithotripsy, and stone extraction.

38. **What is the role of surgery in pain control in CP?**

The role of surgery is reserved for those patients with persistent pain despite medical treatment. Surgery may be offered to drain an obstructed pancreatic duct—similar to endoscopic approaches—and also to resect areas suspicious of malignancy or chronic inflammation. Pain relief is superior to endoscopic approaches, although response rates still vary from 50% to 80% likely due to the chronification of pain that occurs prior to the intervention (e.g., central pain sensitization) and from residual disease remaining in the unresected pancreas.

Several surgical modalities are commonly used:

- Lateral pancreatojejunostomy (modified Puestow procedure) is preferred in patients with distal duct obstruction in the head of the pancreas.
- Pancreatoduodenectomy with pylorus preservation or with antrectomy Whipple procedure is used in patients with pancreatic head-predominant disease, especially when occult malignancy is suspected.
- Duodenum-preserving pancreatic head resection has similar indications as the Whipple procedure, though may be combined with a lateral pancreaticojejunostomy when the pancreatic duct appears obstructed.
- Distal pancreatectomy is preferred for patients with localized small-duct disease usually in the tail of the pancreas; this intervention has lower morbidity compared to pancreatic head surgeries.

Multiple studies have shown that organ-preserving surgeries are better in achieving pain control, likely because of less-extensive (advanced) disease, but there is no change between procedures regarding the preservation of endocrine and exocrine function. Despite surgery, the progression of pancreatitis continues. Several studies have shown that surgery is superior to endoscopic therapy for pain relief, though in practice surgery is often pursued once endoscopic treatments have failed.

39. **What is the role of total pancreatectomy with islet autotransplantation (TPIAT) in CP?**

TPIAT is indicated for debilitating pain secondary to CP. It has been shown to decrease pancreatic pain and opioid use in patients with CP, as well as improve quality of life. However, this procedure results in a very high rate of insulin-dependent diabetes and does not guarantee pain relief, especially when this intervention is deferred to late in the disease course. Most referral centers reserve TPIAT for patients who are poor candidates for partial pancreatic surgical interventions (e.g., small-duct CP), although the landscape is changing as more longitudinal data on the safety and efficacy of TPIAT become available.

CLINICAL VIGNETTE

Available Online

BIBLIOGRAPHY

Available Online

CHAPTER 38

PANCREATIC CANCER

Shajan Peter, MD, Ji Young Bang, MD, MPH and Shyam Varadarajulu, MD

 Additional content available online

1. **How common is pancreatic cancer (PC)?**
   The global annual incidence rate of PC is approximately 8 per 100,000 persons per year. In the United States, of an estimated 62,210 people who are diagnosed with PC annually, approximately 49,830 people die from disease progression. The lifetime risk of developing PC is 1.47% (1 in 64 in men and women), and it is the fourth most common cause of cancer-related deaths after lung, prostate, and colorectal cancer. The incidence is rising at the rate of 0.5%–1% per year and it is predicted to be the second leading cause of cancer death by 2030.

2. **What are the most common types of pancreatic neoplasms?**
   Adenocarcinoma is the most common type of pancreatic neoplasm with almost 90% arising from the ductal epithelium (pancreatic ductal adenocarcinoma [PDAC]). Less common histologic variants of PDAC, which usually present in a similar fashion, include acinar cell adenocarcinoma, adenosquamous carcinoma, and cystadenocarcinoma (serous and mucinous types). The remaining pancreatic neoplasms consist of neuroendocrine tumors and lymphomas.

3. **Where are the cancers located in the pancreas?**
   Sixty to seventy percent of cancers are localized to the head, 5%–10% in the body, and 10%–15% in the tail of the pancreas (Fig. 38.1). The size of cancer in the head ranges from 2.5 to 3.5 cm compared with 5–7 cm for those located in the body and tail.

4. **What are the clinical presentations of PC?**
   Jaundice caused by biliary obstruction is the most common (>50%) presentation among patients with pancreatic head cancer (Table 38.1). Jaundice and/or pruritus may not develop or be a late presentation in cancer located in the body or tail of the pancreas. It also could indicate advanced metastatic disease to the liver. Abdominal pain localized to the upper abdomen or mid- and upper back can be a major symptom and could point to invasion of the celiac or superior mesenteric arteries. Other common reported symptoms such as nausea, weight loss, anorexia, fatigue, and dyspepsia can be seen. New-onset type 2 diabetes mellitus (NOD) or presentation with acute pancreatitis should call attention to PC. Pancreatic exocrine insufficiency caused by ductal obstruction can result in malabsorption with the complaint being diarrhea and/or malodorous, greasy stools. Advanced tumor involvement of the duodenum can result in gastric outlet obstruction. Less common manifestations include panniculitis and depression.

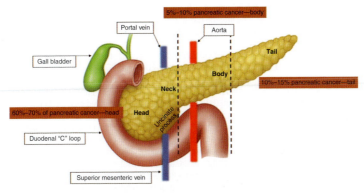

Fig. 38.1 Distribution and location of pancreatic cancer. Tumors of the head of the pancreas are those arising to the right of the superior mesenteric-portal vein confluence. Tumors of the body of the pancreas are defined as those arising between the left edge of the superior mesenteric-portal vein confluence and the left edge of the aorta. Tumors of the tail of the pancreas are those arising to the left of the left edge of the aorta.

Table 38.1 Clinical Presentations in Pancreatic Cancer.

SYMPTOM	PERCENTAGE
Abdominal pain	78–82
Anorexia and early satiety	62–64
Jaundice	56–80
Weight loss	66–84
Diabetes	97
Back pain	48

5. **What are the named clinical signs in PC?**
Courvoisier sign is a palpable, distended, gallbladder in the right upper quadrant in a patient with jaundice resulting from bile duct obstruction secondary to PC. However, this finding is not specific to PC. Patients with distal cholangiocarcinoma or an ampullary mass may present similarly. Trousseau syndrome is a manifestation of PC as superficial or deep vein thrombosis.

6. **What are the identifiable risk factors for PC?**
Smoking is definitely linked to PC, with current smokers having an odds ratio (OR) of 2.2 compared with nonsmokers for developing PC. This OR decreases to 1.2 for ex-smokers and the risk becomes equivalent to that of nonsmokers 10–20 years after smoking cessation. There is some evidence that dietary factors such as consumption of red or processed meat, especially when cooked at high temperatures, and dairy products increase the risk of PC. In addition, contrary to previous thought, there seems to be no protective effect from the consumption of fresh fruits and vegetables or coffee. Alcohol intake (>6 drinks per day) can be an independent increased risk factor for the development of PC by 1.6-fold compared to nondrinking controls. Obesity (body mass index >30 kg/m^2) is associated with an OR of 1.72 and is an independent risk factor for developing PC.

7. **What is the association between diabetes and PC?**
Patients with long-standing diabetes (>3 years) have a 1.5- to 2.4-fold increased risk of developing PC. In addition, gestational diabetes poses a risk for developing PC in later life. On the other hand, the risk of PC is high with NOD (five- to eightfold), suggesting a bidirectional association. Approximately 1% or less of patients with NOD develop PDAC within 3 years. There is also growing evidence that PC can cause paraneoplastic diabetes mellitus or glucose intolerance and this can manifest a few months to 2–3 years prior to the clinical presentation of PC. Diabetes improves after surgical resection of PC. Interestingly, oral hypoglycemic agents such as metformin appear to have a protective relationship.

8. **Is there a risk for developing PC in patients with chronic pancreatitis?**
The pooled relative risk for developing PC among patients with chronic pancreatitis is 13.3 and is estimated to be approximately 2% per decade. The lifetime risk of developing PC in patients with hereditary pancreatitis (autosomal dominant mutation of trypsinogen) is 40%–55%.

9. **What is the association of PC with inherited cancer syndromes?**
Although identification of more than one first-degree relative (FDR) with PC carries a substantial risk for the development of PC, the precise genetic link remains unknown. There is a twofold increased risk in individuals with a single-family member and a sevenfold increase in individuals with multiple family members with PC when compared with the general population. Germline mutations are associated with an increased risk for PC; in particular, *BRAC2* gene mutations account for the highest proportion of known cases among inherited cancer syndromes. Hereditary pancreatitis and the tryptase enzymatic defect carry a potent risk for pancreatic neoplasia by age 70 years in greater than 40% of cases. Peutz-Jeghers syndrome (PJS) is an autosomal dominant polyposis syndrome, in which hamartomatous polyps are found throughout the gastrointestinal tract, but neoplasia risk is greatest outside the gastrointestinal lumen (i.e., in the thyroid, breast, gonads, and especially the pancreas). The familial atypical multiple mole melanoma syndrome is characterized by greater than 50 dysplastic nevi and malignant melanomas in two or more FDRs or second-degree relatives. Other conditions associated with increased risk for PC are listed in Table 38.2.

10. **What are the available serum markers for early detection of PC?**
There is no single marker that has been shown to be ideal for the detection of PC. Carbohydrate antigen (CA 19-9) has been widely used. Using a cutoff of 37 U/mL, the sensitivity and specificity for detection of PC are 86%

Table 38.2 Association Between Pancreatic Cancer and Inherited Syndromes.

ASSOCIATED DISEASE	GENETIC ABNORMALITY	RELATIVE RISK	RISK BY 70 YEARS OF AGE (%)
No history	None	1	0.5
One FDR with PC	?	2.3	1.15
Three FDRs with PC	?	32	16
Familial pancreatic cancer	*BRACA2*, *PALB2*, and *ATM*	2 FDR: 6.4 >3 FDR: 32	2 FDR: 8–12 >3 FDR: 16–38
Peutz-Jeghers syndrome	*STK11/LKB1*	132	36
FAMMM	*CDKN2A/CDK4/P16* Leiden variant	20–34	17
Li-Fraumeni syndrome	*TP53*	2	<5
Hereditary breast-ovarian syndrome	*BRAC1* and *BRAC2*	2 3.5–10	1 5
Hereditary chronic pancreatitis	*PRSS1* and *SPHINK1*	50–80	25–40
Cystic fibrosis	*CFTR*	5.3	<5
Hereditary nonpolyposis syndrome	*hMSH2*, *hMLH1*, and *hPMS1*	1.3	<5
Familial adenomatous polyposis	*APC*	4.6	<5

FAMMM, Familial atypical multiple mole melanoma; *FDR*, first-degree relative; *PC*, pancreatic cancer.

Table 38.3 Tumor Markers in Pancreatic Cancer.

SERUM MARKER	SENSITIVITY (%)	SPECIFICITY (%)
CA 19-9	70–90	90
CEA	16–92	49–93
CA 50	65–90	58–73
CA 125	45–60	76–86
TIMP-1	60–99	50–90

CA, Carbohydrate antigen; *CEA*, carcinoembryonic antigen; *TIMP-1*, tissue metalloprotease 1.

and 87%, respectively, and this increases to 97% and 98% at levels of more than 200 U/mL. Levels of more than 1000 U/mL can be associated with advanced disease. CA 19-9 elevation can also be false positive in the setting of biliary infection (cholangitis), inflammation, or benign obstruction. In addition, CA 19-9 will be undetectable in Lewis antigen-negative individuals. CA 19-9 may be useful as an independent prognostic factor for survival and in monitoring the treatment response. Few other markers are being studied with varying accuracy such as investigational blood-based biomarkers, including circulating tumor DNA and circulating cell-free DNA or exosomes and circulating tumor cells which may be useful for monitoring treatment response and evaluating therapy resistance (Table 38.3).

11. What are the precursors to PC?

There are three known precursors to PC: intraductal papillary mucinous neoplasms (IPMNs), mucinous cystic neoplasms (MCNs), and pancreatic intraepithelial neoplasms (PanINs) (Table 38.4). Majority of PDACs arise from

Table 38.4 Common Features of Pancreatic Precursor Lesions for Pancreatic Cancer.

TYPE OF PRECURSOR LESION	AGE (YEARS)	SEX	CYST-TO-DUCT COMMUNICA-TION	CYST SIZE (CM)	LOCATION	CEA (%)	MUCIN FROM AMPUL-LA	MULTI-FOCAL (%)	RISK OF MALIGNANCY (%)
MCN	40–50	Female > male	Usually not connected	1–3	Body and tail of pancreas	↑80	No	Rare	18
IPMN	60s	Male = female	Connected to MD or BD	<1	Head > tail of pancreas	↑80	Yes	20–30	65 (MD) 40 (BD)
PanIN	↑ With age	Male = female	N/A	Microscopic	Head > tail of pancreas	N/A	No	Often	High grade: unknown Low grade <1

BD, Branch duct; *CEA*, carcinoembryonic antigen; *IPMN*, intraductal papillary mucinous neoplasm; *MCN*, mucinous cyst neoplasm; *MD*, main duct; *N/A*, not available; *PanIN*, pancreatic intraepithelial neoplasia.

pancreatic intraepithelial neoplasia, which progresses through the acquisition of genetic alterations and eventually results in the development of overt PDAC. They are more common in patients with a strong family history of PC. These lesions can cause small-duct obstruction resulting in multifocal atrophy of the pancreas. Computed tomography (CT) scan and endoscopic ultrasound (EUS) are both complementary modalities for diagnosing these lesions. However, imaging, cytologic examination, and serologic examination are limited in their ability to accurately predict the malignant potential, and therefore frequent screening is important. Generally, MCNs are managed by resection and are examined for foci of invasive cancer that portend a poor prognosis. Main-duct IPMN (ductal diameter of ≥10 mm) in young patients or those with high-risk imaging features such as mural nodules, focal masses, or a large unilocular cystic component should be resected.

12. What are the molecular changes that occur in pancreatic intraepithelial neoplasia and progression to PC?

Low-grade pancreatic intraepithelial neoplasias (PanIN 1A and 1B) are characterized by point mutations in the *KRAS* oncogene (found in approximately 90% of PDAC). Grade 2 (PanIN 2) lesions are associated with inactivation of two cyclin-dependent kinase inhibitors, *CDKN2A* (and its encoded protein p16) and *CDKN1A* (and its encoded protein p21). Molecular changes in the later stages of carcinogenesis, representing high-grade pancreatic intraepithelial neoplasias (PanIN 3) include mutations in the critical tumor suppressor gene *TP53* (50%–70% of PDACs), as well as inactivating mutations in *SMAD4* (60%–90%) (Fig. 38.2).

13. What are the common biochemical abnormalities in patients with PC?

Patients with biliary obstruction or metastatic disease can present with elevated serum bilirubin and alkaline phosphatase. Raised white blood cell count and transaminitis can be seen in patients with cholangitis. Serum amylase or lipase is elevated in only 5% of patients as pancreatitis can be an initial presentation. Hyperglycemia is observed in patients with NOD.

14. What imaging modalities are used to diagnose PC?

Transabdominal ultrasound has a sensitivity of 70% for the detection of tumors and has a limited role in diagnosis. The overall sensitivity of multidetector CT (MDCT) for PC is 86%–97% for tumors of any size, but sensitivity of only 77% for smaller (<2 cm) lesions (Fig. 38.3). The recommended dual-phase pancreatic CT protocol includes submillimeter slice thickness, proper timing of arterial and venous imaging, and three-dimensional reconstruction for full vascular assessment (Fig. 38.4). The sensitivity of magnetic resonance imaging (MRI) and integrated positron emission tomogram (PET)-CT is 84% and 73.7%, respectively. These modalities are useful when a CT scan is contraindicated and in determining indeterminate liver lesions. While endoscopic retrograde cholangiopancreatogram (ERCP) with biliary brushings has a low diagnostic yield of 25%–60%, the diagnostic accuracy of EUS-guided fine-needle aspiration () exceeds 85%–90% and is particularly useful for small isodense

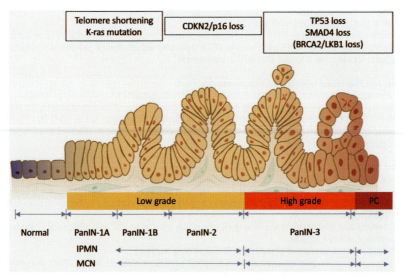

Fig. 38.2 Molecular progression to pancreatic cancer from precursor lesions. *IPMN,* Intraductal papillary mucinous neoplasm; *MCN,* mucinous neoplasm; *PanIN,* pancreatic intraepithelial neoplasia. (Adapted from Laheru D. Pancreatic cancer. In Goldman, L, Cooney, KA, eds. Goldman-Cecil Medicine. 27th ed. Elsevier Limited; 2023. Copyright © 2020 by Elsevier, Inc.)

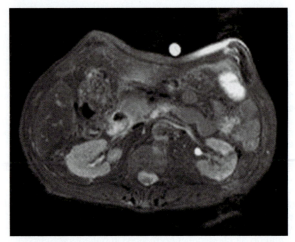

Fig. 38.3 T2-weighted magnetic resonance image with pancreatic head mass.

lesions (Fig. 38.5). Newer imaging modalities such as cholangioscopy, optical coherence tomography, confocal imaging, and contrast-enhanced EUS are still being investigated and could improve the overall diagnostic accuracy.

15. How has EUS influenced the management of patients with PC?

EUS is an important modality for the diagnosis and staging of PC. It is more sensitive than CT for detecting invasion of the portal venous system and its confluence and is inferior to CT for assessing arterial involvement (Fig. 38.6). EUS-FNA of pancreatic tumors has a sensitivity of 85%–90% and specificity of nearly 100%. Tumors smaller than 2 cm are better identified and targeted by EUS. EUS can also be used for the placement of fiducial markers for better targeting of the tumor during radiation therapy and celiac plexus neurolysis for pain relief.

16. What are the histologic features of PDAC on diagnostic EUS-FNA?

Features of PDAC show prominent honeycombing, disorganization, nuclear overlap, and lack of uniform nuclear spacing.

17. What is the double-duct sign in PC?

The double-duct sign, noted on ERCP, demonstrates the presence of stenosis of the distal common bile duct and pancreatic duct in the head of the pancreas (Fig. 38.7). In patients with obstructive jaundice or a pancreatic mass, the double-duct sign has a specificity of 85% in predicting PC.

18. What are the other differential diagnoses for PC?

In the background of chronic pancreatitis, it may be difficult to distinguish PC from chronic pancreatitis. Clinical suspicion and imaging with tissue sampling may enable this differentiation. Autoimmune pancreatitis (AIP) can mimic PC, presenting with similar clinical features such as jaundice, weight loss, and elevated CA 19-9 levels. A finding of increased serum immunoglobulin (IgG4) levels with diffuse pancreatic involvement on CT is supportive of a diagnosis of AIP.

19. What high-risk groups may benefit from screening?

Population-based screening for PC is not currently beneficial due to its relatively low incidence in the United States (3% of new cancers). The CAPS Consortium (International Cancer of the Pancreas Screening Consortium) recommends EUS and/or MRI and magnetic resonance cholangiopancreatography for screening high-risk individuals, who are defined as:

- Individuals who have at least one FDR with PC who in turn also has an FDR with PC (familial PC kindred).
- Carriers of *CDKN2A* variants.
- Patients with PJS (carriers of a germline *LKB1/STK11* gene mutation).
- Patients with known germline variants in *BRCA1, BRCA2, PALB2, ATM, MLH1, MSH2, MSH6*, and one or more affected FDR.

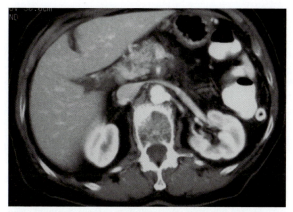

Fig. 38.4 Multidetector computed tomography scan with pancreatic mass encasing the celiac artery.

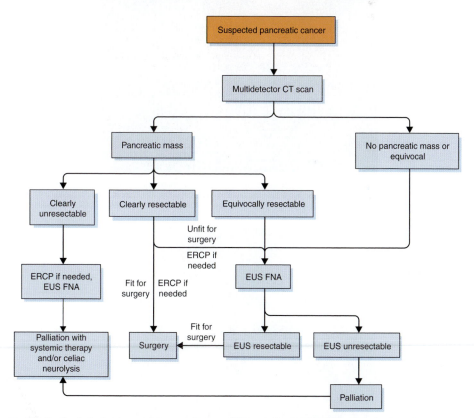

Fig. 38.5 Algorithm for treatment approach to pancreatic cancer. *CT*, Computed tomography; *ERCP*, endoscopic retrograde cholangiopancreatography; *EUS*, endoscopic ultrasound; *FNA*, fine-needle aspiration. (Adapted with permission from Bang JY, Rosch T. EUS and pancreatic tumors. In Varadarajulu, S, Fockens, P, Hawes, RH, eds. Endosonography [E-Book]. Netherlands: Elsevier Health Sciences; 2022.)

20. How is PC staged?

Accurate staging of PC is important, as only 20% of patients are resectable at the time of diagnosis. The American Joint Committee on Cancer staging is the most commonly used system and is based on tumor-node-metastasis staging (Table 38.5). Tumors are classified as resectable, borderline resectable, locally advanced, or unresectable disease.

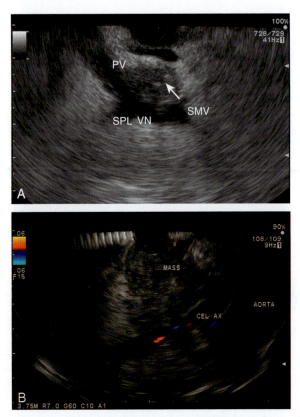

Fig. 38.6 (A) Hypoechoic mass in the head of the pancreas measuring 3 × 2 cm and invading the confluence of the portal vein. Endoscopic ultrasound–guided fine-needle aspiration of the mass revealed adenocarcinoma. (B) Advanced hypoechoic mass in the pancreatic head with celiac artery invasion. *CA*, Celiac artery; *PV*, portal vein; *SMV*, superior mesenteric vein; *SPL VN*, splenic vein.

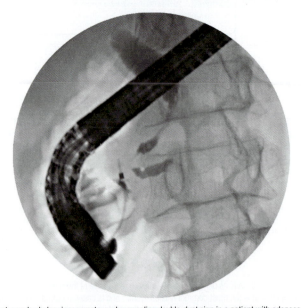

Fig. 38.7 Endoscopic retrograde cholangiopancreatography revealing double-duct sign in a patient with adenocarcinoma.

- "**Curative**" Localized Pancreatic Cancer
  - Resectable (10-15% of newly diagnosed)
    - No vascular involvement
    - Surgical resection → 6 months of postoperative chemotherapy
  - Borderline Resectable (30-35% of newly diagnosed)
    - No vascular involvement
    - Neoadjuvant systemic chemotherapy; surgery for resectable patients; radiation for unresectable patients without distant metastasis
- **Palliative** Advanced Pancreatic Cancer
  - Locally Advanced (30–35% of newly diagnosed)
    - Vascular involvement Encased or > 180 degrees.
    - Neoadjuvant systemic chemotherapy; surgery for resectable patients; radiation for unresectable patients without distant metastasis
  - Metastatic (50–55% of newly diagnosed)
    - Pain control
    - Systemic chemotherapy

21. **What are the staging modalities for PC?**
    The most commonly used modality for the diagnosis and staging of PC is MDCT, which has a high positive predictive value for unresectability. However, MDCT has a lower sensitivity of 25%–50% for predicting

Table 38.5 American Joint Committee on Cancer Classification for Pancreatic Cancer (Eighth Edition).

PRIMARY TUMOR (T)	
TX	Primary tumor cannot be assessed
T0	No evidence of primary tumor
Tis	Carcinoma in situ[a]
T1	Tumor limited to the pancreas, 2 cm or less in greatest dimension T1a: Tumor $\leq$0.5 cm in greatest dimension T1b: Tumor >0.5 cm and <1 cm in greatest dimension T1c: Tumor 1–2 cm in greatest dimension
T2	Tumor limited to the pancreas >2 cm and $\leq$4 cm in greatest dimension
T3	Tumor >4 cm in greatest dimension
T4	Tumor involves the celiac axis or the superior mesenteric artery (unresectable primary tumor)
Regional Lym ph Nodes (N)	
NX	Regional lymph nodes cannot be assessed
N0	No regional lymph node metastasis
N1	Regional lymph node metastasis
Distant Metastasis (M)	
M0	No distant metastasis
M1	Distant metastasis

Stage Grouping
Stage 0 Tis N0 M0: Localized within pancreas
Stage IA T1 N0 M0: Localized within pancreas
Stage IB T2 N0 M0: Localized within pancreas
Stage IIA T3 N0 M0: Locally invasive, resectable
Stage IIB T1, 2, or 3 N1 M0: Locally invasive, resectable
Stage III T4 Any N M0: Locally advanced, unresectable
Stage IV Any T Any N M1: Distant metastases

[a]This includes high-grade pancreatic intraepithelial neoplasia (PanIN-3), intraductal papillary 14/20 mucinous neoplasm with high-grade dysplasia, intraductal tubulopapillary neoplasm with highgrade dysplasia, and mucinous cystic neoplasm with high-grade dysplasia.

resectability. Newer three-dimensional CT imaging techniques are very accurate in detecting vascular invasion: celiac axis (CA), superior mesenteric artery (SMA), and common hepatic artery involvement. The use of MRI or fluorodeoxyglucose–PET-CT scanning may help identify smaller lesions missed on CT. Similarly, EUS is not only helpful in identifying smaller lesions but vital in procuring tissue and therefore is a complementary technique. Because there is a 5%–15% chance that occult metastases will be missed by CT imaging, diagnostic laparoscopy (not done routinely) can help identify these implants (e.g., peritoneal, capsular, or serosal).

22. What are the CT features of unresectability?
PC is deemed unresectable when features of tumor invasion are present such as absence of fat planes in the SMA territory; involvement of the inferior vena cava, aorta, or celiac artery; 180-degree or more of circumferential encasement or occlusion of the SMV–portal venous system; or if distant metastases (e.g., involvement of solid organs or lymph nodes outside the resection zone and peritoneum) are present.

23. Is chemotherapy effective for patients with PC?
Traditional chemotherapy with 5-fluorouracil (5-FU) and folinic acid has an overall response rate of less than 10% with no effect on quality of life or survival. Gemcitabine is preferred to 5-FU because of its favorable toxicity profile, although the overall outcomes are similar. Modified FOLFIRINOX (fluorouracil, irinotecan, leucovorin, and oxaliplatin) is the adjuvant first-line chemotherapy of choice in patients with resectable PC with an anticipated median overall survival of 54.4 months, compared with 35 months for single-agent gemcitabine. For advanced or metastatic disease, multiagent chemotherapy regimens, including FOLFIRINOX, gemcitabine plus albumin-bound (nab)-paclitaxel, and nanoliposomal irinotecan/fluorouracil, all have a survival benefit of 2–6 months compared with a single-agent gemcitabine.

24. Are there specific targetable subtypes or PC for therapy?
Ten to fifteen percent of subtypes of PC have inherited mutations and are potentially susceptible to targeted therapies and therefore are associated with their genetic alterations. For patients with a *BRCA* pathogenic germline variant and metastatic PC, olaparib, a poly(adenosine diphosphate [ADB]-ribose) polymerase inhibitor is a maintenance option that improves progression-free survival following initial platinum-based therapy. PC defective in DNA mismatch repair (MSI) such as Lynch syndrome has been found to be less responsive to 5-FU and gemcitabine and more responsive to FOLFIRINOX. Immune agents such as pembrolizumab, an inhibitor of the immune checkpoint protein PD-1 (programmed cell death protein-1), have been approved for MSI-deficient cancers. Current recommendations advocate testing of all patients diagnosed with PC for germline mutations for high-risk inherited susceptibility genes.

25. What is the median survival after the diagnosis of advanced PC?
PC is associated with a 5-year survival rate of less than 5% and a median survival time of 6 months from the time of diagnosis. Surgical resection is the only curative treatment for PC. However, only 15%–20% of patients are potentially resectable at the time of diagnosis. After surgical resection, median survival is increased by 25–30 months, and when combined with adjuvant chemotherapy, 5-year survival of more than 20% may be achieved. However, the median survival for patients with unresectable PC of head and body is less than 1 year and for those with the involvement of the pancreatic tail, the survival is less than 3 months.

26. What are the poor prognostic factors of PC?
Poor prognostic factors include presentation at a later stage, R1 resection (grossly negative but microscopically positive margins of resection), perineural or vascular invasion, poor performance status, low serum albumin, liver metastases, and elevated CA 19-9 levels. Poor molecular prognostic factors include mutated tumor suppressor genes such as *SMAD4* and *TP53*.

27. What is the surgical procedure adopted for cancer in the body and tail of the pancreas?
Distal pancreatectomy is the procedure of choice for PC in the body and tail; the pancreas is resected from the left of the superior mesenteric vessels. A splenectomy is also conventionally performed.

28. Is there a role for neoadjuvant therapy?
There is no definitive role for neoadjuvant therapy (chemotherapy and/or radiotherapy) in resectable PC. Several ongoing trials comparing surgery-first versus neoadjuvant therapy to determine potential usefulness are being done for this category. A recent meta-analysis showed that preoperative chemoradiation therapy might be beneficial for those patients with borderline resectable or locally advanced unresectable tumors and that downstaging enables resection in up to 30% of patients or improves margin negative resection rates.

29. Is there a role for routine preoperative endoscopic drainage for malignant biliary obstruction?
Currently, there is no evidence to suggest that routine preoperative biliary drainage improves surgical outcomes. It may, however, be reserved for resectable patients with jaundice and significant delay in surgery, those presenting

with acute cholangitis, or borderline resectable patients undergoing neoadjuvant chemoradiation therapy. Metal stents are preferable and if the diagnosis is uncertain or rapid onsite evaluation of EUS-guided FNA/fine-needle biopsy is not available, placing a fully covered metal stent that is easily removable may be considered.

30. What are the endoscopic therapeutic strategies in PC?

Endoscopic biliary stent placement for obstructive jaundice remains the main method of biliary drainage in patients with unresectable PC. Placements of self-expanding metal stents are preferred over plastic stents in patients with longer life expectancy. EUS-guided biliary drainage is an alternative to traditional transpapillary drainage and may be used as a salvage technique after failed ERCP. In patients with gastroduodenal obstruction by a large pancreatic mass, endoscopic placement of an expandable enteral stent bypassing the stricture relieves the obstruction. EUS-guided celiac plexus neurolysis is done to relieve existing pain and also delay onset of pain in asymptomatic patients. This is done by injection of a combination of local anesthetic (e.g., bupivacaine) and highly concentrated alcohol (50%) at the level of the CA. Pain reduction can be expected in 60%–75% of patients within 2 weeks of the procedure.

31. What are other palliative considerations in PC?

As described previously, management for PC requires a multidisciplinary approach including supportive care. Endoscopy helps in palliation of obstructive jaundice, intractable pruritus, treatment of cholangitis, and relieving duodenal obstruction. If endoscopic treatment is not possible, percutaneous transhepatic biliary drainage catheter or stent placement can be performed by an interventional radiologist. If both modalities fail, surgical bypass, such as cholecystojejunostomy or hepaticojejunostomy for biliary drainage or gastrojejunostomy for duodenal obstruction, may be indicated. Other considerations include conventional management of pain using narcotics, treatment of malabsorption or steatorrhea with pancreatic enzyme supplements, nutritional support treatment of hyperglycemia using oral hypoglycemic medications or insulin, and advanced care planning.

BIBLIOGRAPHY

Available Online.

CHAPTER 39

CYSTIC LESIONS OF THE PANCREAS

Robert Moran, MD and Brenda J. Hoffman, MD

 Additional content available online

1. What are pancreatic cystic lesions (PCLs)?

There are two types of PCLs: true pancreatic cysts and pancreatic pseudocysts.

True pancreatic cysts are liquid-filled collection lined by secretory epithelium. Mucinous cysts are lined by ovarian-type stromal cells that secrete mucin. Solid pancreatic neoplasms may contain internal cystic components as seen in pancreatic neuroendocrine tumors and adenocarcinoma. True pancreatic cysts are more commonly referred to pancreatic cystic neoplasms (PCNs).

Pancreatic pseudocysts are fluid-filled collections encapsulated by an inflammatory wall resulting from pancreatitis. Pseudocysts do *not* have a lining of secretory epithelium and the fluid comprised necrotic debris, blood, and pancreatic juice (amylase) if the cyst communicates with the pancreatic duct (PD).

2. What is the clinical importance of PCLs?

Pancreatic cysts can be malignant, premalignant, benign without risks of malignant transformation, or can be a source of symptoms. The management varies greatly from surgical resection to observation without the need for additional testing.

3. How common are PCLs?

PCLs are an increasingly common incidental finding on body imaging with a prevalence of 2.3% in computed tomography (CT) series and 2.4%–13.5% in magnetic resonance imaging (MRI) series. The improved resolution of multidetector CT and MRI scanners allows for the identification of smaller cysts (<1–2 cm). The malignant potential for some cysts requires that all of these lesions be further evaluated with surveillance imaging, cyst fluid analysis, or surgical resection for histopathologic diagnosis.

4. What is the differential diagnosis for PCLs?

The differential diagnosis for PCLs is broad and includes benign lesions without malignant potential, those with malignant potential, and those that are malignant (Table 39.1). Broadly, mucinous cysts have malignant potential, whereas nonmucinous cysts do not. Ninety percent of PCLs are benign, most of which are pseudocysts.

5. What symptoms are associated with pancreatic cysts?

Abdominal pain is the most common indication for body imaging resulting in the finding of pancreatic cysts. It is likely that the majority of these cysts are asymptomatic and truly incidental findings, especially small cysts (<1–2 cm). Single or multiple cysts in the setting of recent acute pancreatitis or an acute exacerbation of chronic pancreatitis are most likely pseudocysts. Large pseudocysts may present as a palpable abdominal mass or cause gastric outlet obstruction-related symptoms such as nausea, vomiting, and early satiety. Pseudocysts may also become infected leading to fever and leukocytosis. Cysts in the head of the pancreas may cause biliary obstruction from either extrinsic compression or invasion of the extrahepatic bile duct.

6. What are the treatment options for pancreatic cysts?

The management of pancreatic cysts has historically been surgical resection with the location of the lesion dictating the type of surgical intervention. Cysts in the head of the pancreas require a pancreaticoduodenectomy (Whipple procedure). Body or tail locations are removed with a distal pancreatectomy. Some cysts may be amenable to enucleation, which is an organ-preserving approach. Resection allows for the treatment of cyst-related symptoms as well as histopathologic diagnosis. Pancreatic pseudocysts may be surgically resected or drained via surgical, endoscopic, or percutaneous techniques. Cyst ablation is a newer therapy aimed at destroying the epithelial lining in mucinous cysts with alcohol or chemotherapy but is only offered at a few select centers.

7. Define a pancreatic pseudocyst.

A pancreatic pseudocyst is a fluid collection encapsulated by a well-defined wall. An acute pancreatic fluid collection takes at least 4 weeks to mature into a pseudocyst. Most pseudocysts resolve over time; however, when there is communication with the PD, they often enlarge or persist as chronic pseudocyst, causing symptoms such as abdominal fullness or pain, early satiety, and gastric outlet obstruction.

Table 39.1 Criteria for Defining Subtypes of Pancreatic Cystic Lesions (PCLs) Into Benign and Malignant Risk Categories.

TYPE OF PCL	CONNECT TO MAIN PD	IMAGING	FLUID AMYLASE	FLUID CEA	FLUID GLUCOSE	SINGLE OR MULTIPLE	MALIGNANCY POTENTIAL
Benign							
Pseudocyst	±	Circumscribed, EUS/anechoic, pancreatitis	High	Low	–	Either	None
SCN	No	Central scar 30%, honeycomb	Low	Low	–	Single	None
Malignant Risk							
SPN	No	Solid cystic tumor	Low	Low		Single	High
CPNT	No	Peripheral rim enhancement	Low	Low		Single	>2 cm moderate
MCN	No	Peripheral calcification, tail of pancreas Uninoculated or septated	Low	High	Low	Single	≥3 cm high
Main-duct IPMN	Yes	PD ≥10 mm	High	High	Low	Either	Very high
Branch-duct IPMN	Yes	Side branch dilation of PD, Grape-like cystic lesion	High	High	Low	Either	Variable risk features[a]

CA, Carbohydrate antigen; *CEA*, carcinoembryonic antigen; *CPNT*, cystic pancreatic neuroendocrine tumor; *EUS*, endoscopic ultrasound; *IPMN*, intrapancreatic neoplasia; *MCN*, mucinous cystic neoplasm; *PD*, pancreatic duct; *SCN*, serous cystic neoplasm; *SPN*, solid pseudopapillary neoplasm.
[a]Variable risk features: presence of mural nodule or solid component, dilation of the main pancreatic duct, pancreatic cyst size ≥3–4 cm, positive pancreatic cytology, or cyst fluid analysis. Other important risk criteria: cyst growth >5 mm/year, elevated CA 19-9, new-onset diabetes mellitus, and acute pancreatitis due to the cystic lesion.
Adapted from Buerlein RCD, Shami VM. Management of pancreatic cysts and guidelines: what the gastroenterologist needs to know. Ther Adv Gastrointest Endosc. 2021;14:1-21.

8. When do you treat pancreatic pseudocysts?

Pseudocysts that are enlarging, infected, or causing symptoms such as pain or gastric outlet obstruction require drainage. Hemorrhagic pseudocysts are a unique circumstance and may require combined surgical and angiographic treatment because of potential vascular involvement.

9. How are pancreatic pseudocyst(s) treated?

Drainage of the cyst into the gastrointestinal lumen has become the preferred intervention with good technical and clinical success. A cystogastrostomy or cystoduodenostomy is created either endoscopically or surgically. Either technique is effective with local expertise dictating the procedure of choice. Delayed drainage procedures of any method (>4 weeks) are associated with improved outcomes. Magnetic resonance pancreatography or endoscopic retrograde cholangiopancreatography (ERCP) are useful studies in determining if the PD communicates with a pseudocyst. ERCP with transpapillary PD stenting is therapeutic in cases in which there is communication between the pseudocyst and PD as primary or adjunctive therapy to transluminal drainage.

10. **Are all cystic lesions of the pancreas malignant?**
No.
 Both serous cystic neoplasms (SCNs) and pancreatic pseudocysts do not carry a risk for malignancy.

11. **What features of PCNs are worrisome for malignancy?**
 - Presence of mural nodule or solid component
 - Dilation of the main PD $\geq$5–10 mm
 - Pancreatic cyst size $\geq$3–4 cm
 - Positive pancreatic cytology or cyst fluid analysis ($\downarrow$glucose and $\downarrow$amylase)
 - Other important criteria: cyst growth $\geq$3 mm/year, elevated carbohydrate antigen (CA) 19-9, new-onset diabetes mellitus, and acute pancreatitis due to the cystic lesion

12. **How prevalent are PCNs?**
Older studies have demonstrated PCNs to be as low as 2.4% in younger population, while more recent studies have demonstrated PCMs at a rate to 50% among older adults, indicating that PMNs are more common with age. Perhaps the two most relevant and recent population studies conducted on PMNs prevalence using MRI from Germany and the Mayo Clinic documented a prevalence of 49% and 41%, respectively. Despite the high overall prevalence of PMNs, few of these lesions are large. A recent review of over 25,000 patients found that the prevalence of PCNs >2 cm to be only 0.8%.

13. **What are the key criteria for characterizing PCNs?**
 - Imaging characteristics (EUS, CT, and MR): vascularity, solid component, location, size, internal scar, honeycomb appearance, or calcification
 - Continuity with main PD
 - Cyst fluid content: carcinoembryonic antigen (CEA), amylase, and glucose
 - Unifocal versus multifocal
     See Table 39.1.

14. **What is the meaning and value of the string sign association with PCN fluid analysis?**
The string sign is performed by placing a drop of the cyst-aspirated fluid between the fingers or between two glass slides and pulling gently apart. If it creates a string >3.5 mm in length, then this is indicative of a mucinous PCN. Although the string sign is a subjective test, it has a sensitivity of 58%, specificity of 95%, and predictive value of 95%.

15. **What are the characteristics of solid pseudopapillary neoplasms (SPNs) of the pancreas?**
These PCNs are mixed solid and cystic lesions that are lined by monomorphic cuboidal mucosa and have a fibrous pseudocapsule. They are more typically seen in young females in their 20s. Since there is no communication with the main PD, fluids from the SPNs are typically low in amylase. Moderate malignant risk and surgery is usually recommended.

16. **What are the typical characteristics of cystic pancreatic neuroendocrine tumors (CPNTs)?**
These PCNs typically have a rich vascular supply, and a bright well-circumscribed peripheral contrast rim enhancement is characteristic. CPNTs are usually located in the head of the pancreas and exhibit low CEA and amylase levels on cyst aspiration. Most CPNTs are nonfunctional and the minority are associated with multiple neuroendocrine syndrome type I.

17. **What are the characteristics of mucinous cystic neoplasms (MCNs)?**
This type of PCN is lined with functional ovarian-type stromal cells which can produce copious amounts of mucus. MCNs are almost exclusively found in middle-aged females and the vast majority are located in the body of the tail of the pancreas. The amylase content in MCNs is low because there is no communication with the PD. CEA levels can be high due to the columnar lining of the MCNs and lesions $\geq$3 cm in size have a high risk of malignancy.

18. **What is the most common type of PCN?**
 - The intraductal papillary mucinous (IPMN) is the most common type of PCN.
 - IPMNs most commonly occur in the head of the pancreas, can be singular or multifocal, and are most commonly found in the fifth to seventh decades of life.
 - There are three subtypes of IPMN:
   - Main-duct (MD) IPMN
   - Branch-duct IPMN
   - Mixed IPMN

Table 39.2 PCM Monitoring Guidelines for Lesions Without "Worrisome" Signs.[a]

PCN SIZE (CM)	2018 ACG GUIDELINE	2018 EUROPEAN GUIDELINE
1–2	MRI in 1 y	MRI or EUS in 6 mo (along with CA 19-9 level)
2–3 cm	MRI or EUS in 6–12 mo	MRI and/or EUS in 6 mo with CA 19-9 level
3–4 cm	MRI or EUS every 6–12 mo at center of excellence	MRI or EUS in 6 mo with CA 19-9

ACG, American College of Gastroenterology; *CA*, carbohydrate antigen; *EUS*, endoscopic ultrasound; *MRI*, magnetic resonance imaging; *PCN*, pancreatic cystic neoplasm.
[a]The US recommendations are stated by the ACG (2018) and the European Guideline (2018).
Adapted from Elta GH, Enestvedt BK, Sauer BG, Lennon AM. ACG clinical guideline: diagnosis and management of pancreatic cysts. Am J Gastroenterol. 2018;113:464-479. https://doi.org/10.1038/ajg.2018.14. Epub February 27, 2018. PMID: 29485131; European Study Group on Cystic Tumours of the Pancreas. European evidence-based guidelines on pancreatic cystic neoplasms. Gut. 2018;67(5):789-804. https://doi.org/10.1136/gutjnl-2018-316027. Epub March 24, 2018. PMID: 29574408; PMCID: PMC5890653.

19. **When should EUS be considered for the evaluation of a PCN?**
As per the American College of Gastroenterology (ACG) 2018 criteria (EUS if any of the following present):
- IPMN or MCN ≥3 cm
- PD ≥5 mm
- Mural nodule or solid component to the cyst
- Monitored increase in cyst size ≥3 mm/year
- Jaundice or pancreatitis due to cyst
- Monitored increase in PD diameter with upstream duct atrophy

20. **Can IPMNs risk for malignancy be stratified by diagnostic criteria?**
Yes.
    Diagnostic criteria that forecast increased malignant risk include the presence of a mural nodule or solid component, dilation of the main PD >5–10≥ mm, pancreatic cyst size ≥3–4 cm, positive pancreatic cytology, or cyst fluid analysis. Other important risk criteria include cyst growth >3–5 mm/year, elevated CA 19-9, new-onset diabetes mellitus, and acute pancreatitis due to the cystic lesion.

21. **What are the surgical indications for PCN resection?**
- First, the patient must meet the 2018 ACG or 2018 European guideline criteria listed below.
- Second, the patient must be an operative candidate, that is, *reasonable* operative survival and *reasonable* life longevity.
- **2018 ACG guideline:** cytology-positive high-grade dysplasia (HGD) or malignancy, mural nodule, all MD-IPMNs, and concerning features on EUS ± fluid analysis.
- **2018 European guideline:**
  - Absolute indications: Cytology suspicious or positive from malignancy or HGD, enhancing mural nodule >5 mm, PD ≥10 mm, solid component, obstructive jaundice with PCN in the head of the pancreas, and symptoms due to PCN.
  - Relative indications: All PCNs ≥4 cm or PCN growth rate ≥5 mm/year, enhancing mural nodule <5 mm, elevated CA 19-9, PD 5–9.9 mm, new-onset diabetes mellitus, and acute pancreatitis due to PCN.

22. **What are the accepted monitoring recommendations for PCNs that do not exhibit worrisome features of malignancy?**
Most advanced centers of therapeutic endoscopy, oncology, and pancreato-biliary surgery will have a collective multidisciplinary approach employing criteria derived from guidelines listed in Table 39.2.

CLINICAL VIGNETTE

Available Online

BIBLIOGRAPHY

Available Online

CELIAC DISEASE

Isabel A. Hujoel, MD and Rupa Mukherjee, MD

CHAPTER 40

 Additional content available online

1. How does celiac disease (CD) manifest?

CD is a systemic immune-mediated condition in which gluten ingestion leads to enteropathy. CD can be symptomatic at diagnosis or have subclinical disease, where symptoms and signs are absent or minimal. Symptomatic disease can be divided into classical (presence of malabsorption) and nonclassical presentation (absence of malabsorption). Both presentations can have gastrointestinal and extraintestinal symptoms and signs (Table 40.1), with the most common gastrointestinal symptoms being diarrhea, bloating, and aphthous stomatitis. While classical disease used to be the most common manifestation, now nonclassical cases are seen in 40%–60% and subclinical in nearly 30%.

Table 40.1 Extraintestinal Manifestations of Celiac Disease.

COMMON	LESS COMMON
• Osteoporosis	• Dermatitis herpetiformis
• Iron deficiency	• Headaches
• Celiac hepatitis	• Infertility and miscarriages
• Arthralgias	• Recurrent pancreatitis
	• Gluten ataxia

2. Which populations are at risk for CD?

CD has an estimated worldwide prevalence of 1.4% and is most prevalent in Europe and Oceania and least prevalent in South America. It is more common in females and those who are younger. Certain populations have a higher risk of CD (Table 40.2).

Table 40.2 Populations at Higher Risk for Celiac Disease.

RISK POPULATION	PERCENTAGE
First-degree relatives of a person with celiac disease	10–15
Down syndrome	10
IgA deficiency	8
Turner syndrome	6
Type 1 diabetes mellitus	5

IgA, Immunoglobulin A.

3. How is CD diagnosed?

The current recommendation is to test for CD when there is a high clinical suspicion (Fig. 40.1). Serologic tests are used for screening, commonly immunoglobulin (Ig) A tissue transglutaminase (tTG) which has an estimated sensitivity greater than 95%. Due to the higher prevalence of IgA deficiency in CD, IgA levels should be checked, and if low, IgG tTG or deamidated gliadin peptide can be tested. Endomysial antibody has high specificity for CD and is helpful when IgA tTG is equivocal. The gold standard for diagnosis is small bowel biopsies. Gross appearance of the duodenum can be normal or suggestive of CD (Fig. 40.2). Four to six biopsies from the second part of the duodenum and two from the bulb should be taken to increase diagnostic yield. The characteristic pathology includes villous atrophy and increased intraepithelial lymphocytes (Fig. 40.3), but severity of damage

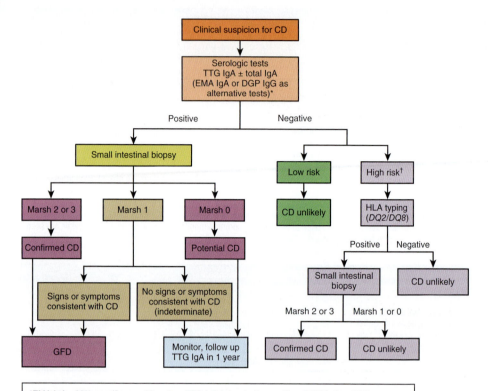

Fig. 40.1 Diagnostic algorithm for celiac disease. *CD*, Celiac disease; *DGP*, deamidated gliadin peptide; *EMA*, endomysial antibody; *GFD*, gluten-free diet; *HLA*, human leukocyte antigen; *Ig*, immunoglobulin; *TTG*, tissue transglutaminase. (From McNally PR. GI/Liver Secrets Plus. 5th ed. Philadelphia, PA: Mosby; 2015 [online color images].)

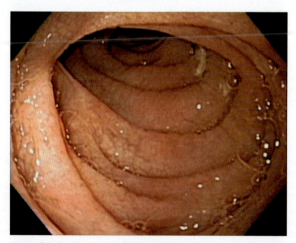

Fig. 40.2 Endoscopic appearance of duodenal mucosa showing characteristic scalloping in celiac disease. (From McNally PR. GI/Liver Secrets Plus. 5th ed. Philadelphia, PA: Mosby; 2015 [online color images].)

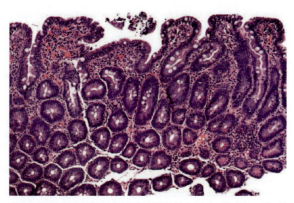

Fig. 40.3 Villous blunting with crypt hyperplasia and increased intraepithelial lymphocytes (tip heavy pattern) in celiac disease. (From McNally PR. GI/Liver Secrets Plus. 5th ed. Philadelphia, PA: Mosby; 2010 and 2015 [online color images].)

can vary and is often described using the Marsh classification. In pediatrics, if serologic titers are high enough, a diagnosis can be made without biopsy; however, in adults, a biopsy is still required for diagnosis.

4. **What are potential complications of CD?**
   - Osteoporosis is a common complication of untreated CD, and people should be screened at diagnosis or 1 year after a gluten-free diet (GFD).
   - Infertility in females can be a complication of undiagnosed CD and improves with a GFD.
   - Untreated CD is associated with mildly elevated aminotransferases that improve on a GFD.
   - Hyposplenism can be seen in untreated CD and may be associated with an increased risk for encapsulated bacterial infections.
   - People with CD have an increased risk for enteropathy-associated T cell lymphoma (EATL) and small bowel carcinoma and appear to have an increased overall cancer risk that resolves with a GFD for some but not all cancers.
   - Untreated CD may be associated with an increased mortality.

5. **How is CD treated? Are there any management options other than a GFD?**
   The only currently available treatment for CD is a lifelong GFD. Access to a dietician with expertise in a GFD is therefore crucial. It is hard to avoid accidental gluten exposure, and this is the leading cause of persistent symptoms in those with CD. In cases of refractory CD (RCD) or celiac crisis, immunosuppressive medications such as corticosteroids (open capsule budesonide or prednisone), mesalamine, or 6-mercaptopurine can be used. There are several ongoing phase II and phase III clinical trials on nondietary therapeutic agents.

6. **What common consequences of GFD do a primary care physician or gastroenterologist need to be aware of?**
   The cornerstone of CD treatment is the GFD. However, GFD has potential inadequacies which can result in constipation, undesirable weight gain, and nutritional deficiencies. As a result, close follow-up with a dietician specializing in CD is an integral part of care, with a focus on healthy food choices, weight maintenance, fiber intake, and nutritional status.
   - Constipation is common, particularly soon after starting GFD. This is often due to the low fiber content of foods used in gluten-free (GF) products. Consequently, initial treatment for constipation should focus on increased dietary fiber and hydration.
   - Another possible consequence of GFD is weight gain and, in some cases, obesity. Body mass index often increases on GFD, especially in those who adhere closely. Multiple factors contribute to weight gain including enhanced intestinal absorption and the hypercaloric content of many GF foods. A few studies have also shown alterations in the lipid panel with a rise in total cholesterol and low-density lipoprotein cholesterol.
   - GF foods often lack B vitamins, iron, and trace minerals, leading to nutritional deficiencies. Patients with CD should be encouraged to eat natural GF foods. Nutritional supplements, including a multivitamin, calcium, and vitamin D, should be recommended for most patients.

7. **How can *suspected* CD be evaluated in patients already on a GFD?**
   Symptom recurrence with gluten exposure or symptom response to a GFD alone cannot be used to diagnose CD. Moreover, celiac serologic testing and intestinal biopsy findings are not reliable to diagnose or exclude CD

in patients already adhering to a GFD given that these tests normalize with sufficient time on a GFD. Celiac gene testing (human leukocyte antigen *DQ2/DQ8*) is recommended if the CD is suspected in someone who is already GF. This has a high negative predictive value (>99%) and can be used to rule out CD. If the gene test is positive for either the *DQ2* or *DQ8* haplotypes, both, or the *DQ2.5* haplotype, the next step is a formal gluten challenge. This involves reintroducing daily gluten (3 g/day or about two slices of bread/day) for several weeks, at least 8 weeks is recommended, followed by an upper endoscopy with multiple duodenal biopsies and repeat celiac serologic testing.

8. What is nonresponsive CD (NRCD) and how is it managed?

Most who are adherent to a GFD have substantial clinical improvement. However, a subset, ranging from 7% to 30%, has NRCD, defined as persistent symptoms, signs, or laboratory abnormalities typical of CD despite a GFD for 6–12 months. The most common cause of NRCD is inadvertent gluten exposure (35%–50% of cases). Other causes include microscopic colitis, irritable bowel syndrome, small intestinal bacterial overgrowth, food intolerances, and RCD. If NRCD is suspected, a systematic approach should be followed to identify the specific cause (Fig. 40.4). It is important to reconfirm the initial diagnosis of CD by reviewing the small intestinal biopsies and confirming serologic findings obtained at diagnosis. Dietary review is also recommended. An endoscopy should be considered if the diagnosis was solely based on serology.

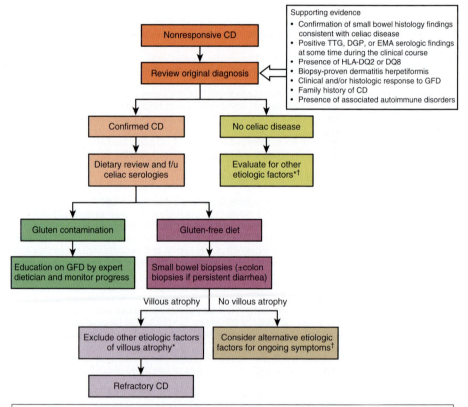

Fig. 40.4 An approach to the investigation of nonresponsive celiac disease. *CD*, Celiac disease; *DGP*, deamidated gliadin peptide; *EMA*, endomysial antibody; *f/u*, follow-up; *GFD*, gluten-free diet; *HLA*, human leukocyte antigen; *SIBO*, small intestinal bacterial overgrowth; *TTG*, tissue transglutaminase. (From McNally PR. GI/Liver Secrets Plus. 5th ed. Philadelphia, PA: Mosby; 2015 [online color images].)

9. **Describe RCD.**

RCD is defined as persistent or recurrent malabsorptive symptoms and villous atrophy despite strict GFD adherence for at least 12 months in the absence of other causes of NRCD and overt malignancy. RCD is a rare condition, affecting around 1%–2% of patients with CD based on case reports from major CD referral centers. RCD affects females more than males, and usually in the fifth decade of life or older. RCD is divided into type I and type II. Type I RCD is more common and has a better overall prognosis. It is characterized by normal intraepithelial lymphocyte phenotype with intact CD3 and CD8 expression, whereas type II RCD is recognized by monoclonal aberrant CD3-positive T-lymphocytes that lack expression of CD8. Treatment for either type includes aggressive nutritional support, budesonide or systemic corticosteroids, and immunosuppressive agents such as azathioprine. Type II RCD is less responsive to treatment and carries a poor prognosis with a high risk for malignant transformation to EATL.

10. **What is the differential diagnosis of villous atrophy of the duodenum or nonceliac enteropathy (NCE)?**

Although a hallmark histopathologic finding in CD, villous atrophy can be seen in various other conditions. NCE refers to the presence of villous atrophy with either negative CD gene testing or negative serology on a gluten-containing diet and lack of histologic response on a GFD. NCE is a rare condition whose clinical symptoms can mimic those of CD. NCEs include the following:

- Autoimmune enteropathy
- Common variable immunodeficiency
- Hypogammaglobulinemia
- Graft-versus-host disease
- Lymphoproliferative diseases: CD4+ indolent lymphomas, EATL (types 1 and 2), and immunoproliferative small intestinal disease
- Chemotherapy
- Radiotherapy
- Infections: Acquired immune deficiency syndrome enteropathy, giardiasis, small intestinal bacterial overgrowth, tuberculosis, Whipple disease, tropical sprue, and *Helicobacter pylori* infection
- Collagenous sprue
- Peptic duodenitis (i.e., Zollinger-Ellison syndrome)
- Crohn disease
- Eosinophilic enteritis
- Drug-induced enteropathy: Angiotensin 2 receptor blockers (e.g., olmesartan), immunosuppressive medications (e.g., methotrexate), and nonsteroidal anti-inflammatory drugs
- Malnutrition

CLINICAL VIGNETTE

Available Online

BIBLIOGRAPHY

Available Online

CHAPTER 41

CROHN'S DISEASE

Mitali Agarwal, MD, Katherine Falloon, MD and Bret A. Lashner, MD

 Additional content available online

DIAGNOSIS

1. **How is Crohn's disease diagnosed?**

   Crohn's disease is an inflammatory disorder that can cause mucosal inflammation in any part of the gastrointestinal (GI) tract, from the mouth to the anus, due to excessive T cell response. Crohn's disease is a clinical diagnosis, that is, the clinician incorporates data from the history and physical, laboratory, endoscopic, histologic, and imaging results to diagnose Crohn's disease. Patients typically experience chronic unexplained diarrhea, abdominal pain, fatigue, fever, weight loss, and growth failure in younger patients. The endoscopic, histologic, and imaging studies usually demonstrate some degree of chronic transmural inflammation of the luminal GI tract. Deep, linear, serpiginous ulcers with discontinuous involvement (skip areas) and strictures, and fistulas may be noted on endoscopy and imaging. Granulomas may be present on biopsy in a minority of patients. Typically, chronic inflammation is noted in pathology. It is the presence of *chronic* inflammation that solidifies the diagnosis of Crohn's disease. Laboratory tests are complementary to the aforementioned studies and aid in assessing the degree of inflammation, anemia, dehydration, and malnutrition. There is no single laboratory test that can be used to make an unequivocal diagnosis of Crohn's disease. Patients with the symptomatic disease should also undergo stool testing to evaluate for fecal pathogens, *Clostridioides difficile*, and inflammation.

2. **What is the role of genetic testing and serologic markers in establishing the diagnosis of Crohn's disease?**

   There are over 200 genetic loci associated with inflammatory bowel disease (IBD) and more than 71 loci are specifically associated with Crohn's disease. Certain genes such as the *NOD2* gene, interleukin (*IL*)-*23* gene, and autophagy-related 16 like 1 (*ATG16L1*) gene have been associated with the susceptibility of Crohn's disease. These genes may play a role in determining the phenotypic expression of Crohn's disease; however, there is no single-genetic variant that has a high enough frequency in the Crohn's disease population to make a diagnosis of Crohn's disease. Thus genetic testing is not indicated for the diagnosis and at present remains a research tool.

   Several serologic markers have been proposed to aid in the diagnosis of Crohn's disease. The best available tests are anti–*Saccharomyces cerevisiae* and perinuclear antineutrophil cytoplasmic antibodies. The accuracy of these markers in differentiating Crohn's disease from ulcerative colitis is limited. Furthermore, serologic markers for Crohn's disease have low sensitivity. Thus routine use of serologic markers to establish diagnosis of Crohn's disease is not indicated.

3. **How do we distinguish ulcerative colitis from Crohn's disease?**

   It may be difficult to distinguish Crohn's disease from ulcerative colitis—especially when Crohn's disease only involves the colon. However, certain clues can support the diagnosis of Crohn's disease versus ulcerative colitis. Table 41.1 provides clues that can help differentiate Crohn's disease from ulcerative colitis.

4. **What diseases can mimic the signs and symptoms of Crohn's disease?**

   The differential diagnosis of Crohn's disease is long and can be divided into infectious and noninfectious causes. The most common mimickers of Crohn's disease are ulcerative colitis, ischemic colitis, diverticulitis, and colorectal cancer. Table 41.2 provides additional differential diagnoses.

5. **What is the natural history of Crohn's disease?**

   Population-based studies from Norway and Minnesota suggest that most patients with Crohn's disease present with ileal, ileocolonic, or colonic inflammation in roughly one-third distribution. Only a minority of patients present with upper GI tract involvement. Furthermore, very few patients have a change in disease location over time (6%–14%). However, over 50% of patients will develop an intestinal complication such as fistula, stricture, or abscess within 20 years of diagnosis. Risk factors associated with progressive disease: young age at diagnosis (<30 years old), extensive involvement at diagnosis (upper GI tract involvement), deep ulceration, perianal or severe rectal disease, cigarette smoking, penetrating or stenotic disease at diagnosis, and prior surgical resection.

   Over 50% of patients require hospitalization at some point in their clinical course. The rate of hospitalization is highest in the first year after diagnosis. Most patients have chronic intermittent symptoms; very few patients

Table 41.1 Clues That Can Aid in Distinguishing Crohn's Disease From Ulcerative Colitis.

CROHN'S DISEASE	ULCERATIVE COLITIS
Discontinuous involvement—skip areas	Continuous involvement
Usually with rectal sparing	Rectal involvement
Perianal involvement	Usually does not have perianal involvement
Deep, linear, and serpiginous ulcers	Shallow and superficial ulceration
Presence of stricture and fistula	Less likely to have strictures and fistula
Granuloma on biopsy (present only in minority of patients)	Cryptitis/crypt abscess on biopsy
Transmural inflammation	Inflammation limited to mucosa
Occasional upper GI tract involvement	Only affects colon and rarely ileum (backwash ileitis)

GI, Gastrointestinal.

Table 41.2 Differential Diagnosis of Crohn's Disease.

LOCATION	INFECTIOUS DIFFERENTIAL DIAGNOSIS	NONINFECTIOUS DIFFERENTIAL DIAGNOSIS
Small bowel	*Coccidioides*	Celiac sprue Common variable immunodeficiency Tropical sprue Intestinal lymphoma
Ileum and cecum	*Histoplasma* *Mycobacterium tuberculosis* *Salmonella* *Yersinia*	Bechet disease
Colon	*Aeromonas* *Campylobacter* *Clostridioides difficile* *Entamoeba histolytica* *Escherichia coli* *Salmonella* *Shigella*	Colorectal cancer Diverticulitis Ischemic colitis Ulcerative colitis
Any location	*Cytomegaloviru*	Irritable bowel syndrome Nonsteroidal anti-inflammatory drug-induced enteropathy Radiation enteropathy Sarcoidosis Radiation enteropathy

have continuously active symptomatic disease or prolonged symptomatic remission. Over 50% of patients will have steroid dependency or steroid resistance in the absence of immunomodulatory or biologic therapy. The 10-year risk of surgical resection has decreased to 30% in the biologic era compared to 40%–55% in the pre–biologic era. Furthermore, the 10-year risk of second resection has also decreased to 30% in biologic era compared to 35% in pre–biologic era.

6. **How do we determine disease activity? What scoring systems are available? How can we score the endoscopic activity of Crohn's disease?**
Disease activity cannot be determined by a single test as disease activity depends on multiple clinical measures, quality of life, complications of disease, and therapy. Crohn's Disease Activity Index (CDAI), Harvey Bradshaw

Index, and patient-reported outcome tools are indices that can help measure disease activity and/or severity. The Montreal classification is a standardized international classification system that takes into account the age of disease onset, location, and disease behavior (stricturing, penetrating, and perianal involvement).

Disease activity can be divided into remission, mild, moderate, or severe. Patients in remission do not have active Crohn's disease on imaging, endoscopy, and pathology. Patients with mild Crohn's disease have mild symptoms: <10% weight loss and no complications (fever, abdominal mass, dehydration, or obstruction). Patients with mild disease have a CDAI <220. Patients with severe disease have significant weight loss and complications such as obstruction, fistula, and abscesses. These patients may need hospitalization. Patients with severe disease have a CDAI >450. Patients with moderate Crohn's disease fit in between mild and severe disease. Patients with moderate-to-severe disease usually require biologic therapy.

The Crohn's Disease Endoscopic Index of Severity and Simple Endoscopic Score for Crohn's disease are both used for scoring the endoscopic activity of Crohn's disease. Rutgeerts' score is used to assess endoscopic activity in patients who have undergone ileocolonic resection (see Question 23).

NATURAL HISTORY

7. **Are patients with Crohn's disease at an increased risk for cancer?**
Patients with Crohn's disease involving the colon are at increased risk for colorectal cancer. Risk factors for colorectal cancer: disease duration of Crohn's disease, extent of colonic involvement, severity of inflammation, family history of colon cancer, and personal history of primary sclerosing cholangitis (PSC). Patients with Crohn's disease involving the small intestine are at increased risk for small intestine adenocarcinoma. The relative risk of small bowel cancer is markedly higher than the general population (at least 18-fold); however, the absolute risk is low. Risk factor for small bowel cancer is long-standing inflammation.

Patients with IBD are at risk for extraintestinal malignancies: cholangiocarcinoma, lymphoma, and skin cancer. There is also an increased risk of lung cancer in patients with Crohn's disease. The increased risk of cancer is due to long-standing inflammation and is related to immunosuppressive therapy.

8. **What are the extraintestinal manifestations (EIMs) of Crohn's disease?**
EIMs are diagnosed in up to 50% of patients with IBD, with one EIM increasing the risk of other EIMs. EIMs are more common in patients with Crohn's disease than in those with ulcerative colitis. They can present at any time, though the majority (75%) present after diagnosis. EIMs can impact almost any organ system in the body, with dermatologic, ocular, neurologic, cardiac, bronchopulmonary, hematologic, hepatobiliary, pancreatic, musculoskeletal, endocrine, renal, and genitourinary manifestations all described in the literature.

Joint EIMs are the most common EIMs and can be broken down into arthralgias (joint pain without inflammation), peripheral arthritis (joint pain with inflammation), and axial arthritis (inflammation involving the sacroiliac joints). Skin EIMs are also common. Erythema nodosum (EN) is the most common skin EIM in Crohn's disease and presents as tender, raised nodules classically on the extensor surfaces of the legs. Pyoderma gangrenosum is more common in ulcerative colitis but can also be seen in Crohn's disease and presents as a pustule that progresses to a burrowing ulcer with violaceous edges. Other skin EIMs include sweet syndrome and metastatic Crohn's disease. Ocular EIMs are rare but important to recognize. Episcleritis is associated with Crohn's disease activity and presents as ocular erythema with associated irritation but no pain or vision changes. Scleritis and uveitis are independent of IBD activity and can present with pain and vision changes. These EIMs are vision-threatening and represent an ocular emergency. Patients who present with possible scleritis or uveitis should be immediately referred to an ophthalmologist. Though classically associated with ulcerative colitis, PSC can also be seen in Crohn's disease. Unfortunately, no effective therapies are available apart from liver transplants in the setting of advanced disease.

9. **Which EIMs parallel disease activity?**
See Table 41.3 for EIM and disease activity.

TREATMENT

10. **What are the general approaches to managing mild-to-moderate Crohn's disease?**
Patients with minimal systemic symptoms, mild endoscopic disease, and low risk of disease progression (see Question 5) can undergo induction of remission with a tapering course of steroids with or without azathioprine. If remission is achieved, then steroid therapy can be stopped, and the patient can be observed with a follow-up endoscopy in 6–12 months. Dietary modification with a specific low carbohydrate diet or Mediterranean diet may be helpful in maintaining remission. Unfortunately, there is a high chance of relapse over 1 year. If the patient does not achieve remission, consider checking azathioprine drug levels and starting biologic therapy.

Table 41.3 Extraintestinal Manifestation (EIM) and Disease Activity.

EIM	MIRRORS IBD ACTIVITY	INDEPENDENT OF IBD ACTIVITY	MAY OR MAY NOT MIRROR IBD ACTIVITY
Arthralgia	+		
Peripheral arthritis			+
Axial arthritis		+	
Erythema nodosum	+		
Pyoderma gangrenosum			+
Episcleritis	+		
Uveitis		+	
Scleritis		+	
Primary sclerosing cholangitis		+	

IBD, Inflammatory bowel disease.

11. **What vaccines are recommended for patients with Crohn's disease?**

Several vaccines are recommended for patients with Crohn's disease. Vaccination should ideally be given prior to starting biologic or immunomodulatory therapy. Patients should avoid live vaccinations after starting biologic therapy. Appropriate vaccinations: COVID-19, pneumococcal polysaccharide vaccine (PPSV23; pneumococcal conjugate vaccine [PCV] 13 or PCV20), hepatitis A/B, inactivated influenza, varicella, human papillomavirus, herpes zoster, and tetanus, diphtheria, pertussis (Tdap). Infants born to mothers on anti–tumor necrosis factor (TNF) therapy should avoid live vaccines for 1 year (e.g., rotavirus vaccine).

12. **Can steroids be used to manage Crohn's disease?**

Corticosteroids were among the earliest available therapeutic agents to be utilized in the treatment of IBD. However, with the emergence of alternative agents with a better safety profile, the role of steroids in the treatment of patients with Crohn's disease has grown far more limited. A substantial body of evidence demonstrates that steroids are not effective agents for long-term treatment, display a number of significant side effects, and even are associated with increased mortality in Crohn's disease. For these reasons, steroids should be used for the induction of remission and in the setting of flares (as a so-called bridge until another agent can take effect) but should not be utilized for the maintenance of remission.

Oral corticosteroids (such as prednisone) are typically used for mild to moderate disease and intravenous formulations (such as methylprednisolone) for moderate to severe disease. In patients with mild-to-moderate Crohn's disease limited to the terminal ileum and/or right colon budesonide (a steroid with some degree of intestinal specificity) may also be considered.

13. **What are immunomodulators, and how can they be used to manage Crohn's disease?**

Immunomodulators are a class of agents that can be used both in the treatment of active Crohn's disease and in conjunction with biologics to decrease immunogenicity. Immunomodulators that are effective for Crohn's disease include azathioprine (oral), 6-mercaptopurine (oral), and methotrexate (oral, subcutaneous, or intramuscular). Due to their slow onset of action (8–12 weeks), these agents are preferred for maintenance rather than induction of remission.

Prior to the initiation of immunomodulators, it is important to counsel patients regarding the side effect profile of these agents. Thiopurine methyltransferase testing is recommended prior to initiation of azathioprine or 6-mercaptopurine and monitoring of blood counts and liver enzymes is required due to risk of dose-dependent myelosuppression and hepatoxicity. Other possible side effects from these agents include pancreatitis, rash, and malignancies (particularly non-Hodgkin lymphoma and non-melanomatous skin cancers). Methotrexate is teratogenic and highly effective contraception is required.

Table 41.4 Anti–Tumor Necrosis Factor (TNF) Therapy Approved for Inflammatory Bowel Disease (IBD).

ANTI-TNF AGENT	STRUCTURE	MODE OF ADMIN-ISTRATION	IBD SUB-TYPE	SELECTED KEY CD TRIALS
Infliximab	Chimeric IgG1 monoclonal antibody—75% human and 25% mouse	IV infusion	CD or UC	ACCENT I and II Trial
Adalimumab	Fully recombinant IgG1 monoclonal antibody	Subcutaneous injection	CD or UC	Classic I and II, Charm, Extend, Adhere
Certolizumab	Humanized Fab' fragment of anti-TNF monoclonal antibodies conjugated to a PEG molecule	Subcutaneous injection	Only CD	PRECiSE Trial
Golimumab	Fully recombinant IgG1 monoclonal antibody	Subcutaneous injection	Only UC	N/A

CD, Crohn's disease; *Ig*, immunoglobulin; *IV*, intravenous; *PEG*, polyethylene glycol; *UC*, ulcerative colitis.

14. **What are the anti-TNF agents? What is their mechanism of action? Which anti-TNF agents are approved for the treatment of Crohn's disease? What labs must be obtained prior to starting anti-TNF therapy?**

    All anti-TNF agents act by blocking some form of TNF, a net proinflammatory cytokine that exists in increased concentrations in the blood, stool, and mucosa of patients with IBD. There are several different classes of anti-TNF agents available to treat Crohn's disease and ulcerative colitis (Table 41.4).

    Of note, due to its unique structure, certolizumab does not cross the placenta, so it is ideal for females seeking to become pregnant.

    Prior to initiation of anti-TNF agents, it is important to check a baseline blood count and liver enzymes. In addition, it is imperative to check for tuberculosis and hepatitis status (particularly hepatitis B) due to the risk of reactivation with initiation.

15. **What are biosimilar anti-TNF agents, and what is their role in managing Crohn's disease?**

    Biosimilar agents are medications that, as the name implies, are quite similar to their originators but of substantially lower cost. Biosimilar may differ slightly in their make-up when compared to the original medication but should have the same safety and efficacy profile, which has been demonstrated in a large non-inferiority trial. According to the most recent American College of Gastroenterology clinical guidelines, biosimilar anti-TNF agents can be used for de novo induction and maintenance therapy, but there are insufficient data regarding switching from one biosimilar to another.

16. **What is the role of therapeutic drug monitoring? How do we interpret drug levels and antibodies?**

    The goal of therapeutic drug monitoring is to optimize dosage and response to biologic agents. This field is still in its infancy, and optimal approach and timing of monitoring remain controversial. However, as a guide drug level in maintenance for infliximab should be 5–10 mg/mL, adalimumab 8–12 mcg/mL, golimumab 1–3 mg/L, certolizumab 13–15 mg/L, vedolizumab 15–20 mg/L, and ustekinumab 1–3 µg/mL.

    While rates of immunogenicity to vedolizumab and ustekinumab are low, antibody formation is common in anti-TNF agents, with rates as high as 60% in those on infliximab. Combination therapy with an immunomodulator can prevent the development of antibodies and help sustain the efficacy of the biologic when antibodies have developed. However, antibody formation decreases the efficacy of the biologic agent and may ultimately warrant discontinuation of the medication.

17. **What are other biologics approved for treatment of Crohn's disease? What is their mechanism of action?**

    See Table 41.5 for additional biologics approved for the treatment of Crohn's disease.

18. **How do we manage perianal and fistulizing Crohn's disease?**

    Perianal and fistulizing Crohn's disease can significantly impact the quality of life for patients and can be challenging to manage for providers. Patients with perianal and fistulizing Crohn's disease should optimally

Table 41.5 Additional Biologics Approved for the Treatment of Crohn's Disease.

BIOLOGIC AGENT	MECHANISM OF ACTION	MODE OF ADMINIS-TRATION	SELECTED KEY CD TRIALS
Vedolizumab	Humanized IgG1 monoclonal antibody to α4β7	IV infusion	GEMINI I and II
Ustekinumab	Humanized IgG1 monoclonal antibody targeting the p40 subunit of IL-12 and IL-23	Subcutaneous injection	UNITI
Risankizumab	Humanized IgG1 monoclonal antibody targeting the p19 subunit of IL-23	Subcutaneous injection	Advance, motivate, and fortify

CD, Crohn's disease; *IgG*, immunoglobulin G; *IL*, interleukin; *IV*, intravenous.

be managed by a multidisciplinary team that includes the gastroenterologist and the colorectal surgeon and depending on the location of the fistula and its associated complications, interventional radiology, gynecology, urology, and infectious disease.

Initial management of perianal and or fistulizing Crohn's disease involves cross-sectional imaging (computed tomography [CT] or magnetic resonance imaging [MRI]) to evaluate the location and extent of the fistula as well as the presence of abscess. Abscesses requiring drainage must be treated prior to the initiation of therapy.

Following this, management depends on the location and severity of the fistula but generally consists of a combination of antibiotics, biologics, and surgical intervention (fistulotomy, mucosal flap, seton, diversion, or even proctectomy with permanent loop ileostomy in the case of severe, medically refractory disease).

The most robust data regarding treatment support the use of the combination of an anti-TNF (infliximab or adalimumab) and an immunomodulator.

19. How do we manage stricturing Crohn's disease?

Up to half of all patients with Crohn's disease will develop a complication, including a stricture, over the course of the disease. Strictures may present anywhere in the GI tract but occur most commonly in the small bowel specifically the terminal ileum.

As in perianal and fistulizing Crohn's disease, cross-sectional imaging (CT or MRI) is important to better characterize the findings, and then a multidisciplinary approach is needed. Medical therapy can be attempted in uncomplicated strictures. The most robust data is for anti-TNF agents, but any biologic could be considered. In patients who are symptomatic with strictures <5 cm, endoscopic balloon dilation can also be attempted. For patients with long, symptomatic strictures not responding to medical therapy, surgery should be pursued. Options include stricturoplasty or resection.

Following surgery, patients are at risk for recurrence. Patients should be closely followed with timing and choice of postoperative biologic therapy tailored to the patient and his/her risk factors (such as smoking, prior surgery, age, and disease phenotype).

PREGNANCY

20. Which IBD medications are contraindicated in pregnancy?

Methotrexate is teratogenic and must be stopped at least 3 months prior to conception. Mesalamines can be continued. However, sulfasalazine requires supplementation with folic acid and should be stopped in males in favor of alternative mesalamine compounds due to the risk of decreased sperm count and reversible infertility.

Steroids should be tapered prior to conception. Should a flare occur during pregnancy, steroids can be used if necessary. Azathioprine can be continued if the patient is already on a stable dose but should not be initiated in pregnancy due to possible side effects.

Biologic therapy is safe and should be continued throughout the pregnancy as the risks of uncontrolled Crohn's disease outweigh the risks associated with the use of these agents.

There are insufficient data regarding small molecules (e.g., tofacitinib, ozanimod, and upadicitinib) and so their use is not advised during pregnancy.

SURGERY

21. What are the indications for surgery in Crohn's disease?

Patients with enteric complications: intestinal perforation, recurrent obstruction, and abscess that is not amenable to drainage, dysplasia, cancer, intractable hemorrhage, or medically refractory disease should be referred for

Table 41.6 Rutgeerts' Score.

RUTGEERTS' SCORE	ENDOSCOPIC CORRELATION
i0	No inflammation and no lesions
i1	≤5 aphthous ulcers proximal to anastomosis
i2a	Isolated anastomotic ulceration
i2b	>5 aphthous ulcers with normal mucosa between the lesions, skip areas of large lesions
i3	Diffuse aphthous ulceration with inflamed mucosa
i4	Diffuse inflammation with large ulcers, nodules, and narrowing

surgery. The most common reason for surgery is small bowel obstruction from fibrostenotic stricture and the second most common reason for surgery is penetrating disease.

22. **What risk factors are associated with postoperative recurrence of Crohn's disease?**
Several risk factors have been identified that increase the risk of postoperative Crohn's disease. The three risk factors associated with the highest risk of recurrence: tobacco smoking, history of penetrating Crohn's disease (fistulas, abscesses, and perforation), and history of two or more prior surgeries. Other risk factors include young age at diagnosis, need for surgery despite aggressive medical treatment with biologics and immunomodulators, short duration of time from diagnosis and need for surgery (<10 years), inflammation located in multiple sites in the GI tract, perianal involvement, severe inflammation, long segment of inflammation, and need for corticosteroids. Patients' risk factors for recurrence must be taken into account when deciding on postoperative treatment.

23. **What is Rutgeerts' score?**
Rutgeerts' score is an endoscopic score used to measure disease activity in patients who have undergone ileocolonic resection. The score assesses inflammation and ulceration proximal to the anastomosis in the ileum. Inflammation proximal to the anastomosis increases the chance of Crohn's disease recurrence postoperatively. Patients with Rutgeerts' score of i2b and above should be treated with biologic therapy (Table 41.6).

CLINICAL VIGNETTE

Available Online

BIBLIOGRAPHY

Available Online

CHAPTER 42

ULCERATIVE COLITIS

Jami A. Kinnucan, MD, FACG, AGAF and Francis A. Farraye, MS, MD, MACG

 Additional content available online

1. What is ulcerative colitis (UC)?

UC is a chronic inflammatory disease of the colon. It is distinct from Crohn disease (CD) of the colon (Crohn colitis) in that the inflammation is restricted predominately to the mucosa and typically only involves the colon. Unlike, Crohn colitis, the rectal segment is almost always involved with UC. Patients can have varying degrees of involvement of the colon including proctitis (rectum), proctosigmoiditis (rectum and sigmoid colon), left-sided colitis (extending to splenic flexure), extensive colitis (extending proximal to the splenic flexure), and pancolitis (involving entire colon including cecum; Fig. 42.1).

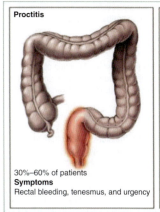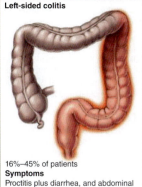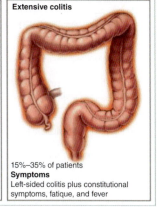

Proctitis	Left-sided colitis	Extensive colitis
30%–60% of patients	16%–45% of patients	15%–35% of patients
Symptoms	**Symptoms**	**Symptoms**
Rectal bleeding, tenesmus, and urgency	Proctitis plus diarrhea, and abdominal cramping	Left-sided colitis plus constitutional symptoms, fatigue, and fever

Fig. 42.1 Ulcerative colitis phenotypes by Montreal classification. (From Ungaro R, Mehandru S, Allen PB, Peyrin-Biroulet L, Colombel J-F. Ulcerative colitis. Lancet. 2017;389(10080):1756-1770.)

2. Define backwash ileitis (BWI).

BWI refers to limited inflammation of the distal few centimeters of the terminal ileum in rare patients with pancolitis. The endoscopic, histologic, and radiologic appearance of BWI is the same as that of UC with superficial continuous inflammation. When deep linear ulcers and strictures are seen in the ileum, a diagnosis of CD with ileal involvement is more likely.

3. What is indeterminate colitis?

As more information is gathered about the pathogenesis of UC and CD, the distinction between these disorders at times can be unclear. In approximately 7% of patients, when the inflammatory process is limited to the colon (without ileal involvement), the endoscopic, histologic, or radiologic findings are insufficiently distinct to separate the two diseases, then the inflammatory bowel disease (IBD) is referred to as indeterminate colitis. Patients can carry the diagnosis of UC for many years until a change in their clinical, radiographic, endoscopic, or histologic presentation becomes more consistent with CD, resulting in a change in the diagnosis. In some patients, the diagnosis of CD of the colon is recognized only after colectomy and the development of recurrent chronic ileitis in the small bowel proximal to an ileostomy or after restorative ileoanal pouch anastomosis (IPAA).

4. Why is it important to distinguish between UC and CD?

While the medical management of the two diseases overlaps significantly, the surgical management differs. UC can be surgically cured by total proctocolectomy with end ileostomy or IPAA. Crohn colitis can also result in total proctocolectomy but in a recent meta-analysis, the risk for small bowel clinical recurrence of disease is about 28% after surgery. At the time of surgery, the correct diagnosis is of the utmost importance to avoid complications, especially after IPAA.

5. What causes UC?

Although the cause of UC is unknown, it appears to be caused by an abnormal intestinal immune response to an external antigen in a genetically predisposed individual. The cause technically remains unknown, although research has clarified that there are genetic, environmental, and immunologic contributions. Approximately 20%–25% of patients with IBD have a first-degree relative with the disease, but the familial association is less in UC than in CD. During the past decade, there have been considerable advances in the understanding of IBD genetics. Since the identification of the first susceptibility gene of IBD (*NOD2*), there are over 240 genetic loci that have been identified in association with IBD. The greatest risk factor is a positive family history. The probability of developing CD in a relative of a patient with UC is increased by twofold, and there is a fourfold risk of UC in a relative of a patient with CD. While only 20%–25% have an identifiable family history of genetic association, the exact environmental link for UC has not been identified. Dietary antigens and bacteria have been proposed as possible triggers to develop IBD and there is ongoing research to better understand these environmental contributors to develop disease. There have been studies looking at the negative impacts of diets higher in fat, refined sugars, animal protein (especially red meat), and lower in fiber and the impact on developing IBD. The incidence of UC is significantly higher in nonsmokers than in smokers and higher still in ex-smokers than in nonsmokers, supporting a protective effect of smoking in UC only. Whether this protective effect is secondary to nicotine or other constituents of cigarettes is not fully understood. There have been several medications linked to increasing the risk of developing IBD including oral contraceptives, exposure to antibiotics, and history of nonsteroidal anti-inflammatory drugs (NSAIDs) use.

6. Who gets UC?

UC equally affects both males and females and, in most patients, onset in the second or third decade of life, however, there may be a second peak in the fifth or sixth decade. UC has been described in all racial and ethnic groups but is more common in Whites than in non-Whites. It is also more common in those of Ashkenazi Jewish descent. This hereditary link is supported by population-based studies.

7. What are the signs and symptoms of UC?

The predominant symptom at the onset of UC is diarrhea, invariably with blood in the stool. If inflammation is confined to the rectum (proctitis), blood may be seen on the surface of the stool; other symptoms include tenesmus, urgency, rectal pain, and passage of mucus without diarrhea. Symptoms are typically consistent with the distribution of disease in the colon (Question 1). More extensive colitis may be accompanied by systemic symptoms such as abdominal pain, weight loss, and malaise in addition to persistent diarrhea with rectal bleeding. Although abdominal pain is not a predominant feature, patients can complain of crampy abdominal discomfort relieved by a bowel movement and may have abdominal tenderness, usually localized to the left lower quadrant. Occasionally patients may present with constipation secondary to the presence of proctitis and resulting rectal spasm; accompanying mucoid rectal discharge might be disclosed by careful history. Although patients may present with extraintestinal manifestations independent of bowel symptoms, more often they parallel the severity of the primary bowel disease. Extraintestinal symptoms can predate the diagnosis of IBD in 26%–30% of patients with the most common extraintestinal symptom peripheral arthritis.

8. How are patients with UC classified?

Truelove and Witts divided patients into those with mild, moderate, and severe disease based on symptoms, physical findings, and laboratory values. In the Montreal classification of UC, the extent of disease can be limited (proctitis, E1) to more extensive (left-sided distal to splenic flexure, E2 or extension proximal to the splenic flexure, E3) (Fig. 42.1). The Mayo score uses frequency of stools, presence of bleeding, endoscopic appearance, and the physician's global assessment (PGA) to arrive at a number for disease activity. The full Mayo score ranges from 0 to 12, with higher scores representing more severe disease. The full score is derived from the partial Mayo score (clinical symptoms and PGA) and the endoscopic Mayo score. Severity can also be further characterized radiologically. A plain film of the abdomen showing any degree of dilation of the colon or ulceration and edema of the mucosa outlined by air (even if not dilated) is indicative of severe disease activity. Although endoscopic appearance does not always correlate well with clinical symptoms, the presence of severe mucosal disease indicates the need for more treatment optimization (Table 42.1). In the 2019 American College of Gastroenterology update on UC, the authors include the use of C-reactive protein (CRP) and fecal calprotectin in the classification of UC disease activity.

9. What are common extraintestinal manifestations of UC?

Extraintestinal manifestations are more commonly seen in patients with CD; however, UC is also associated with these manifestations as well. These manifestations are divided into those that parallel the activity of bowel disease and those that occur independently of bowel disease activity (Table 42.2).

Table 42.1 Ulcerative Colitis Clinical Severity—Montreal Classification.

SEVERITY	STOOLS/DAY	BLOOD IN STOOLS	ESR	SYSTEMIC ILLNESS[a]
Mild	≤4	Present or absent	Normal	Absent
Moderate	4–6	Present or absent	Normal or elevated	Absent
Severe	7–10	Present	Elevated	Present
Fulminant	>10	Present	Elevated	Present

ESR, Erythrocyte sedimentation rate.
[a]Systemic illness: fever, tachycardia, and anemia, ESR >30.

Table 42.2 UC Medication Toolbox as of July 1, 2022.

ORAL MESALAMINE	ORAL STEROID	IMMUNOMODULA-TOR	BIOLOGIC
Sulfasalazine Mesalamine Apriso Colazal Lialda Asacol Pentasa	Prednisone Methylprednisone Budesonide-MMX Uceris	Azathioprine (Imuran) 6-MP Methotrexate	Anti-TNF: Infliximab (Remicade)[a] Adalimumab (Humira)[a] Golimumab (Simponi) Anti-integrin: Vedoli-zumab (Entyvio) Anti-IL-12/23:Ustekinumab (Stelara)
Topical mesalamine	Topical steroid	Small molecule	
Canasa (supp) Rowasa (enema)	Hydrocortisone Anusol (supp) Cortenema Cortifoam Budesonide Uceris foam	JAK inhibitor: Tofacitinib (Xeljanz) Upadacitinib (Rinvoq) S1P receptor modulator: Ozanimod (Zeposia)	

JAK, Janus kinase; *TNF*, tumor necrosis factor; *S1P*, sphingosine 1-phosphate.
[a]Biosimilar availability.

10. What is the arthritis associated with UC?

Arthritis associated with IBD is often classified as a seronegative arthropathy. It is more commonly seen in patients with CD and about 10% of those with UC. Patients often present with joint inflammation of both peripheral small joints and larger joints that migrates from joint to joint. The most affected joints are the knees, hips, ankles, wrists, and elbows. Usually, the joint involvement is asymmetrical and typically responds well to IBD treatment optimization or corticosteroids.

11. Describe the association between UC and ankylosing spondylitis (AS).

Although AS is more commonly associated with CD than UC, patients with UC have a 30-fold increased risk of developing AS than the general population, which does not parallel the colitis activity. AS is a progressive inflammatory arthropathy affecting the sacroiliac joints and the spine. Many patients with early sacroiliitis alone are asymptomatic, and the diagnosis is made on radiographs. Low back pain or central pain along the spine should always be evaluated for an inflammatory etiology in patients with IBD. Treatment can often include the optimization of primary IBD treatment or the addition of additional therapies including corticosteroids, sulfasalazine (SSZ), or immunomodulators. Often these patients are best referred to a rheumatologist for evaluation and management.

12. Discuss the hepatic complications of UC.

Hepatic complications include fatty liver disease, pericholangitis, chronic active hepatitis, cirrhosis, and primary sclerosing cholangitis (PSC). Although most patients with PSC have UC, only a few patients with UC develop PSC and these patients commonly have mild colitis symptoms. PSC is usually suspected with the finding of an abnormally elevated alkaline phosphatase or γ-glutamyl transferase enzyme. PSC is sometimes treated with ursodeoxycholic acid therapy (Actigall); however, its use is controversial. Patients with PSC and UC have a significantly higher risk of developing colorectal neoplasia and cholangiocarcinoma than those without. In those with a progressive course of PSC developing end-stage liver disease, the only treatment would be liver transplant.

13. What are the common ocular manifestations of UC?

Ocular complications occur in less than 10% of patients with IBD. Most concerning complications include scleritis and uveitis which present with severe eye pain, tenderness, and scleral injection (redness) and can be complicated by vision changes/loss. Prompt evaluation and treatment are key. A less severe ocular manifestation is episcleritis which presents with deep injection (redness) of the episclera and is typically associated with active luminal inflammation. Treatment of active inflammation often resolves this extraintestinal manifestation; however, some patients may require topical ocular therapies and occasionally systemic treatments.

14. Describe the association between UC and venous and arterial thromboembolic events

Patients with IBD are at increased risk of both venous and arterial thromboembolic events, most commonly deep venous thrombosis of the lower extremities. The patients at highest risk are those who are hospitalized with severe disease and postoperative patients with IBD. All patients hospitalized with IBD should be placed on thromboprophylaxis. New guidance from international expert consensus to consider extended postdischarge thromboprophylaxis for those patients with IBD with strong risk factors for thromboembolism.

15. How should the practitioner evaluate a patient with UC?

The management of UC depends on the severity and location of disease activity, which are best assessed by a careful clinical history, with emphasis on the duration and severity of symptoms, physical examination, followed by laboratory evaluation and then endoscopic and histologic evaluation to determine the extent and severity of mucosal involvement. Although flexible sigmoidoscopy and biopsy can make a diagnosis and assess the severity of distal disease, a full colonoscopy is essential to determine the extent as well as the full severity. It is important to obtain a detailed history including recent travel, antibiotic, and NSAID use. Laboratory evaluations should include a complete blood count, comprehensive metabolic panel, CRP and stool studies for fecal calprotectin, culture, ova, and parasites (if there is an appropriate history), and *Clostridioides difficile*. *C. difficile* infections have been reported with increased frequency in recent years in patients with IBD. If patients have a known diagnosis of UC, iron studies and a vitamin D level should also be sent and checked at least annually.

These evaluations should provide an indication of severity and extent of disease, which can impact the initial choice of therapy. Factors associated with increased risk for colectomy in UC should be identified (Figs. 42.1 and 42.2). If patients have severe tenderness or tympany on examination, an abdominal x-ray should be performed in flat and upright positions to recognize early or advanced toxic megacolon though in general patients with a worrisome physical examination will undergo computed tomography (CT) abdomen and pelvis. The serologic test perinuclear antineutrophil cytoplasmic antibody has been associated with a diagnosis of UC but has low sensitivity (<50%) and therefore should not be used for the diagnosis of UC. If disease severity is mild to moderate, medical therapy may be commenced on an outpatient basis. However, if the disease is moderate to severe, or not responding to outpatient treatments, hospital admission should be considered.

16. What are treatments commonly used to treat ulcerative colitis?

If patients have mild disease or low-risk disease features, oral and rectal-administered mesalamine-based therapies are typically first-line therapy. In patients who do not respond to mesalamine therapy, budesonide-MMX (Uceris) is an option. If there is no response or intolerance, consider treatment with the oral small molecule therapy ozanimod (Zeposia) in patients with moderate-to-severe UC with or without a corticosteroid bridge

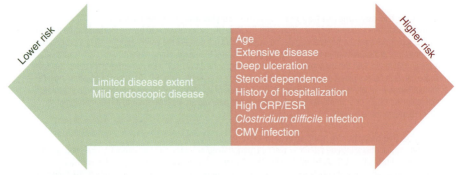

Fig. 42.2 Risk for disease complications/colectomy in patients with ulcerative colitis. *CMV*, Cytomegalovirus; *CRP*, C-reactive protein; *ESR*, erythrocyte sedimentation rate.

to induce remission. However, if patients have features of moderate-to-severe disease or higher-risk disease features, then advanced therapies should be considered first line. Table 42.2 outlines currently available treatments for the treatment of UC. Questions 17–20 will further review treatment options for mild, moderate, and severe UC.

17. What are 5-aminosalicylic acid (5-ASA) products?

SSZ, the first 5-ASA product, has been used successfully for many years in the treatment of mild-to-moderate UC. The 5-ASA molecule is linked to sulfapyridine by a diazo bond that is cleaved by colonic bacteria. The active moiety is the 5-ASA. Given its more systemic properties and sulfa association patients taking SSZ can experience nausea, vomiting, fever, or a rash, all of which are attributable primarily to the sulfapyridine, which is only a carrier molecule. SSZ may also cause agranulocytosis, autoimmune hemolytic anemia, folic acid deficiency, and male infertility secondary to changes in sperm count and morphologic characteristics. Patients on SSZ should supplement with 1 mg of folic acid daily (2 mg if they desire pregnancy). Patients who are intolerant of SSZ can typically tolerate other formation of mesalamine products. Preparations that contain only 5-ASA (mesalamine) are formulated to release in the small bowel or colon based on intestinal pH levels. Mesalamine is currently available in both oral and rectal preparations. Per rectum preparations come as a mesalamine enema (4 g, 60 mL Rowasa) or as a suppository (1 g Canasa). There are multiple oral generic formulations (Table 42.3).

Table 42.3 5-Aminosalicylic Acid (5-ASA) Products.

5-ASA	CARRIER MOLECULE	RELEASE	SITE OF ACTIVITY
Asacol	Eudragit-S	pH >7	Terminal ileum and right colon
Pentasa	Ethylcellulose beads, time release	pH >6	Small bowel and right colon
Olsalazine	Azo bond	Bacteria	Colon (ileum with bacterial overgrowth)
Sulfasalazine	Sulfapyridine	Bacteria	Colon (ileum with bacterial overgrowth)
Lialda	Matrix	Colon pH >6.8	Colon
Apriso	INTELLICOR delayed and extended release	pH ≥6	Colon
Colazal	Diazo bond	Colon	Colon
Dipentum	Dimer	Left colon	Left colon

18. How do I treat proctitis and proctosigmoiditis?

For mild-to-moderate limited UC (proctitis and proctosigmoiditis), rectal therapy may be indicated for both induction and maintenance of remission without the requirement of oral therapy. If the disease is limited to the rectum, a suppository might be all that is required. Mesalamine suppositories can be used once or twice daily, and hydrocortisone suppository (Anusol) can be used once or twice daily. Enema preparations might also be used for proctitis or proctosigmoiditis. Hydrocortisone foam (Cortifoam) or hydrocortisone enemas (Cortenema) also may be used either alone or in alternation with the 5-ASA product. Budesonide foam (Uceris foam) is a rectal steroid-based formulation approved for use in mild-to-moderate colitis extending to 40 cm for induction of remission. For more extensive distal UC (proctosigmoiditis up to 40 cm), the mesalamine enema is effective. Only the mesalamine-based formulations should be used for maintenance when indicated. A combination (oral and rectal) therapy has demonstrated higher rates of remission compared to oral or rectal therapy alone.

19. How do you approach an exacerbation of more extensive mild-to-moderate UC?

When the disease extends more proximally, oral therapies are required in addition to, or instead of, rectal monotherapy. Studies have shown that some patients require a combination of oral and topical therapy to achieve remission. We previously reviewed oral 5-ASA therapy options for mild-to-moderate UC (Table 42.4). Budesonide-MMX (*Uceris) is effective for induction of remission in mild-to-moderate UC and is orally dosed at 9 mg once daily for 8 weeks and can be discontinued without taper. If the disease fails to respond to

Table 42.4 Extraintestinal Manifestations Seen in Ulcerative Colitis.

DEPENDENT ON BOWEL INFLAMMATION	INDEPENDENT ON BOWEL INFLAMMATION
Inflammatory arthropathy (large joint)	Inflammatory arthropathy (small/peripheral)
Pyoderma gangrenosum	Ankylosing spondylitis
Erythema nodosum	Primary sclerosing cholangitis
± Uveitis	± Uveitis
± Episcleritis	± Episcleritis

5-ASA therapy or budesonide-MMX or is moderate to severe in severity at presentation, a short course of oral corticosteroids should be prescribed to achieve clinical remission. The maximal effective oral dose of prednisone prescribed is 60 mg daily though this is associated with more side effects than an induction dose of 40 mg per day. The dose may be tapered to 40 mg/day after 2–7 days if there is improved symptom control. The formula for further tapering of prednisone is individualized to the patient's clinical history and severity of disease. The 5-ASA drugs can be given concurrently with prednisone but be aware that 1%–2% of patients with UC may have an idiosyncratic reaction with worsening of their colitis while on 5-ASA. Prednisone and other systemic corticosteroids are not indicated as maintenance therapy. If a patient has had exposure to steroids >3 months or more than twice in one year, steroid-sparing medical regimens are warranted along with consideration of referral to an IBD specialist.

20. **What advanced therapies are available to manage moderate-to-severe UC in the outpatient setting?**
For mild-to-moderate disease, a 5-ASA product either orally, topically, or both may be all that is necessary. For more moderate-to-severe or recurrent disease, advanced therapy may be required. There are multiple therapies that have been studied and approved for the treatment of moderate-to-severe UC. Table 42.2 provides an overview of all therapies. Beyond mesalamine and previously reviewed small molecule therapies, there are immunosuppressive medications such as 6-mercaptopurine (6-MP)/azathioprine (AZA, Imuran), Janus kinase (JAK) inhibitors (tofacitinib, upadacitinib), and ozanimod. In addition to oral therapies, there are multiple biologic therapy mechanisms, including anti-tumor necrosis factor (anti-TNF), anti-integrin, or anti-IL-12/23 inhibitor. The positioning of therapies can be complex and dependent on patient's severity of disease, prognostic disease factors, response to corticosteroids, preference, comorbidities, and insurance coverage. Recommendations from the newest American Gastroenterological Association (AGA) Clinical Practice Guidelines suggest against the use of thiopurine monotherapy in the treatment of UC. If patients are to be started on thiopurine (azathioprine, 6-mercaptopurine) monotherapy or combination therapy, a thiopurine methyltransferase may be checked prior to initiating therapy and close lab monitoring for laboratory tolerance. Early toxic reactions to these medications include leukopenia, pancreatitis (3%), hepatitis, transaminitis without hepatitis, rash, and fever. Small molecule therapy with JAK inhibition, tofacitinib which inhibits JAK1, JAK3, and upadacitinib which inhibits JAK1 only, requires patients to have previous experience or failure with anti-TNF prior to initiation. This requirement is due to the black box warning (September 2021) due to data showing increased risk for cardiovascular events including heart attack, stroke, cancer, thromboembolic events, and death in patients with rheumatoid arthritis over the age of 50 with one cardiovascular risk factor treated with tofacitinib (upadacitinib carries same warning as same class). There are multiple monoclonal antibodies approved for the treatment of UC. Prior to initiation of biologic therapy, it is recommended that patients are evaluated with Hepatitis B serologic testing (including hepatitis B core Ab) and tuberculosis testing. Monoclonal antibodies that target TNF-α (anti-TNF) therapies approved for UC include infliximab (Remicade and biosimilars), adalimumab (Humira), and golimumab (Simponi). Infliximab is the only anti-TNF given by an infusion; the others are administered by subcutaneous injection. The dosing frequency varies with each therapy. Vedolizumab (Entyvio) is an α4β7 integrin monoclonal antibody that blocks the interaction of memory gut-home T-lymphocytes with intestinal receptors (MAdCAM-1) and is given as IV loading doses and then maintenance every 8 weeks. The most recently approved antagonist to the p40 subunit of IL-12 and -23 is ustekinumab (Stelara). Ustekinumab is administered as a single IV infusion induction dose followed by subcutaneous maintenance every 8 weeks. Several studies have looked at the use of biologics as monotherapy (used alone) as well as combination therapy (used in combination with thiopurine or methotrexate) and based on the AGA UC Practice Guidelines there is weak evidence and recommendations for combination therapy, conditional low recommendation. There are several recommendations that came from AGA UC Guidelines published in 2020 which are outlined in Table 42.5. Of note these guidelines were published prior to the approval of upadacitinib in 2022, readers can assume the same positioning of upadacitinib as tofacitinib.

Table 42.5 Summary of Recommendations From the American Gastroenterological Association (AGA) Clinical Practice Committee for the Management of Moderate-to-Severe Ulcerative Colitis (UC).

RECOMMENDATIONS	STRENGTH OF RECOMMENDATION	QUALITY OF EVIDENCE
1. In adult outpatients with moderate-to-severe UC the AGA recommends using infliximab, adalimumab, golimumab, vedolizumab, tofacitinib, or ustekinumab over to treatment (Medications are ordered based on year of approval by the US FDA)	Strong	Moderate
2a. In adult outpatients with moderate-to-severe UC who are naive to biologic agents, the AGA suggests using infliximab or vedolizumab rather than adalimumab, for induction of remission	Conditional	Moderate
Comment: Patients, particularly those with less severe disease, who place higher value on the convenience of self-administered subcutaneous injection, and a lower value on the relative efficacy of medications, may reasonably choose adalimumab as an alternative		
2b. In adult outpatients with moderate-to-severe UC who are naive to biologic agents, the AGA recommends that tofacitinib only be used in the setting of a clinical or registry study. (No recommendation, knowledge gap)	No recommendation	Knowledge gap
Comment: Updated FDA recommendations (July 26, 2019) on indications for use of tofacitinib in UC recommend its use only after failure of or intolerance to TNF-α antagonists		
2c. In adult outpatients with moderate-to-severe UC who have previously been exposed to infliximab, particularly those with primary nonresponse, the AGA suggests using ustekinumab or tofacitinib rather than vedolizumab or adalimumab for induction of remission	Conditional	Low
3a. In adult outpatients with active moderate-to-severe UC, the AGA suggests against using thiopurine monotherapy for induction of remission	Conditional	Very low
3b. In adult outpatients with moderate-to-severe UC in remission, the AGA suggests using thiopurine monotherapy rather than no treatment for maintenance of remission	Conditional	Low
3c. In adult outpatients with moderate-to-severe UC, the AGA suggests against using methotrexate monotherapy for induction or maintenance of remission.	Conditional	Low
4a. In adult outpatients with active moderate-to-severe UC, the AGA suggests using biologic monotherapy (TNF-α antagonists, vedolizumab, or ustekinumab) or tofacitinib rather than thiopurine monotherapy for induction of remission	Conditional	Low
4b. In adult outpatients with moderate-to-severe UC in remission, the AGA makes no recommendation in favor of or against using biologic monotherapy or tofacitinib rather than thiopurine monotherapy for maintenance of remission	No recommendation	Knowledge gap
5a. In adult outpatients with moderate-to-severe UC, the AGA suggests combining TNF-α antagonists, vedolizumab, or ustekinumab with thiopurines or methotrexate rather than biologic monotherapy	Conditional	Low

Continued

Table 42.5 Summary of Recommendations From the American Gastroenterological Association (AGA) Clinical Practice Committee for the Management of Moderate-to-Severe Ulcerative Colitis (UC). —cont'd

RECOMMENDATIONS	STRENGTH OF RECOMMENDATION	QUALITY OF EVIDENCE
Comment: Patients, particularly those with less severe disease, who place higher value on the safety of biologic monotherapy and lower value on the efficacy of combination therapy may reasonably choose biologic monotherapy		
5b. In adult outpatients with moderate-to-severe UC, AGA suggests combining TNF-α antagonists, vedolizumab, or ustekinumab with thiopurines or methotrexate rather than thiopurine monotherapy	Conditional	Low
6. In adult outpatients with moderate-to-severe UC, the AGA suggests early use of biologic agents with or without immunomodulator therapy rather than gradual step up after failure of 5-ASA	Conditional	Very low
Comment: Patients, particularly those with less severe disease, who place higher value on the safety of 5-ASA therapy and lower value on the efficacy of biologic agents or tofacitinib may reasonably choose gradual step therapy with 5-ASA therapy		
7. In adult outpatients with moderate-to-severe UC who have achieved remission with biologic agents and/or immunomodulators or tofacitinib, the AGA suggests against continuing 5-ASA for induction and maintenance of remission	Conditional	Very low
8. In hospitalized adult patients with ASUC, the AGA suggests using intravenous methylprednisolone dose equivalent to 40–60 mg/day rather than higher doses of intravenous corticosteroids	Conditional	Very low
9. In hospitalized adult patients with ASUC without infection, the AGA suggests against adjunctive antibiotics	Conditional	Very low
10. In hospitalized adult patients with ASUC refractory to intravenous corticosteroids, the AGA suggests using infliximab or cyclosporine	Conditional	Low
11. In hospitalized adult patients with ASUC being treated with infliximab, the AGA makes no recommendation on routine use of intensive vs standard infliximab closing	No recommendation	Knowledge gap

5-ASA, 5-Aminosalicylic acid; *ASUC,* acute severe ulcerative colitis; *FDA,* Food and Drug Administration; *TNF,* tumor necrosis factor; *UC,* ulcerative colitis.

21. **What should I do if my patient's UC is not responding or has progressed from moderate to severe in severity?**

Progression of inflammation beyond mild to moderate in severity requires escalation of therapy (Question 20) and severe disease not responding to outpatient treatment or fulminant disease requires admission to the hospital for IV corticosteroids and fluids. Patients should be monitored carefully by serial physical examination, laboratory tests (including daily CRP), and plain radiographs of the abdomen. Acute severe UC (ASUC) may progress to toxic megacolon or perforation. Progression of disease or fulminant disease on presentation if treated surgically with emergent subtotal colectomy. It is important to consider surgical consultation early in all patients with ASUC. On admission, it is important that patients undergo stool testing for *C. difficile* infection, flexible sigmoidoscopy for disease evaluation, and biopsy for cytomegalovirus colitis as well as receive thromboembolic prophylaxis.

If there is no response to intravenous (IV) corticosteroids within 3–5 days, consideration should be given to the use of rescue management. The more commonly used and studied rescue therapy in steroid-refractory disease include IV cyclosporine, infliximab, or surgery, depending on the urgency of the clinical situation and local experience in the management of this severe complication. In patients who previously have not responded or are allergic to infliximab, off-label high dose tofacitinib has been used as rescue therapy. Rapid deterioration in clinical condition warrants early surgical intervention with ileostomy and subtotal colectomy. An early referral to a specialized IBD center for those with ASUC is recommended. Patients whose disease severity does not warrant hospitalization can be effectively managed with treatment optimization or escalation in the outpatient setting, this was addressed in Question 20.

22. Define toxic megacolon.

Toxic megacolon is defined as a severe attack of colitis with total or segmental dilation of the colon (diameter of transverse colon usually greater than 5–6 cm). It can be recognized by plain radiographs or by CT scan showing the colon to be outlined by air even with a diameter less than 5 cm. Megacolon is considered toxic if two or more of the following criteria are positive in addition to the colon persistently outlined by air:

- Tachycardia with a pulse rate greater than 100 beats per minute
- Temperature greater than 101.5°F
- Leukocytosis greater than 10,000 cells/mm^3
- Hypoalbuminemia less than 3 g/dL

23. If patients reach a state of clinical, endoscopic, or histology remission, how can you prevent disease relapse?

Maintenance therapy should be initiated at the same time or soon after induction therapy and in some cases induction and maintenance therapy are the same. Refer to Table 42.4 for a complete list of therapies used in the treatment of UC for both induction and maintenance of remission in UC. If patients achieve clinical response or remission, it is important to assess disease activity using previously discussed objective measures of disease by defining a target and optimizing therapy until the target is achieved. The STRIDE-II guidelines help providers further implement this "treat-to-target" approach.

24. Are there adjunctive therapies for UC?

One of the adjunctive therapies is Microbiota Therapy.

Probiotics, as defined by the World Health Organization, live microorganisms, which when consumed in adequate amounts confer health and benefit to the host. We know that patients with IBD have less microbial diversity than those without IBD; however, we do not yet fully understand the direct consequences of inflammation. In patients with mild UC on mesalamine, *E. coli Nissile* 1917 has been evaluated in a small study and shown when used as adjuvant therapy in mild disease. In patients with IBD who have undergone IPAA, VSL#3 (Visbiome), which is a combination of *Lactobacillus, Bifidobacterium,* and *Streptococcus* had shown benefits to reduce the incidence and recurrence of pouchitis. Some patients may ask about the benefit of fecal microbiota transplant (FMT) which currently has limited for treatment and to prevent recurrence for those with *C. difficile* infection. There is currently no role for FMT for the primary or adjuvant treatment for UC.

Vitamin and supplements

Vitamin D is a vitamin with immune system effects and up to 79% of patients with IBD are deficient in Vitamin D. Those with low Vitamin D are at increased risk for disease relapse or inadequate response to treatments, supplementation for levels ≤30 ng/mL is indicated. Omega-3 fatty acids have been shown to reduce inflammation and lower rates of UC reported among patients with a diet high in omega-3 fatty acids though the benefits remain unclear, and more studies are indicated. Curcumin (turmeric) has been shown to be anti-inflammatory. In a study looking at 50 patients with UC adding 3000 mg of turmeric as adjuvant therapy to mesalamine was beneficial.

Cannabis

Cannabis use has increased in the IBD population, mainly used for improvement in GI symptoms as the primary indication. Few high-quality studies have been done looking at the impacts of cannabis on UC. Most of the studies have shown no significant impact on clinical response. One small study showed improvement in clinical symptoms and improvement in endoscopic inflammation, however, no improvement in CRP or fecal calprotectin was noted. Overall, there seems to be less perceived benefit in patients with UC when compared to patients with CD.

25. How often should patients have surveillance colonoscopy?

The current recommendations for dysplasia and colorectal neoplasia surveillance begin in patients with UC to a greater extent than proctosigmoiditis 8 years after symptom onset. The current standard of care is the use of colonoscopy at an accepted interval of 1–5 years based on risk factors for colorectal neoplasia. Risk factors for the development of dysplasia or colorectal neoplasia are duration of disease, extent of disease, disease activity, PSC, family history of colorectal cancer, and presence of pseudopolyps (Table 42.6). Those patients with a diagnosis of PSC should begin surveillance colonoscopy at the time of diagnosis and then annually. Current accepted endoscopic techniques include the use of high-definition white light endoscopy with random biopsies throughout the colon in a 4-quadrant fashion with a minimum of 33 biopsies from the colon. Alternative techniques include the use of chromoendoscopy (either dye spray or virtual using narrow band imaging) with targeted biopsies, with or without random surveillance biopsies.

Table 42.6 Factors Associated With Increased Risk for Colorectal Dysplasia and Cancer in Inflammatory Bowel Disease.

Duration of disease
Extent of disease
Active inflammation
Primary sclerosing cholangitis
Family history of colorectal cancer
Pseudopolyposis

26. **What should be done if dysplasia is found during surveillance colonoscopy?**
It depends if the dysplasia is visible or invisible at the time of colonoscopy. Visible lesions should be resected and sent for pathologic analysis. If dysplasia is present, it is recommended that this finding is confirmed independently by a second pathologist. Complete resection of visible lesions should be followed with close surveillance and chromoendoscopy. Partial or unresectable visible lesions should be referred for advanced endoscopic techniques (Endoscopic mucosal resection or endoscopic submucosal dissection) or surgery. Invisible dysplasia (dysplasia found on random colon sampling) should be confirmed by a second pathologist and follow-up chromoendoscopy should be performed (if not done at index colonoscopy) to assess for visible resectable lesion. On a high-quality chromoendoscopy the presence of persistent high-grade or multifocal dysplasia is an indication for surgery. The presence of unifocal low-grade dysplasia would warrant intensive surveillance program including repeat high-quality chromoendoscopy in 6 months.

27. **Is there a role for chemoprevention in UC?**
There is some evidence that long-term mesalamine use may reduce the risk of colon cancer in patients with UC. However, multiple meta-analyses revealed conflicting results about the chemoprotective effects of 5-ASA compounds in the prevention of colorectal cancer in IBD. There is increasing evidence that thiopurines may have protective effects for colorectal cancer in IBD, and this is thought to be related to improved inflammation control. In fact, there is evidence that treatment with the immunosuppressive drug 6-MP is more likely to reduce the risk of colon cancer. The effects of ursodeoxycholic acid and folic acid efficacy have been equivocal. The most important colorectal cancer prevention is adequate inflammation control and appropriate surveillance colonoscopy.

28. **Is diet important in the management of UC?**
We know that patients often feel better when they restrict different foods from their diet, however, this can lead to malnutrition in some. Currently, there is no evidence suggesting that any one diet is beneficial in patients with UC. Most of the studies have researched the impact of dietary intervention in patients with CD. Patients with current active inflammation might tolerate brief dietary changes to avoid increasing symptoms including low residue diet, avoidance of lactose, nonabsorbable sugars, high-fat foods, alcohol, and caffeinated drinks. Ultimately each patient has a different experience with what "trigger" foods to increase symptoms for them. It is important for those patients at risk for malnutrition to partner with GI nutrition team members.

29. **Does stress exacerbate UC?**
There has been a reported association between perceived stress and exacerbation of IBD symptoms. In addition, anxiety and depression are more prevalent in patients with IBD. There are also emerging data regarding the prevalence of posttraumatic stress in patients with IBD which can significantly impact how one navigates medical systems and the management of their disease. Recognition of underlying stressors, coping mechanisms, and comorbid mental health diagnoses are important; therefore screening measures are recommended. Partnering with a gastrointestinal (GI) mental health expert is important in some patients to help patients cope with chronic illness and symptoms and provide therapeutic intervention. Some patients might also require the addition of an anxiolytic agent or an antidepressant.

30. **How does menstruation affect UC and how does UC impact menstruation?**
Studies have shown that female patients with UC have a similar age of menarche, however, poorly controlled inflammation has been associated with a risk for delayed menarche likely secondary to growth failure, use of corticosteroids, or malnutrition. There are reports of increased menstrual abnormalities in females with IBD. In addition, increasing clinical symptoms around the time of menses in particular abdominal discomfort and diarrhea have been reported. If oral contraception is indicated, it is important to partner with a gynecology team to find low estrogen-containing contraceptives or use an intrauterine device to reduce the risk of thromboembolism.

31. Do patients with UC have problems with fertility and pregnancy?

Patients with IBD are less likely to have children due to voluntary childlessness; however, fertility is equal in patients with IBD in remission. However, we do know that active inflammation has been associated with a decreased rate of live births in patients with IBD. Currently, there are no Food and Drug Administration-approved therapies that decrease fertility in female patients with IBD, but several therapies are contraindicated or recommended to avoid due to teratogenicity or inadequate data in pregnancy (methotrexate, tofacitinib, upadacitinib, and ozanimod). SSZ causes reversible defects in sperm morphologic characteristics and motility. It should be replaced with one of the newer 5-ASA products in male patients who are considering family planning. Another impact of IBD on fertility is related to surgery. Females who have undergone IPAA have a threefold increased risk for infertility, however, supported fertility treatments or in vitro fertilization has been effective in achieving pregnancy in these females. Regarding the impacts of IBD in pregnancy and pregnancy on IBD, patients with UC with active disease at the time of conception have a 35% chance of clinical disease relapse during pregnancy. This supports the importance of disease remission prior to planned pregnancy. It is safe to continue most IBD medications throughout pregnancy, see Question 35 for more information. It is important to maintain disease control throughout pregnancy for the best outcomes for both patient and baby.

32. Are IBD medications safe to continue throughout pregnancy?

5-ASA therapies have a long record of safety in pregnancy. If patients are taking SSZ, it is important to supplement with a dose of folic acid of 2 mg during pregnancy. Corticosteroids have also proven to be safe during pregnancy, however, goals to minimize exposure opting for steroid-sparing therapies. We have excellent data from the PIANO registry, a large registry of over 1400 patients with IBD on immunosuppressive therapies in pregnancy showing the safety of these therapies. 6-MP and AZA when used alone or in combination with biologics are safe to continue throughout pregnancy, however, we would avoid newly starting these agents during pregnancy due to the small risk of pancreatitis. All biologic therapies have been studied in patients with UC during pregnancy and have been found to be safe and effective to maintain remission during pregnancy. There are limited data on the use of tofacitinib or upadacitinib in pregnancy, but animal data in tofacitinib in doses 7-73x that were used in patients with IBD showed teratogenic effects. It is currently recommended to discontinue tofacitinib 1 week prior to planned conception. As discussed previously, ozanimod and methotrexate are contraindicated in pregnancy and should be discontinued prior to planned conception. Antibiotics are rarely used in patients with UC but avoiding metronidazole in the first trimester is recommended.

33. What medications are contraindicated in patients with UC?

Evidence suggests that NSAIDs may precipitate exacerbations of the disease and in some cases may even be implicated in the onset of disease. Whenever possible, these drugs should be avoided in patients with IBD. Opioid derivatives should be avoided, when possible, in patients with IBD as they have been associated with increased mortality. Antibiotics should be used when clinically indicated, but antibiotic use is associated with increased risk for *C. difficile* infection in patients with IBD.

34. What are the surgical options for the management of UC?

When medical management fails or complications occur (such as perforation, dysplasia, or cancer), total abdominal colectomy or proctocolectomy with ileostomy or IPAA are options reviewed with the patient. Many patients are frightened by the prospect of having an ileostomy, but education can do much to alleviate their fears. Fortunately, many patients with ileostomies become accustomed to them and continue to lead normal lives without restrictions. The IPAA is a possible alternative to a permanent ileostomy. It consists of a double loop of ileum that is fashioned into a pouch (shaped like a "J") and stapled to a 1- to 2 cm rectal cuff. Disadvantages of IPAA include risk for recurrent inflammation or pouchitis, frequent bowel movements, nocturnal bowel movements or incontinence, and the need for surveillance endoscopy of the rectal cuff. Pouchitis typically responds well to antibiotics in most cases. In patients with recurrent pouchitis, probiotics (Visbiome) can be tried to prevent recurrence. In some cases, 5-ASA products, steroids, immunosuppressives, or biologics may be required. Refractory pouchitis or complications of the pouch may require pouch excision with ileostomy.

CLINICAL VIGNETTE

Available Online

BIBLIOGRAPHY

Available Online

EOSINOPHILIC GASTROINTESTINAL DISEASES AND EOSINOPHILIC ESOPHAGITIS

CHAPTER 43

Cassandra Burger, BA and Nathalie Nguyen, MD

 Additional content available online

1. **How is eosinophilic gastrointestinal disease (EGID) defined?**

   EGID is a global term that describes an increasingly recognized heterogeneous group of gastrointestinal (GI) diseases found in both children and adults. It is characterized by chronic, nonspecific GI symptoms, and a dense eosinophilic inflammatory response that is found in various tissues throughout the GI tract. It can manifest as eosinophilic gastritis (EoG), enteritis (EoN), colitis (EoC), or well-studied eosinophilic esophagitis (EoE). The specific name is determined by the location of the GI tract involvement. Other causes of eosinophilia should be ruled out prior to making the diagnosis of EGID.

2. **What is EoE?**

   EoE is the most common form of EGID. It is a clinicopathologic disorder now recognized as a major cause of feeding difficulties, abdominal pain, vomiting, and failure to thrive in young children and food impactions and dysphagia in adults. EoE is a chronic, allergen-driven inflammatory disease process that is defined by symptoms of esophageal dysfunction and mucosal eosinophilia.

3. **What is the prevalence of EGIDs and EoE?**

   EGIDs are rare disorders with an estimated prevalence of 2.1–8.2 in 100,000, and the overall frequency of EGIDs has increased over the last decade. The incidence of EoE continues to increase, with estimates of 10 cases in 100,000 persons annually and a prevalence of 10–57 in 100,000. The vast majority of patients with EoE are white males, but both of these disease entities have a widespread geographic and ethnic distribution.

4. **What is the role of the eosinophil in the pathogenesis of EGIDs and EoE?**

   EGIDs and EoE are believed to be allergen-mediated, Th-2 cytokine inflammatory responses that develop in genetically susceptible individuals and are associated with GI eosinophilia. With the exception of the esophagus, eosinophils are prominent resident leukocytes within the intestinal mucosa whose precise role in health remains unclear. Although the exact pathogenesis is uncertain and its study is typically limited to superficial mucosal pinch biopsies obtained during endoscopy, EGIDs are thought to be stimulated by exposure to an environmental or food allergen that leads to chemoattraction and recruitment of additional eosinophils to the GI tract. The exact function of eosinophils in the GI tract is unknown, but a number of basic studies support a role in antigen presentation and as effector cells that can release a host of cytotoxic granules, cytokines, chemokines, transforming growth factors, lipid mediators, and neuromediators.

   Gene arrays and genome-wide association studies have identified several key molecules strongly associated with EoE, including thymic stromal lymphopoietin, eotaxin-3, interleukin (IL)-13, IL-4, and IL-5. Familial susceptibility has also been reported in approximately 10% of patients with EGID.

5. **What are some clinical features of EGIDs and EoE?**

   Early descriptions of EGIDs involving the GI tract distal to the esophagus classified the disease based on the identified depth of eosinophilia within the intestinal wall. The mucosal subtype can manifest as GI bleeding, diarrhea, and abdominal pain; the muscular subtype as a partial or complete intestinal obstruction; and the serosal subtype as abdominal distention or ascites (Table 43.1). Recent studies suggest a shift toward the mucosal form of the disease. Up to 75% of patients will report a personal history of atopy, including eczema, food allergies, seasonal allergies, or asthma. Additionally, peripheral eosinophilia can occur in up to 80% of patients with EGID but is variable and can also occur secondary to other comorbid allergic diseases, making this an unreliable biomarker of disease activity.

   Patients with EoE can present with a variety of signs and symptoms of esophageal dysfunction depending on the age of the individual (Table 43.2). Young children often present with feeding difficulties, abdominal pain, food refusal, or reflux-like symptoms such as regurgitation or vomiting. Teenagers and young adults typically present with dysphagia or food impaction. A high index of suspicion is required, as many individuals can develop

Table 43.1 Clinical Features of Eosinophilic Gastrointestinal Disease.

Mucosal	Abdominal pain
	Anemia
	Diarrhea
	GI bleeding
	Nausea
	Protein-losing enteropathy
	Vomiting
	Weight loss
Muscular	Abdominal pain
	Gastric outlet obstruction
	Intestinal dysmotility
	Pancreatitis
	Small intestinal obstruction
Serosal	Eosinophilic ascites
	Eosinophilic peritonitis
	Severe bloating

GI, Gastrointestinal.

Table 43.2 Clinical Features of Eosinophilic Esophagitis.

YOUNG CHILDREN	TEENAGERS AND ADULTS
Abdominal pain	Dysphagia
Chest pain	Food impaction
Gagging	Chest pain
Coughing	
Decreased appetite	
Dysphagia	
Feeding difficulties	
Regurgitation	
Vomiting	
Weight loss	

coping strategies or compensatory behaviors such as using sauces or drinking liquids to lubricate foods, chewing extensively, or avoiding foods they have difficulty swallowing such as meats and breads.

6. What is the natural history of EGIDs?

Three issues regarding the natural history of EoE have become apparent because of broader clinical experiences. First, EoE is a chronic disease in which many patients will respond to standard medical therapies. Second, complications associated with EoE include food impactions, esophageal narrowing, and feeding dysfunction. Who, how, and in whom these develop is uncertain. Third, there does not appear to be any premalignant potential to date, but long-term natural history studies are still required to assess this concern. Finally, there may be other EoE phenotypes based on whether or not patients respond to diet elimination, proton pump inhibitors, and topical steroids.

Because of their relatively low incidence and confounding GI symptoms, there is often a delay in the diagnosis of EGIDs. Based on current studies and clinical experiences, the natural history of EGIDs (except EoE) may include one of three patterns, as patients may suffer from a single occurrence, a recurrent course, or a chronic disease path. Additionally, there are several potential phenotypes based on the depth of intestinal involvement as noted above.

7. How are EGID and EoE diagnosed?

EGIDs are characterized by nonspecific GI symptoms associated with dense GI eosinophilia. The diagnosis is made with mucosal pinch biopsies obtained from upper intestinal endoscopy and/or colonoscopy. What is considered an "abnormal" number of GI eosinophils remains to be defined and is a matter that should be discussed between clinicians and pathologists at local institutions. Diagnostic guidelines have been established for EoE (Box 43.1).

Box 43.1 Diagnostic Criteria for Eosinophilic Esophagitis

Symptoms associated with esophageal dysfunction.
Esophageal biopsy demonstrates eosinophil-predominant inflammation with a peak value of ≥ 15 eosinophils per high-power field.
Secondary causes of esophageal eosinophilia are excluded.

Any patient with a concern for EGID should undergo a thorough evaluation to exclude any other causes of GI eosinophilia. No pathognomonic signs, symptoms, or blood tests exist for defining EGID or EoE. Depending on the specific intestinal organ involved and its accompanying symptoms, there are several approaches.

History and Physical Examination

- Obtain a comprehensive history, including social and family history that accurately outlines all GI and extraintestinal symptoms. This includes timing of onset, duration, progression, aggravating and alleviating factors, associated symptoms (e.g., weight loss), responses to previous medical therapy, travel history, and family history of EGIDs, food impactions, and esophageal dilations. Assess for normal growth and development.
- Inquire about atopic signs or symptoms pertaining to GI, dermatologic, or respiratory reactions to food or environmental antigens.
- Perform a thorough physical examination with particular attention to weight and height, stigmata of atopic disease, and signs of extraintestinal examination findings of other diseases (e.g., skin rash, arthritis, oral lesions, and perianal disease).

Laboratory Tests

- General evaluation: Obtain complete blood count with differential, total immunoglobulin E, erythrocyte sedimentation rate, and stool for infectious evaluation (e.g., ova and parasites, *Helicobacter pylori*).
- Advanced evaluation: If ascites are present, perform paracentesis with cell count and differential. If peripheral eosinophilia is present, consider bone marrow analysis, echocardiogram, serum vitamin B_{12} and tryptase, genetic analysis for FIPL1-PDGFRA mutation, and biopsy and evaluation of other involved tissues.
- Allergy evaluation: Referral to an allergist experienced in the assessment of non–IgE-mediated food allergy is suggested, as unwarranted limitation of foods may lead to malnutrition.

Endoscopy and Histopathologic Examination

- Depending on the location of GI symptoms, an upper intestinal endoscopy or colonoscopy with biopsies is essential to the diagnosis of EGID (Fig. 43.1).
- EoE can be associated with several endoscopic findings such as mucosal edema, esophageal rings, exudate, furrows, crepe paper appearance, small caliber esophagus, and strictures (Fig. 43.2). However, a normal mucosal appearance does not rule out EoE; in fact, one study identified over 15% of patients with suspected EoE and normal endoscopy to have histologic evidence of EoE.
- Endoscopic findings described in EGID with involvement of the stomach include erythema, nodularity, erosions, ulcerations, granularity, thickened gastric folds, and pyloric stenosis. Multiple mucosal pinch biopsies should be obtained because of the limited capture achieved by this technique and because EGIDs and EoE can have a *patchy* distribution. In cases in which deeper involvement is suspected, a surgical full-thickness biopsy may be indicated.

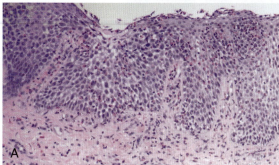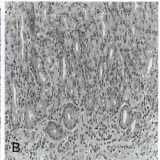

Fig. 43.1 (A) Esophageal biopsy demonstrating eosinophilic esophagitis and (B) gastric antrum biopsy demonstrating eosinophilic gastritis.

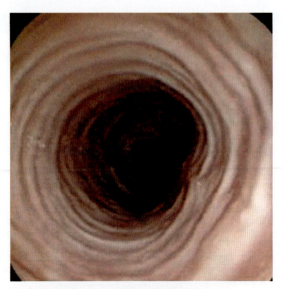

Fig. 43.2 Endoscopic view of rings of the esophagus in eosinophilic esophagitis.

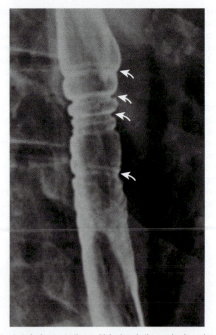

Fig. 43.3 Upper gastrointestinal contrast study demonstrating multiple rings in the proximal esophagus in eosinophilic esophagitis.

Radiologic Evaluation

- Barium esophagram is useful in evaluating patients with dysphagia and may demonstrate mucosal irregularities, long segment narrowing, or focal esophageal strictures that may not be evident during endoscopy (Fig. 43.3).
- Upper GI contrast studies and computed tomography with enteral contrast may demonstrate mucosal irregularities or evidence of obstruction in areas affected by EGID. They can also be used to rule out other etiologic factors such as malrotation and inflammatory bowel diseases.
- Abdominal ultrasound can help identify ascites.

Minimally Invasive Methods of Disease Monitoring
- Trans-nasal endoscopy involves passing an ultrathin endoscope through the nasal passage and into the esophagus where biopsies can be obtained. This procedure is performed without sedation and is a method of disease monitoring in EoE.
- The esophageal string test is a non-endoscopic, minimally invasive method of monitoring disease activity. The patient swallows a capsule with a string that is left in place for one hour. Upon removal, the string can be analyzed for eosinophil-associated biomarkers (eotaxin-3 [Eot3]) and major basic protein-1 concentrations.

8. What is the differential diagnosis of GI eosinophilia?
The differential diagnosis of EGID and EoE includes a host of diseases that also present with GI symptoms and eosinophil-predominant inflammation. Table 43.3 illustrates the breadth of these diseases and the importance of evaluating patients with eosinophils on intestinal biopsy.

9. What are current treatment and management strategies for EGID and EoE?
The treatment of EoE includes dietary elimination, medications including proton pump inhibitors and topical corticosteroids, and esophageal dilation.

Dietary Modification
- Elemental diet (i.e., amino acid–based formula).
- Targeted food elimination based on allergy testing.
- The most common food allergies are dairy, wheat, soy, eggs, nuts, and seafood/shellfish. A step-up approach (2–4–6) to dietary elimination, starting with the most common offending foods has been shown to be effective and practical: step 1 (dairy); step 2 (dairy, wheat); step 4 (dairy, wheat, egg, and soy); and step 6 (all six of the common food allergies).

Table 43.3 Differential Diagnosis of Intestinal Eosinophilia.

PRIMARY EGID	OTHER CAUSES OF INTESTINAL EOSINOPHILIA
Eosinophilic esophagitis	Achalasia Celiac disease Connective tissue diseases (e.g., scleroderma) Crohn disease Drug hypersensitivity Eosinophilic gastroenteritis GERD Graft-versus-host disease Hypereosinophilic syndrome Iatrogenic (e.g., medications) Infection Leiomyomatosis Pemphigus
Eosinophilic gastritis/enteritis	Celiac disease Connective tissue diseases (e.g., scleroderma) Hypereosinophilic syndrome Iatrogenic (e.g., medications) Infection Inflammatory bowel disease Inflammatory fibroid polyps, polyposis Vasculitis (e.g., Churg-Strauss syndrome) Transplant
Eosinophilic colitis	Celiac disease Connective tissue diseases (e.g., scleroderma) Eosinophilic gastroenteritis Hypereosinophilic syndrome Iatrogenic (e.g., medications) Infection Inflammatory bowel disease Juvenile polyps, polyposis, adenomas Vasculitis (e.g., Churg-Strauss syndrome)

EGID, Eosinophilic gastrointestinal disease; *GERD*, gastroesophageal reflux disease.

Medication
- Proton pump inhibitors (e.g., omeprazole and lansoprazole).
- Topical steroids (e.g., fluticasone and budesonide).
- Systemic steroids (e.g., prednisone and methylprednisolone).

Therapeutic Interventions
- Endoscopic dilation (preferably following pretreatment with steroids) for esophageal strictures in EoE.

Because of its low prevalence, prospective, multicenter studies on EGID treatment are lacking, but current management strategies include diet elimination or different formulations of steroids such as systemic steroids or enteral-coated budesonide (Entocort) capsules.

Therapeutic endpoints include normalizing growth and development for children, minimizing symptoms, balancing risks and benefits of treatment with quality of life, and normalization of mucosal findings when possible. Specific treatment strategies should be tailored to the individual, taking into consideration factors such as extent of disease, severity of symptoms, cost, and compliance.

ACKNOWLEDGMENT

The authors would like to acknowledge the contributions of Dr. Glenn Furuta and Shahan Fernando who were the authors of this chapter in the previous edition.

CLINICAL VIGNETTE

Available Online

BIBLIOGRAPHY

Available Online

CHAPTER 44

SMALL INTESTINAL BACTERIAL OVERGROWTH

Roderick Seth Brown, DO and Jack A. Di Palma, MD

 Additional content available online

1. **Define small intestinal bacterial overgrowth (SIBO).**
   The presence of excessive numbers of bacteria in the small bowel causes gastrointestinal symptoms. In regards to objective quantification of bacterial overgrowth, a bacterial colony count $\geq 10^3$ colony-forming units per milliliter (CFU/mL) in a duodenal aspirate is diagnostic. These coliform bacteria are usually only found in the colon.

2. **What is the usual bacterial presence in the gastrointestinal tract?**
   - Oral cavity 200 speciesOral cavity 200 species
   - Stomach $<10^3$
   - Duodenum and proximal jejunum 10^{2-3}/mL
   - Ileum 10^8/mL
   - Colon 10^{10-11}/mL

   The type of species that colonize the small intestine is changed in bacterial overgrowth. In health, small bowel bacteria resemble oropharyngeal flora with Gram-positive, facultative bacteria, which can survive under aerobic or anaerobic conditions. In overgrowth, bacteria are mostly Gram-negative, such as *Escherichia coli*; anaerobic bacteria, including *Clostridia* and *Bacteroides* spp., also predominate (Fig. 44.1).

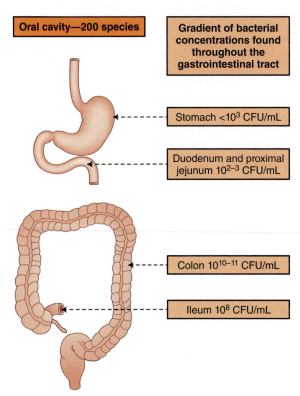

Fig. 44.1 Gradient of bacterial concentrations found throughout the gastrointestinal tract. *CFU*, Colony-forming units.

3. **What are the natural protective mechanisms against SIBO?**
   - Peristalsis
   - Gastric acid
   - Bile acid
   - Pancreatic enzyme activity
   - Small intestinal motility (migrating motor complex)
   - Ileocecal valve

4. **What factors influence small intestinal bacterial proliferation?**
   - Structural lesions
   - Surgically altered anatomy
   - Motility
   - Excessive bacterial load
   - Deficiency in host immune defenses

5. **What kind of abnormalities predispose to bacterial overgrowth?**
   Obstruction to the outflow of luminal contents can occur at the site of surgical anastomosis or with webs, adhesions, or strictures. Surgical diversions and blind loops or neoreservoirs, such as the continent ileostomy, predispose to SIBO. Diverticula and duplications are frequently colonized with colonic-type bacteria, leading to overgrowth. There is an increased prevalence of SIBO in disorders that may result in intestinal failure. There is a frequent association of SIBO with Crohn disease, especially among those who have undergone surgery (Table 44.1).

Table 44.1 Physiologic Abnormalities and Overgrowth.	
Anatomic abnormalities	Surgical anastomosis, webs, adhesions, stricture, small intestinal diverticulosis, blind loop, neoreservoirs, and acute enteric infection
Abnormal communications	Gastrocolic fistula, enterocolic fistula, and ileocecal valve resection
Motility disorder	Scleroderma, diabetes mellitus, pseudoobstruction, opioid use, medications that alter motility, achlorhydria, radiation enteritis, and irritable bowel syndrome
Reduced acid secretion	Medications, atrophic gastritis, and vagotomy
Various mechanisms	Crohn disease, celiac disease, rheumatoid arthritis, obesity, cirrhosis, chronic pancreatitis, chronic kidney disease, cystic fibrosis, amyloidosis, acromegaly, and focal segmental ischemia

6. **How do motility disorders cause bacterial overgrowth?**
   Delayed transit of intestinal contents results in stasis. Overgrowth complicates intestinal pseudoobstruction syndromes. The *intestinal housekeeper* migratory motor complex, when disrupted, is associated with bacterial overgrowth. Paralytic ileus results in bacterial proliferation. SIBO has been identified in 62.5% of patients with scleroderma. Any condition with disordered motility, such as diabetes, irritable bowel syndrome, or medications, predisposes to overgrowth.

7. **How can an excessive bacterial load be delivered to the small bowel?**
   Absence or incompetence of the ileocecal valve and enteric fistula can deliver colonic bacteria to the small bowel in amounts that exceed clearing capacity.

8. **Which impairments of host defenses are important for the development of SIBO?**
   - Acid suppression by surgery or medications (after initial suggestions that proton pump inhibitor use was a risk factor for SIBO, recent work has not found an association)
   - Hypochlorhydria disorders such as pernicious anemia
   - Immune deficiencies, particularly the absence of secretory immunoglobulin A
   - Undernutrition, which can decrease gastric acidity and immune function
   - Cirrhosis, which can lead to abnormal motility and overgrowth with increased incidence of spontaneous bacterial peritonitis

9. **What are the symptoms of bacterial overgrowth?**
   Clinical manifestations vary. Abdominal bloating, pain, gas, distension, flatulence, and diarrhea are the most common symptoms described in SIBO and occur in nearly two-thirds of patients. Patients obstructed by stricture may have bloating and pain. Overgrowth in small intestinal diverticula may present insidiously with metabolic derangements.

10. What is the differential diagnosis of bacterial overgrowth?

Differential diagnosis includes irritable bowel syndrome, lactose and fructose intolerance, celiac sprue, Whipple disease, microscopic colitis, community-acquired *Clostridium difficile* infection, hyper- and hypothyroidism, and medication adverse effects.

11. Why do patients with bacterial overgrowth develop anemia?

Anemia may be megaloblastic and macrocytic as a result of cobalamin deficiency. Microcytic anemia due to iron deficiency results mainly from blood loss or small bowel damage that is *not caused by bacterial overgrowth*. Anaerobic bacteria compete with the host for uptake of cobalamin-intrinsic factor complex, predisposing to vitamin B_{12} deficiency. Whereas luminal bacteria consume cobalamin, folic acid is a product of bacterial substrate fermentation. Thus an important clinical observation in SIBO is the finding of low vitamin B_{12} and high folate levels.

12. What other micronutrient deficiencies are clinically important?

In most cases, micronutrient deficiencies are subtle or undetectable. However, in severe cases, nutritional deficiencies including vitamin B_{12}, vitamin D, and iron deficiencies can occur due to small bowel mucosal derangements with brush border defects and bile acid deconjugation. In addition to iron, calcium, and cobalamin deficiencies, other micronutrient deficiencies include deficiencies of water-soluble vitamins (e.g., thiamine and nicotinamide) and decreased absorption of fat-soluble vitamins (vitamins A, D, E, and K). Trace element malabsorption has not been carefully studied in overgrowth syndromes.

13. How is SIBO diagnosed?

The gold standard for diagnosis is the aspiration of small intestinal fluid and culture. More than 10^3 CFU/mL of duodenal aspirate is diagnostic. See Table 44.2 for the diagnostic approach.

Table 44.2 Diagnosis of Small Intestinal Bacterial Overgrowth.	
History	Prior surgery, older age, medical conditions, or medicines associated with altered motility, evidence of malabsorption or malnutrition such as metabolic bone disease, night blindness, easy bruisability, and tetany
Examination	Evidence of systemic disease: weight loss, malnutrition, and malabsorption
Laboratory values	Hemoglobin (decreased), mean corpuscular volume (increased), vitamin B_{12} (decreased), folic acid (increased), and fecal fat (increased)
Tests	Hydrogen testing with glucose or lactulose, duodenal aspirate for bacterial colony counts and strain identification

14. What testing methods can be used?

- Duodenal intubation for aspiration with bacterial colony counts and stain identification can provide a definitive diagnosis by showing duodenal counts greater than 10^3 CFU/mL. There is a risk of potential contamination by oropharyngeal bacteria contaminating the biopsy channel of endoscopes used to obtain small bowel culture samples. Additionally, bacterial overgrowth can be patchy and thus missed by a single aspiration. Because the test is cumbersome and invasive, most clinicians rely on indirect testing. Duodenal intubation can be performed endoscopically, and protected catheters can be used to obtain more reliable aspirates.
- Radiolabeled breath tests using glycocholic acid or xylose have been used for the diagnosis of overgrowth. Glycocholic acid is released by bacterial deconjugation of radiolabeled bile acids. Xylose is catabolized by Gram-negative aerobes and is absorbed in the proximal small bowel. This technique is no longer used because of safety concerns regarding radiolabeled substrates.
- Fasting breath tests use a carbohydrate substrate (traditionally glucose or lactulose) to assess the production of hydrogen and methane gases. This is based on the premise that human cells are incapable of producing hydrogen and methane gas, thus, signifying the fermentation of carbohydrates by microbes in the gut. An increase in hydrogen concentrations $\geq$20 parts per million (ppm) from baseline within 90–120 minutes is recommended to be diagnostic of SIBO (Fig. 44.2). Methane creates a nomenclature problem when assessing for SIBO as methanogenic archaea in the gut use hydrogen as a substrate in the production of methane. Due to this new proposals have been made for a new term, intestinal methanogen overgrowth. The presence of methane levels >10 ppm is diagnostic of methanogenic overgrowth. *Methanobrevibacter smithii* appears to be the key methanogen responsible for breath methane production.

  In general, hydrogen breath tests are attractive alternatives to intubation tests for bacterial overgrowth. Hydrogen testing, although simple, inexpensive, available, and nonradioactive, has limited sensitivity and specificity.

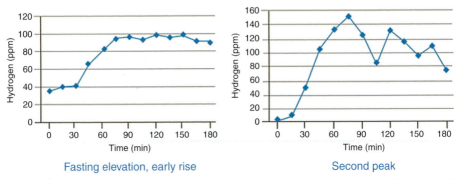

Fig. 44.2 Hydrogen (H2) in parts per million (ppm) ≥20 ppm from baseline within 90–120 min is diagnostic for small intestinal bacterial overgrowth. While not required for diagnosis, a second peak can be observed from colonic bacterial fermentation.

15. **What about other testing methods?**

Quantification of urinary excretion of indican, drug metabolites, and conjugated *para*-aminobenzoic acid does not distinguish overgrowth from other types of malabsorption. An alternative approach to consider is a therapeutic trial of antibiotics. Most patients with SIBO show a symptomatic response within 1 week of initiation of therapy.

16. **What is the treatment for SIBO?**
    - Correction of the underlying condition (if possible)
    - Nutrition
        - Lactose-free, low-residue diet
        - Increase calories
        - Micronutrient supplementation (vitamin B_{12}, fat-soluble vitamins, and trace elements)
    - Antibiotics

17. **What are the antibiotic agents used in the treatment of SIBO?**
    - Amoxicillin-clavulanic acid (875 mg twice daily)
    - Ciprofloxacin (500 mg twice daily)
    - Doxycycline (100 mg twice daily)
    - Metronidazole (250 mg three times daily)
    - Neomycin (500 mg four times daily)
    - Norfloxacin (800 mg daily)
    - Rifaximin (550 mg three times daily)
    - Trimethoprim-sulfamethoxazole (160 mg/800 mg twice daily)
        Rifaximin seems to have superior efficacy and is preferred as it is a nonabsorbable antibiotic.

18. **Do prokinetic agents help?**

Surgery is often impractical or unacceptable, and prokinetic agents can help to relieve stasis and improve the outflow of small intestinal contents. However, standard prokinetic agents are not very effective. In high dosages, the long-acting somatostatin analog, octreotide, can cause steatorrhea, but in low doses, it has been shown to promote motility in normal subjects and patients with slow intestinal motility, that is, scleroderma.

19. **How long should SIBO be treated with antibiotics?**

The objective of antibiotic therapy is not to eradicate the bacterial flora but rather to modify the bacterial milieu in a manner that results in symptomatic improvement. In general, a 7- to 14-day course of antibiotics may improve symptoms for several months in 46%–90% of patients and result in negative breath tests in 20%–75%. After completion of therapy, symptoms should be reassessed. Some patients may require extended therapy, continuous courses, or rotating antibiotic regimens. Prolonged antibiotic therapy poses significant risks, including resistance and enterocolitis (Fig. 44.3).

20. **Can prebiotics be used to treat SIBO?**

Prebiotics are nondigestible, fermentable feeds that stimulate the growth and activity of endogenous colonic bacteria, preferentially *Lactobacillus* and *Bifidobacteria*. There are minimal data regarding their clinical use.

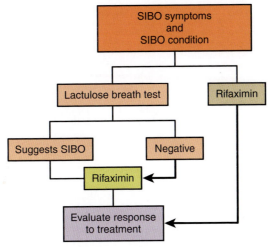

Fig. 44.3 Algorithm to evaluate response to antibiotic treatment. *SIBO*, Small intestinal bacterial overgrowth.

21. **Can probiotics be used to treat SIBO?**
    There is a lack of consistent data to support recommending specific probiotics in the treatment of SIBO.

22. **Is there a role for fecal microbiota transplantation in treating SIBO?**
    There are currently no data to support the use of fecal microbiota transplant in the treatment of SIBO.

CLINICAL VIGNETTE

Available Online

BIBLIOGRAPHY

Available Online

COLON DISORDERS AND COLON CANCER

Carol Rouphael, MD, Carole Macaron, MD and Carol Ann Burke, MD

CHAPTER 45

 Additional content available online

1. **What are the incidence and mortality rates of colorectal cancer (CRC)?**
   In the United States, CRC is the third most commonly diagnosed cancer in males and females. According to data from the Surveillance, Epidemiology, and End Results (SEER) population-based cancer registries, the age-adjusted incidence rate during the period 2015–19 was 37.7 per 100,000 males and females per year. Overall, the lifetime risk of CRC is about 1 in 23 (4.3%) for males and 1 in 25 (4.0%) for females.
   In terms of death rates, CRC is the second leading cause of cancer death in the United States. The age-adjusted mortality rate during the period 2015–19 was 13.4 per 100,000 males and females per year. It is anticipated that 52,580 individuals will die from CRC in 2022.

2. **What is the trend in CRC incidence and mortality rates in the United States in the most recent years?**
   CRC incidence rates established from the most recent data (2010–19) decreased on average by 1.8% per year. Decreases have been largely attributed to increases in the use of CRC screening, removal of colorectal polyps, and lifestyle modification. Observational studies of screening colonoscopy suggest an effect of more than 50% reduction in CRC mortality. Mortality from CRC has also been steadily declining in the United States by 2% per year. This downward trend is mostly in older adults and contrasts with the rising incidence among younger adults observed since the mid-1990s.

3. **How is young-onset CRC defined and what are its implications?**
   Young-onset CRC refers to CRC diagnosed in adults younger than age 50. During the period 2012–16, CRC incidence increased by 2% every year in individuals younger than 50. It is estimated that by 2030, about 1 in 10 colon cancers and 1 in 4 rectal cancers will be diagnosed in patients under age 50. The increasing rate is alarming, and in 2021, the US Preventative Service Task Force (USPSTF) modified their screening recommendation, endorsing starting CRC screening at the age of 45. This was subsequently adopted by the US Multi-Society Task Force (USMSTF) on CRC, which represents the American College of Gastroenterology (ACG), the American Gastroenterological Association, and the American Society for Gastrointestinal Endoscopy.

4. **What is the effect of sex and ethnicity on CRC incidence and mortality?**
   CRC is more common in males than females. Despite improvements in screening and treatment, studies show that racial disparities persist in CRC incidence and mortality. Non-Hispanic Black and non-Hispanic American/Indian Alaska Native males have the highest CRC incidence (52.4 and 52.3 per 100,000, respectively) and mortality (22.7 and 21.3 per 100,000, respectively) compared to Non-Hispanic White males (CRC incidence of 43.5 per 100,000 and CRC mortality of 15.8 per 100,000). Non-Hispanic Asian/Pacific Islanders have the lowest CRC incidence (36.4 and 26 per 100,000 males and females, respectively) and mortality (11.1 and 7.9 per 100,000 males and females, respectively).

5. **Describe the molecular pathways leading to CRC.**
   Three distinct forms of genomic instability have been recognized and constitute three different molecular pathways to colon carcinogenesis:
   - Chromosomal instability is the most common pathway to colon cancer, accounting for 80% of cases. The resulting genomic instability is characterized by loss of heterozygosity by loss of a wild-type copy of a tumor suppressor gene such as *APC*. The colon cancer precursor lesion in this pathway is the adenoma.
   - The microsatellite instability (MSI) pathway is due to the inactivation of a mismatch repair (*MMR*) gene (*MLH1, MSH2, PMS2,* and *MSH6*). The loss of *MMR* gene function causes the inability to repair DNA within the repetitive DNA sequences known as microsatellites.
   - The CpG island methylator phenotype pathway is a cause of approximately 20% of CRC. The serrated neoplasm is the precursor to these cancers.

6. **List the risk factors implicated in the development of sporadic CRC.**
   Several meta-analyses of prospective observational studies have summarized evidence for the associations between dietary factors and the incidence of CRC. A recent umbrella review of 45 published meta-analyses found convincing evidence to support certain direct and inverse associations, as presented in Table 45.1.

Table 45.1 Dietary Factors Implicated in the Development of Colorectal Cancer and Respective Relative Risks.

RISK FACTORS/EXPOSURES	RR	QUALITY OF EVIDENCE
Alcohol		
>4 drinks a day vs. non- or occasional drinkers	1.58 (1.38–1.8)	Convincing, Class I
Red meat		
High vs. low	1.13 (1.08–1.19)	Convincing, Class I
Processed meat		
High vs. low	1.14 (1.07–1.23)	Suggestive, Class III
Dietary calcium		
High vs. low	0.77 (0.73-0.82)	Convincing, Class I
Total dietary fiber		
High vs. low	0.84 (0.78–0.89)	Convincing, Class I

RR, Relative risk.

   Cigarette smoking is a well-established CRC risk factor. Compared to nonsmokers, ever smokers are at an increased risk of CRC and death from CRC, with a pooled relative risk of 1.18 (95% confidence interval [CI], 1.11–1.25) for CRC incidence and 1.25 (95% CI, 1.14–1.37) for CRC mortality.

7. **What is the risk of CRC in patients with inflammatory bowel disease (IBD) and in those with primary sclerosing cholangitis (PSC)?**
   Patients with IBD are at increased risk of CRC with one study demonstrating a 7% risk after 30 years of disease. Surveillance for CRC should occur every 1–3 years depending on the patient's risk. PSC is another independent risk factor for CRC with a stable 2.3% risk at 10 and 20 years. In those with concomitant IBD and PSC, one study showed a 14% and 31% risk of CRC development at 10 and 20 years, respectively. Once PSC is diagnosed, colon cancer screening should begin immediately and surveillance should occur on a yearly basis.

8. **What is the difference between synchronous and metachronous CRC?**
   Synchronous CRC is defined by the presence of more than one tumor at presentation. Metachronous CRC is defined by the subsequent development of another primary colorectal tumor on follow-up.

9. **What are the clinical manifestations of CRC?**
   CRC can present with a variety of symptoms: change in bowel habits, hematochezia or melena, weakness, iron-deficiency anemia, abdominal pain, and weight loss. Streptococcus bovis bacteremia, entero-enteric fistula, and diverticulitis are other unusual presentations of CRC. Left-sided colonic tumors are more likely to present with obstructive symptoms than right-sided colonic tumors. Right-sided colon cancers are more likely to present at an advanced stage because of the large capacity of the cecum and ascending colon.

10. **How is CRC pathologically staged?**
    CRC is classified using the tumor-node-metastasis (TNM) system based on the depth of the primary tumor (T), presence of locoregional lymph node involvement (N), and presence of metastatic disease (M) in other organs. The TNM staging is summarized in Tables 45.2 and 45.3.

11. **What is the relative survival rate for CRC and has it improved over the years?**
    Cancer stage at diagnosis significantly influences the patient's 5-year survival. According to the SEER database, all stages combined, the 5-year relative survival rates for colon and rectal cancer are 64% and 67%, respectively. For localized CRC the 5-year relative survival rate is as high as 90%, and for the advanced stage the 5-year

Table 45.2 Tumor-Node-Metastasis (TNM) Classification of Colon Cancer.

T STAGE	N STAGE	M STAGE
T0: No tumor	N0: No lymph node metastasis	M0: No distant metastasis on imaging
Tis: Adenocarcinoma in situ (tumor limited to the mucosa)	N1: One to three regional lymph nodes are positive, or any number of tumor deposits are present, and all identifiable lymph nodes are negative	M1: Metastasis to one or more distant organs or peritoneal metastasis
T1: Tumor invades the submucosa	N2: N2a: Four to six regional lymph nodes are positive N2b: Seven or more regional lymph nodes are positive	
T2: Tumor invades the muscularis propria		
T3: Tumor invades through the muscularis propria into the pericolorectal tissue		
T4: T4a: Tumor invades visceral peritoneum T4b: Tumor invades or adhere to adjacent organs		

Table 45.3 Tumor-Node-Metastasis (TNM) Stages of Colon Cancer.

TNM STAGE	
I	T1-2, N0, M0
IIA	T3, N0, M0
IIB	T4a, N0, M0
IIC	T4b, N0, M0
IIIA	T1-2, N1, M0 T1, N2a, M0
IIIB	T3-4, N1, M0 T2-3, N2a, M0 T1-2, N2b, M0
IIIC	T4a, N2a, M0 T3-T4a, N2b, M0 T4b, N1-2, M0
IV	Any T, any N, M1

relative survival is as low as 15%. Advances in the diagnosis and treatment of CRC in the past decade have contributed to improved survival from the disease.

12. **Differentiate microsatellite stability (MSS) from MSI: low (MSI-L) and high MSI (MSI-H).**
Defects in the function of MMR proteins in the CRC are usually caused by promoter methylation or bi-allelic pathogenic variants (PVs) or by loss of heterozygosity but can also be caused by germline MMR gene PVs as in Lynch syndrome, resulting in tumor MMR deficiency (MMRd). MMRd alters the length of repetitive DNA sequences in the tumor, called MSI. Tumors with MSI can be classified as either MSI high (MSI-H) or MSI low (MSI-L)

depending on the number of DNA markers showing instability. Using a five-marker panel, MSI-H tumors are those that have two or more of the five markers showing instability, and MSI-L, if only one of the five markers shows instability. Tumors without DNA marker instability are called MSS.

13. What are the prognostic implications of MSI-H tumors?

In most studies, MSI-H tumors have been associated with significant advantages compared with MSS tumors including a survival benefit independent of tumor stage, lower likelihood to metastasize to regional lymph nodes or distant organs, and have lower rates of colon cancer mortality. Treatment with programmed death 1 (PD-1) blockade has been found to be highly effective in MSI-H metastatic CRC that has not responded to standard chemotherapy, with a recent phase 3 open-label trial showing longer progression-free survival when PD-1 inhibitors are received as first-line therapy compared to standard chemotherapy.

14. What is the role of carcinoembryonic antigen (CEA) in the screening, diagnosis, prognosis, and surveillance of CRC?

CEA-related cell adhesion molecule 5, or CEACAM5 (also called CEA), is a high-molecular-weight glycoprotein that belongs to the immunoglobulin superfamily. The National Institutes of Health Consensus Conference and the American Society of Clinical Oncology Expert Panel do not recommend using CEA to screen or diagnose CRC cancer because of its low sensitivity and specificity. A CEA level is recommended preoperatively. If it is high before surgery, it is expected to normalize following successful surgery to remove all of the cancer. A rising CEA level indicates the progression or recurrence of the cancer.

15. How is CRC clinically staged?

Patients with invasive colon cancer require a complete staging workup, including:
- Complete blood count, chemistry profile, CEA
- Computed tomography (CT) scan of chest, abdomen, and pelvis
- Colonoscopy with tumor biopsy

According to the National Comprehensive Cancer Network (NCCN), a positron emission tomography (PET) scan is not routinely indicated at baseline in the absence of synchronous metastatic disease. If suspicious lesions are seen on CT or magnetic resonance imaging, then a PET scan may be appropriate for further delineation.

16. What are the treatment options for early-stage colon cancer?

Surgery is the treatment of choice and offers the best chance of long-term cure. Because pericolic mesenteric lymph nodes are the initial site of metastatic spread, an en-bloc resection of the primary tumor with adequate margins and removal of the regional lymph nodes is recommended. The resection should include the tumor and 5 cm of normal tissue margins on each side of the tumor. A minimum of 12 lymph nodes must be examined to accurately stage colon cancer.

17. When should a follow-up colonoscopy be done after curative surgical resection of CRC?

According to the USMSTF on CRC, patients with curative resection of CRC should undergo a high-quality colonoscopy 1 year after resection and if normal in 3 years, and if normal every 5 years thereafter. If neoplastic polyps are found guidelines for postpolypectomy, and surveillance should be followed. In the case of a patient with an obstructing CRC who did not have a complete clearing colonoscopy preoperatively, the first colonoscopy should be performed 3–6 months after surgery.

18. What are the treatment options for rectal cancer?

The management of rectal cancer involves resection, chemotherapy, and radiation therapy depending on the stage of the disease, with a multidisciplinary treatment approach. Small superficially invasive adenocarcinomas can be removed via polypectomy or local transanal excision if the latter is not feasible. For more invasive tumors, transabdominal excision is recommended. Pre- and/or postoperative chemoradiation or radiation therapy alone is recommended for patients with more advanced disease or depending on the margins of the surgical specimen.

19. At what age should CRC screening begin in average-risk individuals?

Average-risk CRC screening is recommended to begin at age 45 due to the rising incidence and mortality of CRC in individuals under age 50. The recommendation is based upon modeling studies showing benefits of screening outweigh its harms and is endorsed by the ACG, the USMSTF, and the USPSTF.

20. When should CRC screening and surveillance stop?

The USPSTF, USMSTF, and ACG recommend no screening after age 85 due to competing causes of mortality. In patients aged 75–85 years, the decisions to screen should be individualized based on past screening history, comorbidities, and life expectancy. The USMSTF suggests individuals aged 75–85 years with high-risk adenomas may benefit from surveillance but the decision should be individualized based upon aforementioned factors.

21. What are the recommended options for CRC screening?

A variety of average-risk CRC screening options are endorsed by the USPSTF, USMSTF, and ACG. These are elucidated in Table 45.4.

Table 45.4 Screening Options for Average-Risk Colorectal Cancer.

METHOD	INTERVAL	ACG	USMSTF	USPSTF
High sensitivity gFOBT	1 year	Y	No comment	Y
FIT	1 year	Y	Y	Y
MTsDNA[a]	1–3 years	Y	Y	Y
CT colonography	5 years	Y	Y	Y
Flexible sigmoidoscopy	5–10 years	Y	Y	Y
Capsule colonoscopy	5 years	Y	Y	Y
Septin 9		N	N	No comment

ACG, American College of Gastroenterology; CT, computed tomography; gFOBT, guaiac fecal occult blood test; FIT, fecal immunochemical test; MTsDNA, multitarget stool DNA; N, not recommended; USMSTF, US Multi-Society Task Force on Colorectal Cancer; USPSTF, US Preventive Services Task Force.
[a]1–3 years per USPTF, 3 years per ACG and USMSTF.

22. What are the recommended options for CRC screening in individuals with a family history of CRC or advanced polyps?

Such options are shown in Table 45.5.

Table 45.5 Screening Options for Individuals With Family History of Colorectal Cancer or Advanced Polyps.

FAMILY HISTORY	RECOMMENDATION
CRC or advanced polyp in 1 FDR at age <60 years or CRC or advanced polyp in ≥2 FDR at any age	Colonoscopy every 5 years beginning at age 40 or 10 years before the youngest affected relative, whichever is earlier
CRC or advanced polyp in 1 FDR at age ≥60 years	Average-risk screening options beginning at age 40
1 SDR with CRC or advanced polyp	Average-risk CRC screening options

Advanced serrated polyp: serrated polyp ≥10 mm, SSP with dysplasia and traditional serrated adenoma; advanced adenoma: adenoma ≥10 mm, or with villous features, or high-grade dysplasia. CRC, Colorectal cancer; FDR, first-degree relative; SDR, second-degree relative; SSP, sessile serrated polyp.

23. What are the stool-based CRC screening tests?

The stool tests include the guaiac fecal occult blood test (gFOBT), fecal immunochemical test (FIT), and multitarget stool DNA (MTsDNA). FIT measures human hemoglobin and has supplanted gFOBT, with greater patient adherence, not requiring dietary or medication restrictions, and is associated with greater patient adherence with fewer test samples required than gFOBT. FIT has no utility for serrated colorectal lesion detection. The USMSTF recommends a FIT positivity threshold of ≤20 mg/g. The commercially available MTsDNA (known as Cologuard) includes two DNA methylation markers, an assessment of *KRAS* mutations, a marker of total human DNA and a FIT. MTsDNA is approved only in average-risk adults aged 45–85 years.

24. How do fecal occult blood tests identify blood in the stool?

Fecal blood tests are stool-based CRC screening tests designed to detect occult blood loss from colorectal neoplasms. The gFOBT detects blood through the pseudoperoxidase activity of heme or hemoglobin which converts the colorless guaiac to a blue color. The FIT test is an antibody that reacts with human globin.

25. Compare the diagnostic accuracy of MTsDNA with FIT.

The landmark trial comparing MTsDNA and FIT showed a sensitivity for CRC and advanced adenomas and sessile serrated polyps (SSPs) ≥10 mm of 92.3% and 42.4% versus 73.8% and 23.8% ($P = .002$ and $P < .001$), respectively. The specificity for CRC for MTsDNA and FIT were 86.6% and 94.9% ($P < .001$), respectively.

26. **What are some of the key quality indicators for high-quality colonoscopy?**
    These quality indicators are shown in Table 45.6.

Table 45.6 Quality Indicators for High-Quality Colonoscopy.

METRIC	BENCHMARK
Adequate bowel preparation including photodocumentation	≥95% in outpatients ≥85% in inpatients
Complete to cecum including photodocumentation	≥95% in outpatients ≥90% in inpatients
Adenoma detection rate: screening and surveillance examinations	≥30% in males ≥20% in females
Adenoma detection rate in FIT-positive individuals	≥45% in males ≥35% in females
Colonoscope withdrawal time	≥6 minutes
Recommended colonoscopy interval followed	≥90%

FIT, Fecal immunochemical test.

27. **What is postcolonoscopy CRC (PCCRC)?**
    The term postcolonoscopy colorectal cancer is recommended to be used to define a CRC occurring after a colonoscopy when no CRC was diagnosed. The subtypes of PCCRC include interval (identified before the next recommended colonoscopy) and noninterval (identified at or after the next recommended colonoscopy. Seventy percent of PCCRCs are attributed to missed (52%) and incompletely resected lesions (19%).

28. **What are the different serrated lesions?**
    Serrated lesions of the colorectum include hyperplastic polyps (HPs) and SSPs also known as sessile serrated lesions or sessile serrated adenomas and TSAs. The prevalence of HPs is 20%–40%, SSPs 5%–9%, and TSAs <1%. In a recent study, PCCRC was significantly lower when performed by endoscopists with a clinically significant serrated polyp (TSA or SSP of any size, HP ≥1 cm, or HP >5 mm proximal to the sigmoid colon) detection rate of ≥3 versus <3%.

29. **According to the USMSTF consensus update on CRC, what are the recommendations for surveillance colonoscopy in average-risk patients with history of adenomas?**
    The recommendations for surveillance colonoscopy in average-risk patients with history of adenomas are summarized in Table 45.7.

Table 45.7 US Multi-Society Task Force Recommendations for Surveillance Colonoscopy in Patients With History of Adenomas.

MOST ADVANCED ADENOMAS ON BASELINE COLONOSCOPY	RECOMMENDED SURVEILLANCE INTERVAL (YEARS[a])
<3, <10 mm TA	7–10
3–4, <10 mm TA	3–5
5–10, <10 mm TA	3
≥10 mm TA	3
Adenoma with villous features or high-grade dysplasia	3
>10 adenomas	1
Piecemeal resection adenoma ≥20 mm	6 months[a]

TA, Tubular adenoma.
[a]Unless specified otherwise.

30. **What is the prevalence of a germline pathogenic variant in patients with CRC undergoing multigene panel testing?**
The prevalence of germline PVs varies according to age. High and moderate or low penetrance genes were found in 34%, 20%, and 10% of individuals with CRC under age 35, under age 50, and over age 50, respectively.

31. **Should colonoscopy be performed after an episode of diverticulitis to search for CRC?**
A meta-analysis of over 50,000 patients demonstrated a 1.9% pooled prevalence of colon cancer in patients with diverticulitis; 8% in patients with complicated diverticulitis and 1.3% in patients with uncomplicated diverticulitis (1.3%). Colonoscopy is recommended 6–8 weeks after an episode of complicated diverticulitis or a first episode of uncomplicated diverticulitis but may be deferred if a high-quality colonoscopy was performed within the last year. Colonoscopy should be considered sooner if alarm symptoms are present.

32. **According to the USMSTF consensus update on CRC, what are the recommendations for surveillance colonoscopy in average-risk patients with history of serrated polyps?**
The recommendations for surveillance colonoscopy in average-risk patients with history of serrated polyps are summarized in Table 45.8.

Table 45.8 US Multi-Society Task Force Recommendations for Surveillance Colonoscopy in Patients With History of Serrated Polyps.

MOST ADVANCED SERRATED POLYPS ON BASELINE COLONOSCOPY	RECOMMENDED SURVEILLANCE INTERVAL (YEARS[a])
≤20 HPs <10 mm	10
1–2, <10 mm SSP	5–10
3–4, <10 mm SSP	3–5
5–10, <10 mm SSP	3
SSP ≥10 mm	3
SSP with dysplasia	3
HP ≥10 mm	3–5
TSA	3
Piecemeal resection of SSP ≥20 mm	6 months[a]

HP, Hyperplastic polyp; *SSP*, sessile serrated polyp; *TSA*, traditional serrated adenoma.
[a]Unless specified otherwise.

33. **List the hereditary colorectal cancer syndromes with their respective pathogenic variants, mode of inheritance, and disease features.**
The hereditary colorectal cancer syndromes are summarized in Table 45.9.

34. **What is serrated polyposis syndrome (SPS)?**
SPS is the most common polyposis syndrome diagnosed by either of two 2019 World Health Organization criteria (1) ≥5 serrated polyps proximal to the rectum, all being ≥5 mm in size with 2 of them ≥10 mm in size or (2) >20 serrated polyps of any size throughout the colon with ≥5 being proximal to the rectum and is inclusive of the cumulative lifetime number of HPs, sessile serrated lesions or traditional serrated polyps. More than 80% of SPS patients have adenomas. The etiology is believed to be related to environmental factors and germline pathologic variants in *RNF43* are rarely detected in some families with SPS.

35. **What is Lynch syndrome?**
Lynch syndrome is an autosomal-dominant cancer syndrome caused by a PV in an *MMR* gene or *EPCAM* gene. Lynch syndrome is the most common hereditary cause of CRC and increases the risk for many extracolonic cancers.

36. **What is the molecular signature of Lynch-associated cancers?**
The molecular signature of Lynch-associated tumors is MMRd which can be detected by high levels of MSI-H or loss of expression in the MMR proteins *MLH1*, *MSH2*, *MSH6*, or *PMS2* on immunohistochemistry.

Table 45.9 Hereditary Colorectal Cancer Syndromes.

SYNDROME	PATHOGENIC VARIANT	MODE OF INHERITANCE	MAIN FEATURES (IN ADDITION TO CRC)
Non-Polyposis CRC Syndromes			
Lynch syndrome	MLH1, MSH2, MSH6, PMS2, EPCAM	Autosomal dominant	Endometrial, ovarian, urothelial, gastric, small bowel, pancreaticobiliary, and brain cancers (usually gliobastomas); sebaceous skin neoplasms/cancer
CMMRD	MLH1, MSH2, MSH6, PMS2	Autosomal recessive	Brain, gastric, small bowel, skin, breast, bladder, Wilms (and other kidney) and hematologic cancers; sarcoma; café au lait spots
Adenomatous Polyposis Syndromes			
Classic FAP	APC	Autosomal dominant	Duodenal, gastric, and colorectal adenomas and cancers; hepatoblastoma; thyroid cancer; congenital hypertrophy of the retinal pigment epithelium; dental abnormalities; osteomas; desmoid tumors; soft tissue tumors
Attenuated FAP	APC	Autosomal dominant	Desmoid tumors, thyroid cancer, and duodenal and gastric adenomas and cancer similar to classic FAP but colorectal polyposis and cancer attenuated
MYH-associated polyposis	MUTYH	Autosomal recessive	Duodenal, gastric, and colorectal adenomas and cancer attenuated compared to classic FAP; thyroid cancer
NTHL1-associated polyposis	NTHL1	Autosomal recessive	Colorectal adenomas; breast, endometrial, and urothelial cancers; meningioma
Polymerase proofreading–associated polyposis	POLE, POLD1	Autosomal dominant	Colorectal adenomas; endometrial, ovarian, and brain cancers
MSH3-associated polyposis	MSH3	Autosomal recessive	Colorectal and duodenal adenomas; gastric and brain cancer
MLH3-associated polyposis	MLH3	Autosomal recessive	Colorectal adenomas; breast cancer
AXIN2-associated polyposis	AXIN2	Autosomal dominant	Oligodontia, ectodermal dysplasia; duodenal and colorectal adenomas; hepatocellular, breast, lung and prostate cancers
Hamartomatous Polyposis Syndromes			
Juvenile polyposis syndrome	SMAD4 BMPR1A	Autosomal dominant	GI hamartomas; gastric cancer; SMAD4–HHT
Peutz-Jeghers syndrome	STK11	Autosomal dominant	Mucocutaneous pigmentation; GI hamartomas; breast, GI, pancreatic, ovarian, endometrial, cervical, and testicular cancers
PTEN Hamartoma tumor syndrome	PTEN	Autosomal dominant	GI hamartomas; esophageal glycogen acanthosis, skin lesions; macrocephaly; breast, thyroid, renal, and endometrial cancers

CMMRD, Constitutional mismatch repair deficiency syndrome; CRC, colorectal cancer; FAP, familial adenomatous polyposis, GI, gastrointestinal; HHT, hereditary hemorrhagic telangiectasia.

37. What are the surveillance recommendations for patients with Lynch syndrome?

The screening recommendations for individuals with Lynch syndrome vary according to MMR PV and include colonoscopy, gynecologic, upper gastrointestinal, and urothelial screening with varying levels of evidence to support their benefit. Recommendations by the NCCN are summarized in Table 45.10.

Table 45.10 National Comprehensive Cancer Network Screening Recommendations for Patients With Lynch Syndrome.

CANCER SITE	AGE TO BEGIN SCREENING (YEARS)	EXAMINATION	SCREENING INTERVAL
Colorectum	20–25 (*MLH1, MSH2*, and *EPCAM*) 30–35 (*PMS2* and *MSH6*)	Colonoscopy	1–2 years
Uterus and ovaries Prophylactic TAHBSO should be considered	30–35 After childbearing	Transvaginal ultrasound and endometrial biopsy	1 year
Stomach	30–40 <30 based on family history (history of UGI cancers or high-risk findings like intestinal metaplasia or gastric adenomas)	EGD Noninvasive *Helicobacter pylori* testing once Lynch syndrome is diagnosed for all patients	2–4 years <2 years based on family history (history of UGI cancers or high-risk findings like intestinal metaplasia or gastric adenomas)
Urinary tract	30–35	Urinalysis	1 year

EGD, Esophagogastroduodenoscopy; *TAHBSO*, total abdominal hysterectomy with bilateral salpingo-oophorectomy; *UGI*, upper gastrointestinal.

38. What are the surveillance recommendations for patients with familial adenomatous polyposis (FAP)?

The surveillance recommendations are summarized in Table 45.11.

Table 45.11 National Comprehensive Cancer Network Screening Recommendations Screening Recommendations for Patients With Familial Adenomatous Polyposis.

SURVEILLANCE SITE	AGE TO BEGIN SCREENING (YEARS)	EXAMINATION	SCREENING INTERVAL
Colorectum Retained colon and rectum)	10–15	Colonoscopy	1 year
If colectomy and IRA		Sigmoidoscopy	6–12 months
If TPC with IPAA		Pouchoscopy	1 year
Duodenum and papilla	20–25	EGD with visualization of the papilla	1–3 years based on Spigelman staging system
Stomach	20–25	EGD	1–3 years
Thyroid	Late teenage years	Ultrasound	1 year or longer depending on findings

EGD, Esophagogastroduodenoscopy; *IPAA*, ileal pouch-anal anastomosis; *IRA*, ileorectal anastomosis; *TPC*, total proctocolectomy.

39. **Is there adjunct to colonoscopy to decrease the polyp burden in patients with FAP?**

   No chemopreventive agents are currently approved for colorectal polyposis control in FAP. Sulindac at a dose of 150 mg twice daily, celecoxib 400 mg twice daily, eicosapentaenoic acid (2 g daily), and erlotinib (75 mg daily) were shown in randomized controlled trials to reduce the number and size of colorectal polyps compared to placebo.

40. **Does Aspirin prevent CRC in patients with Lynch syndrome?**

   There are data showing that the daily use of Aspirin 600 mg for at least 2 years decreases the risk of CRC in individuals with Lynch syndrome. The dose and duration of Aspirin use have not been established yet with ongoing studies investigating the optimal dose and duration of Aspirin.

CLINICAL VIGNETTE

Available Online

BIBLIOGRAPHY

Available Online

CONSTIPATION AND FECAL INCONTINENCE

Adil Ghafoor, MD and Satish S.C. Rao, MD, PhD, FRCP

 Additional content available online

1. How is constipation defined?

Constipation is a bowel disorder that is often misunderstood and misinterpreted. The Rome IV criteria define this as symptoms of difficult, infrequent, or incomplete defecation, as these are the predominant symptoms of constipation. Most patients endorse excessive straining or incomplete stool evacuation than infrequent stool evacuation. Other symptoms of constipation include abdominal fullness, bloating, and use of manual maneuvers to facilitate defecation (Table 46.1). Chronic constipation (CC) is now considered part of a spectrum of disorders that includes slow transit constipation, constipation-predominant irritable bowel syndrome (IBS-C), and evacuation disorders due to the overlap in symptomatology between the three disorders and the possibility of patients transitioning from one disorder to the other.

Table 46.1 Rome IV Criteria for Chronic Constipation and Constipation-Predominant Irritable Bowel Syndrome.

CHRONIC CONSTIPATION	CONSTIPATION-PREDOMINANT IRRITABLE BOWEL SYNDROME

Two or more of the following criteria must be present for ≥3 months with symptom onset at least 6 months prior to diagnosis:
1. Must include two or more of the following:
  a. Fewer than three spontaneous bowel movements per week
  b. Straining occurring more than one-fourth (25%) of defecations
  c. Lumpy or hard stools (BSFS 1–2) more than one-fourth (25%) of defecations
  d. Sensation of anorectal obstruction/blockage more than one-fourth (25%) of defecations
  e. Sensation of incomplete evacuation more than one-fourth (25%) of defections
  f. Manual maneuvers to facilitate more than one-fourth (25%) of defections (e.g., use of a digit and pelvic floor support)
2. Loose stools are rarely present without the use of laxatives
3. Insufficient criteria for irritable bowel syndrome
	Symptoms must be present for ≥3 months with symptom onset at least 6 months prior to diagnosis: Recurrent abdominal pain, on average, ≥1 day per week in the last 3 months, associated with ≥2 of the following:
	1. Related to defecation
	2. Associated with a change in stool frequency
	3. Associated with a change in stool form or appearance
	At least 25% of stools should be considered hard/lumpy *or* less than 25% of stools are considered loose/watery to diagnose constipation predominance

BSFS, Bristol Stool Form Scale.

2. What is the difference between primary and secondary constipation?

Primary constipation can be subdivided into slow-transit constipation, evacuation disorders, and IBS-C. Secondary constipation is caused by factors that are not intrinsic to problems of the colon or anorectal function as seen in primary constipation. Such causes can include lifestyle, diseases, or medications (most common cause) and others (Table 46.2). Secondary causes should be considered before diagnosing a patient with primary constipation.

3. Identify the prevalence and impact of constipation.

North American studies estimate that 2%–27% of the population experience constipation. CC is highly prevalent and is estimated to have a pooled prevalence of 14%, ranging from 11% to 18% worldwide. This wide range is likely a result of the heterogeneity of the definition. It is twice as common in females. Other risk factors include increasing age and lower socioeconomic status. Constipation poses a significant economic burden, through both direct health care and indirect (e.g., work loss) costs.

4. Which populations are at increased risk for experiencing constipation?

Risk factors for constipation are listed in Table 46.3.

Table 46.2 Causes of Secondary Constipation.

CATEGORY	EXAMPLES
Medications	Analgesics (especially opioids and NSAIDs), anticholinergics, antidiarrheals, loop and thiazide diuretics, antihistamines, antidepressants, antipsychotics, anticonvulsants, antacids (containing calcium or aluminum), calcium channel blockers, metallic ions, hydralazine, clonidine, monoamine oxidase inhibitors, antiparkinson agents, resins, and chemotherapeutic agents (e.g., vinca derivatives)
Structural	Stricture, external compression, rectal prolapse, rectocele, and colorectal cancer
Metabolic	Hypocalcemia and hypercalcemia, hypomagnesemia, chronic kidney disease, and dehydration
Endocrine	Diabetes mellitus, hypothyroidism, hyperparathyroidism, panhypopituitarism, pregnancy, and pheochromocytoma
Neurogenic	Stroke, spinal cord injury, Parkinson disease, multiple sclerosis, dementia, autonomic neuropathy, POTS, Hirschsprung disease, colonic pseudoobstruction, and paraneoplastic syndromes
Myopathic	Ehlers-Danlos syndrome, scleroderma, myotonic dystrophy, and amyloidosis
Other	Depression, anorexia, and physical inactivity

NSAIDs, Nonsteroidal anti-inflammatory drugs; *POTS,* postural orthostatic tachycardia syndrome.

Table 46.3 Risk Factors for Constipation.

Demographic	Advanced age
	Female sex
	Low socioeconomic status
	Low income or education
	Non-White ethnicity
Lifestyle	Dehydration
	Immobility
	Travel
	Low-fiber diet
Medical	Recent abdominal surgery or pelvic surgery
	Critical Illness
	Malnutrition
	Medications (Table 46.2)
	Polypharmacy

5. What are the potential causes of acute constipation?

Patients who present with acute constipation should be evaluated for such causes as mechanical bowel obstruction, small bowel ileus, colonic pseudoobstruction, trauma, new painful anorectal, abdominal or pelvic conditions, and dietary changes.

6. What are the subtypes of primary constipation?

Primary constipation can be subdivided into slow-transit constipation, evacuation disorders, and IBS-C. It is important to note, however, that significant overlap of subtypes exists.

7. Describe normal colonic motility.

Neural control of the colon is mediated by complex interactions between luminal wall mechano- and chemoreceptors that are a part of the autonomic and enteric nervous systems as well as the interstitial cells of Cajal, which function as pacemaker cells. Alterations in colonic motor function can be caused by dysfunction of the nerves, the smooth muscle, or any of the chemical signals between them leading to motility and bowel disorders. Contractions in the colon can be nonpropagated, segmental bursts, or can be propagated throughout the colon. Propagated contractions of high amplitude are responsible for mass movements that generally occur upon awakening and after meals. The term gastrocolonic response reflex refers to the postprandial increase in colonic motor activity. Average colonic transit time is approximately 36 hours.

8. **Describe the normal mechanisms of defecation.**

The major muscles involved in defecation are the puborectalis muscle and the internal and external anal sphincters (Fig. 46.1) and abdominal and rectal muscles. Resting tone is provided primarily by the internal anal sphincter (approximately 80%). The puborectalis maintains tonic contraction at rest. When stool is present in the rectal vault, the internal anal sphincter relaxes via a reflex known as the rectoanal inhibitory reflex (RAIR), and the external anal sphincter contracts under voluntary mechanisms mediated by the pudendal nerve. During the process of defecation the abdominal and rectal muscles contract, puborectalis relaxes, facilitating a straightening of the rectoanal angle and subsequent pelvic floor descent. With voluntary relaxation of the external anal sphincter, often in addition to increased abdominal pressure, stool is allowed to pass.

9. **What is dyssynergic defecation (DD) or pelvic floor dyssynergia?**

Pelvic floor dyssynergia refers to a defecatory disorder in which there is inadequate relaxation or paradoxical contraction of the anorectal muscles while attempting to pass a bowel movement or inadequate rectal push effort. In two-thirds of cases, it appears to be an acquired disorder that can arise from a number of causes, including excessive straining, pregnancy, and psychological stress. Patients with DD may also have delayed transit. It is important to investigate any form of defecatory dysfunction prior to assessing colonic transit.

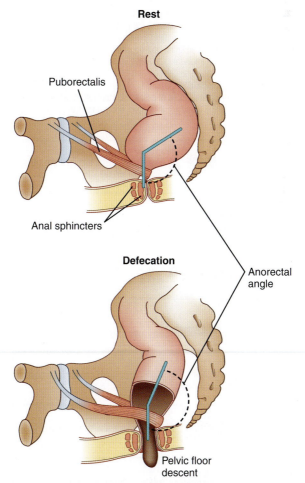

Fig. 46.1 At rest the puborectalis muscle acts as a sling that provides tonic anterior traction on the rectum. This creates the anorectal angle (between 80 and 110 degrees) that inhibits spontaneous, involuntary passage of stool. During the act of defecation the puborectalis, the pelvic floor, and the external anal sphincter muscles relax. In a synchronous fashion, the anorectal angle straightens about 15 degrees, the perineum descends 1.0–3.5 cm, and the external sphincter relaxes resulting in the passage of stool.

10. **What is DD?**
    DD is a common type of evacuation disorder that is an acquired behavioral disorder characterized by the inability to coordinate abdominal and pelvic floor muscles to evacuate stool. There are three main mechanisms associated with DD: paradoxical anal sphincter relaxation, impaired anal sphincter relaxation, and inadequate abdominal and rectal propulsive forces that facilitate stool evacuation. The disorder can arise from several causes, including excessive straining, pregnancy, and psychological stress. Patients with DD may also have delayed transit. It is important to investigate any form of defecatory dysfunction prior to assessing colonic transit.

11. **What is a rectocele?**
    A rectocele is an anterior outpouching of rectal wall through a weakened rectovaginal septum (the fascial wall that separates the rectum and the vagina) with rare occurrences of posterior outpouching. Presence of a rectocele, enterocele, or excessive perineal descent may lead to symptoms of obstructive defecation. It is common among females with certain risk factors including aging, obesity, obstetric injury, multiple vagina deliveries, and the presence of DD.

12. **What questions are important to ask a patient with constipation?**
    A thorough history should reveal the onset and duration of symptoms, stool frequency and consistency, presence of the urge to defecate, feelings of incomplete evacuation, and the need for straining or manual maneuvers for disimpaction. Ask about other gastrointestinal (GI) complaints, such as nausea and vomiting, abdominal or rectal pain, dysphagia, blood in the stool, weight loss, fever, family history of GI cancers, loss of appetite, presence of rectal prolapse, and history of iron-deficiency anemia. A thorough review of systems is needed to evaluate for potential secondary causes of constipation. The patient's medications, including over-the-counter medications and dietary supplements, should be reviewed. In an appropriate setting and with a plan to support the patient, soliciting a history of abuse may also be important.

13. **What is the Bristol Stool Form Scale?**
    The Bristol Stool Form Scale is a validated method of assessing stool consistency in patients with constipation (Fig. 46.2). Patients are asked to rate the quality of their stool according to the chart's depictions. The Bristol

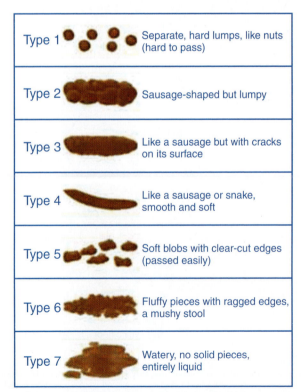

Fig. 46.2 Bristol Stool Form Scale. (From Lewis SJ, Heaton KW. Stool form scale as a useful guide to intestinal transit time. Scand J Gastroenterol.1997;32:920-924.)

Stool Form Scale has been shown to correlate with stool transit time in patients with constipation and is a key component of the defecation history.

14. **What important physical examination characteristics should be assessed in patients with constipation?**

A thorough systemic examination, including abdominal and neurologic examination, and musculoskeletal examination (joint hypermobility) should be performed to help rule out secondary causes of constipation. The perineal and digital rectal examinations should be detailed, as described in Table 46.4.

Table 46.4 Components of the Digital Rectal Examination, Technique, Expected Findings, and Grading of Responses.

DIGITAL RECTAL EXAMINATION	TECHNIQUE	FINDINGS AND GRADING OF RESPONSE(S)
1. Inspection of the anus and surrounding tissue	Place patient in the left lateral position with hips flexed to 90 degrees. Inspect perineum under good light	Skin excoriation, skin tags, anal fissure, scars or external hemorrhoids, gaping anus, prolapsed hemorrhoids or rectum, and condyloma
2. Testing of perineal sensation and the anocutaneous reflex	Stroke the skin around the anus in a centripetal fashion (toward anus), in all four quadrants, by using a stick with a cotton bud	Normal: brisk contraction of the perianal skin, the anoderm, and the external anal sphincter Impaired: no response with the soft cotton bud, but anal contractile response seen with the opposite (wooden) end Absent: no response with either end
3. Digital palpation	Slowly advance a lubricated and gloved index finger into the rectum and feel the mucosa and surrounding muscle, bone, uterus, prostate, and pelvic structures	Tenderness, mass, stricture, or stool and the consistency of the stool (BSFS) Examine prostate for nodules, mass, and tenderness Evaluate for retroverted uterus and rectocele
4. Maneuvers to assess anorectal function and dysfunction		
Resting tone	Assess strength of resting sphincter tone	Normal, weak (decreased), or increased
Squeeze maneuver	Ask the patient to squeeze and hold as long as possible (up to 30 s)	Normal, weak (decreased), or increased
Sphincter defects	Palpate anal sphincter muscle for defects during rest or squeeze maneuver	Describe as present or absent and degree of sphincter loss using a clock or in quadrants
Push and bearing down maneuver	In addition to the finger in the rectum, place the other hand over the patients' abdomen. Ask the patient to push and bear down as if to defecate and assess changes in abdominal muscle tightening, perineal descent, and contraction or relaxation of anal sphincter and puborectalis	1. Abdominal push effort: normal, weak (decreased), and excessive 2. Anal relaxation: normal, impaired, and paradoxical contraction 3. Puborectalis relaxation: normal, impaired, and paradoxical contraction 4. Perineal descent: normal, excessive, and absent 5. Rectal mucosal intussusception/prolapse: presence or absence
Anorectal pain assessment	Palpate coccyx (bidigital) and palpate levator ani muscle in all four quadrants	Presence or absence of tenderness over coccyx and/or levator ani muscle. If present, grade intensity on a scale of 0–10, and whether sensation(s) experienced at home is reproducible

BSFS, Bristol Stool Form Scale.

From Rao SSC. Rectal exam: yes, it can and should be done in a busy practice! Am J Gastroenterol. 2018;113(5):635-638.

15. **Which laboratory studies should be checked in a patient with constipation?**
    Constipation alone does not require specific laboratory testing. In fact, in the absence of alarm signs and symptoms, it is recommended to proceed with treatment. Alarm features include new onset or sudden change in bowel habits, GI bleeding, weight loss, anemia, obstructive symptoms, or family history of colorectal cancer. When high suspicion exists for a secondary cause of constipation, laboratory studies should be targeted toward the suspected disorders.

16. **When should referral to a gastroenterologist be considered in a patient with constipation?**
    Fig. 46.3 depicts an algorithmic approach to the evaluation of constipation in adults. Initial evaluation often occurs at the primary care physician's office. Referral may be warranted in more refractory cases or when specialized studies, such as colonoscopy or anorectal manometry (ARM), are indicated.

17. **Which patients with constipation should get a colonoscopy?**
    Colonoscopy should be reserved for patients with alarm features present. Alarm signs include age ≥45, change in stool caliber, blood in stool, unintended weight loss, fever, abdominal mass, family history of GI cancer, iron-deficiency anemia, recent onset constipation, and loss of appetite. Routine colonoscopic cancer screening should always be considered a separate issue.

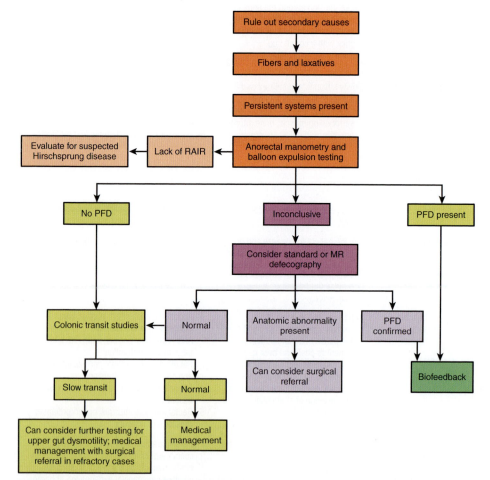

Fig. 46.3 Diagnostic algorithm for the evaluation of constipation. *MR,* Magnetic resonance; *PFD,* pelvic floor disorder; *RAIR,* rectoanal inhibitory reflex. (Adapted from Bharucha AE, Dorn SD, Lembo A, Pressman A. American Gastroenterological Association medical position statement on constipation. Gastroenterology. 2013;144(1):211-217.)

Normal push

Dyssynergic pattern

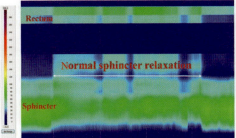
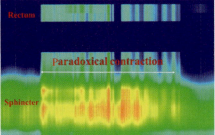

Fig. 46.4 Manometric findings of normal push effort versus dyssynergic defecation.

18. **What is ARM (anorectal manometry), and how is it used?**

    ARM is a test that allows for the recording and simultaneous measuring of intraluminal pressure changes at multiple levels and coordination of the pelvic floor muscles that control defecation. Pressure measurements allow for assessing anorectal motor function at rest and during maneuvers that simulate physiologic activities including squeeze, defecation maneuver, Valsalva, and retention effort. During the procedure, a probe with a balloon attached is inserted into the patient's rectum. The patient is then asked to squeeze, as if trying to hold in a bowel movement, and then bear down, as if attempting to defecate. Graded inflation of the attached balloon helps assess rectal sensation as well as the RAIR (recto and inhibitory reflex). ARM helps to assess DD and is now considered a first-line test for patients with constipation refractory to medications. Refer to Fig. 46.4 for manometric findings of normal push effort versus DD.

19. **What is balloon expulsion testing?**

    Balloon expulsion testing is a simple, office-based test indicated as a first-line screening option for assessing the ability to defecate. It is commonly performed alongside ARM and involves inflating a balloon in the rectum with 50 mL of water or using a special device and then asking the patient to mimic defecation into a commode. Delay in expelling the balloon (typically >1 minute) has been thought to indicate DD, although the sensitivity and specificity of this test are variable, ranging from 68% to 94% and 71% to 81%, respectively.

20. **What important finding might be seen on ARM in a patient with Hirschsprung disease?**

    Patients with Hirschsprung disease lack RAIR. This important reflex allows relaxation of the internal anal sphincter with the presence of stool in the rectal vault. Although an uncommon finding, Hirschsprung disease is an important diagnosis as treatment is primarily surgical.

21. **What other tests might be performed in a patient with constipation?**

    Testing used for constipation is detailed in Table 46.5.

22. **Describe some dietary and lifestyle modifications that patients with constipation can adopt to improve their symptoms.**

    Patients with mild constipation may benefit from increasing dietary fiber and fluid intake. Patient should also work to increase their daily physical activity and exercise. Additionally, they should be encouraged to allow sufficient time for a bowel movement. Though increased activity is encouraged, there is little evidence to support its recommendation for the treatment of constipation.

23. **What is the appropriate use of fiber supplementation?**

    Patients should be taught to increase their fiber intake to 25–35 g daily. This increase should be gradual, however, to avoid bloating and flatulence. Patients with severe constipation may develop worsening constipation with fiber. Similarly, overdosing on fiber may also aggravate constipation and cause bloating. Additionally, patients should maintain adequate hydration throughout the day. The exceptions to a high-fiber diet recommendation are patients who have true colonic inertia and those who have terminal reservoir syndrome or problems with megarectum and impaction. These patients may benefit from a low-residue diet.

24. **Describe potential pharmacologic treatments for constipation.**

    Multiple pharmacologic therapies are available and are detailed in Table 46.6.

Table 46.5 Testing Used in the Evaluation of Constipation.

TEST	HOW PERFORMED	PURPOSES AND USES
HR-ARM	Anorectal catheters with more sensors than traditional non–high-resolution catheters are placed in the anorectal region. Patients perform maneuvers including squeeze, cough, and simulated evacuation. Anorectal pressures are recorded during these maneuvers to assess these maneuvers that are under voluntary control of striated muscle. Metrics including rectoanal gradient and defecation index are the most useful	Used to evaluate sensorimotor function of the anorectum by assessing intraluminal pressure changes at multiple levels at rest and squeeze Evaluates patterns of dyssynergic defecation Evaluates rectoanal inhibitory, retention effort, defecation maneuvers, and Valsalva reflex Assesses rectal sensation and compliance
Balloon expulsion testing	Preferably nonlatex balloon inflated with 50 mL warm water that is attached to a plastic catheter is inserted into the rectum while patient is lying in left lateral position with hips and knees flexed Then seated on a commode in privacy, patient asked to expel balloon and record the time taken to expel the balloon Usually performed in conjunction with ARM	Considered best test to assess inability to expel solid stool First-line screening investigation for dyssynergic defecation Sensitivity and specificity for dyssynergic defecation is 69%–94% and 71%–81%, respectively Generally accepted limit for balloon expulsion is 1 minute. Longer times indicate an evacuation disorder
Abdominal radiography	Can be performed upright or in lying position	Assists in evaluation of ileus, obstruction, and impaction
Colonic transit (Sitzmarks)	Single versus multiple capsules with radiopaque markers are ingested. Serial abdominal x-rays over 5–7 days are performed and retention of the markers is recorded	Assesses colonic transit delay through use of ingested radiopaque markers tracked radiographically over time. Has historically been the most common test for colon transit assessment
Wireless motility capsule	Patients ingest the capsule at an office visit after eating a standard meal Should not be performed in patients with or suspicion of strictures, luminal obstruction, altered anatomy, or severe pyloric stenosis	Ingested capsule that records and measures pH, pressure, and temperature throughout the intestinal tract Measures gastric emptying, small bowel, colonic, and whole-gut transit
Colonic scintigraphy	A radioisotope (commonly indium) is delivered to the cecum or terminal ileum via capsule that dissolves at pH of 7.2–7.4	Allows for accurate and quantitative results for colonic transit time Takes 48 hr to complete Can also be used to measure transit in each tract of the gut including stomach and small bowel
Standard or MR defecography	Performed in the sitting position after 150 mL of barium paste is placed in the patient's rectum. Under fluoroscopy, the patient is asked to simulate defecation. Can also be performed using MR	A dynamic fluoroscopy study of evacuation used to help in diagnosing evacuation disorders Can also provide useful information on structural changes of the anorectal region including rectoceles, rectal prolapse, intussusception, descending perineum syndrome, and dyssynergic defecation Use of MR can help evaluate pelvic floor anatomy (anal sphincters, levator ani muscle, and surrounding tissue) while simultaneously assessing stool evacuation Often used in conjunction with balloon expulsion time, anorectal manometry, or in patients with normal manometry but prolonged expulsion time

Table 46.5 Testing Used in the Evaluation of Constipation.

TEST	HOW PERFORMED	PURPOSES AND USES
Colonic manometry and barostat testing	Manometry can be performed with barostat that entails placement of a 10 cm-long highly compliant balloon under colonoscopic and fluoroscopic guidance in the middescending colon. The balloon is connected to the manometer and air is either pumped into or withdrawn. The manometer measures muscle tone, compliance, and distention of the colon and rectum	Provides a comprehensive evaluation of colonic motility and motor patterns Barostat allows the study of muscle tone and sensory and motor responses to distention of the rectum and colon

ARM, Anorectal manometry; *HR-ARM,* high-resolution anorectal manometry; *MR,* magnetic resonance.

Table 46.6 Medications and Devices Currently Used for Constipation.

CLASS	DRUG	DOSE	MECHANISM OF ACTION	RECOMMENDATION GRADE
OTC Medications				
Osmotic laxatives	PEG 3350	8.5–34 g/day	Increases water into the intestines, softens stool, and allows for easier passage of stool	A
	Sorbitol	30 g/day		C
	Glycerin	1 rectal suppository daily for 15 minutes		C
Stimulants	Senna	2–4 tablets (8.6 mg) 1–2 times per day	Through direct contact activation of enteric neurons, they stimulate bowel movement and intestinal water secretion	A
	Bisacodyl	10–30 mg oral, 10 mg suppository per day		B
	Sodium picosulfate	5–10 mL daily		B
	Cascara	20–30 mg/day		C
Magnesium	Magnesium oxide	25 mL/day	Magnesium acts as an osmotic laxative by increasing water movement into intestines due to its poor absorption. Also activates NO synthase and release of cholecystokinin increasing motility	B

Continued

Table 46.6 Medications and Devices Currently Used for Constipation.—cont'd

CLASS	DRUG	DOSE	MECHANISM OF ACTION	RECOMMENDATION GRADE
	Magnesium sulfate	10–20 g up to twice per day		B
	Magnesium citrate	200 mL/day		B
	Magnesium-rich water	No official dose		B
	Magnesium hydroxide	400–1200/mL mg up to twice daily		C
Surfactants/ stool softeners	Docusate sodium	100 mg twice per day	Acts to decrease surface tension of the stool to allow increased water and lipids to penetrate the stool and thus softening stool for easier passage	C
	Docusate calcium	240 mg daily		C
Soluble fibers	Psyllium	1 tablespoon up to three times per day	Stimulate water and mucous secretion to create a gel with resistant to dehydration that normalize stool form	B
	Polydextrose	4–12 g daily		Insufficient
	Inulin	20–40 g/day		Insufficient
Insoluble fibers	Methylcellulose	4 caplets (500 mg) up to three times per day	Stool bulking and softening	C
	Bran	20–25 g/day		C
Mixed fibers	SupraFiber	5 g twice daily	Components of both soluble and insoluble fiber	B
Prescription Medications				
Osmotic laxatives	Lactulose	10–20 g (15–30 mL) every other day, up to twice per day	Increases water into the intestines, softens stool, and allows for easier passage of stool	A
	Lactitol	10–20 g/day		B
IBAT inhibitor	Elobixibat (undergoing clinical trials)	5–15 mg/day (not FDA approved, available in Japan)	Inhibits enterohepatic bile acid circulation which leads to more bile spilling into the colon and accelerated colonic transit and laxation	A
Serotonin receptor agonists	Prucalopride	1 or 2 mg/day (depending on age, renal and hepatic function)	5-HT4 receptor agonist stimulate colonic motility and laxation	A

Table 46.6 Medications and Devices Currently Used for Constipation.

CLASS	DRUG	DOSE	MECHANISM OF ACTION	RECOMMENDATION GRADE
Opioid receptor antagonists	Methylnaltrexone	1 dose of 12 mg subcutaneous injection daily, 450 mg oral daily	Peripheral mu-opioid receptor antagonists which reverse opioid-induced constipation without affecting analgesia	A
	Naloxegol	12.5–25 mg daily		A
	Naldemedine	0.2 mg daily		A
Prosecretory agents	Lubiprostone	24 µg twice a day	Chloride channel 2 agonist. Activates chloride channels leading to chloride, water, and bicarbonate secretion into lumen and laxation	A
	Linaclotide	145 µg/day	GC-C receptor agonist causes increased cGMP and ultimately the activation of CFTR channels to increase chloride and intestinal fluid secretion and laxation	A
	Plecanatide	3 mg/day		A

5-HT4, 5-Hydroxytryptamine receptor 4; *CFTR*, cystic fibrosis transmembrane conductance regulator; *cGMP*, cyclic guanosine mono-phosphate; *FDA*, US Food and Drug Administration; *GC-C*, guanylate cyclase-C; *IBAT*, ileal bile acid transporter; *NO*, nitric oxide; *OTC*, over-the-counter.

25. What nonpharmacologic therapies can be used to treat constipation?

In addition to dietary (increasing fiber) and lifestyle modification (increasing physical exercise), for patients with constipation due to pelvic floor dysfunction and DD, biofeedback is considered the best treatment option. Biofeedback is a form of behavioral training based on the theory of operant conditioning in which patients are taught how to retrain their anorectal muscles and restore normal coordination involved in defecation or maintaining continence. This treatment is the preferred treatment for those with pelvic floor disorders, defecatory disorders, and fecal incontinence (FI). Biofeedback has shown benefit in up to 70%–80% of patients with a sustained response up to at least 1 year after treatment. Additionally, vibrating capsule taken daily, five times a week has been recently approved for the treatment of chronic constipation.

26. When should surgical referral be considered in a patient with constipation?

Surgical referral is rarely required and should be reserved for patients with refractory symptoms who have already seen a gastroenterologist or those with colonic inertia, Hirschsprung disease, or anatomic abnormalities. Surgeries may include forms of colectomy with or without ileorectal anastomosis. However, studies have shown long-term surgical complications and increased emergency department visits. The decision to proceed with surgery should be decided by a well-informed patient who has been evaluated by both a gastroenterologist and colorectal surgeon.

27. What are the potential complications of constipation?

Complications can include hemorrhoids, anal fissures, fecal impaction, rectal prolapse, stercoral ulcers, and rectal bleeding, among others.

28. How is FI defined?

FI is defined as the inability to prevent stool from leaking out through the anus or the involuntary passage of stool and may occur with either mucus, liquid, or solid stool.

29. What causes FI?

FI can occur from anal sphincter injury, neurologic conditions, and conditions that affect the compliance and accommodation of the rectum. Common causes of anal sphincter injury that occur because of childbirth include forceps delivery, prolonged second stage of labor, and large child birth weight. Sphincter injury can also result from anal dilatation, lateral sphincterotomy, anorectal fistula, perineal trauma, and pelvic fracture. Muscle-related injury can also occur from myopathic conditions including muscular dystrophy, myasthenia gravis, radiation, and internal sphincter degeneration. Neurologic causes can be central or peripheral. Common central nervous system conditions include multiple sclerosis, dementia, stroke, brain tumors, and spinal cord lesions. Common peripheral neurologic causes include cauda equina lesions, diabetic neuropathy, and alcohol-related neuropathy. Common conditions that affect compliance and accommodation of the rectum and lead to FI include radiation-induced inflammation and fibrosis, Crohn disease, and ulcerative colitis.

30. **What are the prevalence and effect of FI?**
   FI is a very common disorder but is often underreported. It is also the second leading cause for nursing home placement. It is estimated to have a prevalence of 7%–15% in adults that are not hospitalized or in a nursing home. It is estimated to be prevalent in up to 33% of hospitalized adults and 70% of adults in nursing homes. FI prevalence in females after vaginal childbirth has declined from 13% to 8% over the past 20 years which may reflect improvements in obstetrical care.

31. **Which populations are at increased risk for suffering from FI?**
   Increased rates are seen in older adults and institutionalized populations. In addition, FI can frequently be seen in patients with neurologic disorders, diabetes mellitus, obesity, or decreased mobility. Additionally, the rate of FI immediately after vaginal childbirth in primiparous females has declined from 13% to 8%, which may be attributed to improvements in obstetrical care including decrease in instrumented vaginal delivery (use of forceps and vacuum extraction) and more selective use of episiotomy. Among females with FI, Caucasian ethnicity, depression, chronic diarrhea, and urinary incontinence (UI) are independent risk factors for the development of FI. In males, UI is the only independent risk factor. Furthermore, rectal urgency is the strongest predictor associated with the development of FI.

32. **What questions are important to ask a patient with FI?**
   Patients with incontinence are often embarrassed to discuss their problem, so you must ask them directly if they have ever had involuntary loss of stool. Once this is established, patients should be asked about sensations of urge to defecate, passage of solid or liquid stool, awareness of the episodes, duration and frequency, and presence of tenesmus and nocturnal symptoms. Additional history regarding diarrhea should be obtained. Patients should be asked about urinary or sexual complaints as many of the causes of FI can affect the entire pelvic floor. Questions regarding self-esteem, isolation, travel limitations, and day planning can also give insight in the severe impact FI is causing the patient. A thorough medical history, including history of diabetes, neurologic disease, prior anorectal trauma or surgery, and a complete obstetric history, should be obtained. Ask specific questions about prior deliveries, including type, use of forceps, length of labor, size of baby, and need for episiotomy. Finally, medications should be reviewed, including over-the-counter medications and dietary supplements, such as sorbitol (an osmotic laxative).

33. **What are the important physical examination characteristics to look for in patients with FI?**
   Overall examination should include an assessment of cognitive and other neurologic deficits as well as signs of endocrinopathies and systemic inflammatory conditions. As with patients with constipation, a detailed perineal and digital rectal examination should be performed (Table 46.4). Careful attention should be paid to identifying anatomic abnormalities, such as rectal prolapse.

34. **Which laboratory studies should be checked in a patient with FI?**
   There are no laboratory tests that need to be performed routinely in these patients. Causes of diarrhea should be pursued when appropriate.

35. **What other tests might be performed in a patient with FI?**
   Useful tools in evaluating FI include high-resolution ARM (HRM), endoanal ultrasound, standard or magnetic resonance defecography, and nerve conduction studies including translumbosacral anorectal magnetic stimulation (TAMS). HRM can be useful in quantifying pressures of the external and internal anal sphincters or puborectalis muscle as well as sensory thresholds of the rectum. Endoanal ultrasound is used to identify anatomic defects of the anal sphincters. TAMS is a safe and well-tolerated procedure that allows to comprehensively assess pelvic anorectal neuropathy. Prior to TAMS, anal electromyography and pudendal nerve terminal motor latency (PNTML) were the only methods available to measure neuromuscular integrity between the terminal portion of the pudendal nerve and anal sphincter. However, TAMS is superior to PNTML testing in assessing lumbosacral neuropathy which is often a cause of FI. Furthermore, endoscopy can be useful in detecting inflammation or evaluating causes of diarrhea.

36. **Name some pharmacologic treatments for FI.**
   Fiber supplementation can help bulk stools. There is weak evidence to show that medications including loperamide, cholestyramine, clonidine, topical phenylephrine, and oral valproate may benefit FI. Other medications

that slow transit time include atropine and diphenoxylate. Tricyclic antidepressants can lead to the side effect of constipation, so they can be used in incontinence for this effect.

37. What nonpharmacologic therapies can be used to treat FI?

Biofeedback therapy is a safe and effective behavioral treatment for FI to entail a therapist working with a patient to improve anal sphincter strength, improve coordination between abdominal, gluteal, and anal sphincter muscles during voluntary squeeze, and during rectal balloon distention that improve sensation and sensorimotor coordination during voluntary squeeze. It has shown to be efficacious in up to 80% of patients with FI. Furthermore, injection of bulking agents into the anal canal, such as dextranomer in stabilized hyaluronic acid or silicone elastomers, provide for barrier augmentation for the treatment of FI. Intra-anal dextranomer microsphere injection was shown to be effective in a large, multicenter, sham-controlled randomized controlled trial (RCT). Therapy using sacral nerve stimulation (SNS) or percutaneous tibial nerve stimulation may be offered, similar to patients with constipation. In SNS, patients begin with a temporary stimulator, and given positive results, a permanent stimulator can be placed. Studies regarding radiofrequency ablation are based on the premise that thermal lesions created in muscles below the mucosa aid in remodeling and tightening during healing. Outcomes appear conflicting with some promising short- and long-term results, with larger studies and a sham RCT needed. Finally, plug devices have been tried, but they are poorly tolerated, and study sizes are too small to indicate efficacy. A novel treatment is translumbosacral neuromodulation therapy that uses repetitive magnetic stimulation of the lumbar and sacral plexus nerves has recently been shown to be efficacious in the treatment of FI.

38. When should surgical referral be used in a patient with FI?

Referral to surgery should be used in refractory patients or in those with anatomic defects, such as an external anal sphincter disruption. Unfortunately, there are few RCTs comparing the various surgical techniques to their nonsurgical alternatives, and long-term results can vary. Furthermore, anal sphincter repair or sphincteroplasty does not appear to be effective in the long term. Colostomy can be offered to those not candidates for barrier devices, perianal bulking injection, SNS, or sphincteroplasty and who have failed medical management. Surgical options available to patients are described in Table 46.7.

39. Describe some particular concerns regarding FI in older adults.

FI is common in older adults and can stem from diarrhea or constipation. It is highly prevalent but underreported. Fecal impaction with overflow should be ruled out. Cognition plays a role in continence; thus, dementia in older patients can be a contributing factor to incontinence. In those with cognitive impairment, therapies that require active participation, such as biofeedback, may be more difficult. In addition, limited mobility in some older patients may make incontinence particularly difficult to treat. Finally, management of decubitus ulcers and perineal skin in bedbound patients is essential to avoid infection.

Table 46.7 Surgical Options for the Management of Fecal Incontinence.

PROCEDURE	DESCRIPTION AND USES
Sphincteroplasty	Reconstructs the anal sphincter Used specifically in those with distinct sphincter defects
Dynamic graciloplasty	Transposes the gracilis muscle around the anal canal along with electrical stimulation to the muscle. Used to enhance sphincter tone
Artificial anal sphincter	Similar purposes as dynamic graciloplasty, with use of an artificial device
Anterior levatorplasty	Ligates the two sides of the levator muscle to improve pelvic floor function. Often performed in conjunction with other procedures
Total and postanal pelvic floor repair	Postanal repair involves plication of several pelvic floor muscles, to improve overall function; rarely performed Total repair combines postanal repair and anterior levatorplasty
Rectal augmentation	Creates a side-to-side ilcorectal pouch Increases rectal capacity and compliance
Fecal diversion	Creates a stoma for severe, debilitating symptoms or recurrent infections in areas of skin breakdown
Antegrade continence enema	Irrigates the colon with large volume enemas via an ostomy site Primarily used in children, but can be used in adults with overflow incontinence caused by constipation

ACKNOWLEDGMENTS

The authors would like to thank the National Institute of Diabetes, Digestive and Kidney Diseases (NIDDK) for research support with U01DK115575-01 and R01DK121003-01 for Dr. S. Rao. We would also like to thank Ms. Helen Smith for superb secretarial assistance.

BIBLIOGRAPHY

Available Online

CHAPTER 47

DIVERTICULITIS

Tomoki Sempokuya, MD and Peter Mannon, MD, MPH

 Additional content available online

1. What is the clinical presentation of colonic diverticulitis?

The most common symptom is acute to subacute onset of left lower quadrant abdominal pain. Other signs and symptoms include fever, leukocytosis, bowel habitus changes, nausea without vomiting, and elevated C-reactive protein (Table 47.1). Diagnostic accuracy based on clinical symptoms alone is 40%–65% as diverticulitis can also present with atypical symptoms.

Table 47.1 Diagnositic Approach for Acute Diverticulitis.

History and Physical Examination
- Left lower quadrant tenderness and unremitting abdominal pain
- Fever
- Leukocytosis

Differential Diagnosis

ELDERLY PATIENTS	MIDDLE-AGED AND YOUNG PATIENTS	OTHER
Ischemia	Appendicitis	Amebiasis
Carcinoma	Salpingitis	Collagen vascular disease
Volvulus	IBS	Infectious colitis
Obstruction	Penetrating ulcer	Postirradiation
Proctosigmoiditis	Urosepsis	Prostatitis
Penetrating ulcer		IBS
Nephrolithiasis/urosepsis		

Qualifiers
Extremes of age (more virulent)
Asian ancestry (right-sided symptoms)
Immunosuppresive drugs and chronic renal failure (abdominal examination insensitive)

Evaluations

Plain x-rays	Good initial first step. May show ileus, obstruction, mass effect, ischemia, and perforation for other diseases.
CT scan	Very helpful in staging the degree of complications and evaluating them. Should be considered in all cases of suspected diverticulitis.
Ultrasound	Can be a safe and helpful noninvasive test to evaluate acute diverticulitis. Over 20% of examinations are suboptimal because of intestinal gas; highly operator dependent.
Contrast enema	Generally no longer used as routine diagnostic test. However, it can be useful in selected cases of stricture, fistula, and perforating disease when other investigations are unclear.
Endoscopy	A full colonoscopy during an attack of acute diverticulitis is generally contraindicated. However, a cautious flexible sigmoidoscopy with minimal air insufflation may be useful when the diagnosis is in doubt (rectal bleeding and anemia) to exclude ischemic bowel, Crohn disease, carcinoma, and other possibilities.

CT, Computed tomography; *IBS,* inflammatory bowel disease.
Adapted from Freeman SR, McNally PR. Diverticulitis. Med Clin North Am. 1993;77:1152.

2. **What is the difference between uncomplicated and complicated diverticulitis?**
Uncomplicated diverticulitis has features of colonic wall thickening and pericolonic inflammation. Complicated diverticulitis, occurring in 12% of diverticulitis cases, presents with abscess, obstruction, peritonitis, strictures, perforations, and/or fistula.

3. **What is the differential diagnosis?**
For elderly patients the differential diagnosis includes ischemic bowel, volvulus, inflammatory bowel disease, colorectal carcinoma, nephrolithiasis, and bowel obstruction (depending on the aspects of presentation). For younger patients, the differential diagnosis includes appendicitis, inflammatory bowel disease, salpingitis, and nephrolithiasis. Atypical manifestations of other diagnoses include irritable bowel disease, infectious colitis, amebiasis, radiation colitis, and prostatitis (Table 47.1).

4. **What is the diagnostic test of choice for diverticulitis?**
A computed tomography (CT) scan of the abdomen and pelvis with intravenous (IV) and oral contrast is the diagnostic test of choice to confirm the presence of diverticulitis and to assess for complications. CT scan has an excellent positive and negative likelihood ratio for diagnosing diverticulitis. CT scan is also useful to assess those who failed to respond to therapy, patients with immunocompromised status, and those with multiple recurrences, particularly to detect diverticulitis with perforating complications like abscess formation. Although it is operator dependent, abdominal ultrasonography may be an alternative means to assess for diverticulitis while avoiding IV contrast administration and radiation exposure.

5. **How is sigmoid diverticulitis classified?**
The most widely known surgical classification of sigmoid diverticulitis remains perhaps the Hinchey classification (Table 47.2). Hinchey III and IV indicate diffuse peritonitis, which is associated with significant morbidity and approximately 20% mortality. It is important to point out that the Hinchey classification was originally established based on intraoperative findings and is therefore not completely applicable to cases of sigmoid diverticulitis not requiring surgery, which make up the majority.

Table 47.2 Hinchey Classification of Sigmoid Diverticulitis.

	HINCHEY CLASSIFICATION
Stage I	Pericolic abscess confined by the mesentery of the colon
Stage II	Pelvic abscess resulting from a local perforation of a pericolic abscess
Stage III	Generalized peritonitis resulting from rupture of pericolic/pelvic abscess into the general peritoneal cavity
Stage IV	Fecal peritonitis results from the free perforation of a diverticulum

6. **What is the management of uncomplicated diverticulitis?**
Outpatient management with supportive care (monitoring for worsening of symptoms, adequate nutrition, and hydration) with reevaluation within 7 days is reasonable for patients without comorbidities (such as elderly, morbid obesity, uncontrolled diabetes, underlying cardiopulmonary, and renal disease) who can tolerate oral intake. For patients with significant comorbidities or unable to tolerate oral intake, inpatient management with IV fluid and analgesics are indicated. Antibiotics should be given to high-risk patients such as immunocompromised or elderly individuals.

7. **Is the use of antibiotics indicated in all patients with diverticulitis?**
Antibiotics administration should be used selectively only on these patients with complicated diverticulitis, or immunosuppressed patients. Double-blind, placebo-controlled randomized trial showed noninferiority of placebo over antibiotics in the management of acute uncomplicated diverticulitis regarding the length of stay and 30-day readmission rates. The DINAMO study also showed noninferiority of antibiotic-free outpatient management for mild acute diverticulitis, defined as good symptom control without signs of sepsis at the emergency department, compared to antibiotic treatment.

8. **What are the antibiotic options for treating diverticulitis in outpatient and inpatient settings?**
Possible treatment options include broad-spectrum penicillin, a combination of either fluoroquinolone, cephalosporin, or trimethoprim-sulfamethoxazole with metronidazole and clindamycin (Table 47.3). For immunocompetent individuals, the typical duration of antibiotic treatment is 4–7 days. For immunosuppressed individuals, the duration is 10–14 days.

Table 47.3 Antibiotic Options in the Treatment of Sigmoid Diverticulitis.

OUTPATIENT ANTIBIOTIC TREATMENT OPTIONS	INPATIENT ANTIBIOTIC TREATMENT OPTIONS
Fluoroquinolone + antianaerobic agent	*Fluoroquinolone + antianaerobic agent*
Ciprofloxacin 500 mg PO q 12 hr *plus* metronidazole 500 mg PO q 6–8 hr	Ciprofloxacin 400 mg IV q 12 hr or levofloxacin 500 mg IV + metronidazole 500 mg IV q 6 or q 8 hr
Penicillins	*Penicillins*
Amoxicilin-clavulanate 875/125 mg PO q 12 hr	Ampicillin-sulbactam 3 g IV q 6 hr piperacillin-tazobactam 3.375 g IV q 6 hr
Cephalosporins	*Cephalosporins*
Cephalexin 500 mg PO q 12 hr *plus* metronidazole 500 mg PO q 6–8 hr	Ceftriaxone 1 g IV q 12 hr
Others	*Carbapenems*
Trimethoprim-sulfamethoxazole 800/160 mg PO q 6 hr + metronidazole 500 mg PO q 6–8 hr	Imipenem-cilastatin 500 mg IV q 6 hr
Clindamycin 450 mg PO q 6 hr	Meropenem 1 g IV q 8 hr
	Ertapenem 1 g IV q 12 hr

IV, Intravenous; *PO,* per os.

9. **How should an inpatient be managed?**
   Orders for patients admitted for acute sigmoid diverticulitis should include nothing by mouth and rehydration with IV fluids, while also receiving IV antibiotics. In this respect, possible agents include broad-spectrum penicillins or cephalosporins. A combination of a fluoroquinolone and metronidazole is a widely used alternative, particularly in patients allergic to penicillin. Rarely used but acceptable alternatives, especially in the critically ill patient, include carbapenems (Table 47.3).

10. **What is the natural history of diverticulitis following the first attack of uncomplicated disease?**
    Most hospitalized patients experience improvement in their condition during the first 48 hours following admission. Serial clinical examinations and monitoring laboratory values are critical to promptly identify patients unresponsive to medical management. Once the patient recovers from the first uncomplicated disease attack managed conservatively, up to 20% of patients may experience recurrent diverticulitis after 10 years.

11. **What are the indications for colonoscopy after diverticulitis?**
    If a high-quality colonoscopy was not done within a year, patients diagnosed with their initial diverticulitis and complicated diverticulitis should undergo colonoscopy to rule out underlying malignancy, depending on age, and underlying comorbidities.

12. **When will you perform a colonoscopy after diverticulitis?**
    At least 6–8 weeks after the diagnosis, or until complete resolutions of symptoms, whichever is longer.

13. **What is the role of surgery in the management of diverticulitis?**
    Complicated diverticulitis with sepsis may require surgical source control. For recurrent diverticulitis and/or ongoing complaints, a 5-year follow-up of DIRECT trial showed elective sigmoidectomy yielded a higher quality of life score than conservative management. However, 11% of the operation group had complications with anastomotic leakage. The LASER trial also showed a higher quality of life score after laparoscopic elective sigmoidectomy to treat recurrent, complicated, or persistent diverticulitis. However, it showed a similar major complication rate of 10%.

14. **What is the rate of persistent diverticulitis managed nonoperatively?**
    Among patients with diverticulitis managed nonoperatively, 8.2% experienced persistent diverticulitis, defined as the need for retreatment within 60 days from the initial episode. Immunosuppression (such as chronic steroid, chemotherapy, immunosuppressive medications, and primary or acquired immunodeficiency), younger age, and abscess were associated with persistent diverticulitis. Patients with persistent diverticulitis had a higher incidence of recurrent diverticulitis and sigmoid colectomy.

15. **What are the risk factors associated with recurrent diverticulitis?**
    Risk for recurrent diverticulitis includes complicated diverticulitis, family history of diverticulitis, female sex, younger age of onset, current smoking, and obesity.

16. **What is the dietary recommendation to reduce the risk of developing diverticulitis?**
    A diet high in fiber from vegetables, fruits, and whole grains and low in red meat and legumes is associated with a lower risk of diverticulitis. Consumption of nuts, seeds, or corn is not associated with increased risk and may be protective.

17. **What is the management strategy for acute perforated purulent diverticulitis?**
    Based on the long-term follow-up of the SCANDIV trial, there were no differences in quality of life scores and severe complication rates between the laparoscopic saline lavage group and the primary resection group. The lavage treatment group had higher rates of any reoperation, including stoma reversal and diverticulitis recurrence. However, the long-term stoma prevalence was lower than the primary resection group.

18. **What are the most important complications of sigmoid diverticulitis?**
    Stricture, fistula, abscess, and peritonitis are the most important complications of sigmoid diverticulitis. It is generally accepted that bleeding is not associated with acute colonic inflammation. Phlegmon has been mentioned as an example of complicated diverticulitis but remains a somewhat arbitrary definition. Although a stricture can require surgery because of acute large bowel obstruction, surgery can also be indicated in the absence of obstructive symptoms when malignancy cannot be safely ruled out as the cause of a sigmoid stricture (Fig. 47.1). More rarely, the sigmoid inflammation can extend into the retroperitoneum and cause ureteral obstruction, most commonly on the left side.

19. **Which are the target organs of complicated fistulizing sigmoid diverticulitis?**
    All the organs surrounding the sigmoid colon can become a fistulizing target: bladder (Fig. 47.2), vagina, small bowel (Fig. 47.3), uterus, and skin (Fig. 47.4). Prior hysterectomy increases the risk for diverticulitis-related colovaginal fistula.

20. **What are the considerations for immunosuppressed individuals with diverticulitis?**
    Immunosuppressed patients may present with complications such as perforations, so a CT scan to assess for complications should be considered. For uncomplicated diverticulitis, immunosuppressed patients may have progression to complicated disease or sepsis, so broad-spectrum antibiotics with anaerobic coverage should be started promptly.

21. **What is the treatment strategy for patients with diverticulitis with isolated pericolic air?**
    The ACCSENT study and the DIABOLO trial suggest that Hinchey 1A diverticulitis with isolated pericolic air may undergo initial nonoperative therapy with IV antibiotic administration. However, clinical deterioration, such as the development of an acute abdomen or sepsis, may necessitate surgical intervention.

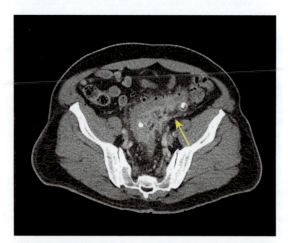

Fig. 47.1 Computed tomography scan demonstrating Ambrosetti mild sigmoid diverticulitis. Large arrow demonstrates sigmoid diverticulitis with colonic thickening and straining. (From Stocchi L. Current indications and role of surgery in the management of sigmoid diverticulitis. World J Gastroenterol. 2010;16:804-817.)

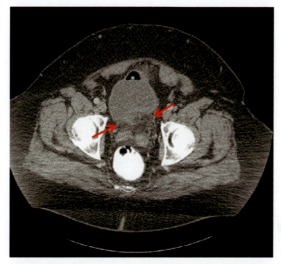

Fig. 47.2 Computed tomography scan demonstrating colovesical fistula. Note the air in the bladder (*) and colovesicular inflammation (*arrows*).

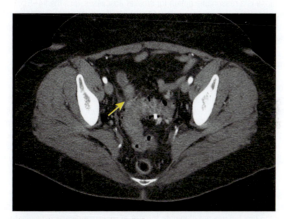

Fig. 47.3 Computed tomography scan demonstrating a coloenteric fistula (*arrow*).

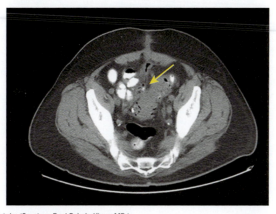

Fig. 47.4 Colocutaneous fistula. (Courtesy Ravi Pokala Kiran, MD.)

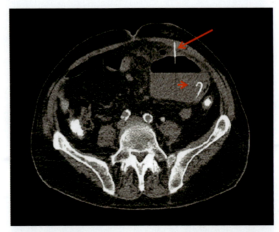

Fig. 47.5 Computed tomography scan demonstrating percutaneous catheter (*arrows*) drainage of the diverticular abscess.

22. **How do you manage diverticular abscess?**
    A trial of antibiotics alone is a reasonable option for smaller abscesses, less than 4–5 cm. For larger abscesses, patients may undergo percutaneous drainage (Fig. 47.5), typically via CT guidance along with antibiotic treatment. Surgical intervention may be necessary if the external approach is too challenging or if a deteriorating clinical status suggests advancing infection despite percutaneous drainage.

23. **What are the management options in patients with peritonitis caused by perforated diverticulitis?**
    Patients with peritonitis complicated by diffuse fecal spillage intra-abdominally are usually managed with resection of the sigmoid and a (usually) temporary colostomy associated with rectal stump, an operation referred to as a Hartmann procedure. When the level of peritoneal contamination is less severe, it is permissible to perform a restorative sigmoid resection associated with primary colorectal anastomosis and proximal stoma diversion, usually by means of a diverting loop ileostomy. The creation of a diverting ileostomy is associated with a much greater probability of having the stoma eventually taken down. On the other hand, a colostomy created during a Hartmann procedure becomes permanent in approximately one-third of patients, usually because of patient comorbidities.

24. **Should patients with recurrent diverticulitis undergo surgical resection?**
    Decisions for surgical resection should be individualized and should not rely solely on the number of recurrences. Surgery may reduce the risk but will not eliminate the risk of recurrent diverticulitis. Factors to consider for such surgical management are comorbidities, patients' preferences, severity and complications of diverticulitis, and operative risk.

CLINICAL VIGNETTE

Available Online

BIBLIOGRAPHY

Available Online

SURGICAL CONSIDERATIONS IN INFLAMMATORY BOWEL DISEASE AND BENIGN ANORECTAL PATHOLOGIES

Samuel H. Lai, MD and Jon D. Vogel, MD

 Additional content available online

SURGICAL CONSIDERATIONS IN ULCERATIVE COLITIS

1. **At what age group(s) do patients usually first present with ulcerative colitis (UC)?**
   Two age groups:
   - 15–30 years old
   - 55–65 years old

2. **Is Crohn disease and UC always distinguishable from each other?**
   No. Ten to fifteen percent of colitis cases referred for surgical considerations are termed indeterminate colitis as they cannot be definitively characterized as Crohn disease or UC.

3. **How should the extent of UC be classified?**
   Anatomically via the Montreal classification:
   E1—Ulcerative proctitis: involvement limited to the rectum
   E2—Left-sided UC: involvement limited to distal to splenic flexure
   E3—Extensive UC/pancolitis: involvement extends proximal to the splenic flexure

4. **What are the elective surgical options for UC?**
   - Total abdominal colectomy with ileorectal anastomosis
   - Total proctocolectomy with end ileostomy
   - Total proctocolectomy with continent ileostomy reservoir (Kock pouch)
   - Total proctocolectomy with ileal pouch-anal anastomosis (IPAA)

5. **What are the typical first-line treatments for patients hospitalized with UC flare?**
   - Intravenous (IV) methylprednisone (40–60 mg daily)
   - Continued on diet as tolerated
   - Venous thromboembolism (VTE) prophylaxis

6. **What workups should patients hospitalized with UC flare undergo?**
   - Abdominal plain films to assess for megacolon (transverse colon diameter 6 cm or greater) and toxic megacolon
     - Diagnosis of *toxic* megacolon is based on clinical findings. Plain films are only able to diagnose megacolon.
   - Endoscopy with flexible sigmoidoscopy to assess disease severity
   - Testing for cytomegalovirus and *Clostridoides difficile*

7. **What is the typical rescue therapy for UC flares if first-line treatments are not effective?**
   If no significant improvement is seen after 3–5 days from initiation of corticosteroid, the use of IV infliximab or IV cyclosporine is considered for rescue therapy.

8. **How does fulminant colitis present clinically?**
   Clinically: Severe form of acute colitis with
   - 10+ bloody stools per day
   - Anemia (hemoglobin <10.5 g/dL), blood transfusion requirements
   - Erythrocyte sedimentation rate >30 mm/hr
   - Fever
   - Tachycardia
   - Abdominal pain with distension

9. **When should surgical consultation be obtained for patients hospitalized with UC flare?**
   - Surgical consultation should be obtained early on and if patients do not show signs of improvement within 72 hours of initiating IV therapy.
   - Early surgical consultation and intervention have been associated with decreased postcolectomy complications.

10. **What are the indications for surgery in UC and what factors should be considered?**
   - Indications:
     - Intractability or failure of medical management to control colitis
     - Fulminant colitis, toxic megacolon, severe refractory disease, or colonic perforation
     - Hemorrhage
     - Presence of invisible high-grade dysplasia, invisible multifocal low-grade dysplasia, or visible dysplasia not amenable to endoscopic excision
     - Treatment of carcinoma
   - Other factors to consider:
     - Patient-specific preferences
     - Previous medical therapy including exposure to monoclonal antibodies
   - Risk factors for requiring total abdominal colectomy:
     - Age of diagnosis less than 40
     - Extensive colitis
     - Severe endoscopic disease with spontaneous bleeding and deep ulcerations
     - Previous hospitalization for colitis
     - Elevated C-reactive protein
     - Low serum albumin

11. **What type of procedure should be performed for patients who are acutely worsening and at risk of developing fulminant colitis or toxic megacolon?**
   Total abdominal colectomy with end ileostomy.

12. **What dose of preoperative corticosteroid is associated with increased postoperative complications?**
   Twenty milligrams or more of prednisone equivalents per day.

13. **Should patients on high-dose preoperative corticosteroids undergo total proctocolectomy with IPAA as initial surgery?**
   No. To reduce the risk of anastomotic leak and pelvic sepsis, patients on high-dose steroids should undergo total abdominal colectomy with end ileostomy as the initial procedure. The creation of IPAA should be delayed until steroids can be weaned, in addition to resolution of anemia and improvement in preoperative nutritional status.

14. **Should patients receive postoperative VTE prophylaxis postoperatively even if discharged from the hospital?**
   Yes. Patients with inflammatory bowel disease (IBD), including patients with UC, are at high risk for VTE and should receive extended VTE prophylaxis postoperatively (e.g., 28 days postoperatively).

15. **What type of ileal pouches are used?**
   - Majority of ileal pouches are J-pouch due to relative technical ease in creation compared to other ileal pouches (W-pouch or S-pouch) with similar or better functional results. Higher-volume reservoirs (e.g., W-pouch) are generally not recommended due to poor emptying. S-pouches are mainly used only when there is mesenteric length limitation preventing a J-pouch from reaching the anus.
   - Comprehensive preoperative considerations and intraoperative judgment on selecting and creating the optimal ileal pouch are paramount due to the detrimental effects of pouch complications (e.g., pelvic sepsis) on long-term pouch function.

16. **Describe the different possible staged approaches involved in a pouch surgery.**
   - **One staged**:
     - Less often performed and generally not recommended due to the risk of anastomotic leak and infection
     - Total proctocolectomy with IPAA creation without diverting ileostomy at index procedure
   - **Traditional two staged**:
     - Typically used in the elective setting
     - Stage 1: Total proctocolectomy with IPAA and diverting ileostomy creation
     - Stage 2: Diverting ileostomy closure (in general, 6–8 weeks after initial operation)

- **Three staged:**
  - Used most often in urgent/emergent setting in hospitalized patients with severe UC
  - Stage 1: Total abdominal colectomy with end ileostomy and rectal remnant
  - Stage 2: Completion proctectomy and IPAA and diverting ileostomy creation
  - Stage 3: diverting ileostomy closure
- **Modified two staged:**
  - Stage 1: Total abdominal colectomy with end ileostomy and rectal remnant
  - Stage 2: Completion proctectomy and IPAA creation without diverting loop ileostomy

17. **Is there a difference in minimally invasive (laparoscopic or robotic) versus open approach in IPAA surgery?**
Generally, minimally invasive approaches are preferred due to improved short-term outcomes (shorter length of stay, decreased surgical site infection, and less interoperative blood loss) without compromising long-term outcomes (i.e., pouch failure or functional outcomes).

18. **Describe possible long-term complications of proctectomy and pouch formation that may be related to pelvic dissection.**
    - Males: urinary symptoms (urgency, increased frequency, or incontinence), sexual dysfunction (10%–20%), and increased stool frequency and seepage
    - Females: infertility (up to 26%), vaginal dryness, dyspareunia, urinary symptoms, sexual dysfunction, increased stool frequency and seepage, and increased incidence of cesarean section

19. **What is pouchitis?**
    - Pouchitis, one of the most frequent long-term complications of IPAA, is a nonspecific acute or chronic inflammation of the reservoir.
    - Pouchitis occurs in up to 40% of patients with IPAA; it presents with watery, bloody stools, urgency, frequency, abdominal pain, fever, malaise, and possible exacerbation of extraintestinal manifestations of IBD.
    - The cause is uncertain, but the risk is greater in chronic UC than in familial polyposis. Pouch stasis, bacterial overgrowth, dysbiosis, ischemia, pelvic sepsis, oxygen-derived free radicals, altered immune status, and lack of mucosal trophic factors have been proposed as etiologic factors.
    - Despite a preoperative diagnosis suggestive of UC and not Crohn disease, a subset of patients (~10%) will develop Crohn disease, like pouchitis with characteristics of a penetrating or fibrostenotic phenotype. However, definition of Crohn disease of the pouch remains widely heterogeneous.

20. **What is the main treatment for pouchitis?**
    - Successful treatment regimens include metronidazole or ciprofloxacin and other antianaerobic antibiotics (10- to 14-day course for acute pouchitis) as well as steroid or 5-aminosalicylate enemas. Topical volatile fatty acids and glutamine have been used with variable success.
    - Maintenance with the probiotic VSL#3 has been reported to help prevent recurrences.
    - Monoclonal antibody therapy may have limited efficacy and may be considered in patients with antibiotic refractory pouchitis.
    - In Crohn disease, like pouchitis, aggressive management with biologics or immunomodulators may be required to promote mucosal healing as antibiotics are generally not highly effective.
    - Although half of patients with pouchitis at some time suffer a recurrence, very few develop medically refractory pouchitis that requires surgery. Surgical treatment includes intestinal diversion or pouch excision.

21. **What are the risk factors for developing colorectal cancer (CRC) in UC?**
    - Younger age of diagnosis of UC and longer duration of UC
    - Increased anatomical extent of disease
    - Increased severity of disease
    - Having a family history of CRC, with the risk further increased when diagnosed prior to 50 years
    - Presence of primary sclerosing cholangitis (PSC)

22. **When should a patient start surveillance colonoscopy after being diagnosed with UC?**
Patients should undergo screen colonoscopy within 8 years of initial onset of symptoms!

23. **What is the recommended colon cancer screening surveillance schedule for high-risk and low-risk patients with UC?**
    - High-risk patients: Annual colonoscopy. This includes patients with PSC, active inflammation, a first-degree relative with CRC or dysplasia, and/or presence of a stricture.
    - Average risk patients: Every 1–3 years.

24. **Do patients who have undergone colectomy and with a rectal remnant need to undergo continued surveillance?**
Yes, regular endoscopic surveillance is warranted since rectal stump is still at risk for developing neoplasm in 3%–10% of patients.

25. **What is the recommended intervention for patients with visible lesions/dysplasia found during colonoscopy screening?**
   - Endoscopic en bloc excision (either endoscopic dissection [ESD] or endoscopic mucosal resection [EMR]) with subsequent close endoscopic surveillances.
   - Lesions that cannot be removed endoscopically (or lesions that are not visible) should undergo colectomy.

26. **How often should patients with UC with IPAA undergo pouch surveillance?**
   - Initially, surveillance at 1 year after surgery, then every 3–5 years thereafter.
   - If patient underwent proctocolectomy and IPAA creation for neoplasm or was found to have neoplasm on the surgical specimen, then pouch surveillance should be considered every 1–3 years.

SURGICAL CONSIDERATIONS IN CROHN DISEASE

27. **What classes of medical therapy are currently available for Crohn disease?**
   - Glucocorticoids
   - Immunomodulators
     - Methotrexate, 6-mercaptopurine, and azathioprine
   - Monoclonal antibodies
     - Anti–tumor necrosis factor (anti-TNF) (infliximab, adalimumab, and certolizumab)
     - Anti-integrin (vedolizumab)
     - Anti-interleukin (ustekinumab)

28. **When should surgical intervention be considered in patients with Crohn disease?**
   - Elective setting:
     - In patients who have medically refractory disease (obstruction, fistulae, and abscess), are nonadherent to medical therapy, or cannot tolerate medical therapy due to medication side effects.
   - Acute setting:
     - Patients with impending or actual perforations, fulminant colitis.
     - Patients who present with obstructive symptoms suggestive of high-grade or total obstruction should first undergo nonoperative management with nasogastric tube decompression and bowel rest. If patients fail nonoperative management, then surgery is warranted.
     - Other indications include intra-abdominal infections that cannot be controlled with antibiotics or percutaneous drains, or rare instances of bowel ischemia or infarction.

29. **Patients with less than 100 cm of small bowel remaining after small bowel resection are at risk for developing what complication(s)?**
Short gut syndrome.

30. **What is the general size cutoff for intra-abdominal abscess when considering whether to treat with antibiotics or percutaneous drainage (PD)?**
   - Initial management of intra-abdominal abscess in Crohn disease depends on the size of the abscess. In general, abscess less than 3 cm may be treated with antibiotics alone.
   - Abscess greater than 3 cm is generally treated with antibiotics and PD together.
   - The utilization of preoperative PD and antibiotics treatment first improves postoperative outcomes compared to using surgical management as initial treatment.

31. **Does the presence of enteric fistula necessitate surgical intervention?**
   - No. The mere presence of enteric fistula does not always mandate surgery. Surgical considerations should be prompted when patients present with significant malabsorption, intractable diarrhea, recurrent infection, persistent fistula despite medical therapy, or significant quality of life concerns.
   - In patients with intra-abdominal abscess due to penetrating Crohn disease and enteric fistulas, the abscess should be first controlled through antibiotics and PD. If uncontrollable, the patient should be considered for surgery with resection of the involved diseased bowel or proximal diversion alone depending on intraoperative findings. Noninflamed bowel or other internal organs that may be involved in the fistula may not require resection and can often be repaired primarily.

32. **What are the different types of intestinal strictures and their preferred first-line treatment in Crohn disease?**
    - Inflammatory:
      - Medical therapy (steroids, immunomodulators, or anti-TNF monoclonal antibodies)
    - Fibrostenotic:
      - Endoscopic dilation or surgical repair:
        - General indications for endoscopic dilation include the stricture being limited in length (<5 cm), without associated abscess, fistula, dysplasia, or cancer.

33. **What type of surgical intervention is generally available for small bowel strictures that are not amenable to medical treatment or endoscopic dilation?**
    Resection or strictureplasty.

34. **When should strictureplasty be considered over resection when considering surgical treatment for small bowel strictures?**
    - Strictureplasty is generally used when patients have multiple strictures that are not near each other anatomically. Strictureplasty performed under this setting can preserve small bowel length that would otherwise be removed if the patient were to undergo resection.
    - Strictureplasty can also be performed in areas where resection of the bowel carries high risk (e.g., duodenum).
    - Oftentimes, strictureplasty is utilized in combination with bowel resection to optimize patient outcome and bowel preservation.

35. **What are the types of strictureplasty and when are they utilized?**
    For the types of strictureplasty, see Fig. 48.1.
    - Heineke-Mikulicz
      - Strictures <10 cm in length
    - Finney
      - Strictures 10–25 cm in length
    - Michelassi (isoperistaltic side-to-side)
      - Strictures >25 cm in length

36. **Are strictures in the colon managed similarly to strictures in the small intestine?**
    - No. Due to concern for potential malignancy, colorectal strictures generally are not recommended to undergo strictureplasty.
    - Colonic strictures should be evaluated for malignancy or dysplasia. If the stricture does not allow for endoscopic evaluation, the patient should undergo standard oncologic resection.

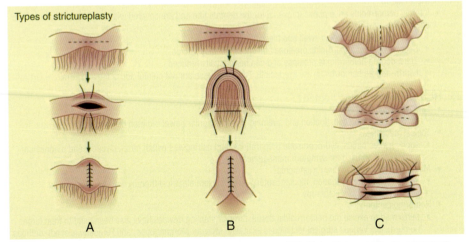

Types of strictureplasty

A   B   C

Fig. 48.1 Illustration of types of strictureplasty: (A) Heineke-Mikulicz, (B) Finney, and (C) side-to-side isoperistaltic. (From Chaudhri S, Rooney PS. Surgical management of inflammatory bowel disease. Surgery. 2008;26(8):352-356.)

37. **When should patients with Crohn disease typically start surveillance for colon cancer?**
Screen colonoscopy should be performed within 8 years of initial diagnosis. Patients diagnosed with PSC should undergo screening colonoscopy at the time of diagnosis due to increased risk for malignancy.

38. **What is the recommended treatment for patients with Crohn disease found to have single visible dysplasia on screen colonoscopy?**
   - If the visible dysplasia (confirmed by two different pathologists) is amenable to endoscopic resection, then endoscopic en bloc excision (ESD or EMR) is preferred.
   - If the visible dysplasia is not amenable to endoscopic excision, then individualized decision-making is required to determine the extent of colectomy that best balances the oncologic risks with potential complications of colectomy and preservation of unaffected colonic segments.

SURGICAL CONSIDERATIONS IN BENIGN ANORECTAL PATHOLOGIES

39. **What are anal fissures?**
A generally painful rip or tear in the sensitive anoderm of the anal canal. Most anal fissures are located in the posterior (90%) or anterior (10%) midline of the anal canal.

40. **What disorders should be considered in patients with laterally situated anal fissures?**
Crohn disease, syphilis, tuberculosis, leukemia, carcinoma, and acquired immunodeficiency syndrome.

41. **How are acute fissures managed?**
   - Conservative treatment consists of stool softeners and bulk agents to avoid hard bowel movements, sitz baths to help decrease sphincter spasm, topical anesthetics, and topical steroids.
   - In chronic fissures, topical nitroglycerin or nifedipine ointment reduces anal spasm. Injection of botulinum toxin has also been used to temporarily relax the anal sphincter.

42. **What are the signs of a chronic anal fissure?**
A chronic anal fissure can be identified by the presence of a sentinel pile (skin tag or hemorrhoid), anal ulcer (with fibropurulent material or visible internal sphincter muscle in the base), and a hypertrophied anal papilla arising from the dentate line.

43. **Which surgical procedures are available for the treatment of a chronic anal fissure?**
Open or closed lateral internal sphincterotomy, excision (ulcerectomy), excision, and Y-V or other anoplasty.

44. **Differentiate external from internal hemorrhoids.**
   - External hemorrhoids originate distal to the dentate line of the anus and are covered by squamous epithelium. External hemorrhoids may thrombose or become filled with clotted blood. Typically, these are painful, involving the anoderm.
   - Internal hemorrhoids arise above (proximal to) the dentate line and are covered with transitional and columnar epithelium.
     - First-degree hemorrhoids swell and bleed.
     - Second-degree hemorrhoids prolapse and spontaneously reduce.
     - Third-degree hemorrhoids prolapse and can be manually reduced.
     - Fourth-degree hemorrhoids are irreducible. Typically, these are not painful above the anoderm.

45. **How are hemorrhoids treated?**
   - Lifestyle management:
     - aimed at reducing constipation and straining through regular bowel regimen or fiber intake
   - Topical medicines:
     - such as anesthetics, hydrocortisone preparations, and astringents (witch hazel, glycerin, and magnesium sulfate) can be used for symptom management
   - Minimally invasive outpatient treatments:
     - include rubber band ligation, bipolar cautery, direct current electrical therapy, infrared coagulation, sclerotherapy, and cryotherapy
   - Hemorrhoidectomy:
     - performed to excise the hemorrhoidal tissue. Circular stapling devices have also been used to treat larger hemorrhoids. Various surgical techniques exist with Milligan-Morgan (open) and Ferguson (closed) methods being the two major techniques:
       - Open technique: wound bed being left open and allow to heal by secondary intention
       - Closed technique: hemorrhoidectomy wound is closed with absorbable sutures (e.g., chromic)

- Doppler-guided transanal hemorrhoidal dearterialization (THD):
  - a more recent surgical approach in the treatment of symptomatic internal hemorrhoids using Doppler guidance to identify hemorrhoidal arteries with subsequent ligation. THD may be less painful with faster recovery time compared to hemorrhoidectomy

46. How is an acute thrombosed external hemorrhoid best treated?
- If presented within 72 hours of onset, excision of the clot and involved hemorrhoidal complex (as opposed to incision alone) can be performed to best prevent future recurrence at the same site.
- Thrombosed external hemorrhoids that present after 72 hours of symptom onset can be observed without surgical intervention as the pain and discomfort associated with hemorrhoidectomy may outweigh that of the thrombosed hemorrhoid, which generally will resolve over the next 2–3 weeks.

47. Explain the cause of anorectal abscesses and fistulas.
- A cryptoglandular origin seems to provide the best explanation. Four to 10 anal glands enter the anal canal at the level of the crypts in the dentate line. The glands extend back into the internal sphincter two-thirds of the time and into the intersphincteric space half the time. Blockage of the gland leads to an overgrowth of bacteria with resultant pressure necrosis and abscess formation.
- An abscess or infection that causes an abnormal communication between two epithelialized surfaces (such as the anal canal and perianal skin) creates a fistula.

48. List the various types and locations of anorectal abscesses.
Types and locations are submucosal, intersphincteric, perianal (anal verge), ischiorectal (perirectal), and supralevator (Fig. 48.2).

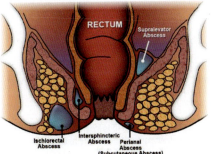

a: superficial fistula
b: intersphincteric fistula
c: transsphincteric fistula
d: supraspincteric fistula
e: extrasphincteric fistula

Fig. 48.2 Illustration of types of anal fistula and abscesses. (From American Society of Colon and Rectal Surgeons. Abscess and fistula expanded information. In American Society of Colon and Rectal Surgeons Patient Brochure. Available at: https://fascrs.org/patients/diseases-and-conditions/a-z/abscess-and-fistula-expanded-information.)

49. What is the best treatment for an anorectal abscess?
- Prompt incision and drainage. There is little or no role for antibiotics (exceptions are immunocompromised patients, patients with prosthetic heart valves, severe cellulitis, or evidence of systemic infection) and no reason to wait for the abscess to *point* or become fluctuant before surgical treatment.
- Most acutely presenting anorectal abscesses are diagnosed based on clinical findings and will not need further imaging confirmation or surgical consult prior to incision and drainage.
  - Exceptions include patients who present with occult abscesses, complex anal fistula, or perianal Crohn disease. These patients should be considered for computed tomography scan, ultrasound, magnetic resonance imaging, or fistulography.
- Incision should be as close to the anal verge as possible to minimize the length of any fistula that may occur as a result. Incision size should allow for adequate drainage of the abscess.
- Packing of the abscess cavity/wound may not be necessary if abscess has been adequately drained as it may promote unnecessary pain without significant improvement in abscess resolution or healing time.

50. What is the Goodsall rule?
- Goodsall rule is used to predict the path/direction of anorectal fistula based on the location of the external fistula opening (Fig. 48.3).
- Goodsall rule is divided based on the location of the external opening to the transverse anal line (anterior or posterior):

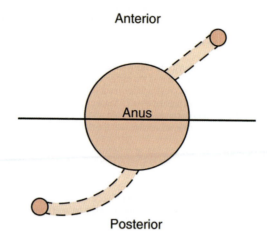

Fig. 48.3 The Goodsall rule helps predict the location of the internal opening of an anal fistula based on the site of its external opening. Accurately determining the criminal crypt of fistula origin on the dentate line is important at the time of surgical treatment, generally fistulotomy. If the anus is divided into imaginary anterior and posterior halves in the coronal plane, posterior fistulas tend to curve into the posterior midline. Anterior fistulas shorter than 3 cm tend to proceed radially to the dentate line, whereas anterior fistulas longer than 3 cm may track back to the posterior midline.

- In fistula with anterior external openings, the fistula tract generally runs directly into the anal canal
  - Exception: if the anterior opening is more than 3 cm from the anus, the fistula may have a curved trajectory, similar to posterior fistulas, that opens into the posterior midline of the anal canal.
- In fistula with posterior external openings, the fistula tract generally curves toward the posterior midline of the anal canal.

51. What is a seton?
- A seton is a drainage device used to control and treat an anal fistulous abscess. It is inserted through and through a fistula tract and secured to itself, thus making a circle about some portion of the anal sphincter muscle. It serves as a cutting device to exteriorize the fistula slowly.
- Typical seton used include Penrose drains, Silastic vessel loops, or silk sutures.

52. What are the common indications for inserting a seton?
- High fistulous abscesses involving greater than one-half the length of the anal canal muscle
- Anterior fistulas in a female
- IBD
- Older adult patients or patients with multiple previous anorectal surgeries

53. List treatment options for anorectal fistulas.
- Fibrin sealant glues
- Collagen plug
- Monoclonal anti-TNF antibodies for Crohn fistulas
- Surgery such as ligation of intersphincteric fistula tract (LIFT) procedure and fistulotomy with excision and debridement of the fistula tract, muscle repair, and advancement flap coverage

54. When is anorectal suppurative disease especially dangerous?
In the presence of neutropenia, as associated with chemotherapy. Unfortunately, surgery and even anorectal digital examination may be contraindicated. Often bacterial infection is widespread without the formation of purulence or a classic abscess.

55. What is Fournier gangrene?
- Fournier gangrene is a necrotizing soft tissue infection of the perineum. Although rare, it can present as a suspected perirectal abscess, so a high index of suspicion must be maintained. Treatment is prompt surgical debridement.

- Local signs—crepitance, bullae, and cellulitis.
- Systemic signs—altered mental status, hypotension, and oliguria.

56. What is perianal Paget disease?
- Perianal (extramammary) Paget disease is characterized by a scaly, inflamed dermis resembling eczema.
- Biopsy reveals typical Paget cells with round, pale, vacuolated, mucin-positive cytoplasm with an eccentric reticular nucleus.
- It is often a chronic condition, but underlying carcinoma must be ruled out as invasive anorectal cancer may be associated with Paget disease.

57. Which patient characteristics are associated with rectal prolapse?
- Chronic constipation
- Deep pouch of Douglas
- Neurologic disease
- Patulous anus
- Female sex
- Diastasis of the levator ani muscles
- Nulliparity
- Lack of fixation of the rectum to the sacrum
- Redundant rectosigmoid colon
- Previous anorectal surgery

58. What surgical options are available for rectal prolapse?
- Resection (open or laparoscopic approach) of redundant colon and rectum is generally associated with the best long-term results in patients who are fit for a major operation.
- For patients at higher risk for major surgery, the Altemeir procedure (perineal proctectomy) offers an alternative surgical approach.

CLINICAL VIGNETTE

Available Online

BIBLIOGRAPHY

Available Online

COLITIS: *CLOSTRIDIOIDES DIFFICILE* INFECTION, MICROSCOPIC COLITIS, AND RADIATION PROCTITIS/PROCTOPATHY

Stephen M. Vindigni, MD, MPH and Christina M. Surawicz, MD

 Additional content available online

CLOSTRIDIOIDES DIFFICILE COLITIS

1. What is *Clostridioides difficile*?

First isolated in 1935 and named for its difficult isolation from the feces of infants, *Bacillus difficile* is an anaerobic, Gram-positive, spore-forming, toxin-producing bacteria spread by the fecal-oral route. By the 1970s this *Bacillus* was renamed *Clostridium difficile* and its toxins were implicated as a major cause of diarrhea and as the cause of pseudomembranous colitis. More recently in 2016, the bacterium has been renamed *Clostridioides difficile*. *C. difficile* infection (CDI) has historically been precipitated by the use of broad-spectrum antibiotics that disrupt the normal intestinal microbiome allowing for the overgrowth of *C. difficile*. There is an increasing prevalence of sporadic and community-acquired cases occurring in healthy hosts without prior antibiotic exposure. Some healthy individuals are asymptomatic carriers. Patients with CDI can experience a spectrum of symptoms, ranging from a self-limited course of diarrhea to severe cases with ileus, toxic megacolon, and even death.

2. How does CDI cause disease?

C. difficile infects the colon when its normal microbiome is disrupted. This is most commonly due to antibiotic exposure but can be related to other conditions, such as immune suppression, older age, inflammatory bowel disease (IBD), cirrhosis, and chronic kidney disease. *C. difficile* grows in the colon and causes disease by the production of two toxins, A and B. Toxins A and B cause mucosal damage and inflammation of the colon by disrupting the actin cytoskeleton of the intestinal epithelial cells while triggering an inflammatory cascade. *C. difficile* strains that do not produce toxins are not pathogenic.

3. What are the risk factors for CDI?

The most common risk factors for CDI include antibiotic exposure (usually within the prior 2 months), recent hospitalization (especially surgical patients, intensive care unit patients, and posttransplant patients), age older than 65, comorbidities, long-term care facility exposure, and immunosuppression. Colonization at the time of hospital admission increases the risk of developing CDI sixfold. Among community-acquired CDI cases, risk factors include prior antibiotic exposure, cardiac or renal disease, and the presence of IBD. Hospital settings remain an important reservoir, in part, because the spores of the anaerobic *C. difficile*, can survive for up to 5 months if sporicidal cleaning agents are not used.

4. Which antibiotics are most commonly implicated?

Clindamycin, cephalosporins (especially third generation), and fluoroquinolones are most commonly associated with CDI. However, CDI can occur with any antibiotic, even single-dose preoperative antibiotics.

5. Why do some people develop *C. difficile* diarrhea and others are simply colonized?

From 7% to 18% of healthy adults are carriers of *C. difficile* without symptoms; in newborns and healthy infants, the carriage rate is as high as 84%. Colonization is more common following a recent hospitalization (21%) and residence in a long-term care facility (30%). Among patients with colonization, about half may carry toxigenic strains, but still do not mount CDI. Studies of patients with *C. difficile* colonization have shown that serum levels of immunoglobulin G antibody against toxin A have been associated with protection from disease expression and prevention of recurrences. Treatment is not recommended in asymptomatic colonized patients.

6. What are the current epidemiologic characteristics of CDI?

CDI is the most common nosocomial infection of the gastrointestinal tract. Since the early 2000s the morbidity and mortality of CDI have been increasing with epidemics reported in the United States, Canada, Europe, and Japan. In 2011 the estimated incidence of CDI in the United States was 453,000 cases annually with about 14,000 deaths due to the infection. More recent data from 2011 to 2017 have shown fewer infections

(~24% decrease) due to improved preventive efforts and fewer health care–associated infections; similar improvement has been seen in long-term care facilities.

The marked increase of CDI around the year 2000 has been attributed, in part, to the evolution of hypervirulent strains, such as the NAP/027/BI (North American Pulsed Field type 1, polymerase chain reaction [PCR] ribotype 027, restriction-endonuclease analysis group BI). This strain carries two genes of interest. The first gene, *tcdC*, has an 18-base pair deletion; this mutation renders the *tcdC* gene ineffective in inhibiting the production of toxins A and B, which may explain its pathogenicity. The second gene encodes a *C. difficile* binary toxin (CDT) similar to the iota toxin found in *Clostridium perfringens*, but it is not known if it contributes to pathogenicity. Patients infected with this strain have higher rates of severe CDI with higher rates of colectomy and mortality. This strain also has higher rates of fluoroquinolone and clindamycin resistance. Recent surveillance data suggest infections with this strain have been declining; however, other hypervirulent strains have been identified.

7. How is CDI diagnosed?

There is no single perfect test to diagnose CDI. Some tests are very sensitive, others are specific. In general, testing strategies should include both sensitive and specific tests to distinguish colonization from active CDI (Table 49.1). A sensitive test identifies the presence of the organism but does not identify if it is producing toxin. Toxin causes the disease.

Table 49.1 Tests for the Diagnosis of *Clostridioides difficile* Infection.

TEST	SENSITIV-ITY (%)	SPECIFICITY (%)	COMMENTS
Nucleic acid amplification tests (PCR or LAMP)	95–96	94–98	Detects gene for toxin B. Good negative predictive value. If positive, requires a test for toxin
GDH	94–96	90–96	Good negative predictive value. If positive, requires a confirmatory test
EIAs for toxins A and B	57–83	99	Detects the presence of toxin, thus distinguishes carrier/colonization from active infection

EIAs, Enzyme immunoassays; *GDH,* glutamate dehydrogenase; *LAMP,* loop-mediated isothermal amplification; *PCR,* polymerase chain reaction.

There are two sensitive tests: nucleic acid amplification tests (NAATs) and glutamate dehydrogenase (GDH). NAAT includes PCR and loop-mediated isothermal amplification testing for *C. difficile* toxin genes. NAAT is a common test in clinical laboratories. While NAAT is highly sensitive, its flaw is that it does not clarify if the gene is actively producing toxin, so a follow-up toxin test is needed if NAAT is positive. For example, asymptomatic colonized patients may have a positive NAAT only with negative toxin testing leading to CDI overdiagnosis. The second sensitive test is GDH. This test identifies an enzyme in both toxigenic and nontoxigenic strains of *C. difficile*. As it is very sensitive, it has a negative predictive value but also requires additional confirmatory testing. NAAT and GDH are good screening tests given their sensitivity, but both require follow-up confirmatory tests to evaluate for active infection.

Enzyme immunoassay (EIA) tests for toxins A and B are specific, but they are not sensitive enough to be stand-alone tests. Therefore a two-step algorithmic approach is recommended for CDI diagnosis. A common approach is to initially screen with either NAAT (usually PCR) or GDH and if there is a positive result, confirm with EIA toxin testing.

In summary:
- Positive NAAT/GDH and positive EIA = active CDI
- Positive NAAT/GDH and negative EIA = suggests colonization
- Negative NAAT/GDH = no *C. difficile* present and no further testing recommended

8. Who should be tested for *C. difficile*?

Only patients with diarrhea should be tested. Diarrhea is defined as three or more unformed stools in the prior 24 hours. This can be challenging as patients may have other reasons for loose stools. Repeat testing is discouraged as a negative test is positive less than 5% of the time on testing of a second stool. Additionally, because diagnostic tests may stay positive for up to a month, a test of cure is not advised. Of note, regardless of testing modality, if the patient presents with severe illness and concern for CDI is high, empiric antibiotic therapy should be initiated, even if *C. difficile* tests are negative. Additionally, if testing is negative, a broad differential for diarrheal stools should be considered. Lack of response to vancomycin in mild or moderate cases further supports

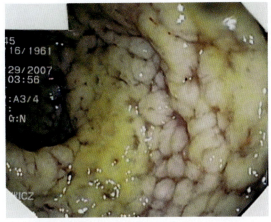

Fig. 49.1 Endoscopic findings of confluent pseudomembranes in the colon of a patient with pseudomembranous colitis. (Reprinted from Knight CL, Surawicz CM. *Clostridium difficile* infection. Med Clin N Am. 2013;97:523-536, with permission from Elsevier.)

that CDI is less likely and another explanation for diarrhea should be pursued. Severe CDI cases may not respond as quickly to vancomycin and so lack of a robust response does not rule out CDI.

9. **What are the typical findings on colonoscopy?**
   Colonoscopy may be normal or show nonspecific colitis. With severe disease, the colon mucosa has creamy white-yellow plaques (pseudomembranes) (Fig. 49.1). Although it is a sign of severe CDI, pseudomembranes can also sometimes be seen with ischemic colitis. Histologic studies show that the pseudomembrane usually arises from a point of superficial ulceration, accompanied by acute and chronic inflammation of the lamina propria. The pseudomembrane is composed of fibrin, mucin, debris of sloughed mucosal epithelial cells, and polymorphonuclear cells.

10. **What are the hallmarks of severe CDI?**
    Severe CDI is defined as leukocytosis (white blood cell count >15,000 cells/mm^3) and serum creatinine >1.5 mg/dL. Low serum albumin is often present and is associated with poor outcomes. There are several scoring systems aimed at assessing the clinical severity of CDI cases, although none have been very useful in daily practice beyond recognizing the previously discussed factors, which often correlate with severity.

11. **What are the hallmarks of fulminant CDI?**
    Patients with fulminant CDI are critically ill with an increased risk of mortality. Clinical features can include fever and shock with hypotension. Inflammatory markers, such as C-reactive protein and stool calprotectin (>2000 µg/g), may be elevated. Ileus may also be present. Severe colitis can result in toxic megacolon and progress to colonic perforation and/or death with multiorgan failure.

12. **How do we treat CDI?**
    Implicated antibiotics should be discontinued, if possible. Do not use antidiarrheals because the number of stools must be monitored to determine response to treatment. Clinical suspicion should prompt empiric treatment in patients with severe illness while awaiting test results. Two oral drugs are used for therapy: vancomycin and fidaxomicin, a poorly absorbed antibiotic. In nonsevere CDI, vancomycin or fidaxomicin are the recommended treatments. Oral metronidazole may be used as a first-line option only in low-risk patients with mild disease if there is a resource-limited setting without access to vancomycin. In severe CDI cases, oral vancomycin or fidaxomicin should be used. The typical treatment course is 10 days. In fulminant CDI, higher doses of oral vancomycin are recommended with consideration of adding intravenous (IV) metronidazole and vancomycin enemas if an ileus is present. Patients with fulminant disease who do not respond to maximal medical therapy may require surgical consultation with surgical options that include total colectomy with end ileostomy or diverting loop ileostomy with colon lavage of intraluminal vancomycin postoperatively. Fecal microbiota transplantation (FMT) can be considered in patients with severe and fulminant CDI that is refractory to antibiotics, particularly if the patient is a poor surgical candidate. For a summary of CDI treatments, see Table 49.2.

Table 49.2 Antibiotic Treatment Options for *Clostridioides difficile* Infection (CDI).

CDI SEVERITY OF DISEASE	DRUG AND DOSE	COMMENT
Nonsevere (no signs of severe disease below)	Vancomycin 125 mg PO qid × 10 days Or Fidaxomicin 200 mg PO bid × 10 days	1. In patients with IBD, vancomycin is recommended 2. In low-risk patients, one can consider metronidazole 500 mg PO tid × 10 days if resource limited
Severe (WBC >to 15,000 cells/mm³ and/or serum creatinine >1.5 mg/dL)	Vancomycin 125 mg PO qid × 10 days Or Fidaxomicin 200 mg PO bid × 10 days	Do not use metronidazole
Fulminant (severe and hypotension or shock or ileus or megacolon)	Vancomycin 500 mg PO qid	1. Can add metronidazole 500 mg IV q 8 hr 2. If ileus, consider vancomycin enemas, 500 mg qid 3. Surgery should be considered in cases not responding to maximal medical therapy. FMT can also be considered
Recurrent CDI first recurrence	Vancomycin pulse/taper regimen Or Fidaxomicin 200 mg PO bid × 10 days If initial course was fidaxomicin, vancomycin pulse/taper regimen	Second recurrence: FMT via colonoscopy preferred. If not a candidate, long-term low-dose suppressive vancomycin can be used

FMT, Fecal microbiota transplantation; *IBD,* inflammatory bowel disease; *IV,* intravenous; *PO,* by mouth; *qid,* four times daily; *tid,* three times daily; *WBC,* white blood cell.

13. When should you expect a response to treatment?

Response to treatment usually occurs within 3–5 days. There is no evidence to support stool testing for cure; therefore this should not be done. Both toxins A and B EIA may remain positive for as long as 30 days, including in patients with resolution of symptoms; false positives may further complicate patient care.

14. What is recurrent CDI (rCDI) and how do you treat a first recurrence?

Despite therapy, approximately 20% of patients have CDI recurrence, likely due to the altered intestinal microbiome. Moreover, spores may persist in the environment despite the initial elimination of the *C. difficile* bacteria leading to reexposure. rCDI is defined as a recurrence of diarrhea and a confirmatory diagnostic test (either NAAT or EIA) within 8 weeks of treatment of the initial infection. Patients who have one recurrence are at increased risk of additional recurrences. The recommended treatments for initial rCDI are a tapered, pulse-dosed vancomycin regimen or fidaxomicin if the initial treatment was vancomycin (Table 49.2).

15. What if there are further recurrences of CDI?

The goal of CDI has been focused on the eradication of the pathogen with antibiotic treatment; however, with a persistently altered microbiome, there is an adjunct treatment—FMT. FMT is the transfer of *healthy bacteria* from a healthy donor to a recipient with an altered microbiome, such as in the case of CDI. The goal of FMT is to reestablish the diverse normal microbiome within the large intestine. FMT repopulates bacteria relatively quickly, and the effect persists. It is recommended that FMT be considered in patients who have a second recurrence of CDI. Colonoscopy is the preferred mode of delivery. FMT is viewed as a success if the patient does not have a CDI recurrence within 8 weeks. Multiple studies and systematic reviews have described high levels of success with FMT, with response rates of up to 98%. If the patient is determined not to be a good candidate for FMT, a long-term, low-dose suppressive vancomycin regimen can be used.

16. Are there any special considerations for patients with IBD?

Patients with IBD, especially with ulcerative colitis or Crohn colitis, are at increased risk of CDI. This risk is increased regardless of age or IBD medication. Any patients with IBD who display a change in symptoms or concerns for flare should be tested for *C. difficileC. difficile.* Treatment in these patients should be with oral vancomycin (125 mg orally four times daily × 14 days); fidaxomicin and metronidazole are not recommended. Immunosuppressive therapy should be continued and not held due to infection. It is often important to consult with an IBD expert on these cases.

17. **How can we control** *C. difficile* **epidemics in hospitals?**
    In health care settings, one core prevention strategy is the isolation of patients with confirmed or suspected CDI; patients should have personal bathrooms until their diarrhea resolves and patient rooms should have dedicated equipment. Contact enteric precautions should be initiated; *C. difficile* spores have been cultured from patient bathrooms, bedpans, stethoscopes, and blood pressure cuffs. Staff should use isolation gowns and gloves and engage in hand hygiene with soap and water. Once patients depart from their isolation rooms, these rooms should be cleansed with an Environmental Protection Agency sporicidal agent. As increasing antibiotic resistance remains a concern, antibiotic stewardship is recommended. There has not been a benefit demonstrated with the prophylactic use of probiotics.

18. **What is bezlotoxumab?**
    Bezlotoxumab is a medication containing a fully humanized monoclonal antibody that binds *C. difficile* toxin B. The binding of toxin B neutralizes the toxin thereby limiting damage to the colon. The Food and Drug Administration (FDA) has approved this medication for *C. difficile* with a single 10 mg/kg dose IV over a 60-minute infusion. It is very expensive and thus is recommended for patients who are at an increased risk of recurrence. Thus bezlotoxumab is an adjunct to antibiotic therapy as it has been shown to prevent *C. difficile* recurrence (up to 10% compared to placebo) with greater efficacy in patients with more risk factors for rCDI. Of note, a risk of heart failure has been demonstrated with the use of this drug, particularly in patients with underlying cardiac disease.

19. **What other treatment options are available or under development and investigation?**
    Although research is underway, one hypothesis is that patients with rCDI have an altered immune response contributing to disease recurrence. Thus there are active investigations into the development of a *C. difficile* vaccine. There are also novel therapeutics, including newer antibiotics and oral spore-containing formulations for rCDI. Among antibiotics, teicoplanin is an oral antibiotic used in Europe that has shown efficacy in the elderly; ridinilazole is in clinical trials as another antibiotic with efficacy against *C. difficile* without producing significant alteration of the microbiome. There are several microbiota replacement spore-containing agents under evaluation with two approved by the FDA: SER-109 (administered orally) and RBX2660 (administered rectally).

MICROSCOPIC COLITIS

20. **What is microscopic colitis (MC)?**
    MC is a chronic inflammatory disease of the colon, characterized by chronic, nonbloody, watery diarrhea with grossly normal-appearing colonic mucosa, and abnormal histology on colorectal biopsy. It usually presents in middle-aged people and is more common in females. There are two forms: collagenous colitis (CC) and lymphocytic colitis (LC). Both have similar symptoms but different changes in colorectal biopsy.

21. **What are the clinical features of MC?**
    The most common clinical symptoms are chronic, nonbloody diarrhea (95%), weight loss (91%), abdominal pain (40%), urgency (29%), and nocturnal diarrhea (22%). These symptoms can be severe in some patients. Clinically, CC and LC are indistinguishable.

22. **How are patients with MC distinguished from patients with irritable bowel syndrome (IBS)?**
    The gold standard is colorectal biopsy, which is normal in patients with IBS. There is considerable overlap of symptoms between MC and IBS. Studies have shown that as many as 33% of patients with biopsy-proven CC or LC will have a prior diagnosis of IBS and that as many as half of the patients diagnosed with MC will also meet the diagnostic criteria for IBS.

23. **Are there any laboratory tests or imaging studies that can help establish the diagnosis of MC?**
    Laboratory tests and radiographic imaging are generally nondiagnostic; therefore there is no role for imaging studies in the diagnosis of MC, unless indicated for other reasons. Fecal leukocytes may be present, but stool cultures are negative. C-reactive protein levels, erythrocyte sedimentation rates, and stool calprotectin may be elevated; anemia may be present. Colonoscopy typically is normal, but there can be subtle mucosal changes in the colon.

24. **How common is MC?**
    Studies show CC incidence rates of 2.6–10.8 per 100,000 people and LC incidence rates of 2.2–14 per 100,000 people. Cases have been identified in the United States, Europe, Canada, Africa, Asia, Australia, and Latin America,

suggesting worldwide distribution. The highest incidence has been in northern countries (the United States, Denmark, and Canada) suggesting a north-south gradient, although this is not uniformly consistent. Additionally, MC tends to be more common in older adults, with an average age of diagnosis at 65. Overall, MC is more common in females.

25. **Which parts of the colon are most commonly affected?**
MC can be diffuse or can involve the colon discontinuously. Thus, it is important to biopsy both the left and right colon for diagnosis. In one prior study, the highest yield was from biopsies of the transverse colon.

26. **What agents are associated with the pathogenesis of MC?**
Nonsteroidal anti-inflammatory drugs (NSAIDs) are thought to be a pathogenic factor in some patients. A case-controlled study showed that patients with CC were three times more likely to take NSAIDs. LC has been associated with the use of sertraline. Other potential medications associated with the development of MC include aspirin, acarbose, clozapine, entacapone, flavonoid, proton pump inhibitors (especially lansoprazole), ranitidine, and ticlopidine. Of note, many of these drugs have an adverse effect of chronic diarrhea; therefore attributing a drug as the cause of MC is more challenging. Although the contribution of environmental factors is not clear, smoking has been associated with MC, including with the development of disease 10 years earlier than nonsmokers. In one study, previous or current smoking had an odds ratio of 2.4 for CC and 1.6 for LC, see Table 49.3.

27. **Are there associated conditions in patients with MC?**
A wide variety of associated conditions are described in case reports, including thyroid disease, celiac disease, diabetes, rheumatoid arthritis, and asthma and allergies in up to 40%–50% of patients with MC. If a patient with celiac disease treated with a gluten-free diet continues to have diarrheal symptoms, colonoscopy should be considered to evaluate for concurrent MC, see Table 49.3.

Table 49.3 Etiologic Factors Associated With Microscopic Colitis.

FACTORS	EXAMPLES
Medications	NSAIDs and aspirin PPIs, especially lansoprazole H2 blockers Statins SSRIs Clozapine Acarbose
Social habits	Smoking
Diseases (autoimmune)	Celiac disease Thyroiditis Type 1 diabetes mellitus, nonerosive oligoarticular arthritis
Genetics	*HLA-DR3-DQ2* haplotype

H2, Hydrogen; *NSAIDs*, Nonsteroidal antiinflammatory drugs; *PPIs*, proton-pump inhibitors; *SSRIs*, selective serotonin reuptake inhibitors.

28. **What is the natural history of MC?**
The natural history is not known. Often the disease is insidious but may have an acute onset in up to 40% of patients. In one study, 505 patients with MC experienced resolution of their symptoms after 3 years. However, as many as 30% of patients treated for MC will experience persistent diarrhea 10 years after diagnosis. The clinical course may be complicated by the patient's response to medication. There is no increased risk of malignancy associated with MC.

29. **What are the treatment options?**
Initially, patients with MC can make dietary changes (avoid caffeine, alcohol, and possibly dairy products) and stop any medications that have been associated with MC. Some patients do well on antidiarrheal agents (loperamide) or on cholestyramine alone. A meta-analysis has shown that oral budesonide (9 mg daily) for 6–8 weeks has been effective in decreasing symptoms in 81% of patients with CC; however, symptoms recurred in 60%–80% of patients with the cessation of budesonide. These patients responded to retreatment with budesonide and often required subsequent slow tapers. Budesonide has also been shown to be effective in treating LC. There are no evidence-based alternatives to budesonide. Bismuth subsalicylate and sulfasalazine or mesalamine have shown

efficacy in a few studies. Probiotics offered no benefit over placebo in studies. Some patients require stronger immunosuppressants, such as methotrexate, 6-mercaptopurine, or azathioprine; there is ongoing research to determine the utility of anti–tumor necrosis factor therapy with infliximab and adalimumab. In rare cases, patients may require surgery, such as diverting ileostomy or colectomy, for severe and refractory disease.

RADIATION PROCTITIS/PROCTOPATHY

30. What is the spectrum of radiation injury to the distal colon?
Radiation injury of the rectum from pelvic radiation can be acute or chronic. Acute radiation proctitis is better called proctopathy because there is little or no inflammation. There are two types of chronic injury: radiation-associated vascular ectasias (RAVE) and radiation proctopathy, where there is mucosal injury, but minimal to no inflammation.

31. What are the symptoms of acute injury?
Acute radiation injury to the colon typically occurs within 6 weeks of radiation exposure and is manifested by abdominal or pelvic pain, diarrhea, mucus discharge, tenesmus, and rarely bleeding. These symptoms are self-limited and typically resolve in 2–6 months without therapy.

32. What are the symptoms of chronic injury?
Symptoms of chronic radiation proctopathy can occur 9–12 months following radiation therapy but can be delayed after the initial radiation exposure. The primary symptom is rectal bleeding and associated iron-deficiency anemia due to RAVE. Other symptoms include fecal urgency, change in stool caliber and/or consistency, constipation, and overflow diarrhea.

33. What is the role of colonoscopy and biopsy?
Endoscopic features in the acute phase may be normal, or nonspecific. Endoscopy may be normal or may show telangiectasias, pallor, and friable mucosa. On biopsy, there may be vascular ectasias, with dilated capillaries, and hyalinized lamina propria around the vessels. In chronic injury, late changes commonly involve fibrosis with obliterative endarteritis resulting in chronic ischemia, stricture formation, and bleeding. Endoscopy may show telangiectasias and/or strictures. On biopsy, there may be fibrosis of the lamina propria and crypt distortion but minimal or no inflammatory cell infiltrate or ulcers.

34. What can be done to prevent radiation damage?
The extent of radiation colitis depends on the cumulative radiation dose, fraction size, technique of radiation delivery, amount of tissue exposed, and presence of other treatments, such as surgery or chemotherapy. Of those listed, radiation dose appears to be the most significant factor. Radiation damage can be reduced by limiting the dosage and area of exposure while shielding adjacent tissues.

35. How can symptoms of acute and chronic radiation be managed?
For acute injury, supportive therapy may be all that is needed. When symptoms are bothersome, sodium butyrate enemas have been shown to induce remission.

For chronic injury, sucralfate enemas may decrease symptoms of pain, tenesmus, and/or bleeding.

36. What is the role of endoscopic therapy for bleeding?
Endoscopic therapy can help treat persistent rectal bleeding due to telangiectasias. Argon plasma coagulation, heater probe, bipolar cautery, and radiofrequency ablation have all been used. Patients should be transfused with blood as needed and take oral iron.

37. How are chronic, radiation-induced bowel strictures managed?
Patients with mild obstructive symptoms often benefit from the use of stool softeners. Endoscopic dilation of the stricture may be helpful if the stricture is short. Patients with long or angulated strictures may benefit from surgery as these lesions are more likely to perforate with dilating procedures. Recurrent strictures may be treated with steroid injections. Colonic stents have also been used but increase the risk of bowel perforation.

BIBLIOGRAPHY

Available Online

UPPER GASTROINTESTINAL HEMORRHAGE

Geoffrey Bader, MD and John Gancayco, MD

 Additional content available online

1. What is the definition and burden of upper gastrointestinal (UGI) bleeding?

UGI bleeding refers to bleeding from sites in the esophagus, stomach, or duodenum proximal to the ligament of Treitz. Nearly 80% of patients visiting emergency departments (EDs) for UGI bleeding are admitted to the hospital, resulting in over 300,000 admissions annually with a mortality of 3.5%–10%.

2. What are the signs, symptoms, and risk factors of UGI bleeding?

Overt UGI bleeding is mostly typically present with melena (black, tarry stool), which can be produced with as little as 50 mL of blood. Patients may also manifest with hematemesis (vomiting of red blood or coffee ground emesis) and/or hematochezia. Aside from hematemesis, no feature is specific to UGI bleeding. Melena is the feature most suggestive of a UGI bleed (likelihood ratio [LR] 25) but can be seen with distal small bowel and right-sided colonic bleeding. Other features suggestive of a UGI bleed rather than lower GI bleed include a blood urea nitrogen (BUN)/creatinine ratio of more than 30 (LR 7.5), and a report of melena (LR 5.1–5.9). While hematochezia more typically indicates a lower GI bleeding source, it can occur with large volume bleeding from a UGI bleeding source and is typically associated with hemodynamic instability. Additional signs (e.g., ascites and spider angiomata) and symptoms (e.g., abdominal pain and heartburn) may also be present and guide suspicion for an underlying etiology. Table 50.1 summarizes important presenting features in patients with UGI bleeding.

3. What are the most common etiologies of UGI bleeding?

Peptic ulcer disease (PUD) is by far the most common etiology of UGI bleeding (20%–50%), followed by gastroduodenal erosions (8%–15%), esophagitis (5%–15%), complications of portal hypertension (5%–20%), Mallory-Weiss tears (8%–15%), and vascular malformations (5%). Other less common causes such as aortoenteric fistulas and GI tumors make up the remaining cases with an identifiable etiology.

4. What are the best clinical features to risk stratify the severity of suspected UGI bleeding?

The primary goal of the initial assessment is to risk stratify patients who need urgent intervention versus those who can undergo nonurgent endoscopy, or even be discharged from the ED for outpatient care. Numerous factors are a part of this process, including patient history, vital signs and physical examination, and initial tests. High-risk features include a history of malignancy, cirrhosis, hematemesis on presentation, hemoglobin <8 mg/dL, and abnormal vital signs. Mild to moderate blood loss (500–1000 mL) results in resting tachycardia, whereas loss of 1000 mL will produce orthostatic changes. Loss of 2000 mL or more of blood will produce shock. Fig. 50.1 outlines the appropriate algorithmic approach to UGI bleeding upon presentation to the ED.

5. What are the validated scoring systems to risk stratify the severity of suspected UGI bleeding?

The Glasgow-Blatchford score (GBS) is the recommended risk assessment tool to identify very-low-risk patients who can be discharged from the ED with outpatient follow-up (Table 50.2). Patients with a GBS score of 0–1 have a ≤1% risk of transfusion, hemostatic intervention, or death. Additional prediction scores include the AIMS-65 (albumin, international normalized ratio [INR], mental status, systolic blood pressure, age >65 years) to predict in-hospital mortality and the Rockall score to predict mortality after incorporating endoscopic findings.

6. What role is there for nasogastric (NG) tube lavage?

A bloody NG lavage has been shown to increase the likelihood of high-risk lesions at the time of endoscopy (positive predictive value 32%–45%). However, NG lavage is not necessary for diagnosis, prognosis, or visualization and is very painful and poorly tolerated by patients. Therefore it is *not routinely* recommended in patients with suspected UGI bleeding!

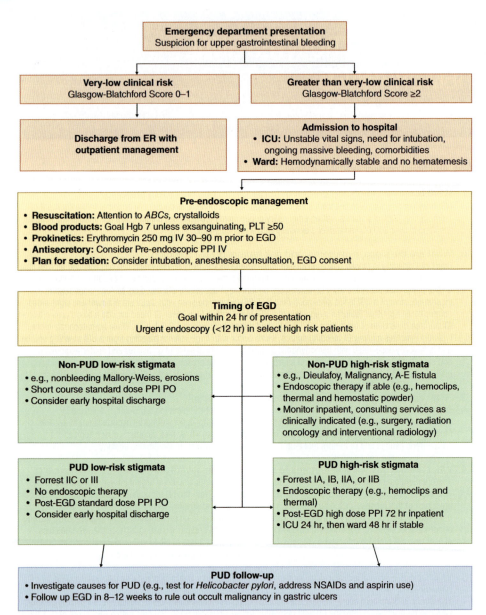

Fig. 50.1 Algorithm for the management of nonvariceal upper gastrointestinal bleeding. *ABCs,* Airway, breathing, circulation; *A-E fistula,* aortoenteric fistula; *EGD,* esophagogastroduodenoscopy; *Hgb,* hemoglobin; *ICU,* intensive care unit; *IV,* intravenous; *NSAIDs,* nonsteroidal anti-inflammatory drugs; *PLT,* platelets; *PO,* by mouth; *PPI,* proton pump inhibitor; *PUD,* peptic ulcer disease. (Data from Laine L, Barkun AN, Saltzman JR, Martel M, Leontiadis GI. ACG clinical guideline: upper gastrointestinal and ulcer bleeding. Am J Gastroenterol. 2021;116:899-917.)

7. **What are the first steps in the management of UGI bleeding?**

The initial care of patients with UGI bleeding is focused on the patient's *ABCs* (airway, breathing, circulation). Patients with large volume hematemesis or altered mental status should be considered for intubation for airway protection. Adequate vascular access is critical, including two large-bore (≥18 gauge) peripheral intravenous (IV) catheters, and potentially a central venous line. Volume replacement with crystalloid fluids is central to

Table 50.1 Risk Factors, Symptoms, and Signs of Upper Gastrointestinal (UGI) Bleeding.

RISK FACTORS	HISTORY	EXAMINATION
Medications (aspirin, NSAIDs, and corticosteroids) Stress (trauma, burns, and CNS injury) Intubation ≥48 hr Coagulopathy (PLT <50 or INR >1.5) Alcohol abuse Chronic liver disease *Helicobacter pylori* infection	Melena Hematemesis Hematochezia Dizziness Syncope Acid reflux (esophagitis) Dyspepsia Vomiting prior to bleeding episode (Mallory-Weiss tear) Aortic aneurysm repair (aortoenteric fistula) Prior UGI bleeding	Orthostasis Tachycardia Hypotension Melena or hematochezia on rectal examination Nasogastric tube aspirate positive for blood or *coffee grounds* Abdominal tenderness Stigmata of chronic liver disease

CNS, Central nervous system; *PLT*, platelets; *INR*, international normalized ratio; *NSAID*, nonsteroidal anti-inflammatory drug; *UGI*, upper gastrointestinal.

Table 50.2 Glascow-Blatchford Score

CLINICAL PARAMETERS AT PRESENTATION	THRESHOLDS	SCORE
Systolic blood pressure (mm Hg)	≥ 110	0
	100 to 109	1
	90 to 99	2
	< 90	3
Blood urea nitrogen (mg/dL)	< 18	0
	18 to 22	1
	22 to 28	2
	28 to 69	3
	> 70	6
Hemoglobin for men (g/dL)	≥ 13	0
	12 to 12.9	1
	10 to 11.9	3
	< 10	6
Hemoglobin for women (g/dL)	≥ 12	0
	10 to 11.9	1
	< 10	6
Other variables at presentation	Pulse > 100	1
	Melena	1
	Syncope	2
	Hepatic disease	2
	Cardiac failure	2
	Maximum score	**23**

The risk of requiring endoscopic intervention increases with a higher score. A Blatchford score of zero to one is associated with a low likelihood of the need for urgent endoscopic intervention.
Adapted from Blatchford O, Murray WR, Blatchford M. A risk score to predict need for treatment for upper gastrointestinal hemorrhage. Lancet. 2000;356:1318-1321.

resuscitation, particularly in the presence of active bleeding or abnormal vital signs. Initial laboratories include a complete blood count, creatinine, BUN, prothrombin time (PT), partial thromboplastin time, and a blood type and screen. Patients with active bleeding and hemodynamic instability should have units of packed red blood cells (RBCs) cross-matched for urgent use.

8. **What are the recommended hemoglobin transfusion goals in patients with UGI bleeding?**
   In a landmark trial, patients with acute UGI bleeding randomized to a *restrictiverestrictive* hemoglobin goal of 7 g/dL had a significantly better survival rate than those managed with a goal of 9 g/dL. It is important to note that patients with preexisting cardiovascular disease and those with exsanguinating UGI bleeding were excluded from such trials. It is reasonable that patients with hypotension with preexisting cardiovascular disease receive packed RBC transfusion before hemoglobin levels drop below 7 g/dL and to target a hemoglobin threshold of 8 g/dL.

9. **What are the goal platelet and coagulation factors in patients with UGI bleeding?**
   Best practices regarding correction of platelets and coagulation factors remain controversial, driven largely by a paucity of data. Expert opinion recommends a goal platelet count of greater than 50,000 prior to endoscopy, regardless of prior antiplatelet therapies. Historically, a goal INR of less than 1.5–2.0 was recommended, though the benefit of this recommendation has been called into question, particularly given the shift to direct oral anticoagulants (DOACs) from warfarin. The use of antithrombotic medications requires careful multidisciplinary discussion, as the risks of cardiopulmonary or neurologic thromboembolic events are usually more devastating than ongoing UGI bleeding. Regardless of the cause, endoscopy should not be delayed for the correction of coagulopathy.

10. **What is the role for *reversing* coagulopathy among patients with cirrhosis and UGI bleeding?**
    It is critical to note that in patients with cirrhosis the PT does not reflect bleeding tendency, and correction of INR with fresh-frozen plasma (FFP) or recombinant activated factor VII to *correct* INR does not improve outcomes and is not recommended.

11. **What is the role and benefit of pre-endoscopic proton pump inhibitors (PPIs) in patients with UGI bleeding?**
    Despite near universal clinical use, the data supporting the role of pre-endoscopic PPI are relatively modest and limited in its clinical outcomes. The primary benefit of PPIs is driven by their ability to increase gastric pH, thus optimizing platelet aggregation and clot formation. Omeprazole infusion has been shown to reduce the rate of high-risk stigmata and need for endoscopic intervention. To date, pre-endoscopic PPI has not been demonstrated to reduce bleeding or mortality.

12. **What is the role of prokinetic medications in patients with UGI bleeding?**
    The use of prokinetic agents is based on their theoretical ability to propel blood and clot distally to aid in adequate endoscopic visualization of bleeding stigmata. Guidelines recommend the infusion of 250 mg IV erythromycin 20–90 minutes prior to endoscopy, based in large part on a meta-analysis demonstrating significant reductions in hospital length of stay and the need for second-look endoscopy.

13. **When should upper endoscopy be performed?**
    Timing of endoscopy is a clinical judgment, dependent on the assessment of severity and adequate resuscitation, as early endoscopy in patients with hemodynamic instability or significant comorbidities can result in harm. Guidelines recommend endoscopy be performed within 24 hours of presentation. More urgent endoscopy (within 12 hours) may be considered for select high-risk patients, such as those with hematemesis or persistent hemodynamical compromise after initial resuscitation.

14. **What endoscopic findings guide risk stratification and treatment?**
    Endoscopy is effective at diagnosing and management of most causes of UGI bleeding, along with guiding medical therapies and disposition. The Forrest classification of peptic ulcers is a widely used system to standardize lesion descriptions, predict rebleeding and mortality risk, and guide treatment (Table 50.3). Other notable high-risk endoscopic features for rebleeding include size (i.e., >1–2 cm) and location such as the posterior duodenal wall.

15. **What are the endoscopic techniques for managing nonvariceal UGI bleeding?**
    There are numerous endoscopic therapies, which can broadly be categorized as mechanical (e.g., clips) or thermal (e.g., multipolar catheters) (Table 50.4). There is no definitively superior modality, thus the choice is at the discretion of the endoscopist based on the type and location of the lesion, along with endoscopist expertise. Subcutaneous epinephrine should be used in combination with another hemostatic modality, not as monotherapy. Over-the-scope clips (OTSCs) are currently recommended for patients with recurrent ulcer bleeding after previous successful endoscopic hemostasis. Endoscopic hemostatic powder spray TC-325 can be considered for actively

Table 50.3 Forrest Classification of Peptic Ulcers.

FORREST CLASSIFICATION	STIGMATA OF HEMORRHAGE	PREVALENCE (%)	TREATMENT	REBLEEDING RATE WITHOUT ENDOSCOPIC THERAPY (%)	MORTALITY WITHOUT ENDOSCOPIC THERAPY (%)
IA	Spurting blood	12 (spurting + oozing)	IV PPI bolus + infusion, endoscopic treatment	55 (spurting and oozing)	11
IB	Oozing blood		IV PPI bolus + infusion, endoscopic treatment		
IIA	Nonbleeding visible vessel	8	IV PPI bolus + infusion, endoscopic treatment	43	11
IIB	Adherent clot	8	IV PPI bolus + infusion, consider endoscopic treatment	22	7
IIC	Flat pigmented spot	16	Oral PPI	10	3
III	Clean-based ulcer	55	Oral PPI	5	2

IV, Intravenous; *PPI,* proton pump inhibitor.
Adapted from Laine L, Jensen DM. Management of patients with ulcer bleeding. Am J Gastroenterol. 2012;107(3):345-360.

bleeding lesions as a temporizing method if the use of other modalities is precluded by lesion characteristics (e.g., poor visibility), with plans for a repeat endoscopy for definitive intervention.

16. **What are the basic management principles for non-PUD etiologies found on endoscopy?**
While PUD is the most common etiology of UGI bleeding, additional lesions have characteristic findings and unique management principles.
   - Mallory-Weiss tears are lacerations of the gastroesophageal junction, gastric cardia, or distal esophagus, often occurring as a result of excessive emesis and typically with self-limited bleeding. Endoscopic therapy is reserved for lesions with ongoing or severe bleeding, with endoscopic techniques similar to PUD and dependent on the location and endoscopist expertise; short-term (2–4 weeks) oral standard-dose PPI is typically recommended.
   - Dieulafoy lesions are ruptured dilated aberrant submucosal arteries without associated ulceration that typically occur in the stomach but may occur through the GI tract. Combination endoscopic modalities similar to PUD management are effective; given these lesions can be difficult to identify without active hemorrhage, adjacent tattoo placement is recommended to facilitate retreatment if recurrent bleeding is suspected.
   - Aortoenteric fistulas are a medical emergency, typically presenting with a self-limited *herald* bleed followed by massive UGI hemorrhage. Clinical suspicion should be prompted by history (such as a prior aortic surgery) and requires emergent contrasted computed tomography imaging and surgical consultation.

17. **How is nonvariceal UGI bleeding that is refractory to initial endoscopic managed?**
Index endoscopic therapy with appropriate PPI therapy is successful in controlling bleeding in 80%–90% of patients with nonvariceal UGI bleeding. Among patients with recurrent bleeding, repeat endoscopic therapy has been shown to achieve hemostasis in over 70% of patients after a second attempt, as well as fewer complications compared with surgery; there is evidence supporting the use of OTSCs in this setting. For patients who continue to bleed despite endoscopic attempts, transcatheter arterial embolization by interventional radiology should be considered and surgical consultation should be obtained.

Table 50.4 Endoscopic Techniques for the Management of Nonvariceal Bleeding.

TECHNIQUE	USAGE
Epinephrine (1:10,000) injected in four quadrants around the lesion	Not effective as monotherapy for hemostasis; useful temporizing measure requiring combination with another endoscopic technique
Thermal contact therapy (bipolar probes and heater probes)	Decrease further bleeding, need for surgery, and mortality; ideal practice is 10 Fr probe when possible, firm pressure for 8–10 s at 15 W, for 4–5 pulses
Through-the-scope endoclip	Decrease bleeding and need for surgery; can be technically challenging in certain locations (e.g., posterior duodenal wall) and lesion characteristics (e.g., fibrosis and large ulcer size)
Over-the-scope clips	Consider for select cases, typically persistent bleeding from PUD despite standard therapy or large, fibrotic ulcer beds not amendable to hemoclips or when thermal therapy is ineffective
Hemostatic powder spray (TC-325)	Consider in cases of massive bleeding with poor visualization, for salvage therapy, and diffuse malignancy–associated bleeding
Other: APC, Nd:YAG laser, monopolar thermal probe, thrombin/fibrin glue, sclerosant (e.g., absolute alcohol and 5% ethanolamine)	Not first-line (limited data, less availability, and cost issues), sclerosants have risk of tissue necrosis

APC, Argon plasma coagulation; Fr, French; Nd:YAG: neodymium-doped yttrium aluminum garnet; *PUD*, peptic ulcer disease; *W*, watts. Data from Mullady DK, Wang AY, Waschke KA. AGA clinical practice update on endoscopic therapies for non-variceal upper gastrointestinal bleeding: expert review. Gastroenterology 2020;159(3):1120-1128. ISSN 0016-5085. https://doi.org/10.1053/j.gastro.2020.05.095.

18. **What is the non-endoscopic management of PUD?**
Patients who underwent successful endoscopic therapy of a high-risk ulcer should receive high-dose PPI therapy given continuously (80 mg IV bolus followed by 8 mg/minute infusion) or intermittently (80 mg IV bolus followed by 40 mg twice daily, orally if feasible) for 3 days in the hospital. These patients can then be considered for discharge and continued on twice-daily PPI; the total duration of PPI therapy is controversial, with guidelines offering a conditional recommendation of at least 2 weeks therapy after endoscopy based on limited data, but many patients clinically receive 8–12 weeks therapy based on convention. Patients with low-risk PUD do not require inpatient high-dose PPI and can be considered for early discharge post-endoscopy and oral standard-dose PPI.

19. **What post-endoscopic workup is required for PUD?**
All patients with PUD should be assessed for contributing etiologies, including *Helicobacter pylori* testing (via gastric biopsies at the time of index endoscopy and/or urea breath test or stool antigen once off PPI for at least 2 weeks). Among patients with idiopathic PUD, indefinite standard-dose PPI should be considered. Follow-up endoscopy is also recommended for gastric PUD (see Question 20).

20. **What is the management of antithrombotic agents in the setting of acute GI bleeding?**
Recent guidelines have changed the management of antithrombotic agents in the setting of acute GI bleeding. DOACs and vitamin K antagonists should be held in the setting of acute GI bleeding. For patients taking vitamin K antagonists, the administration of FFP or vitamin K is not recommended. In cases of life-threatening UGI bleeding for patients taking vitamin K antagonists, prothrombin complex concentrate (PCC) is recommended over FFP or vitamin K. For patients on DOACs, PCC and reversal agents, such as idarucizumab and andexanet alfa, are not recommended due to limited data on efficacy and cost. Patients on antiplatelet agents admitted for UGI bleeding should not be given platelets. Patients with UGI bleeding who are on aspirin for secondary prevention of cardiovascular disease should have aspirin continued. If aspirin is withheld for patients on presentation, aspirin should be restarted on the day hemostasis is achieved.

21. **When should patients receive follow-up after their episode of nonvariceal UGI bleeding?**
Patients should follow-up with their primary care physician within 1–2 weeks after hospitalization to screen for recurrent bleeding. For the majority of patients with gastric ulcers, a follow-up endoscopy is recommended

after 8–12 weeks of medical therapy to ensure endoscopic healing and to exclude gastric cancer; notably, false-negative biopsy rates of 2%–5% have been reported of malignant gastric ulcers on index endoscopy. Duodenal ulcers and most etiologies of non-PUD GI bleeding, such as Mallory-Weiss tears and Dieulafoy lesions, do not require dedicated follow-up endoscopy.

22. When should one suspect a variceal bleed?

Despite advances in care, variceal hemorrhage remains a uniquely life-threatening event for patients with cirrhosis, with a 6-week mortality rate of 10%–20%. A high index of suspicion and rapid diagnosis facilitate numerous unique adjunctive medical therapies and resuscitation principles that improve outcomes among patients with variceal hemorrhage. Risk factors for chronic liver disease (e.g., excessive alcohol use and viral hepatitis), stigmata of chronic liver disease on physical examination (e.g., spider angiomata, palmar erythema, and jaundice), and hematemesis, with hematochezia and hemodynamic compromise, make a variceal bleed more likely.

23. What pre-endoscopic therapies should be considered in the management of suspected variceal bleeding?

- Among patients with cirrhosis who experience GI bleeding, over 50% develop bacterial infections, which has been shown to be an independent risk factor for failure to control bleeding, high risk of rebleeding, and increased mortality. Early antibiotic prophylaxis with antibiotics (e.g., IV ceftriaxone 1 g every 24 hours) for a maximum of 7 days is first-line; treatment can be discontinued once hemorrhage has resolved, and use should not be extended after hospital discharge.
- An IV splanchnic vasoconstrictor (only octreotide is available in the United States) to decrease portal pressure acutely should be started as soon as possible, as early administration is associated with improved survival. Typical dosing of octreotide is a 50 mcg IV bolus followed by a continuous infusion of 50 mcg/hr, to be continued for 2–5 days.
- It is important to remember that patients with cirrhosis are still at risk of bleeding from nonvariceal sources, which collectively account for approximately 50% of UGI bleeds in patients with cirrhosis. Thus pre-endoscopic PPIs should be considered.
- Fig. 50.2 outlines the appropriate algorithmic management of suspected variceal hemorrhage.

24. What endoscopic therapies are available to control esophageal variceal bleeding?

Once the patient has been stabilized, preparation for endoscopy should be completed. Endoscopy should be performed as soon as safely possible (<12 hours), as endoscopy >15 hours from presentation has been associated with increased mortality. Variceal hemorrhage is defined by the presence of a bleeding varix, a clot, a white nipple sign, or if varices are present and no other source is identified. When a variceal source is confirmed, endoscopic variceal band ligation (EVL) should be performed, as it has been shown to be superior to sclerotherapy in rebleeding rates (26% vs. 44%), mortality (24% vs. 31%), and complication rates (11% vs. 25%). Cyanoacrylate glue is not recommended.

25. What is the role of transjugular intrahepatic portosystemic shunt (TIPS) in esophageal variceal bleeding?

Despite appropriate antibiotics, vasoconstrictors, and EVL, 10%–15% of patients will experience persistent bleeding or early rebleeding. First-line rescue therapy is TIPS, connecting the hypertensive portal vein to the normotensive inferior vena cava, which results in rapid decrease in portal pressures, and thus decreases in bleeding. Of note, there is also a role for *early* preemptive TIPS for high-risk esophageal variceal bleeding among select patients with Child-Pugh class C (score less than 14) cirrhosis or class B with active bleeding.

26. What other techniques are available for rescue therapy in esophageal variceal bleeding?

In patients with uncontrolled bleeding who are not TIPS candidates or when TIPS is anticipated to be delayed, placement of a balloon tamponade (e.g., Sengstaken-Blakemore) can be considered as a temporary (maximum of 24 hours) bridge to definitive treatment. Self-expanding esophageal metal stents have been similarly utilized and have the advantage that they can remain in place for 7 days. Endoscopic hemostatic powder spray TC-325 has also been described in the acute control of variceal hemorrhage, though follow-up EVL would still be needed.

27. How is gastric variceal bleeding treated?

Although esophageal varices are more prevalent and bleed more frequently, gastric variceal hemorrhage tends to be more severe and associated with higher mortality rates. Management for gastric varices is nuanced and highly dependent on location, underlying vascular supply, and proceduralist expertise. For gastric varices on the lesser curvature of the stomach, band ligation can offer definitive therapy. Cardiofundal gastric varices are best managed endoscopically with cyanoacrylate injection; band ligation may be temporizing in this location, but is rarely definitive, while sclerotherapy has poor hemostasis rates and high incidence of rebleeding and complications. TIPS has been shown to reduce rebleeding compared to cyanoacrylate injection but is generally less effective than

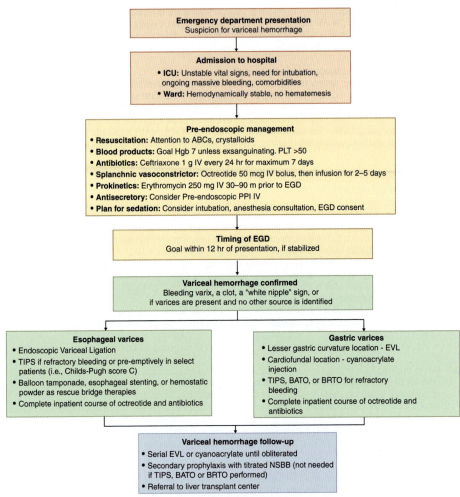

Fig. 50.2 Algorithm for the management of variceal upper gastrointestinal bleeding. *ABCs*, Airway, breathing, circulation; *BATO*, balloon-occluded anterograde transvenous obliteration; *BRTO*, balloon-occluded retrograde transvenous obliteration; *EGD*, esophago-gastroduodenoscopy; *EVL*, endoscopic variceal ligation; *Hgb*, hemoglobin; *ICU*, intensive care unit; *IV*, intravenous; *NSBB*, nonselective beta-blocker; *PLT*, platelets; *PPI*, proton pump inhibitor; *TIPS*, transjugular intrahepatic portosystemic shunt.

when utilized for esophageal varices. Balloon-occluded retrograde transvenous obliteration or balloon-occluded anterograde transvenous obliteration are alternative radiologic procedures increasingly used for the management of gastric variceal bleeding in patients with hepatic encephalopathy, or contraindications to TIPS, in the presence of a gastrorenal shunt.

28. **What follow-up considerations are there for patients after a variceal bleed?**
    Combined therapy with nonselective beta-blockers with repeat EVL is the cornerstone of prevention of rebleeding. Current evidence supports the use of propranolol or nadolol titrated to achieve a resting heart rate of 55–60 beats per minute without inducing a systolic blood pressure of <90 mm Hg. For patients who underwent EVL, repeat endoscopy with EVL is recommended every 1–4 weeks until the varices are eradicated, after which they should complete a follow-up endoscopy in 3–6 months and then every 6–12 months thereafter. Short-term use of PPI (~10 days) could be considered post-EVL to decrease postbanding ulcer size, though data are lacking to support a decrease in bleeding complications. Patients who underwent successful TIPS do not require repeat endoscopy, though they should be monitored for complications such as hepatic encephalopathy with consideration for prophylactic rifaximin. Perhaps most importantly, variceal hemorrhage is a decompensating event, and patients should establish care with a liver transplant center.

ACKNOWLEDGMENT

The authors would like to acknowledge the contributions of Drs Davinder Sandhu and Lisa Strate, who were the authors of this chapter in the previous edition.

CLINICAL VIGNETTE

Available Online

BIBLIOGRAPHY

Available Online

CHAPTER 51

LOWER GASTROINTESTINAL TRACT BLEEDING

Richard Bower, MD and Joseph G. Cheatham, MD

 Additional content available online

1. **Define lower gastrointestinal bleeding (LGIB).**
   Overt bleeding that originates from any site distal to the ileocecal valve. Bright red blood per rectum, termed hematochezia, typically, but not always, signifies a lower gastrointestinal (GI) bleeding source.

2. **How common is LGIB?**
   The annual incidence of LGIB is approximately 20 per 100,000 population.

3. **Are there known LGIB risk factors?**
   Age is the strongest risk factor with a 200-fold increased incidence between the third and ninth decades of life. Nonsteroidal anti-inflammatory drugs (NSAIDs), low-dose aspirin, moderate to high alcohol use, and nonaspirin antiplatelet drugs are independent risk factors for diverticular bleeding. Anticoagulants are associated with an increased risk of diverticular bleeding.

4. **What is the mortality associated with LGIB?**
   Most cases of LGIB (65%–85%) are self-limited and uncomplicated. Overall, mortality is low, ranging from 2.4% to 3.9%, and is related to patient comorbidities but increases to approximately 23% if the bleeding occurrs after hospitalization.

5. **Name the signs and symptoms defining severe LGIB.**
   Overt hematochezia accompanied by hemodynamic instability or orthostatic hypotension continued bleeding after hospitalization, recurrent bleeding after 24 hours of stability, a decrease in hemoglobin of at least 2 g/dL, or transfusion of at least 2 units of packed red blood cells (PRBCs).

6. **What is considered life-threatening LGIB?**
   Major overt hematochezia with shock or severe hypotension requiring pressors, a decrease in hemoglobin of >5 g/dL, or requiring transfusion of ≥5 units of PRBCs.

7. **Are current risk scoring systems helpful in predicting outcomes?**
   Validated predictive risk stratification scores for adverse outcomes of LGIB include ABC Strate, NOBLADS, Sengupta, BLEED, Birmingham, SALGIB, the HAKA, and others (see Konstantinos T, Gkolfakis P, Gralnek IM, Oakland K, Manes G, Radaelli F, et al. Diagnosis and management of acute lower gastrointestinal bleeding: European Society of Gastrointestinal Endoscopy (ESGE) Guideline. Endoscopy. 2021;53(8):850-868 for acronyms). Additionally, some risk scoring systems initially developed for upper GI bleeding have shown predictive ability for adverse outcomes in LGIB (AIM65, Glasgow-Blatchford and Rockall scores). Alternatively, the Oakland score (Table 51.1) was developed to predict safe discharge. Oakland score (≤8) has a 95% probability of safe discharge. No score accounts for all potential adverse or positive outcomes, thus scoring tools if utilized should augment clinical judgment.

8. **What are some helpful bleeding characteristics in assessing a patient with LGIB?**
   Such characteristics are shown in Table 51.2.

9. **Name the most common causes of severe and life-threatening hematochezia.**
   Diverticular, angiodysplasia, post polypectomy ulcer, severe colonic ischemia, and an upper GI source (~15% of patients presenting with hematochezia and hypotension/tachycardia have an upper source).

Table 51.1 Oakland Score for Predicting Safe Discharge in Acute Lower Gastrointestinal Bleeding.

VARIABLE	SCORE
Age (years)	
• <40	0
• 40–69	1
• >70	2
Sex	
• Female	0
• Male	1
Previous LGIB Admission	
• No	0
• Yes	1
Digital Rectal Examination Findings	
• No blood	0
• Blood	1
Heart Rate (beats per minute)	
• <70	0
• 70–89	1
• 90–109	2
• >110	3
Systolic Blood Pressure (mm Hg)	
• 50–89	5
• 90–119	4
• 120–129	3
• 130–159	2
• >160	0
Hemoglobin (g/dL)	
• 3.6–6.9	22
• 7.0–8.9	17
• 9.0–10.9	13
• 11.0–12.9	8
• 13.0–15.9	4
• >16.0	0

https://www.mdcalc.com/10042/oakland-score-safe-discharge-lower-gi-bleed

10. **Do all patients with LGIB need endoscopic evaluation in the hospital?**

Patients with self-limited bleeding and no adverse clinical features can be considered for outpatient management. An Oakland score of ≤8 can help aid but not replace the clinicians' overall assessment.

11. **What can help differentiate between an upper and a lower source of bleeding?**
Characteristics of a upper gastrointestinal (UGI) source include the following:
• History of an UGI ulcer, chronic liver disease, or use of aspirin or NSAIDs
• Nausea, vomiting, hematemesis, and/or epigastric pain
• Serum blood urea nitrogen (BUN)/creatinine ratio greater than 30 is highly suggestive
• Melena on digital rectal examination (DRE)
    Characteristics of an LGI source include the following:
• Absence of UGI symptoms or risk factors
• Hematochezia or maroon blood per rectum
• History or previous LGIB

Table 51.2 Clinical Characteristics and Historical Features in Suspected Lower Gastrointestinal Bleeding.

| BLEEDING SOURCE | APPEARANCE OF BLOOD | | | VOL-UME | BLEEDING ONSET | SIGNS/SYMPTOMS ASSOCIATIONS |
	BRB	MA-ROON	ME-LENA			
Diverticular	4+	2+	1+	4+	Acute	Painless and NSAIDs?
Colitis (UC, Crohn disease)	4+	2+	1+	2+	Chronic	Diarrhea, ABD pain, and tenesmus
Malignancy or polyps	3+	2+	2+	1+	Chronic	Painless, weight loss, and stool changes
Angiodysplasia	4+	3+	1+	3+	Acute/I	Painless, Heyde syndrome, and prostate/cervical radiationn
Hemorrhoidal	4+	1+		1+	Acute/I	Blood around stool on tissue and dripping in toilet
Ischemic	4+	1+		1+	Acute	Hypotension and bleeding preceded by ABD pain
Postpolypectomy	4+	2+		3+	Acute	History of polypectomy in the past 14 days
Infectious	3+	1+		1+	Acute/SA	Diarrhea, fevers, and acutely ill
Aortoenteric fistula	4+	1+		4+	Acute	History of AAA repair
UGIB	1+	3+	4+	4+	Acute	Abdominal pain, NSAIDs, and + NG lavage

AAA, Abdominal aortic aneurysm; *ABD,* abdominal; *BRB,* bright red blood; *I,* intermittent; *NG,* nasogastric; *NSAID,* nonsteroidal anti-inflammatory drug; *SA,* subacute; *UC,* ulcerative colitis; *UGIB,* upper gastrointestinal bleeding.

12. What are the first steps taken in the management of a patient with a severe LGIB?
- Stabilize and resuscitate with lactate Ringer or normal saline through a large bore IV.
- Order laboratory tests: complete blood count, electrolytes, BUN, creatinine, international normalized ratio (INR) in patients suspected of having a coagulopathy (liver disease or on warfarin), and type and cross for packed RBCs.
- Obtain an electrocardiogram for those with known arteriosclerotic heart disease or older than 50 years.
- Perform a history (time of bleeding onset, pain, upper GI symptoms, recent endoscopy, current and recent medications; and indications for antiplatelet, anticoagulation if taking, prior bleeding history, history of liver disease, prior aortic aneurysm repair). Perform a focused physical examination: vital signs, cardiopulmonary, abdominal, and a DRE.
- Note: DRE is mandatory for all patients with LGIB to help evaluate for active bleeding and to characterize the color and consistency of blood and stool.

13. How can continued or recurrent LGIB be determined?
Serial monitoring of the patient's hematocrit should be performed. Take into account volume contraction and dilution effects before and after resuscitation Hemodynamic parameters should be monitored for signs of worsening volume depletion, especially in the setting of adequate volume resuscitation.

14. What are the most common causes of LGIB?
The most common cause is diverticular bleeding, accounting for 30% of LGIB. Anorectal, colitis, and post polypectomy bleeding make up the majority of the remaining causes of LGIB (Fig. 51.1).

15. What is the natural history of LGIB from diverticulosis?
- Bleeding occurs in 17% of patients with colonic diverticular disease.
- Approximately 80% of patients stop bleeding spontaneously.

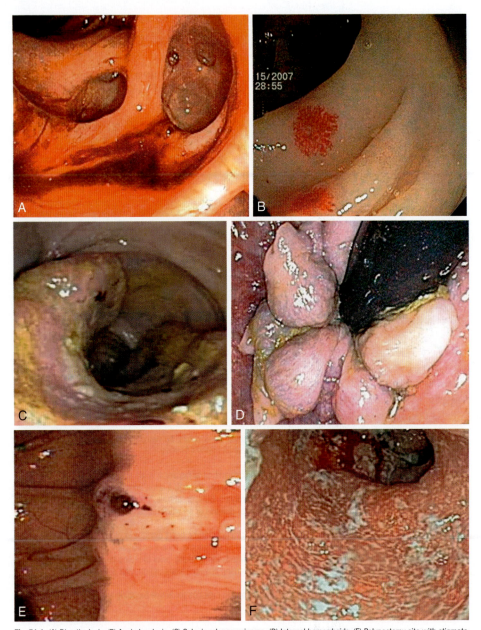

Fig. 51.1 (A) Diverticulosis. (B) Angiodysplasia. (C) Colonic adenocarcinoma. (D) Internal hemorrhoids. (E) Polypectomy site with stigmata of recent bleeding. (F) Ulcerative colitis.

- ~ 70% will not rebleed.
- ~ 30% will rebleed and may require treatment.

16. **Should antiplatelet and anticoagulation be held in the setting of LGIB?**
    Acetylsalicylic acid (ASA) for primary cardiovascular prophylaxis should be withheld and considered for permanent discontinuation. See Table 51.3 for conditional recommendations of specific agents.

Table 51.3 Antiplatelet and Anticoagulation Management Conditional Recommendations in Lower Gastrointestinal Bleeding (LGIB).

| DRUG | SEVERITY OF LGIB | | | | | | HELD? WHEN TO RESTART |
| | SELF-LIMITED | | SEVERE | | LIFE THREATENING | | |
	HOLD	REVERSE	HOLD	REVERSE	HOLD	REVERSE	
ASA for first prevention	Yes	No platelets	Yes	Platelets not recommended	Yes	Platelets not recommended	Consider discontinue
ASA for second prevention	No	No platelets	No	Platelets not recommended	Consider	Platelets not recommended	After hemostasis is achieved
P2Y₁₂ inhibitor (Clopidogrel)	No	No platelets	No	Platelets not recommended	Yes and cardiology consult	Platelets not recommended	Collaboration with cardiology
Vit K antagonist (warfarin)	No	No PCC No FFP No Vit K	Yes	PCC is not necessary in most Vit K if supratherapeutic No FFP	Yes	Consider PCC, Vit K if supratherapeutic FFP if PCC is not available	As soon as clinically possible
Antifactor Xa (Apixaban and Rivaroxaban)	No	No	Yes	Andexanet alpha not recommended Possible PCC	Yes	Consider Andexanet alpha with hematology consult Possible PCC	As soon as clinically possible
Direct thrombin inhibitor (Dabigatran)	No	No	Yes	Idarucizumab not recommended Possible PCC	Yes	Consider idarucizumab with hematology consult Possible PCC	As soon as clinically possible

ASA, Acetylsalicylic acid; *FFP*, fresh frozen plasma; *PCC*, prothrombin complex concentrate; *Vit K*, vitamin K.

17. Do all angiodysplasias cause LGIB?

The answer is no. Asymptomatic angiodysplasias are frequently found during routine colonoscopy. Most (75%) bleeding colonic angiodysplasia is found in the right colon. Endoscopic treatment with argon plasma coagulation (APC) should be attempted if they are actively bleeding or are thought to be the source of significant bleeding or recurrent anemia requiring transfusion. Endoscopic treatment of these lesions, especially in the thin-walled right colon, can result in perforation or brisk bleeding. Some experts recommend saline injection lift prior to treating with APC.

18. What role does urgent colonoscopy have in the diagnosis of LGIB?

Ileo-colonoscopy, following a large-volume (4–6 L) polyethylene glycol bowel purge, is the diagnostic method of choice for LGIB. The use of a nasogastric tube combined with an antiemetic agent may facilitate bowel preparation in patients who are intolerant of oral intake. This can establish a diagnosis in 70%–90% of cases. To date, there are no high-quality studies that show urgent colonoscopy improves clinical outcomes or lowers costs when compared with routine elective colonoscopy. Therefore it is reasonable to perform an ileo-colonoscopy at some point during a patient's hospitalization for LGIB.

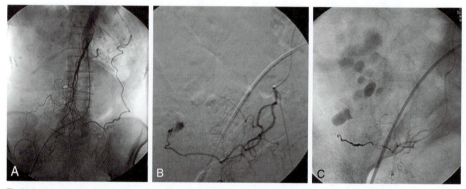

Fig. 51.2 (A) Angiography of superior mesenteric artery with evidence of bleeding (*circle, bottom left*). (B) Subselective angiography of ileocolic artery with (C) deployed coils for embolization. (Courtesy COL Kenneth H. Cho, MD.)

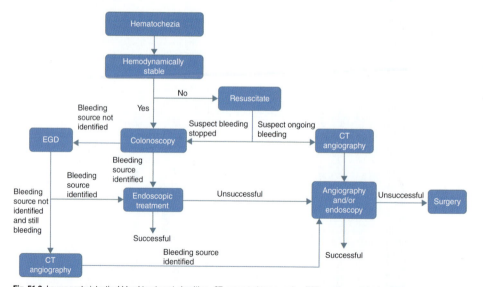

Fig. 51.3 Lower gastrointestinal bleed treatment algorithm. *CT*, computed tomography; *EGD*, esophagogastroduodenoscopy.

19. **What is the role of nuclear medicine scintigraphy, CT angiography (CTA), catheter angiography (CA) in the diagnosis, and treatment of LGIB?**

All represent second-line tests (and therapy in the case of CA), following a nondiagnostic upper and lower endoscopy in a hemodynamically stable patient suspected of ongoing bleeding. CTA and CA's localization and therapeutic yield increase significantly in patients with hemodynamic instability and suspicion of ongoing bleeding. Nuclear medicine scintigraphy is no longer routinely recommended if other modalities are available due to its relatively low accuracy in localizing the bleeding source.

Please see Fig. 51.2 for angiographicdemonstration of bleeding ileo-colonic artery treated with subselective angiography and coil embolization.

20. **What endoscopic methods are available for hemostasis?**

Diverticular bleeding can be treated with submucosal injections of dilute epinephrine, followed by contact electrocautery devices, through the scope or over cap hemostatic clip placement, or band ligation but weigh the risk of right side colon perforation with band ligation. Angiodysplasias can be treated with contact electrocautery, APC, or clips. Consider saline injection lift prior to treatment with APC or electrocautery on the right side of the colon. Visible vessels and post polypectomy bleeding can be managed with electrocautery and hemostatic clips. Hemostatic topical agents can be used as a salvage therapy in LGIB. See Table 51.3 for antiplatelet/anticoagulation management considerations.

21. **What is the role of surgery in LGIB?**

Surgery is rarely necessary and is associated with significant morbidity and mortality. In the rare case of recurrent bleeding despite other attempted therapies, surgery for definitive therapy may become necessary (Fig. 51.3).

CLINICAL VIGNETTE

Available Online

BIBLIOGRAPHY

Available Online

CHAPTER 52

OCCULT AND OBSCURE GASTROINTESTINAL BLEEDING

Mitchell S. Cappell, MD, PhD

 Additional content available online

1. **What is occult gastrointestinal (GI) bleeding and how does it differ from overt GI bleeding?**
   Occult GI bleeding is microscopic blood loss from the GI tract that is not overtly or grossly apparent. It is typically detected by a guaiac test or fecal immunologic test (FIT; see Question 5).

2. **How is occult GI bleeding usually detected?**
   Occult GI bleeding is typically detected by obtaining a stool sample, smearing the stool sample on a guaiac-impregnated card, and applying a reagent solution to the card. A positive test is indicated by the change in the color of the impregnated card from colorless to bright blue because of the presence of peroxidase (or pseudoperoxidase) in the stool. As little as 2–5 mL of blood per rectum per day can produce a positive guaiac test.

   Occult blood in the stool can also be detected by FIT. In this test the presence of blood in stool can be detected by antibodies against human blood. The FIT test is more specific and accurate than the guaiac test but is more expensive to perform and generally must be performed in a laboratory as opposed to the guaiac test which can be performed at the bedside.

3. **What are the difficulties with guaiac testing for fecal occult blood?**
   The sensitivity of three guaiac tests obtained on 3 consecutive days is moderately high (up to 80%) for detecting colon cancer. It is recommended to test for stool guaiac on three consecutive days because colon cancers typically bleed only intermittently.

   Additional weaknesses of guaiac testing for colon cancer include the following:

   False positivity may be due to recent ingestion of fresh fruits and uncooked vegetables, especially cruciferous vegetables (cabbage, cauliflower, and broccoli) that can catalyze the colorimetric reaction because of the presence of pseudoperoxidase in this produce; or recent ingestion of red meat, especially steak, that contains residual blood from cows or other mammals that can catalyze the reaction. Recent ingestion of iron- or bismuth-containing medications (e.g., Pepto-Bismol) can cause stools to appear dark blue to black and result in a false-positive stool guaiac test reading. Recent aspirin or nonsteroidal anti-inflammatory drug (NSAID) use can cause microscopic GI bleeding without any intrinsic lesion in the GI tract. A dried stool specimen can lead to a falsely negative guaiac test, whereas rehydration of a dried specimen can lead to a falsely positive test. Individuals who are colorblind may not be able to recognize a positive guaiac test due to their inability to recognize the blue color.
   - Adenomatous colon polyps usually do not bleed and often are not detected by a guaiac test.
   - Microscopic bleeding from the upper GI tract—ulcer, gastritis, esophagitis, and so on—can cause the guaiac test to be positive.
   - A positive stool guaiac test cannot distinguish bleeding from the colon versus an upper GI source.
   - Approximately 5%–10% of all guaiac tests are falsely positive.

4. **How should guaiac tests be ideally performed to detect fecal occult blood?**
   - Stool specimens should be collected over 3 consecutive days.
   - Guaiac testing should be performed on a fresh specimen (<7 days).
   - Dried stool specimens should be rehydrated to increase test sensitivity.
   - Patients should refrain from eating red meat (steak) and cabbage, cauliflower, or broccoli because ingesting these foods can cause a spurious guaiac-positive test.
   - Avoid taking aspirin or NSAIDs for several days before the test because these drugs can cause microscopic amounts of blood in the stool that can produce guaiac-positive test results (without an intrinsic GI lesion).

5. **What test for fecal occult blood is superior to guaiac testing but is considerably more expensive to use?**
   In FIT, antibodies to human hemoglobin are collected from venipuncture of rabbits previously exposed to human blood and are coupled to fluorescent proteins for easy detection. These antibodies attach to human blood (hemoglobin) in stool and are detected by their fluorescence. The FIT test is superior to guaiac tests for the detection of colon cancer and colonic adenomatous polyps. In Japan, all patients over 45 years old, undergo a FIT

test as screening for colon cancer, with patients with a positive FIT screening test then undergoing colonoscopy as the diagnostic test.

Advantages of FIT test.
- Specific for human hemoglobin. Does not recognize cow or other mammalian hemoglobin (e.g., ingested steak).
- Cabbage, cauliflower, or broccoli do not cause a falsely positive FIT test.
- Hemoglobin released from upper GI tract bleeding is digested, and usually not immunologically reactive to FIT. Therefore upper GI tract bleeding usually does not produce a positive FIT test.

6. **Is testing a nasogastric (NG) aspirate for fecal occult blood clinically useful?**
   No. This test is frequently falsely positive because of incidental microscopic bleeding from nasopharyngeal or esophageal trauma during NG tube insertion.

7. **What is fecal genetic testing and can this test be used to replace the standard guaiac test for occult blood to screen for colon cancer?**
   Passage of stool through the colon leads to the shedding of microscopic amounts of colonic tissue containing cellular DNA that remain viable in stool for many days. Genetic mutations present in microscopic amounts in this tissue can be detected by polymerase chain reaction of stool samples. An array of genetic tests is performed to detect genetic mutations associated with colon cancer, such as *APC* mutation (a molecular marker for adenomatous polyps), and *BAT* mutation (a marker for mismatch repair gene mutations). The sensitivity of a single fecal DNA test is reportedly approximately 80% for colon cancer but is much lower for advanced adenomas, a characteristic that currently limits its clinical applicability. Even so, it has a higher sensitivity than guaiac testing for detecting advanced adenomas. It is hoped that future identification of novel genetic mutations in colonic carcinogenesis will yield additional genetic tests to place in the genetic array to increase fecal genetic test sensitivity, especially for detecting colonic adenomas.

8. **What is the sensitivity and specificity of guaiac testing for fecal blood?**
   The sensitivity of guaiac testing depends on the specific brand used. Several guaiac reagents are marketed. The most sensitive brand is the Hemoccult II-SENSA test. The sensitivity also depends on the lesion to be detected. It is not a good test for detecting colonic adenomas because adenomas infrequently bleed. It is moderately (up to 80%) sensitive at detecting colon cancer when performed on 3 consecutive days to account for intermittent bleeding from colon cancer. Guaiac testing can detect microscopic bleeding in the stool from non-neoplastic lesions, such as gastric or duodenal ulcers or inflammatory bowel disease. As discussed in Question 3, listed above, guaiac testing can be falsely positive due to ingested foods. Guaiac testing has reduced sensitivity if the stool specimen is dried, and dried stool specimens should be rehydrated when this situation occurs.
   The specificity of guaiac testing is only approximately 20%–30% for detecting significant colonic lesions. The yield of colonoscopy performed for a guaiac-positive test is 3%–4% for colon cancer and colonic 15%–20% for colonic adenomas in patients (or somewhat higher in elderly patients).

9. **How is a patient with a positive fecal occult blood test (FOBT) evaluated?**
   The evaluation of a positive FOBT depends somewhat on the clinical situation.
   Asymptomatic persons with positive FOBT and iron-deficient anemia require a colonoscopy. If colonoscopy is negative for a source of FOBT or anemia, then esophagogastroduodenoscopy (EGD) should be performed.

10. **How do patients with iron-deficiency anemia present clinically in terms of symptoms, signs, and laboratory abnormalities?**
    - Pica (swallowed non-nutritive objects) is sometimes associated with iron-deficiency anemia
    - Pallor (due to decreased hemoglobin concentration in body tissue)
    - Weakness (attributed to decreased hemoglobin concentration in blood)
    - Palpitations (due to decreased blood perfusion)
    - Koilonychia (spoon nails that appear scooped out in the center of the nail)
    - High-output congestive heart failure (due to decreased blood volume in intravascular space)
    - Dyspnea on exertion (due to decreased oxygen-carrying capacity of blood)
    - Orthostatic symptoms (due to decreased intravascular blood volume)
    - Microcytic, hypochromic indices for erythrocytes
    - Percent of iron saturation <16%

11. **How should young menstruating women with iron-deficiency anemia be evaluated?**
    The evaluation of iron-deficiency anemia in pregnant or relatively young menstruating females is individualized according to clinical presentation and menstrual and obstetric history. Iron deficiency during pregnancy is common. In a series of 186 menstruating women, 12% had a clinically important lesion detected by endoscopy.

The most common cause of bleeding was peptic ulcer disease in 3%, and gastric cancer in 3%. On multivariate analysis, independent predictors of a significant lesion at endoscopy included a positive FOBT, hemoglobin <10 g/dL, and abdominal symptoms. Menstruating females with a positive FOBT, who have iron-deficiency anemia out of proportion to menstrual blood loss, abdominal symptoms, are ≥35 years old, or have a family history of GI malignancy should be strongly considered for GI endoscopy.

12. **How often is iron-deficiency anemia caused by underlying chronic GI blood loss?**
Approximately 60% of persons with iron deficiency will have an identifiable cause detected by EGD and colonoscopy: However, 40% of persons will not have an identifiable cause.
- EGD demonstrates upper GI pathology in 36% (11% duodenal ulcer, 5% gastric ulcer, and 3% anastomotic ulcer).
- Colonoscopy demonstrates lower GI pathology in 25% (colon cancer being a not infrequent cause).
- Diagnostic investigations should always be directed by symptoms and signs.
- Non-GI causes should be considered as a potential cause of iron-deficiency anemia:
- Pregnancy
- Hematuria
- Celiac disease
- Menstrual bleeding
- Nutritional deficiencies.

13. **What do the terms upper GI bleeding (UGIB), lower GI bleeding (LGIB), and middle GI bleeding (MGIB) mean?**
The categorization of gastrointestinal bleeding terms is shown in Table 52.1. Although this categorization is appealingly simplistic, sometimes clinically suspected MGIB, based on one negative EGD and one negative colonoscopy, turns out to be UGIB that was missed on an initial EGD or LGIB that was missed on an initial colonoscopy. This initial misdiagnosis can occur in up to 20% of cases of suspected MGIB.

14. **What is meant by obscure GI bleeding?**
Obscure GI bleeding, sometimes referred to as GI bleeding of obscure origin (GIBOO), is defined as recurrent or persistent GI bleeding without an identifiable source despite EGD, colonoscopy, and a radiologic examination of the small bowel. The obscure bleeding may be acute and gross or occult and microscopic. Obscure GI bleeding constitutes approximately 5% of all GI bleeding.
    This definition of GIBOO is becoming outdated because of improved detection by capsule endoscopy and a variety of small bowel endoscopic techniques (such as single-balloon or double-balloon endoscopy).

15. **What radiologic tests are available for patients with obscure GI bleeding (GIBOO) and what is their yield?**
- Small bowel series: Yield is only approximately 10%. Disadvantages: misses arteriovenous malformations (AVMs) which cannot be seen radiologically but are readily detected visually by GI endoscopy. The presence of radiographic contrast in the gut from a small bowel series obscures AVM detection and precludes angiography.
- Enteroclysis: Yield is approximately 15%. Disadvantages: misses angiodysplasia, and contrast in the gut obscures and precludes angiography. More expensive than a small bowel series. Both a small bowel series and

Table 52.1 Categorization of Gastrointestinal Bleeding Terms.

LOCATION	DEFINITION	METHOD OF EVALUATION
UGIB	Esophagus, stomach, and duodenum to the ligament of Treitz	EGD
LGIB	Colon from the ileocecal valve to the anus	Colonoscopy (usually) Nuclear medicine studies or arteriography (special situations)
MGIB	Small bowel from ligament of Treitz to the ileocecal valve (jejunum and ileum)	Capsule endoscopy, enteroscopy (push-type, single balloon, or double balloon) Radiologic (contrast enterography) consisting of small bowel series and enteroclysis Nuclear medicine studies or arteriography (special situations)

EGD, Esophagogastroduodenoscopy; *LGIB*, lower gastrointestinal bleeding; *MGIB*, middle gastrointestinal bleeding; *UGIB*, upper gastrointestinal bleeding.

enteroclysis have become relatively obsolete because of advances in abdominal computed tomography (CT) and CT enterography.

- Abdominal CT: Method is superior for detecting extraintestinal lesions within the abdomen but is inadequate sensitive in detecting intrinsic GI lesions (see, CT enterography given below).
- CT enterography: Method is good for outlining abnormal anatomy and mucosal pathology of small bowel in diseases such as Crohn disease, other inflammatory small bowel disorders, or small bowel tumors. Test disadvantages: misses angiodysplasia, and the presence of radiographic contrast in the gut obscures the intestinal lumen and precludes angiography.
- Nuclear medicine bleeding scan: 99 m technetium is attached to autologous erythrocytes ex vivo and then blood with this attached radioactive marker is reintroduced intravenously. Extravasated blood in the bowel lumen, detected by its radioactive marker of 99 m technetium, confirms active bleeding. Active GI bleeding as low as 0.1–0.5 mL/min can be detected, but localization is generalized to abdominal regions and may be difficult to accurately localize.
- Mesenteric angiography: Yield is approximately 20%. A bleeding scan is often performed first to confirm that the GI bleeding is active, followed by a mesenteric angiography if the bleeding scan is positive. Bleeding is recognized by extravasation of blood or an abnormal vascular pattern. Angiography may, moreover, be therapeutic. Actively bleeding GI lesions can be arrested by embolization with gelfoam or metal coils delivered via the angiographic catheter. The major risk of therapeutic embolization is mesenteric ischemia, which has decreased to <1% with super-selective cannulation. Also, angiographic therapy may fail to arrest the bleeding (in about 10% of cases).

16. **When a patient is referred to a tertiary center for obscure GI bleeding, is it worthwhile for the specialized tertiary care gastroenterologist at this center to repeat another EGD or colonoscopy before performing specialized small bowel examinations?**
Patients referred to a tertiary center for obscure GI bleeding usually undergo repeat EGD and colonoscopy despite having undergone an initial EGD and colonoscopy before referral. The yield on repeat EGD is approximately 10%. Commonly identified lesions on the repeat EGD include Cameron ulcers (ulcers within a hiatal hernia), peptic ulcers, vascular angiodysplasia, gastric antral vascular ectasia, and Dieulafoy's lesions. Esophageal varices that were thought to be incidental findings on the first EGD may be recognized as the bleeding source on repeat EGD by finding stigmata of recent hemorrhage on the varices, such as wale bites or red streaks. When a cause of iron-deficiency anemia is not identified, normal-appearing duodenal mucosa should be biopsied to exclude possible celiac disease.

Repeat colonoscopy is especially important when the initial procedure was hampered by a technically incomplete colonoscopy or poor bowel preparation. Commonly identified lesions at repeat colonoscopy (initially missed lesions) include colon cancer, angiodysplasia, diverticular bleeding, and Crohn colitis.

17. **How is small bowel capsule used for endoscopy of the small bowel in patients with obscure GI bleeding?**
The most widely available and most commonly performed test to evaluate the small bowel for obscure GI bleeding is small bowel capsule endoscopy. Capsule endoscopy primarily supplies images of the small bowel but can also supply limited images of the esophagus, stomach, and cecum. A recorder is usually worn by the patient to receive the transmitted images. The capsule battery generally permits the transmission of endoscopic images for approximately 8 hours. The capsule is swallowed with water and passively traverses the alimentary tract by peristalsis. Patients fast overnight before the procedure and should receive a liquid polyethylene glycol–3350 bowel preparation shortly before the procedure to evacuate luminal debris and provide a clear fluid interface.

Several small bowel capsule brands are commercially available. The PillCam is the latest model. It has a variable frame rate, ranging from two frames per second when stationary up to six frames per second when moving quickly. Other brands include the EndoCapsule by Olympus Corporation (Allentown, Pennsylvania), and the MiRoCam capsule marketed by Medivators, Inc. (Minneapolis, Minnesota).

18. **What other endoscopic tests are available to evaluate the small bowel in patients with obscure GI bleeding?**
Various long endoscopes permit diagnosis and potential treatment of small bowel lesions in the jejunum or ileum.
- Push enteroscopy uses an enteroscope that is similar, but substantially longer than a standard upper GI endoscope (esophagogastroduodenoscope). The longer enteroscope allows intubation more distally, typically into the proximal jejunum, approximately 50 cm beyond the ligament of Treitz.
- Spiral enteroscopy uses a 118-cm-long overtube with a soft, raised, spiral helix at its distal end (Spirus Medical Inc., Stoughton, Massachusetts) that is placed over a long enteroscope. The overtube is affixed to the enteroscope via a coupling device that permits rotation of the overtube. The spiral ridge of the overtube engages the small bowel plicae circulares (folds) during clockwise rotation like a screw into wood. The enteroscope is advanced by rotating the overtube clockwise, which pleats the small bowel onto the overtube.

The most common complication is self-limited mucosal trauma from spiraling over mucosal folds. Spiral enteroscopy has limited clinical applicability because this superficial mucosal trauma occurs frequently. The rate of major complications is low at 0.4%, including a 0.3% rate of GI perforation.

- Double-balloon enteroscopy uses a 200-cm-long enteroscope with a latex balloon at its tip, and a 145-cm-long soft overtube with another latex balloon at its tip, and pumps to inflate both balloons. This enteroscope is advanced during repetitive cycles of inflation and deflation of the individual balloons coupled with alternating advancement of the enteroscope or overtube. The diagnostic yield for this endoscope for the indication of obscure bleeding ranges from 40% to 80%. An expert can frequently intubate the entire small bowel up to the ileocecal valve. The rate of major complications is approximately 0.7%, with a 0.4% rate of GI perforation. The double-balloon enteroscope is resource intensive and costly because it generally requires two endoscopic operators and takes a much longer time to perform than a colonoscopy. The double-balloon enteroscope is an important modality, but its use is generally limited to tertiary endoscopy centers. It is generally not performed by nonacademic, community-based gastroenterologists.
- Single-balloon enteroscopy uses a 140-cm-long overtube and a 200-cm-long enteroscope. The overtube is equipped with an inflatable balloon at its tip to aid in endoscope advancement through the small bowel by pleating of small bowel on the overtube. The average depth of small bowel insertion ranges from 150 to 250 cm. Single-balloon enteroscopy has a yield somewhat lower than double-balloon enteroscopy, with a diagnostic yield of 40%–65%. Complications include abdominal pain, pyrexia, mucosal tears, aspiration pneumonia, and cardiovascular events. The rate of GI perforation is approximately 0.4%. Unlike a double-balloon enteroscopy, single-balloon enteroscopy requires only one endoscopist and requires much less time to perform than double-balloon enteroscopy.

19. What are the common causes of obscure GI bleeding as determined by capsule endoscopy?
Capsule endoscopy identifies a source for obscure GI bleeding in about 56% of cases:
- Small bowel angiodysplasia in 22%
- Small bowel ulcers in 10%
- Small bowel tumors in 7%
- Small bowel varices in 3%
- Luminal blood without identifiable lesion in approximately 8%
- Esophageal or gastric source of bleeding in approximately 8%
- Colonic angiodysplasia in 2%

20. What are the advantages, disadvantages, and contraindications of capsule enteroscopy?

Advantages
- Approximately 60% yield of diagnosis for GI bleeding of obscure etiology.
- Much better diagnostic yield than push enteroscopy and small bowel series or enteroclysis.
- Relatively high diagnostic yield for small bowel tumors, ulcers, and Crohn disease.

Disadvantages
- Capsule retention occurs in up to 1% (usually at the site of pathologic obstruction or partial obstruction such as a stricture) or less likely at a fistula, ulcer, or mass.
- Crohn disease is the most common cause of capsule retention.

Contraindications
- Esophageal stricture
- Zenker diverticulum
- Known intermittent or partial small bowel obstruction
- Not approved for use during pregnancy

    In a patient with a high likelihood of small bowel stricture or partial obstruction, a patency capsule test should be performed before capsule endoscopy. The patency capsule is identical in size and shape to the PillCam capsule but contains barium within a lactose shell that will dissolve within 2 days of ingestion. A plain radiograph is obtained 24–30 hours after patency capsule ingestion. Small bowel luminal patency is suggested by the passage of the capsule into the colon or toilet. Capsule endoscopy is contraindicated if the patency capsule is retained in the small bowel at 24–30 hours after ingestion.

21. What are angiodysplasia?
Normally arteries are connected to veins via intervening capillaries. Arteries are exposed to high pressure because they directly receive blood pumped from the heart and have a relatively thick, muscular wall to contain blood under high pressure without bursting or leaking. The very narrow capillaries between arteries and veins

normally dissipate the high pressure occurring in the arterial system through friction to produce a low pressure in the venous system. Veins typically have thin walls because they are exposed to low intravascular pressures. Angiodysplasia is a vascular tuft or tangle of vessels with a central feeding artery directly connected to veins without intervening capillaries. Angiodysplasia is sometimes called AVM to describe this vascular anomaly. In angiodysplasia, the veins distal to the feeding artery are exposed to abnormally high pressure because of the absence of intervening capillaries (which would normally dissipate the high pressure through friction) and can become leaky usually manifesting subclinically as occult GI bleeding or infrequently clinically as gross GI bleeding.

22. **How do angiodysplasia appear at endoscopy?**
At endoscopy angiodysplasia appears as a dense macular, reticular network of vessels (vascular tuft) which is typically 2–8 mm wide and is composed of intensely bright, red lesions resulting from the presence of oxygenated, *arterialized* blood within vessels directly supplied by an artery without an intervening capillary. Without capillaries the oxygen attached to hemoglobin is not released and the veins are not deoxygenated. A prominent feeding artery or draining vein is occasionally noted. Angiodysplasias are differentiated from mucosal erosions or hemorrhages from endoscopic trauma because angiodysplasias, unlike traumatic lesions, have a fine internal vascular structure often resembling a starburst, stellate, or arachnoid network. Angiodysplasia is also found before intubating a GI region because they are not caused by trauma during endoscopic intubation.

23. **How do angiodysplasia appear at angiography?**
Angiodysplasia appears as a vascular tuft or tangle of vessels resulting from a local mass of irregular vessels, best visualized in the arterial phase. It demonstrates early and intensely filling veins because of direct communication of the artery to the veins without intervening capillaries. It typically shows persistent opacification beyond the normal venous phase (slowly emptying vein) likely from tortuosity (ectasia) of the draining vein. At angiography, bleeding angiodysplasia shows extravasation of blood in which the blood is seen to actively pool near the vascular tuft. Angiodysplasias typically bleed only intermittently and demonstrate extravasation of contrast in only approximately 10% of cases at angiography.

24. **What are common risk factors for angiodysplasia?**
Sporadic angiodysplasias most commonly occur as (acquired) lesions in older adults. They are believed to arise as degenerative lesions of aging caused by chronic, intermittent, and low-grade obstruction of veins and capillaries. They most commonly occur in the cecum or proximal right colon. This predilection is explained by the greater cecal mural tension owing to its larger luminal diameter, according to Laplace's law. Exposure to greater mural tension tends to stretch the vessel wall and promote angiodysplasia.
Angiodysplasias are sometimes associated with the following syndromes or diseases:
- Hereditary hemorrhagic telangiectasia (HHT): HHT is a genetic vascular disorder caused by mutations of the endoglin *(ENG)* gene (type 1 HHT), or the *ACVRLI* gene (type II HHT). These mutations impair blood vessel endothelial growth and repair, which results in tortuous blood spaces lined by a single layer of endothelial cells. These mutations lead to the widening of small vessels that eventually create angiodysplasia. Because these patients have a diathesis for angiodysplasia, they can develop extensive and large angiodysplasia in several organs, most commonly the nasal mucosa, GI mucosa, oropharynx, and lips. Nasal angiodysplasia may present as recurrent epistaxis (nosebleeds) that are difficult to treat because of the extensiveness of these angiodysplasia. Oropharyngeal angiodysplasia may be identified on physical examination of the oropharynx or lips. GI angiodysplasias tend to bleed significantly and repeatedly because of their thin and fragile vascular wall that lacks a muscular coat. Patients often present with the clinical triad of telangiectasia, recurrent epistaxis, and a compatible family history of epistaxis and bleeding GI angiodysplasia. Patients with HHT are differentiated from sporadic angiodysplasias by clinical presentation at a much younger age, multiplicity of GI lesions, positive family history, chronic epistaxis, and frequent episodes of GI bleeding from angiodysplasia.
- Chronic renal failure: Patients with chronic renal failure have a significantly higher frequency of GI bleeding from angiodysplasia than the general population.
- Collagen vascular disease: A number of case reports have associated GI angiodysplasia with scleroderma or related disorders such as calcinosis cutis, Raynaud phenomenon, esophageal dysfunction, sclerodactyly, and telangiectasia syndrome.
- Aortic stenosis: Although somewhat controversial, numerous studies have associated aortic stenosis with chronic GI bleeding from angiodysplasia. The bleeding may not reflect an increased risk of developing angiodysplasia in patients with aortic stenosis, but an increased tendency of bleeding from preexisting angiodysplasia caused by destruction of multimers of von Willebrand factor from high shear forces across a stenotic aortic valve.

25. **How can GI angiodysplasia be treated at endoscopy or at angiography to avoid surgical resection for chronic GI bleeding?**
Angiodysplasias that are actively bleeding, oozing, unusually large, or otherwise a likely cause of recent or chronic GI bleeding may be treated at endoscopy or angiography. Angiodysplasia can be ablated at endoscopy

using high energy delivered via argon plasma coagulation (APC), electrocoagulation (e.g., Bicap or Gold Probe), thermocoagulation (e.g., Heater Probe), or injection sclerotherapy (e.g., sodium tetradecyl sulfate). APC has a very high rate of success at preventing rebleeding from angiodysplasia (up to 99% effective) and is relatively easy to perform at endoscopy with a low complication rate. At angiography, bleeding angiodysplasias are identified by extravasation of contrast. The catheter is snaked close to the angiodysplasia by super-selective catheterization and metal coils or gelfoam are released from the catheter to embolize the vessel feeding the angiodysplasia.

When encountering numerous angiodysplasias at endoscopy performed for recent GI bleeding, the practitioner should treat *only* those angiodysplasias that are actively bleeding or oozing, that have stigmata of recent hemorrhage (e.g., an adherent clot), or are unusually large. Angiodysplasias that are small, not actively bleeding, and do not have any stigmata of recent hemorrhage generally do not require endoscopic therapy.

26. How can lesions identified by capsule endoscopy be further defined before performing surgery?

Capsule endoscopy often does not permit an ideal view of intestinal mucosal lesions because the capsule tumbles through the small bowel naturally by peristalsis without any opportunity to manually adjust capsule position to obtain a better view. Moreover, capsule endoscopy also does not permit biopsy or brushing of the lesion for cytologic or pathologic analysis. It is solely diagnostic and not therapeutic. Single-balloon or double-balloon enteroscopy can better view small intestinal lesions identified by capsule endoscopy. Lesions can be biopsied or ablated at double-balloon enteroscopy.

27. What is a Meckel diverticulum, how does it clinically present, and what test is standardly used to diagnose it?

A Meckel diverticulum is a congenital diverticulum or outpocketing of the small intestinal mucosa that typically occurs in the middle-to-distal ileum, approximately 150 cm proximal to the ileocecal valve. It occurs in approximately 2% of the population. This congenital anomaly is clinically important because of its propensity to cause obscure GI bleeding, especially in children. The bleeding is secondary to intestinal ulceration from acid secreted by ectopic (oxyntic) gastric mucosa lining the diverticulum. The bleeding typically occurs in children who present with painless LGIB. However, Meckel diverticulum is also in the differential diagnosis of obscure, painless, LGIB in adults, especially young adults. Patients usually present with dark red or burgundy (maroon) stools.

Meckel diverticular bleeding is diagnosed by a Meckel scan, see Chapter 70. A Meckel scan is approximately 90% sensitive and 90% specific for bleeding from a Meckel diverticulum in children. However, it is less accurate in adults.

28. How often does GI bleeding occur in patients with coronavirus disease (COVID-19) infection?

What is the role of EGD or colonoscopy to evaluate GI bleeding in patients infected with COVID-19? Do patients with COVID-19 with obscure GI bleeding require endoscopic evaluation, either EGD or colonoscopy? Do patients with COVID-19 infection require capsule endoscopy or balloon enteroscopy for suspected small bowel GI bleeding?

A. As of March 2022, more than six million people have died from COVID-19 infection and many hundreds of millions of people have contracted the infection. Mortality is related to older age, obesity, diabetes, numerous comorbidities, and immunodeficiency due to underlying diseases or immunosuppressive therapy. It is important and timely to review clinically significant considerations about GI bleeding in patients infected with COVID-19.

B. GI bleeding is not very common but is also not rare in patients with COVID-19, with an overall rate of about 5% in hospitalized patients with COVID-19 infection. The rate of overt GI bleeding is relatively low despite the frequent presence of ACE receptors in the small bowel. About 30% of patients with COVID-19 infection pass mRNA of COVID-19 in their stool. Patients infected with COVID-19 have a much lower rate of GI bleeding than diarrhea.

C. Most GI bleeding in patients infected with COVID-19 is low-grade and self-limited, related to local mucosal inflammation associated with the viral infection. Often the patients manifest superficial mucosal erosions without ulcers. Occasionally GI bleeding is overt and severe, most often related to severe COVID-associated pneumonia with respiratory failure. Such patients often have gastric or duodenal (stress) ulcers associated with respiratory failure, severe multiorgan failure, and intensive care unit stay. Patients also have an increased incidence of mesenteric ischemia/ischemic colitis due to a hypercoagulable state and microthrombi which may present initially with mild GI bleeding. Infected patients can paradoxically have GI bleeding due to anticoagulation prophylaxis to prevent thromboses in the GI tract or elsewhere in the body.

D. Most patients with GI bleeding associated with COVID-19 infection can be managed conservatively without GI endoscopy because the bleeding is typically self-limited. Occasionally GI bleeding requires endoscopy for severe bleeding causing cardiovascular compromise or overt, active, bleeding for which therapeutic endoscopy is contemplated. Transmission of COVID-19 infection to endoscopy personnel is possible but can be minimized by the use of personal protective equipment, including gowns impervious to water, use of eye guards and N95 masks, and other precautions. It is currently not felt necessary to intubate most patients infected with

COVID-19 undergoing EGD, although some centers may do this prophylactically in certain circumstances. A concern in intubating patients infected with COVID-19 prophylactically for EGD is the potential difficulty of extubating them if they have COVID-19 pneumonia and potential respiratory compromise.

There are little or no data on the use of capsule endoscopy, single-balloon or double-balloon enteroscopy to evaluate obscure GI bleeding in patients with COVID-19. These tests should currently be considered investigational in patients infected with COVID-19.

BIBLIOGRAPHY

Available Online

CHAPTER 53

EVALUATION OF ACUTE ABDOMINAL PAIN

John S. Goff, MD

 Additional content available online

1. Provide a useful clinical definition of an acute abdomen.
This clinical scenario is characterized by abrupt onset of severe pain caused by infarction, perforation, inflammation, obstruction, or organ rupture. Surgical intervention is usually required.

2. What are the four types of stimuli for abdominal pain?
1. Stretching or tension—visceral nociception
2. Inflammation—mediated by kinins, histamine, prostaglandins, and so on
3. Ischemia—similar to inflammation
4. Neoplasm—nerve invasion

3. What are the three categories of abdominal pain (Fig. 53.1)?
1. Visceral pain occurs when noxious stimuli affect an abdominal viscus. The pain is usually dull (cramping, gnawing, or burning) and poorly localized to the ventral midline because the innervation to most viscera is multisegmental. Secondary autonomic effects such as diaphoresis, restlessness, nausea, vomiting, and pallor are common.
2. Parietal pain occurs when noxious stimuli irritate the parietal peritoneum. The pain is more intense and more precisely localized to the site of the lesion. Parietal pain is likely to be aggravated by coughing or movement.
3. Referred pain is experienced in areas remote from the site of injury. The remote site of pain referral is supplied by the same neurosegment as the involved organ; for example, gallbladder pain may be referred to the right scapula and pancreatic pain may radiate to the midback.

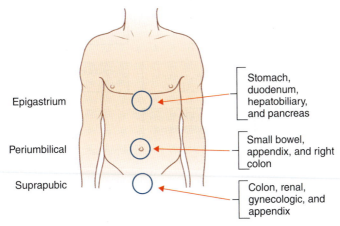

Epigastrium — Stomach, duodenum, hepatobiliary, and pancreas

Periumbilical — Small bowel, appendix, and right colon

Suprapubic — Colon, renal, gynecologic, and appendix

Fig. 53.1 Location of visceral pain.

4. How does the character of the abdominal pain help in the evaluation?
Most pain tends to be midline because of bilateral innervations, with the exception of pain from the kidneys, ureters, abdominal wall, gallbladder, and the ascending or descending colon, which tend to lateralize (Table 53.1).

Table 53.1 Classification of Pain by the Rate of Development.

Explosive and excruciating (instantaneous)	Myocardial infarction Perforated ulcer Ruptured aneurysm Biliary or renal colic (passage of a stone)
Rapid, severe, and constant (over minutes)	Acute pancreatitis Complete bowel obstruction Mesenteric thrombus
Gradual and steady pain (over hours)	Acute cholecystitis Diverticulitis Acute appendicitis
Intermittent and colicky pain (over hours)	Early subacute pancreatitis Mechanical small bowel obstruction

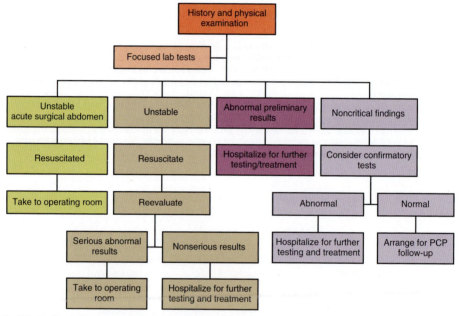

Fig. 53.2 Algorithm for the assessment of acute abdominal pain. *PCP,* Primary care physician.

5. **What are the important historical questions to ask (see Fig. 53.2 for an algorithm of the assessment of acute abdominal pain)?**
   - What is the location of the pain, and does it radiate?
   - What is the chronology of the pain—sudden onset, slowly over hours, intermittent.
   - What are the exacerbating and alleviating factors? What are the effects of eating or drinking, activity, position, coughing, passage of gas or stool, or urination?
   - What associated symptoms are there? Assess for nausea, vomiting, no passage of gas or stool, diarrhea, constipation, bloody stools or emesis, dysuria, dysmenorrhea, dyspareunia, fever, or chills.
   - Especially important previous medical history questions are conditions that might mute the early symptoms of an acute abdominal process such as immunosuppression, diabetes, chronic renal failure, or steroid use.
   - Obtain a social history of drug use, alcohol abuse, smoking, and sexual behavior.
   - Obtain a history of medication use, including prescribed, over-the-counter, and birth control pills.
   - Obtain a menstrual history.

6. **What are the important components of the physical examination for patients with acute abdominal pain?**
   - **General status:** Is the patient hemodynamically unstable? Does he or she need immediate hemodynamic resuscitation and emergent laparotomy (e.g., ruptured spleen, ruptured hepatic tumor, aneurysm, ectopic pregnancy, or mesenteric apoplexy)?
   - **Inspection:** Visually evaluate for distention, hernias, scars, and hyperperistalsis.
   - **Auscultation:** Hyperperistalsis suggests obstruction; absence of peristalsis (no bowel sounds heard over 3 minutes) suggests peritonitis (silent abdomen); bruits suggest the presence of an aneurysm.
   - **Percussion:** Tympany suggests either intraluminal or free abdominal air.
   - **Palpation:** Start the examination away from the area of tenderness and be gentle. Abdominal pain with voluntary coughing suggests peritoneal signs. Deeply palpating the abdomen only diminishes patient trust and cooperation. The enlarged gallbladder will be missed on aggressive, deep palpation. Inspiratory arrest during light palpation of the right hypochondrium suggests gallbladder pain (Murphy sign). Localized pain suggests localized peritonitis (e.g., appendicitis, cholecystitis, diverticulitis).
   - **Pelvic and rectal examination:** These examinations should be done in *all* patients with abdominal pain. A painful examination may be the only sign of pelvic appendicitis, diverticulitis, or tubo-ovarian pathologic conditions. Bimanual examination is critical to exclude an obstetric or a gynecologic cause.
   - **Iliopsoas test:** With the legs fully extended in a supine position, the patient is requested to raise the legs unilaterally. Pain occurs when the right psoas muscle is inflamed (e.g., appendicitis).
   - **Obturator test:** This test is performed by flexing the patient's thigh at right angle to the trunk and then rotating the leg externally. Inflammation of the obturator internus muscle causes pain (e.g., tubo-ovarian abscess or pelvic appendicitis).

7. **Which laboratory tests should be obtained in patients with acute abdominal pain?**
   Although laboratory tests are helpful in confirming the evolution of a disease process, they are frequently not helpful in localizing the cause of abdominal pain.
   - Obtain a complete blood count. Elevation of the white blood cell count suggests inflammation; however, the absence of leukocytosis may be misleading early in the course of the disease. A low hematocrit with a normal mean corpuscular volume (MCV) suggests acute blood loss, whereas a low hematocrit with a low MCV suggests iron deficiency from chronic gastrointestinal (GI) blood loss or malabsorption.
   - Amylase and lipase elevations may suggest pancreatitis, but amylase can come from various other sources, including salivary glands, lungs, intestines, and ovaries.
   - Liver enzyme elevations may be suggestive of hepatobiliary causes of pain. Elevations of aspartate or alanine aminotransferase suggest hepatocyte injury. Alkaline phosphatase or γ-glutamine transferase elevations suggest canalicular or biliary injury. Total bilirubin elevations greater than 3 mg/dL suggest common bile duct obstruction or associated intrahepatic cholestasis, but if bilirubin elevation is predominantly unconjugated and not associated with liver enzyme elevations, it may be due to Gilbert syndrome.
   - Evidence of pyuria on urinalysis suggests urinary tract infection but also may be seen in nephrolithiasis prostatitis or even pelvic appendicitis.
   - Chemistry analysis can be helpful in the global assessment of patient health, kidney function, hyperglycemia, acidosis, and electrolyte disturbances.
   - Pregnancy tests (beta–human chorionic gonadotropin [HCG]) should be ordered for all premenopausal females.
   - Stool examination for occult blood may be useful.
   - Electrocardiography is performed for all patients with possible myocardial infarction or older than 50 years.

8. **Which radiologic tests should be ordered to evaluate the patient with acute abdominal pain?**
   The selection of tests depends on the likelihood of the pretest clinical diagnosis and the ability of the radiologic test to confirm clinical suspicion.
   - **Plain radiographs** of the abdomen are quick and readily available and can be done at the bedside. They can detect bowel obstruction (dilated loops of bowel with air/fluid levels), volvulus, and viscus perforation (free air). Occasionally, they may suggest stone disease ($\approx$20% of gallbladder stones, and $\approx$80% of renal stones are calcified) or ruptured aortic aneurysm (separation of aortic wall calcium and mass effect). Calcium in the area of the pancreas might suggest pancreatitis as the cause of pain. A gasless abdomen, air in the bowel wall, or air in the portal venous system suggests bowel infarction or severe infection. Free intra-abdominal air is best detected with the patient in the left lateral decubitus position for 10 minutes, but a computed tomography (CT) scan is more sensitive to small amounts of air (see Chapter 69).
   - **Ultrasound (US)** of the abdomen is quick, noninvasive, and can be performed at the bedside. The disadvantages of US include variable operator expertise and suboptimal examination in the obese or gaseous abdomen. US is excellent for evaluating the gallbladder, bile ducts, liver, kidneys, appendix, and pelvic organs (see Chapter 69).

- **CT of the abdomen** provides a detailed view of the anatomy. Oral and intravenous contrast agents increase the accuracy. CT has become an extension of the physical examination and the single most helpful radiologic examination of the patient with acute abdominal pain. CT is better than US for evaluation of the pancreas but often lacks the spatial resolution to identify biliary stone disease (see Chapter 69).
- **Magnetic resonance imaging** does not offer any diagnostic advantage over CT scan and often cannot be used if the patient has metal implants.
- **Hepatobiliary Iminodiacetic Acid (HIDA)** scan is the most accurate test for acute cholecystitis (see Chapter 70).

9. **Pain referred to the abdomen can be confusing. What are the common extra-abdominal causes of referred abdominal pain?**
   - **Thoracic:** Pneumonia, pulmonary embolism, pneumothorax, myocardial infarction or ischemia, esophageal spasm, or perforation
   - **Neurogenic:** Radicular pain (spinal cord compression from tumor, abscess, or compression), varicella zoster infection, or Tabes dorsalis
   - **Metabolic:** Uremia, porphyria, acute adrenal insufficiency, and ketoacidosis
   - **Hematologic:** Sickle cell anemia, hemolytic anemia, and Henoch-Schönlein purpura
   - **Toxins:** Insect bites (scorpion bite–induced pancreatitis), lead or arsenic poisoning, cocaine, and amphetamines

10. **What are some common causes of nonserious abdominal pain?**
    - Mesenteric adenitis
    - Irritable bowel syndrome
    - Viral and bacterial enteritis
    - Pre-eruptive shingles
    - Abdominal migraine
    - Costochondritis
    - Gastroesophageal reflux disease

11. **List the common causes of acute abdominal pain in gravid females.**
    - Appendicitis
    - Ovarian cysts complicated by torsion, rupture, and hemorrhage
    - Ectopic pregnancy
    - Gallbladder problems (acalculous cholecystitis, cholecystitis, or choledocholithiasis)

12. **What is the most common cause of acute abdominal pain in older adult patients?**
    Biliary tract disease is responsible for 25% of all cases of acute abdominal pain in older adult patients requiring hospitalization. Bowel obstruction, gastric volvulus, and incarcerated hernia are the next most common, followed by appendicitis.

13. **What symptoms are helpful in evaluating for appendicitis?**
    It is decidedly uncommon for acute appendicitis to present with nausea, vomiting, or diarrhea before abdominal pain. Usually, acute appendicitis is heralded by pain and often followed by anorexia, nausea, and sometimes single-episode vomiting. Acute appendicitis should be first on the differential diagnosis list in any patient with acute abdominal pain without a prior history of appendectomy. A simple scoring system of clinical parameters and laboratory tests, the Alvarado score, has been validated to be very predictive of acute appendicitis (Table 53.2), but recent studies suggested that the Appendicitis Inflammatory Response (AIR) score (https://www.mdcalc.com/appendicitis-inflammatory-response-air-score) based on vomiting, rebound tenderness, right iliac fossa pain, fever, polymorphonuclear leukocytosis, and elevated C-reactive protein performed even better for diagnosis of appendicitis.

14. **Discuss atypical forms of appendicitis.**
    When the appendix is retro-cecal or retro-ileal in location, the inflamed appendix is often shielded from the anterior abdomen. The pain is often less pronounced, and localizing signs on physical examination are uncommon. Symptoms and signs of appendicitis in older patients are subtle. Pain is often minimal, fever is only mild, and leukocytosis is unreliable. A high index of suspicion is essential.

15. **Describe the US findings of acute appendicitis.**
    The appendix appears as a round target with an anechoic lumen, surrounded by a hypoechoic and thickened (greater than 2 mm) appendiceal wall. This finding with the reproduction of pain under the transducer has a diagnostic accuracy of 95% and a negative predictive value of 97%. Although US evaluation for appendicitis has the advantage of bedside portability and lack of radiation, CT has been shown to have superior sensitivity, accuracy, and negative predictive value (96% vs. 76%, 94% vs. 83%, and 94% vs. 76%, respectively).

Table 53.2 Alvarado Score.

SYMPTOMS	SCORE
Migration of pain to right iliac fossa	1
Anorexia	1
Nausea and vomiting	1
Signs	
Raised temperature, >37.3°C	1
Rebound pain	1
Tenderness in the right iliac fossa	2
Laboratory Findings	
Elevated leukocyte counts	2
Neutrophil left shift (>75%)	1
Total	**10**

Score = 5–6 possible appendicitis; score = 7–8 probable appendicitis; score = 9–10 very probable appendicitis.

16. **When laparotomy is performed for presumed appendicitis, what is the acceptable false-negative rate? How often is another cause identified in this setting?**
A false-negative laparotomy rate of 10%–20% is reported. In roughly 30% of these cases, some other cause of abdominal pain is identified, such as mesenteric lymphadenitis, Meckel diverticulum, cecal diverticulitis, pelvic inflammatory disease, ectopic pregnancy, or ileitis.

17. **What is the single best test to evaluate patients infected with human immunodeficiency virus (HIV) infection who complain of acute abdominal pain?**
Because of the variety of causes of abdominal pain in such patients, it has been argued that CT scan is the single best test.

18. **What are the cardinal features of a ruptured tubal pregnancy?**
   - Amenorrhea (missed period or scant menses)
   - Abdominal and pelvic pain
   - Unilateral, tender adnexal mass
   - Signs of blood loss without blood in the GI tract

19. **What are the characteristics of acute intestinal obstruction?**
   - Nausea and vomiting
   - Failure to expel flatus
   - Prior abdominal surgery or presence of hernia
   - Peristaltic pain (colicky pain—every 10 minutes for jejunal obstruction and every 30 minutes for ileal obstruction)

20. **List the clinical characteristics and causes of large bowel obstruction.**
   - Most patients are older than 50 years of age.
   - Lower abdominal cramping pain is gradual in onset.
   - Abdominal distention is a prominent feature.
   - Dilated loops of bowel with haustra distinguish the colon from the small bowel on abdominal x-rays or CT scans (see Chapters 66 and 69).
   - Causes include obstructing neoplasm, diverticulitis, hematoma (trauma or bleeding disorder), and cecal or sigmoid volvulus.

21. **List the clinical characteristics of diverticulitis.**
Right-sided diverticulitis occurs in only 1.5% of patients in Western countries but is more common among Asians. Up to 75% of these patients present with right lower quadrant pain, often misdiagnosed as acute appendicitis.

- Age older than 50 years (mean age 63 years)
- Localized left lower abdominal pain (often for several days' duration)
- Palpable mass in left lower quadrant (20%)
- Bowel movement change (50% constipation, 30% diarrhea), bleeding is rare
- Urinary urgency (10%–15%)
- Low-grade fever and leukocytosis (note 45% may have normal white blood cell count)

22. **What are the characteristic CT findings of diverticulitis?**
For the characteristic CT findings of diverticulitis, see Chapter 69.
    Note: In 10% of patients, diverticulitis cannot be distinguished from carcinoma and a gentle and cautious endoscopic examination may need to be performed.
- Increased soft tissue density within pericolic fat, secondary to inflammation (98%).
- Colonic diverticula (84%).
- Bowel wall thickening (70%).
- Soft tissue masses representing phlegmon and pericolic fluid collections, representing abscesses (35%).
- In 10% of patients, diverticulitis cannot be distinguished from carcinoma and a gentle and cautious colonoscopy may be needed.

23. **List the clinical hallmarks of acute cholecystitis.**
- Patients often give a history of prior episodes of milder abdominal pain.
- Abdominal pain usually arises after a meal, especially after a large or fat-containing meal.
- Pain typically crescendos over 20–30 minutes and then plateaus.
- Pain lasting longer than 1–2 hours is usually accompanied by gallbladder wall inflammation.
- Associated nausea occurs in 90% of patients; vomiting may follow the onset of pain in 50%–80% of patients.
- Radiation of pain to the back is common; pain radiates to the right scapula in 10% of cases.
- Low-grade fever is common.
- Right hypochondrium tenderness is generally present. Inspiratory arrest during gentle palpation of the right upper quadrant (RUQ) (Murphy sign) suggests acute cholecystitis.
- Diagnostic tests include HIDA scan or US.

24. **What is the differential diagnosis of RUQ pain besides acute cholecystitis?**
- Liver: severe hepatitis with swelling and stretching of the liver capsule, liver metastasis, Fitz-Hugh-Curtis syndrome, congestive hepatopathy (hepatic vein thrombosis—Budd-Chiari syndrome), and hepatoma or liver adenoma with infarction or internal bleeding
- Pancreas: pancreatitis and pseudocyst
- GI tract: peptic ulcer disease with or without perforation and acute appendicitis (retro-cecal)
- Kidney: pyelonephritis and nephrolithiasis
- Lung: pneumonia, pulmonary embolism, and pleurisy
- Heart: myocardial infarction and pericarditis
- Pre-eruptive varicella zoster

25. **When should a patient undergo surgery for an acute abdomen?**
Surgery should be performed when, in the judgment of the surgeon, a problem will be identifiable or treatable by surgical intervention. There is no substitute for good surgical judgment and intuition.

26. **What conditions can result in an acute abdomen in patients infected with HIV?**
Patients with HIV can have any of the usual causes of an acute abdomen; all non-HIV-specific diagnoses must be considered. Perforation is most often due to cytomegalovirus (CMV) infection in the distal small bowel or colon; this is the most common cause of the acute abdomen in late-stage HIV infection. CMV infection of the vascular endothelial cells leads to mucosal ischemic ulceration and perforation. HIV-associated lymphoma and Kaposi sarcoma also can lead to perforation, but this finding is rare. Acquired immune deficiency syndrome cholangiopathy, papillitis, and drug-induced pancreatitis (e.g., pentamidine, sulfamethoxazole-trimethoprim [Bactrim], didanosine, and ritonavir) are unique causes of abdominal pain in patients with HIV.

27. **Are patients with systemic lupus erythematosus (SLE) at increased risk for intra-abdominal catastrophe?**
Approximately 2% of patients with SLE develop lupus vasculitis, one of the most devastating complications of SLE. The fatality rate is greater than 50%. Small vessels of the bowel wall are affected, leading to ulceration, hemorrhage, perforation, and infarction.

28. **How common are severe GI manifestations of polyarteritis nodosa (PAN)?**
PAN is a vasculitis that may have visceral involvement. GI bleeding from intestinal ischemia is seen in 6% of cases, bowel perforation in 5%, and bowel infarction in 1.4%. Acalculous cholecystitis occurs in up to 17% because of direct vasculitic involvement of the cystic artery and gallbladder.

29. **What are some rare causes of acute abdominal pain?**
   - Eosinophilic gastroenteritis
   - Epiploic appendagitis
   - Familial Mediterranean fever
   - Hereditary angioedema
   - Addison disease (acute adrenal insufficiency)
   - Diabetic ketoacidosis (DKA)
   - Porphyria
   - Sickle cell crisis

CLINICAL VIGNETTE

Available Online

BIBLIOGRAPHY

Available Online

WEBSITES

Available Online

CHAPTER 54

ACUTE DIARRHEA

John W. Lee, MD, John Westhoff, MD, MPH, FACEP, FACOEM, FAWM, Mark D. Riddle, MD, DrPH, FISTM and Patrick E. Young, MD, MACP, FACG, FASGE

 Additional content available online.

EPIDEMIOLOGY

1. **What is acute diarrhea?**
   The World Health Organization defines diarrhea as the passage of three or more loose or liquid stools per day (or more frequent passage than is normal for the individual). Importantly, the passage of frequently formed stool is not diarrhea but rather hyperdefecation. Some authors define diarrhea based on stool weight, but this is impractical outside of a research setting. Acute diarrhea is diarrhea lasting for fewer than 14 days.

2. **How frequently does acute diarrhea caused by infection occur in the United States?**
   The National Institute of Diabetes and Digestive and Kidney Disease estimates that there are 179 million cases of acute diarrhea in the United States annually. While most cases are mild, self-limited, diarrhea prompts nearly 2.5 million office visits and nearly 1.2 million emergency department visits annually in the United States. Approximately 9.4 million cases of foodborne illness, 56,000 hospitalizations, and more than 1300 deaths occur annually in the United States and are attributable to known pathogens. Norovirus, *Salmonella*, preformed toxins, and *Campylobacter* spp. cause the majority of illnesses. An additional 38.4 million illnesses with 72,000 hospitalizations occur annually presumably as a result of an unidentified pathogen.

3. **Which bacterial organisms produce preformed toxins that cause acute diarrhea?**
   Symptoms that occur rapidly (<12 hours) after ingestion and include nausea, vomiting, or diarrhea are consistent with the ingestion of a preformed toxin. Some of these toxins are heat stable and persist despite cooking. Heat-stable *Staphylococcus aureus* enterotoxin, *Bacillus cereus* enterotoxins (often associated with rice), and *Clostridium perfringens* (rewarmed meats such as ham) cause the majority of cases. Symptoms are generally self-limited. Point source outbreaks with multiple cases associated with one recent meal are typical. Additionally, ciguatera and scombroid seafood poisoning, caused by heat-stable toxins from bioaccumulation and spoilage, respectively, are common and can present with diarrhea as part of their syndromes.

4. **What is persistent diarrhea?**
   Persistent diarrhea is that which lasts for 14–28 days. The differential diagnosis of persistent diarrhea differs somewhat from acute diarrhea. In terms of infection, bacterial enteric pathogens, parasites, and protozoa are more likely to result in persistent disease whereas viral pathogens are less common. Of course, conditions that will go on to produce chronic diarrhea (such as inflammatory bowel diseases [IBDs]) will also pass through a phase where they qualify as persistent. One should consider the following organisms in the differential diagnosis of persistent diarrhea:
   - Bacteria: *Campylobacter, Vibrio, Escherichia coli, Shigella, Salmonella, Clostridioides difficile, Treponema pallidum*, and *Chlamydia trachomatis* (lymphogranuloma venereum that may cause tenesmus and mimic IBD).
   - Parasites (helminths): *Strongyloides* infection may lead to colitis.
   - Protozoa: *Giardia, Isospora, Cyclospora,* and *Cryptosporidium.*

5. **What are the characteristics of noninflammatory and inflammatory diarrhea syndromes?**
   Noninflammatory diarrhea consists of a syndrome of watery, nonbloody, nonpurulent diarrhea, and often lacks prominent systemic signs and symptoms such as fever or myalgias. Specific etiologic factors often go undiagnosed and the course is often self-limited. Inflammatory diarrhea consists of frequent, smaller volume, mucoid or bloody stools, often associated with tenesmus, fever, and more prominent or severe abdominal pain. On laboratory evaluation, inflammatory diarrhea may exhibit positive fecal leukocytes and positive stool lactoferrin and calprotectin, though these are not required in the diagnosis and generally do not impact management in acute cases.

6. **What disorders and infections are associated with inflammatory diarrhea?**
   Inflammatory diarrhea is generally associated with disorders that cause mucosal disruption. Mucosal compromise may be due to a primary (IBD) or secondary (invasive infectious organism) process. Invasive infectious agents associated with diarrhea include *Salmonella, Shigella, Campylobacter*, enterohemorrhagic *E. coli* (EHEC; 0157: H7), enteroinvasive *E. coli*, and other Shiga toxin–producing *E. coli* (STEC), *C. difficile, Entamoeba histolytica*, and

Yersinia enterocolitica. Noninfectious causes of inflammatory diarrhea include ulcerative colitis, Crohn disease, radiation enteritis, ischemic and vascular diseases, and diverticulitis.

7. What disorders and infections are associated with noninflammatory diarrhea?

Most noninflammatory diarrhea is infectious in origin with noninvasive pathogens that generate toxins or use other means to promote a secretory process. Causative agents include *Vibrio cholerae*, enterotoxigenic *E. coli* (ETEC), staphylococcal and clostridial toxins, viruses, protozoa, *Cryptosporidium*, and Giardia.

8. Who is most at risk (morbidity and mortality) from acute diarrheal illness?

The very young, older adults, and the immunocompromised are most at risk for morbidity and mortality from acute diarrheal illness. Other risk factors include travel to developing countries, daycare exposure, and recent antibiotic exposure. Among the young and healthy mortality is extremely rare. Children younger than the age of 5 in developing countries, mainly sub-Saharan Africa and Asia, suffer disproportionately from diarrheal disease. Annually, 800,000 pediatric deaths are attributable to diarrheal diseases, and they are the second leading cause of death in children under 5 accounting for one in nine deaths worldwide. Meanwhile, travelers' diarrhea affects upward of 20 million people per year and is the most common illness to affect travelers.

9. What vaccine-preventable viral pathogen is a major cause of pediatric diarrhea?

Rotavirus infection is a major cause of outbreaks and sporadic diarrhea worldwide. Among children and older adults, outbreaks of rotavirus diarrhea result in significant morbidity and mortality. Based on a recent review of 101 articles from 47 countries, rotavirus vaccination has been associated with a 59% relative risk reduction in hospitalizations and a 36% reduction in the combined endpoint of hospitalization and death. The introduction of rotavirus vaccines led to a 50% reduction in the rotavirus stool carriage rate in children under age 5.

10. What is the most common cause of outbreak and sporadic cases of acute infectious gastroenteritis and diarrhea in Western countries?

Norovirus infection remains the most common cause of acute sporadic and outbreak-associated diarrhea and gastroenteritis in Western countries. Experts estimate that in the United States, 21 million cases of Norovirus gastroenteritis occur annually leading to 2.2 million clinic visits, 465,000 emergency department visits, and 109,000 hospitalizations. Noroviruses are members of the Calicivirus family and fall into five genogroups (G.I through G.V). Although some genogroups can infect and are present in both humans and animals, most outbreaks result from human-to-human transmission. The majority of pandemic strains have been G.II.4 subtypes.

11. What organisms are most likely to present with bloody diarrhea or acute dysentery?

Invasive bacterial pathogens, and to a lesser extent amoebae, are more likely to present with diarrhea accompanied by fever or dysentery. Among bacterial pathogens *Shigella* spp., nontyphoidal *Salmonella*, *Campylobacter* spp., STEC, and EHEC variants are the most common. *E. histolytica*, the agent of amebic dysentery, may also cause bouts of watery or bloody diarrhea with colitis. Importantly, climate change may have a significant impact on the range of dysenteric illnesses as warmer temperatures favor the proliferation of *Shigella* and *Salmonella* spp.

12. What are the subtypes of diarrheagenic *E. coli*?

There are five major pathotypes of diarrheagenic *E. coli*:
- ETEC produces either heat-labile and/or heat-stable toxins and causes watery diarrhea—a classic cause of travelers' diarrhea.
- Enteropathogenic *E. coli* (EPEC) has a characteristic *attaching and effacing* effect in the small bowel. It is the classic cause of infantile diarrhea in the developing world but increasingly recognized as a common cause of travelers' diarrhea.
- Enteroinvasive *E. coli* (EIEC) invades the mucosal lining causing a dysentery syndrome clinically similar to shigellosis.
- Enteroaggregative *E. coli* (EAEC) causes persistent diarrhea in children and in patients with human immunodeficiency virus (HIV)—also an increasingly common cause of travelers' diarrhea.
- STEC are also called EHEC because they often cause bloody diarrhea. O157:H7 is the most common serotype worldwide—and the only pathogenic strain that you can readily identify via nonmolecular testing, that is, using Sorbitol-MacConkey agar. Classically, the transmission source is contaminated beef, but many other foods can carry it. The use of antibiotics in STEC/EHEC infection is controversial as meta-analysis suggests this may be associated with an increased risk of hemolytic uremic syndrome (HUS).

13. What are the epidemiologic features and species most commonly associated with shigellosis?

Shigellosis is an important cause of both watery diarrhea and (less commonly) dysentery among travelers, but children under four in endemic settings bear most of the burden of the disease. In the United States, shigellosis is often associated with children in daycare settings and men who have sex with men. *Shigella flexneri* is the leading cause of endemic diarrhea in developing countries. *Shigella sonnei* is the leading cause of endemic diarrhea in high-income countries. *Shigella dysenteriae* is associated with outbreaks caused by natural disasters or massive social disruption.

14. **What antibiotic class should one avoid when treating acute diarrhea associated with travel to Southeast Asia?**
    Antibiotic resistance among international travelers is a growing problem, in part due to the self-administration of antibiotics. The high rate of *Campylobacter* resistance to quinolones in Southeast Asia in particular makes them a poor choice for the empiric treatment of travelers' diarrhea there. In addition, emerging quinolone resistance for *Shigella, Salmonella*, ETEC, and EAEC exists in most of the world. Azithromycin is the agent of choice for empiric treatment of febrile travelers' diarrhea, particularly when one notes blood, pus, or mucus in stool. You can manage milder cases without antibiotics.

15. **What agents of acute diarrhea can one contract when ingesting raw oysters?**
    Oysters and other filter-feeding bivalves, whether farmed or harvested from the wild, can harbor and concentrate both viral and bacterial enteric pathogens. *Vibrio parahaemolyticus* and Norovirus are the most common pathogens acquired when one ingests raw oysters. Contamination via runoff from nearby human populations likely contributes to the risk.

16. **What specific unique etiologic factors exist for acute diarrheal illness in immunocompromised hosts?**
    Host factors such as the type of cellular or humoral immune deficiency play an important role in the risk for specific diarrheal pathogens. Organ transplantation, IgA deficiency, hypogammaglobulinemia, and ongoing immunosuppressive therapy are among the most common scenarios of concern. Patients with HIV not taking highly active antiretroviral agents are also at risk. In addition to the usual causes of acute diarrhea, immunocompromised hosts are particularly vulnerable to cytomegalovirus (CMV) and parasites like *Cryptosporidium, Cyclospora*, and *Isospora*. Noninfectious factors such as antiretroviral, cytotoxic, or molecularly targeted pharmaceuticals, monoclonal antibodies, immunotherapy agents, and graft-versus-host disease can also cause or contribute to acute diarrhea. See Chapter 56 for further discussion of diarrhea in immunocompromised hosts.

17. **What infectious agents are associated with acute and persistent diarrheal illness in patients with HIV?**
    The pathogens responsible for diarrhea in the general population are also common in patients with HIV. In contrast to immunocompetent hosts, bacteria like *S. flexneri, Salmonella enteritidis*, and *Campylobacter jejuni* sometimes cause persistent diarrhea in those with HIV. In general, the likely infectious agents vary significantly with the degree of immune compromise. In addition to common pathogens, patients with CD4 counts less than 200 cells/mm^3 are susceptible to opportunistic infections, including a host of bacterial (e.g., *Mycobacterium*), parasitic (e.g., *Cryptosporidium, Microsporidia, Isospora*, and *Cyclospora*), viral (e.g., CMV), and rarely—fungal (e.g., histoplasmosis) infections. With the advent of highly active antiretroviral therapies, diarrhea caused by opportunistic infections has decreased while the incidence of noninfectious causes, for example, antiretroviral-associated diarrhea, has increased among patients with HIV worldwide.

18. **What are the common causes of acute diarrheal illness among solid organ transplant patients?**
    Diarrhea from both infectious and noninfectious causes is common after solid organ transplant. *C. difficile* is a common bacterial pathogen in transplant patients. CMV and norovirus are common viral causes. Other infectious agents are similar to those found in the general population with some key differences; symptoms tend to be more severe, there is a higher incidence of opportunistic infections, and chronic infections or prolonged shedding are more frequent, for example, with norovirus.

19. **Which bacterial agent of acute diarrhea has humans as its most important reservoir and is more likely to spread and cause disease outbreaks from person-to-person contact?**
    Shigella is the primary bacterial cause of endemic diarrhea, in part, because humans serve as a major reservoir. Outbreaks often originate from person-to-person contact, via childcare or school settings, and through direct contamination of food.

20. **What presentation and historical features are useful in defining the etiologic factors of acute diarrhea syndromes?**
    Travel and contact history, acuity, presence of fever, volume, quality, and presence of blood or mucus in stool are useful clues to etiology. Host factors such as age, immune status, and socioeconomic status are also helpful. Table 54.1 pairs diarrheal syndromes with the most common pathogens for developed and developing countries.

Table 54.1 Prevalence and Infectious Causes of Common Infectious Diarrhea by Syndrome Type.

PRESENTATION	ESTIMATED PREVALENCE (%)	DEVELOPED COUNTRIES	DEVELOPING COUNTRIES
Watery diarrhea	90	Viral and preformed toxins	*Escherichia coli, Campylobacter jejuni, Salmonella*, and *Shigella*
Dysentery (fever with mucoid or bloody stools)	5–10	*Shigella*, enteroinvasive *E. coli*, and *Campylobacter*	*Shigella*, enteroinvasive *E. coli, C. jejuni*, and *Entamoeba histolytica*
Persistent diarrhea	3–4	Enterpathogenic *E. coli, Giardia, Yersina*, and *Campylobacter*	Enteropathogenic *E. coli* and *Giardia*
Large volume/rice-water stool	1	*Salmonella* and enterotoxigenic *E. coli*	*Vibrio cholerae* and enterotoxigenic *E. coli*
Hemorrhagic colitis (abdominal pain with bloody diarrhea and no fever)	<1	Enterohemorrhagic *E. coli*	Enterohemorrhagic *E. coli*

21. **What is the most common cause of travelers' diarrhea?**
Bacterial infections are responsible for 80%–90% of cases of travelers' diarrhea, and *E. coli* continues to be the most common cause. Previously, we thought ETEC was the most prevalent strain, but EPEC and EAEC now appear to be more common. Parasites are responsible for approximately 10% of cases, and approximately 2%–15% of cases are viral.

22. **What tests can you use to diagnose infectious diarrhea?**
Although routine stool cultures for common bacterial agents (*E. coli, Salmonella, Shigella*, and *Campylobacter*) and microscopy (for ova and parasites) can be useful in clinical practice, newer tests have emerged that are faster, more sensitive, and less labor-intensive. Enzyme immunoassays (EIAs) for pathogenic antigens have become the tests of choice for many protozoa, viruses, and some bacterial products. Testing for viral pathogens is rarely necessary because of the self-limited nature of the infection. Polymerase chain reaction (PCR) techniques have become widespread for a number of pathogens, and the US Food and Drug Administration recently approved kits that perform PCR assays for multiple pathogens from a single specimen (multiplexed PCR). These may become the test of choice for undifferentiated diarrhea (Table 54.2).

23. **When should you obtain stool cultures?**
The overuse of stool cultures in clinical practice is a source of misspent time and money. Bacteria that are commonly tested include *Salmonella* spp., *Campylobacter* spp., *Shigella* spp., and STEC. They are positive in only approximately 1.5%–5% of samples submitted. Stool cultures are clinically useful in nonhospitalized patients who have had diarrheal illnesses lasting for more than 5 days, cases suspicious for dysentery or severe diarrhea, or in cases of outbreaks. One should not submit stool cultures for patients hospitalized for more than 3 days.

24. **How does one differentiate IBD from acute infectious diarrhea?**
The initial presentation of IBD can be difficult to distinguish from some forms of acute infectious diarrhea. One can consider IBD in patients with persistent bloody diarrhea (>7 days) with a negative infectious workup and lack of response to empiric therapy. Patients with a history of recurrent or chronic gastrointestinal (GI) complaints, patients 20–30 years of age, and those with extraintestinal manifestations of IBD (aphthous ulcers, uveitis, arthralgias, erythema nodosum, and pyoderma gangrenosum) have a higher likelihood of IBD. Lower endoscopy may help distinguish between these diagnoses, although the endoscopic findings are quite similar in the early phases of each disease. Inflammatory markers are also nonspecific.

25. **When should one be concerned about a systemic infection from a non-enteric pathogen in a patient presenting with diarrhea?**
Most enteric pathogens present with a diarrhea-predominant clinical syndrome, although other symptoms (headache, myalgias, fever, and malaise) may also be present. Most of these infections are self-limited and resolve within a few days. Stool studies generally readily identify those that can cause more severe illness (*Shigella*, STEC, *C. difficile*). Many other non-enteric infectious agents and systemic illnesses can present with diarrhea. One should consider these potential etiologic factors when a patient has persistent diarrhea with negative stool studies

Table 54.2 Sensitivity and Specificity for Common Microbiological Tests Used in the Evaluation of Infectious Diarrhea.

STOOL TEST	SENSITIVITY (%)	SPECIFICITY (%)
Clostridioides difficile cytotoxic assay	93	98
C. difficile PCR assay	77–100	92–100
C. difficile EIA (toxin A and B)	29–86	91–100
C difficile EIA (GDH)	83–100	88–100
C. difficile LAMP assay	92	94
Campylobacter EIA	75–100	97–98
Shiga toxin EIA	92–100	98–100
Giardia EIA	94–99	100
Entamoeba histolytica EIA	82	99
Multiplexed PCR assays	87–100	93–100

EIA, Enzyme immunoassay; *GDH,* glutamate dehydrogenase; *LAMP,* loop-mediated isothermal amplification; *PCR,* polymerase chain reaction.

or develops symptoms that are not typically seen with infectious diarrhea syndromes (high fever [>103°F], jaundice, cough, altered mental status, etc.).

26. Is endoscopy useful in evaluating acute infectious diarrhea?

Endoscopy should not be part of the routine evaluation of acute diarrhea but may help in select situations such as evaluating for IBD in patients with persistent bloody diarrhea and a negative infectious workup who do not respond to empiric therapy. When there is a strong suspicion of *C. difficile* and stool tests are negative or not available, flexible sigmoidoscopy may reveal characteristic pseudomembranes. Finally, endoscopy may also be useful for immunocompromised patients to evaluate for CMV colitis, which frequently requires a histologic diagnosis.

27. What is the best test to evaluate for *C. difficile* infection?

Traditionally, one diagnosed *C. difficile* infection with EIA tests and confirmatory toxigenic cultures or cytotoxic assays. Unfortunately, EIA tests are labor intensive and have limited sensitivity, prompting the development of more rapid and reliable tests. PCR tests are now the test of choice as they are rapid (within hours) and highly sensitive and specific. Loop-mediated isothermal amplification assays are even faster (1 hour) and simpler than PCR and may play a future role. The Infectious Diseases Society of American guidelines from 2010 still recommend a two-step procedure with an initial EIA test for glutamate dehydrogenase followed by a confirmatory toxigenic culture assay or cell culture cytotoxin B assay. Endoscopy is an insensitive, invasive, and expensive means of diagnosis and one should not routinely employ it.

28. When is a *test of cure* necessary for acute infectious diarrhea?

In most cases of acute infectious diarrhea, resolution of symptoms is enough. There are no indications for tests of cure with *C. difficile* in patients whose symptoms have resolved. Many health departments require that restaurant workers with *Salmonella* infections have a stool test to demonstrate that they are no longer carrying the bacterium before they return to work, but there are no official guidelines from academic societies or the federal government. Providers should consult their local health department agencies regarding this matter.

29. Describe the initial treatments for *C. difficile* infection.

The first treatment for *C. difficile* infection is to stop any offending antibiotics, if possible. If symptoms persist, treatment depends on the clinical context. For mild to moderate infections, one may begin by using either oral vancomycin (125 mg four times daily for 10 days) or fidaxomicin (200 mg twice daily for 10 days). If these are unavailable, metronidazole 500 mg three times daily for 10 days is acceptable. In severe, but not fulminant, infection, the initial treatment is the same. For fulminant infection, one should ensure adequate volume resuscitation, and begin vancomycin 500 mg orally every 6 hours for the first 48–72 hours. For complicated severe infection, one may add intravenous (IV) metronidazole (500 mg every 8 hours).

30. **What is the role of oral rehydration solution (ORS) for acute infectious diarrhea?**
ORS has revolutionized the treatment of acute infectious diarrhea worldwide. ORS takes advantage of the fact that sodium and glucose are cotransported in the jejunum, a mechanism unaffected by pathologic increases in intestinal secretion that leads to enhanced water absorption. Numerous trials have shown that ORS decreases morbidity in adults and both morbidity and mortality in children. Head-to-head trials show ORS to be equivalent to IV hydration for acute gastroenteritis therapy in children. Because it decreases diarrheal volume, hypo-osmolar ORS is preferred.

31. **How should one dose ORS?**
The dose depends on the degree of dehydration. For mild dehydration (3%–5% decrease in body weight), 50 mL/kg taken in 2–4 hours is appropriate. For moderate dehydration (6%–9% decrease in body weight), the dosage should be increased to 100 mL/kg taken over the same period. If the dehydration is more severe, one should use initial treatment with IV rehydration followed by ORS at 100 mL/kg in 4 hours.

32. **What is the role of antimotility agents (AMAs) in the treatment of acute infectious diarrhea?**
Most episodes of acute diarrhea are self-limited, lasting less than 24 hours, and do not require AMAs. For longer-lasting diarrheal illnesses, these agents may decrease total diarrhea duration, thus improving quality of life. In general, AMAs are safe for use in adults with the following caveats: one should not use AMAs if the patient is critically ill or has a known or suspected *C. difficile* or *E. coli* 0157:H7 infection, fever, or dysentery. Children younger than 3 years should not receive AMAs because of an increased number of adverse events in this population. When combined with antimicrobials for travelers' diarrhea, AMAs can shorten illness duration from 3 to 5 days to less than 24 hours, particularly if the patient has more frequent diarrheal episodes.

33. **Do antiparasitic agents (APAs) play a role in the treatment of acute diarrhea?**
For immunocompetent patients in the developed world, empiric APAs play no role in the management of acute diarrhea. In patients in the developing world or those who are immunosuppressed, treatment should be guided based on the results of testing as there is not a one-size-fits-all APA (Fig. 54.1).

34. **What are the indications for antibiotics in acute infectious diarrhea?**
Antibiotic use for acute diarrhea depends largely on the infectious agent. In the developed world, most acute diarrhea is self-limited and viral, rendering antibiotics moot. If a particular pathogen is confirmed or highly suspected based on clinical presentation (*C. difficile*, *Giardia*, EHEC, ETEC, EIEC, *Shigella* spp., *Isospora*, *Microsporidia*, *Cyclospora*, *E. histolytica*) antibiotics are reasonable. For nontyphoidal *Salmonella*, antibiotics lend no benefit and prolong clearance of the pathogen. An empiric quinolone is reasonable in adults with inflammatory diarrhea not thought to be from STEC. Most clinical microbiology labs can readily rule out Shiga toxin production.

35. **How does antibiotic use affect the risk of HUS?**
In the United States, STEC 0157:H7 infection, generally from contaminated ground beef, causes the majority of diarrhea-associated HUS. In several series the use of antibiotics appears to increase the risk of HUS in children younger than 10 years old. Although the data regarding adults are less clear, there is no evidence that the use of antibiotics shortens the duration of illness or decreases symptoms, and thus one should avoid them in these cases.

LONG-TERM CONSEQUENCES AND SEQUELAE OF DIARRHEAL ILLNESS

36. **What sequelae have been associated with acute enteric infections?**
A growing list of long-term and other sequelae have been associated with enteric infections. A strong link has been established mechanistically, epidemiologically, and from animal models between enteric infection and autoimmune phenomena like the Guillain-Barré syndrome (GBS) and reactive arthritis. During the last decade, epidemiologic evidence from outbreaks and large cohort studies has established a heightened risk of development of irritable bowel syndrome and other disorders of gut-brain interaction after enteric infection. Most recently, emerging evidence is shedding light on the global impact of early childhood infections in low- and middle-income populations on chronic enteric dysfunction, growth stunting, and poor cognition.

37. **Which bacterial agent of acute diarrhea is most likely to result in bacteremia and distant ectopic foci of infection?**
Nontyphoidal strains of *Salmonella* are invasive and may lead to bacteremia after enteric infection. Among older patients, endocarditis or other septic foci of infection have been reported after salmonellosis. Salmonella infections, both typhoidal and nontyphoidal, are situations in which bacteremia is common but highest culture yield is from bone marrow aspirate.

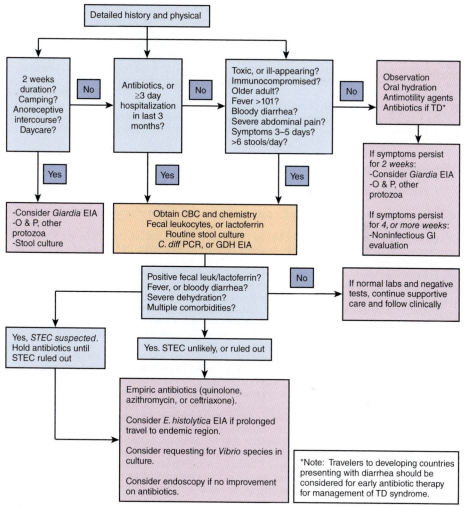

Fig. 54.1 Diagnostic algorithm for diarrhea management. *CBC,* Complete blood count; *EIA,* enzyme immunoassay; *GDH,* glutamate dehydrogenase; *GI,* gastrointestinal; *O & P,* ova and parasites; *PCR,* polymerase chain reaction; *STEC,* Shiga toxin–producing *Escherichia coli; TD,* travelers' diarrhea.

38. What enteric infection has been associated with GBS?

Respiratory and intestinal infections, vaccinations, and other immunologic influences have been associated with GBS, an autoimmune demyelinating or axonal peripheral neuropathy usually manifesting as progressive ascending weakness and paralysis. *C. jejuni* infection is the most common infection associated with GBS and is usually of an axonal subtype. Molecular mimicry of the bacterial lipopolysaccharide and ganglioside moieties on peripheral nerves appears to be a dominant mechanism. In the developing world, it is estimated that one-third of all cases of acute flaccid paralysis are GBS caused by *Campylobacter.*

39. What enteric pathogens are associated with reactive arthritis?

Several enteric bacterial pathogens may be associated with postinfectious autoimmune arthritis syndromes. *Salmonella, Yersinia, Campylobacter,* and *Shigella* are most commonly associated. More recently, *E. coli* and *C. difficile* infections have been associated with arthralgia or arthritis syndromes as well. In addition to asymmetric oligoarthritis, some patients may develop conjunctivitis or skin eruptions (keratoderma blennorrhagica or erythema nodosum). Management includes the treatment of the inciting infection and then judicious use of anti-inflammatory therapies (nonsteroidal anti-inflammatory drugs, disease-modifying antirheumatic drugs, steroids).

40. **What role do prebiotics and probiotics play in the treatment of acute diarrhea?**

The use of probiotics for the treatment of acute diarrhea remains controversial. The rationale is based on the idea that probiotic organisms compete for binding sites and also may produce metabolites and acids harmful to enteric pathogens. Evidence for and against the approach is difficult to evaluate because of the variety of probiotics and formulation types in existence (*Saccharomyces*, *Lactobacillus acidophilus*, Bifidobacterium, etc.) as well as methodological factors. A Cochrane review published in 2020 included 82 studies and showed no difference in duration of diarrhea, chances diarrhea would last ≥48 hours or risk of hospitalization.

41. **What are the primary risk factors for foodborne illness in the United States?**

The most common causes of foodborne illness are norovirus, *Salmonella, Clostridium perfringens, Campylobacter,* and *S. aureus*. The top five risk factors contributing to foodborne illness in the United States are follows:
- Food from unsafe sources
- Inadequate cooking
- Improper hot/cold holding temperatures
- Contaminated equipment
- Poor personal hygiene

42. **What counseling is appropriate for patients on the prevention of acute diarrhea from domestic sources?**

It is recommended by the US Centers for Disease Control and Prevention that individuals follow four simple steps—Clean, Separate, Cook, and Chill—to prevent foodborne illness at home. These four simple steps can be expanded in explanation as follows:

1. **Clean:** Wash your hands and surfaces often. Germs that cause food poisoning can survive in many places and spread around your kitchen. Wash hands for 20 seconds with soap and water before, during, and after preparing food and before eating. Wash your utensils, cutting boards, and countertops with hot, soapy water after preparing each food item. Rinse fresh fruits and vegetables under running water. Do not wash meat, chicken, turkey, or eggs as this can contaminate surfaces in your kitchen.
2. **Separate:** Do not cross-contaminate one food with another. Raw meat, poultry, seafood, and eggs can spread germs to ready-to-eat foods—unless you keep them separate. Use separate cutting boards and plates for raw meat, poultry, and seafood. When grocery shopping, keep raw meat, poultry, seafood, and juices away from other foods. Keep raw meat, poultry, seafood, and eggs separate from all other foods in the refrigerator.
3. **Cook to the right temperature:** Food is safely cooked when the internal temperature gets high enough to kill germs that can make you sick. The only way to tell if food is safely cooked is to use a food thermometer. You cannot tell if food is safely cooked by checking its color and texture (except for seafood). Use a food thermometer to ensure foods are cooked to a safe internal temperature depending on the type of food.
4. **Chill:** Refrigerate promptly. Bacteria can multiply rapidly if left at room temperature or in the "Danger Zone" between 40°F and 140°F. Keep your refrigerator at 40°F or below, your freezer at 0°F or below, and know when to throw food out. Divide warm foods into several clean, shallow containers so they will chill faster. Refrigerate perishable food within 2 hours. If the food is exposed to temperatures above 90°F (like a hot car or picnic), refrigerate it within 1 hour. Thaw frozen food safely in the refrigerator, in cold water, or in the microwave. Never thaw foods on the counter because bacteria multiply quickly in the parts of the food that reach room temperature.

Finally, patients should be reminded to report suspected cases of foodborne illness to their local health department. Calls from citizens are key to the early detection of outbreaks and to understand risks to individuals and populations.

CLINICAL VIGNETTE

Available Online

BIBLIOGRAPHY

Available Online

WEBSITES

Available Online

CHAPTER 55

CHRONIC DIARRHEA

Lawrence R. Schiller, MD

 Additional content available online

1. **Define chronic diarrhea.**

   Diarrhea is defined as an increase in the frequency and fluidity of stools. For most patients, diarrhea means the passage of loose stools. The Bristol Stool Form Chart can be used to categorize stool form: types 6 and 7 (mushy or completely liquid stools) constitute diarrhea. Although loose stools often are accompanied by an increase in the frequency of bowel movements, most patients do not classify frequent passage of *formed* stools as diarrhea. However, many investigators use the frequency of defecation of loose stools as a quantitative criterion for diarrhea. By this standard, passage of more than two loose bowel movements per day is considered abnormal (Table 55.1). Some authors also incorporate stool weight in the definition of diarrhea. Normal stool weight averages approximately 80 g/day in females and 100 g/day in males. The upper limit of normal stool weight (calculated as the mean plus two standard deviations) is approximately 200 g/day. Normal stool weight depends on dietary intake, and some patients on high-fiber diets exceed 200 g/day without reporting that they are having diarrhea. Thus stool weight by itself is an imperfect criterion for diarrhea.

Table 55.1 Criteria for Diagnosis of Diarrhea.

CRITERION	NORMAL RANGE	DIARRHEA, IF
Increased stool frequency	3–14 stools/week	>2 stools/day
More liquid stool consistency	Soft—formed stools	Loose—unformed
Increased stool weight Males Females	 0–240 g/24 hr 0–180 g/24 hr	 240 g/24 hr >180 g/24 hr

2. **What other disorder may be described as diarrhea?**

   Occasionally patients with fecal incontinence describe that problem as diarrhea, even when stools are formed. Physicians must be careful to distinguish fecal incontinence from diarrhea because incontinence is usually due to problems with the muscles and nerves regulating continence and not just to passage of unusually voluminous or liquid stools.

3. **What is the basic mechanism of all diarrheal diseases?**

   Diarrhea is due to the incomplete absorption of fluid from luminal contents. Normal stools are approximately 75% water and 25% solids. Normal fecal water output is approximately 60–80 mL/day. An increase in fecal water output of 50–100 mL is sufficient to cause loosening of the stool. This volume represents approximately 1% of the fluid load entering the upper intestine each day; thus malabsorption of only 1%–2% of fluid entering the intestine may be sufficient to cause diarrhea (Fig. 55.1).

4. **What pathologic processes can cause diarrhea?**

   Excessive stool water is due to the presence of some solute that osmotically obligates water retention within the lumen. This solute can be some poorly absorbed, osmotically active substance, such as magnesium ions, or can be an accumulation of ordinary electrolytes, such as sodium or potassium, that normally are absorbed easily by the intestine. When excess stool water is due to the ingestion of a poorly absorbed substance, the diarrhea is called osmotic diarrhea. Examples of this include lactose malabsorption and diarrhea induced by osmotic laxatives. When excessive stool water is due to the presence of extra electrolytes resulting from the reduction of electrolyte absorption or stimulation of electrolyte secretion, diarrhea is known as secretory diarrhea. Causes of secretory diarrhea include infection, particularly infections that produce toxins that reduce intestinal fluid electrolyte absorption, reduction of mucosal surface area resulting from disease or surgery, absence of an ion transport mechanism, inflammation of the mucosa, ingestion of drugs or poisons, endogenous secretagogues such as bile acids, dysfunction caused by abnormal regulation by nerves and hormones, and tumors producing circulating secretagogues.

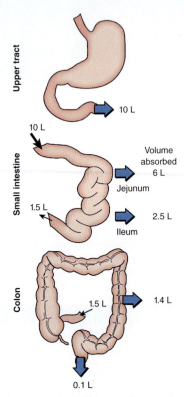

Fig. 55.1 Fluid loads through the intestine. Each day approximately 9–10 L of fluid passes into the jejunum. This consists of approximately 2 L of ingested food and drink, 1.5 L of saliva, 2.5 L of gastric juice, 1.5 L of bile, and 2.5 L of pancreatic juice. The jejunum absorbs most of this load as nutrients are taken up, and the ileum absorbs most of the rest. The colon absorbs more than 90% of the fluid load reaching it, leaving only 1% of the original fluid entering the jejunum excreted in stool. Substantial fluid malabsorption in the small bowel can overwhelm colonic absorptive capacity and may result in diarrhea. Less severe disruption of colonic absorption can lead to diarrhea because of the lack of any more distal absorbing segment. A reduction of absorptive efficiency of only 1% for the total intestine can result in diarrhea.

5. **List three classifications of diarrheal diseases.**
   Because the symptom of diarrhea has such a broad differential diagnosis, it is useful to classify the type of diarrhea to restrict the differential diagnosis to a more manageable number of conditions. Three helpful classification schemes include as follows:
   - acute versus chronic (4 weeks or longer),
   - epidemiologic criteria (traveler's, epidemic or outbreak, acquired immune deficiency syndrome [AIDS], and institutional), and
   - stool characteristics (watery, fatty, and inflammatory).
      Watery stools are typically runny and lack blood, pus, or fat. Watery diarrhea is subdivided into secretory and osmotic types, depending on stool electrolyte concentrations. Fatty stools have an excess of fat, which can be shown by qualitative testing with the Sudan stain or by quantitative analysis of a timed stool collection for fat. Inflammatory diarrheas typically contain blood or pus. If not grossly evident, these characteristics can be detected by a fecal occult blood test or by staining the stool for neutrophils. Classifying diarrheas by stool characteristics enables the physician to sort quickly through more likely and less likely diagnoses (Table 55.2). This scheme is thus very useful in chronic diarrheas in which the construction of a reasonable differential diagnosis can lead to more appropriate testing and more rapid diagnosis.

6. **What are the likely causes of diarrhea, according to epidemiologic characteristics?**
   Traveler's diarrhea
   - Bacterial infection (mostly acute)
   - Protozoal infection (e.g., amebiasis and giardiasis)
   - Tropical sprue

Table 55.2 Tests for Evaluation of Systemic Diseases Associated With Chronic Secretory Diarrhea.

CATEGORY	CONDITIONS	DIAGNOSTIC TESTS
Endocrine diseases	Hyperthyroidism Addison disease Panhypopituitarism Diabetes mellitus	Thyroid-stimulating hormone, T4 ACTH-stimulation test, cortisol ACTH-stimulation test, TSH Blood glucose, and glycosylated hemoglobin
Endocrine tumor syndromes	MEN-1 (Wermer syndrome) Hyperparathyroidism Pancreatic endocrine tumors Pituitary tumors (also may have adrenal cortical tumors and thyroid adenomas) MEN-2a (Sipple syndrome) Medullary thyroid cancer Pheochromocytoma Hyperparathyroidism MEN-2b (same as MEN-2a + neuromas and Marfanoid phenotype)	Parathormone Gastrin, VIP, insulin, and glucagon Prolactin, growth hormone, and ACTH Calcitonin Urine metanephrine Parathormone
Hematologic diseases	Leukemia and lymphoma Multiple myeloma	Complete blood count Serum protein electrophoresis
Immune system disorders	AIDS Amyloidosis Common variable immunodeficiency IgA deficiency	HIV serology Mucosal biopsy Immunoglobin levels
Heavy metal poisoning		Heavy metal screen

ACTH, Adrenocorticotropic hormone; *AIDS*, acquired immune deficiency syndrome; *HIV*, human immunodeficiency virus; *Ig*, immunoglobulin; *MEN*, multiple endocrine neoplasia; *T4*, thyroxine; *TSH*, thyroid-stimulating hormone; *VIP*, vasoactive intestinal polypeptide.

Epidemics and outbreaks
- Bacterial infection
- Viral infection (e.g., rotavirus and norovirus)
- Protozoal infections (e.g., cryptosporidiosis)
- Brainerd diarrhea (epidemic idiopathic secretory diarrhea)

Patients with AIDS
- Opportunistic infections (e.g., cryptosporidiosis, cytomegalovirus, herpes, and *Mycobacterium avium* complex)
- Drug side effect
- Lymphoma

Institutionalized patients
- *Clostridioides difficile* toxin–mediated colitis
- Food poisoning
- Ischemic colitis
- Fecal impaction with overflow diarrhea
- Tube feeding
- Drug side effect

7. **What are the likely causes of osmotic watery diarrhea?**
   Osmotic laxatives (e.g., Mg^{2+}, PO_4^{3-}, and SO_4^{2-}) and carbohydrate malabsorption.

8. **List the likely causes of secretory watery diarrhea.**
   - Bacterial toxins
   - Ileal bile acid malabsorption

- Inflammatory bowel disease (ulcerative colitis, Crohn disease, microscopic colitis [lymphocytic and collagenous colitis], and diverticulitis)
- Vasculitis
- Drugs and poisons
- Stimulant laxative abuse
- Disordered motility or regulation (postvagotomy diarrhea, postsympathectomy diarrhea, diabetic autonomic neuropathy, amyloidosis, and irritable bowel syndrome)
- Endocrine diarrhea (hyperthyroidism, Addison disease, gastrinoma, vasoactive intestinal polypeptide tumor [VIPoma], somatostatinoma, carcinoid syndrome, medullary carcinoma of the thyroid, and mastocytosis)
- Other tumors (colon cancer, lymphoma, and villous adenoma)
- Idiopathic secretory diarrhea (epidemic secretory [Brainerd] diarrhea and sporadic idiopathic secretory diarrhea)
- Congenital syndromes (e.g., congenital chloridorrhea)

9. List the likely causes of inflammatory diarrhea.
- Inflammatory bowel disease (ulcerative colitis, Crohn disease, diverticulitis, and ulcerative jejunoileitis)
- Infectious diseases (pseudomembranous colitis, invasive bacterial infections [tuberculosis and yersiniosis], ulcerating viral infections [cytomegalovirus and herpes simplex], and invasive parasitic infections [amebiasis and strongyloidiasis])
- Ischemic colitis
- Radiation colitis
- Neoplasia (colon cancer and lymphoma)

10. List the likely causes of fatty diarrhea.
Malabsorption syndromes
- Mucosal disease (celiac disease and Whipple disease)
- Small bowel bacterial overgrowth
- Chronic mesenteric ischemia
- Short bowel syndrome
- Postgastrectomy syndrome

Maldigestion
- Pancreatic exocrine insufficiency
- Orlistat ingestion
- Inadequate luminal bile acid concentration

11. Summarize the initial approach to patients with chronic diarrhea.
The scheme in Fig. 55.2 is based on obtaining a careful history, looking for specific physical findings, and obtaining simple laboratory data to help classify diarrhea as watery, fatty, or inflammatory. The value of obtaining a quantitative (as opposed to a spot) stool collection is debated among experts. A quantitative collection over 48 or 72 hours permits a better estimation of fluid, electrolyte, and fat excretion but is not absolutely necessary for the appropriate classification of diarrhea.

12. How are secretory and osmotic watery diarrhea distinguished?
The most useful way to differentiate secretory and osmotic types of watery diarrhea is to measure fecal electrolytes and calculate the fecal osmotic gap. In many diarrheal conditions, sodium and potassium along with their accompanying anions are the dominant electrolytes in stool water. In secretory diarrhea, there is a failure to completely absorb electrolytes or actual electrolyte secretion by the intestine; sodium, potassium, and their accompanying anions are responsible for the bulk of osmotic activity in stool water and the retention of water within the gut lumen. In contrast, in osmotic diarrhea, ingestion of poorly absorbed, osmotically active substances is responsible for holding water within the gut lumen; electrolyte absorption is normal and thus sodium and potassium concentrations can become quite low (Fig. 55.3). The fecal osmotic gap calculation takes advantage of these distinctions to differentiate the two conditions.

13. How is the fecal osmotic gap calculated?
Fecal osmotic gap represents the osmotic activity in stool water *not* due to electrolytes. The sum of the concentrations of sodium and potassium in stool water is multiplied by 2 to account for the anions that are also present, and this product is subtracted from 290 mOsm/kg, the approximate osmolality of luminal contents within the intestine. (This number is a constant in this calculation because the relatively high permeability of the intestinal mucosa beyond the stomach means that osmotic equilibration with plasma will have taken place by the time that luminal contents reach the rectum.) As an example, let us assume that a patient with watery diarrhea has a sodium concentration of 75 mmol/L and a potassium concentration of 65 mmol/L in stool water.

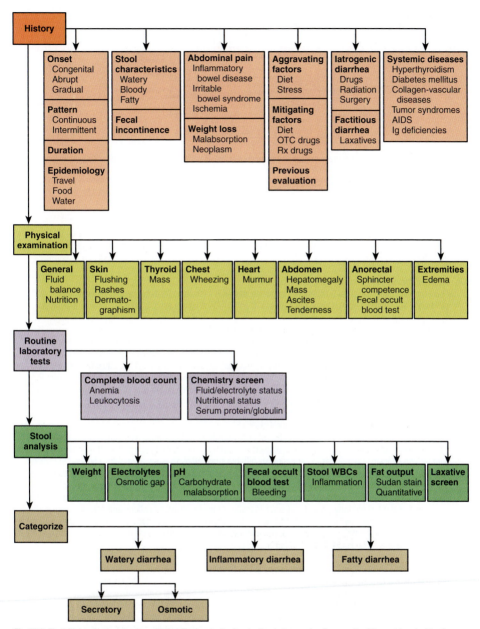

Fig. 55.2 The initial evaluation plan for patients with chronic diarrhea is aimed at assessing the severity of the problem, looking for clues to cause, and classifying the diarrhea as watery (with subtypes of osmotic and secretory diarrhea), inflammatory, or fatty. *AIDS*, Acquired immune deficiency syndrome; *Ig*, immunoglobulin; *OTC*, over the counter; *Rx*, prescription; *WBC*, white blood cell. (From Fine KD, Schiller LR. AGA technical review on the evaluation and management of chronic diarrhea. Gastroenterology. 1999;116:1464–1486.)

Adding these together yields a concentration of 140 mmol/L. Doubling this to account for anions means that electrolytes account for 280 mOsm/kg of stool water osmolality. Subtracting this from 290 mOsm/kg yields an osmotic gap of 10 mOsm/kg. In contrast, if stool sodium was 10 mmol/L and potassium concentration was 20 mmol/L, the combined contribution of cations and anions in stool water would be only 60 mOsm/kg, yielding

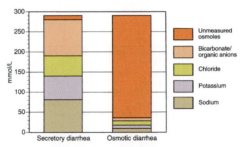

Fig. 55.3 Electrolyte patterns differ between osmotic and secretory diarrhea. In secretory diarrhea, electrolytes account for the bulk of the osmotic activity of stool water. In contrast, in osmotic diarrhea electrolyte absorption is normal and therefore electrolyte concentrations are very low; most of the osmotic activity is due to unmeasured osmoles. (Bicarbonate concentrations are *virtual* and are not directly measurable in most circumstances because of reaction with organic acids generated by fermentation by colonic bacteria.)

a fecal osmotic gap of 230 mOsm/kg. This represents the amount of some unmeasured substance that is contributing to fecal osmolality, presumably some poorly absorbed substance that is being ingested but not absorbed.

14. How is the fecal osmotic gap interpreted?
Fecal osmotic gaps less than 50 mOsm/kg correlate well with secretory diarrheas caused by incomplete electrolyte absorption. Fecal osmotic gaps greater than 50 mOsm/kg are associated with osmotic diarrheas.

15. What precautions are necessary when measuring fecal osmotic gaps?
Be certain that the stool has not been contaminated with either water or urine. Dilution by water or hypotonic urine will falsely lower fecal electrolyte concentrations and will elevate the calculated osmotic gap. This can be detected by actually measuring fecal osmolality; values that are substantially less than 290 mOsm/kg indicate dilution. Contamination with hypertonic urine may also affect fecal electrolyte concentrations but is harder to detect unless the concentration of creatinine in stool water is measured or the sum of measured cations and assumed anions is much greater than 290 mmol/L.

16. How does one evaluate osmotic diarrhea?
Osmotic diarrheas are typically due to ingestion of poorly absorbed cations, such as magnesium, or anions, such as sulfate. In addition, carbohydrate malabsorption, such as that caused by ingestion of lactose in a patient with lactase deficiency, and ingestion of poorly absorbable sugar alcohols, such as sorbitol, can lead to osmotic diarrhea. Measuring stool pH can help to distinguish between osmotic diarrheas caused by poorly absorbed cations and anions and those caused by ingestion of poorly absorbed carbohydrates and sugar alcohols. Carbohydrates and sugar alcohols are fermented by colonic bacteria, reducing fecal pH below 5 because of the production of short-chain fatty acids. In contrast, ingestion of poorly absorbed cations and anions does not affect stool pH much and stool pH is typically 7 in these circumstances. Once acidic stools have been discovered, check the diet and inquire about food additives and osmotic laxative ingestion. Specific testing for magnesium and other ions in stool is readily available to confirm any suspicions (Fig. 55.4).

17. Describe the evaluation of chronic secretory diarrhea.
Because there are many causes of chronic secretory diarrhea, an extensive evaluation is necessary (Fig. 55.5). Rare cases of infection should be excluded by multiplex PCR or by bacterial culture, examination of stool for parasites, and tests for protozoal antigens. Stimulant laxative abuse is best excluded by looking for laxatives in the urine or stool. Structural disease and internal fistulas can be evaluated with small bowel radiography or computed tomography (CT) scanning of the abdomen and pelvis. Endoscopic examination of the upper gastrointestinal tract and colon is routine and should include biopsy of even normal-appearing mucosa, looking for microscopic evidence of disease. Systemic diseases such as hyperthyroidism, adrenal insufficiency, and defective immunity can be evaluated with appropriate tests (Table 55.2).

18. When should neuroendocrine tumors be suspected as a cause of chronic secretory diarrhea?
Neuroendocrine tumors are uncommon causes of chronic secretory diarrhea. For example, one VIPoma might be expected per 10 million people per year. Table 55.3 lists these tumors and their markers. Because of the rarity of these tumors as a cause of chronic diarrhea, other causes of secretory diarrhea should be considered first. If the tumor is visualized by CT scan or if systemic symptoms (e.g., flushing) are present, evaluation for neuroendocrine

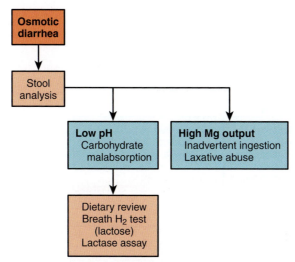

Fig. 55.4 Once a diagnosis of osmotic diarrhea is made, evaluation is fairly straightforward; only a few causes are possible. H_2, Hydrogen; Mg, magnesium. (From Fine KD, Schiller LR. AGA technical review on the evaluation and management of chronic diarrhea. Gastroenterology. 1999;116:1464-1486.)

tumors may have a better yield. Blanket testing for tumor-associated peptides is likely to yield many more false positives than true positives and therefore can be very misleading.

19. **What is Bayes theorem? How does it relate to the diagnosis of peptide-secreting tumors?**
Bayes theorem links the prevalence of the diagnosis to the positive predictive value of a diagnostic test. The positive predictive value of a test depends on the likelihood of the condition in the population to be tested, not only on the accuracy of the test. For example, peptide-secreting tumors are rare causes of chronic diarrhea with prevalences ranging from 1 per 5,000 to 1 per 500,000 patients with chronic diarrhea, depending on tumor type. Bayes theorem can be expressed in the following simplified formula:

$$\text{Post test odds of diagnosis} = \text{Pretest odds} \times \text{Likelihood ratio}$$

where the likelihood ratio = probability of true-positive result/probability of true-negative result.
   Because the pretest odds of a peptide-secreting tumor are so long and the false-positive rate of serum peptide assays for that diagnosis is so high (approximately 45%), the positive predictive value for serum peptide assays is substantially less than 1%. An abnormal test result would be misleading more than 99% of the time if applied to all patients with chronic diarrhea.

20. **What is the likely outcome in patients with chronic secretory diarrhea in whom a diagnosis cannot be reached?**
Diagnostic testing may fail to reveal a cause for chronic diarrhea in up to 25% of patients with chronic diarrhea depending on referral bias and the extent of evaluation.
   Some patients with chronic secretory diarrhea that evades a serious diagnostic evaluation have a similar history of previous good health with the sudden onset of diarrhea, often accompanied by acute, but not progressive, weight loss. Although the acute onset suggests an acute infectious process, patients have negative microbiologic studies and do not respond to empiric antibiotics. Diarrhea usually persists for 12–30 months and then gradually subsides. This condition can be sporadic or can occur in epidemics. The epidemic form (Brainerd diarrhea) seems to be associated with ingestion of potentially contaminated food or drink, but no organism has been implicated. Management consists of the effective use of nonspecific antidiarrheals until the process subsides.
   In other patients with chronic undiagnosed secretory diarrhea, a diagnosis will become apparent in time. Once a thorough evaluation has been concluded, it is, therefore, preferable to treat patients with undiagnosed secretory diarrhea symptomatically and follow them at intervals rather than endlessly repeat diagnostic testing.

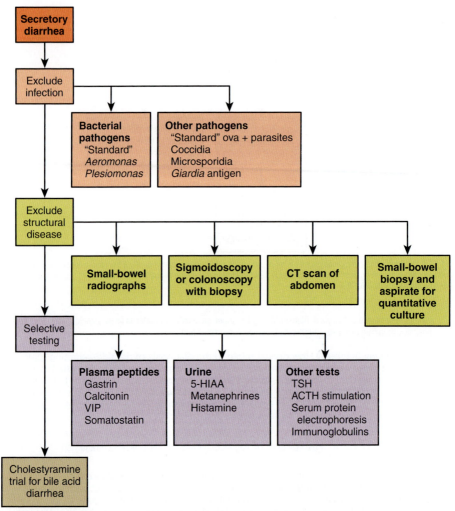

Fig. 55.5 Evaluation of secretory diarrhea can be very complex. This scheme can be used to guide the evaluation, depending on the specifics of each case. Not every test needs to be done on every patient. *5-HIAA*, 5-Hydroxyindoleacetic acid; *ACTH*, adrenocorticotropic hormone; *CT*, computed tomography; *TSH*, thyroid-stimulating hormone; *VIP*, vasoactive intestinal polypeptide. (From Fine KD, Schiller LR. AGA technical review on the evaluation and management of chronic diarrhea. Gastroenterology. 1999;116:1464-1486.)

21. **Describe the evaluation of chronic fatty diarrhea.**

Chronic fatty diarrhea is due to either maldigestion or malabsorption. Maldigestion can occur with pancreatic exocrine insufficiency, with ingestion of the lipase inhibitor orlistat, or if there is a bile acid deficiency, which reduces fat emulsification. Malabsorption typically is due to mucosal diseases such as celiac disease, small intestinal bacterial overgrowth, or small bowel fistula or resection.

Pancreatic exocrine insufficiency can be evaluated with a secretin test or measurement of chymotrypsin or elastase in the stool. Because these tests are not widely available or have poor specificity and sensitivity, clinicians often resort to a therapeutic trial of pancreatic enzymes. If this is done, the patient should be treated with a high dose of enzymes and the effect of this treatment on stool fat excretion as well as symptoms should be assessed.

Bile acid deficiency is a rare cause of maldigestion and is best assessed by direct measurement of duodenal bile acid concentration postprandially. Tests showing excess bile acid excretion in stool (radiolabeled bile acid excretion or total bile acid excretion tests) do not directly assess duodenal bile acid concentration, but if fecal

Table 55.3 Neuroendocrine Tumors Causing Chronic Diarrhea and Their Markers.

TYPICAL SYMPTOMS	TUMOR	MEDIATOR AND TUMOR MARKER
Gastrinoma	Zollinger-Ellison syndrome: pancreatic or duodenal tumor, peptic ulcer, steatorrhea, and diarrhea	Gastrin
VIPoma	Verner-Morrison syndrome: watery diarrhea, hypokalemia, achlorhydria, and flushing	Vasoactive intestinal polypeptide
Medullary thyroid carcinoma	Thyroid mass and hypermotility	Calcitonin and prostaglandins
Pheochromocytoma	Adrenal mass and hypertension	Vasoactive intestinal polypeptide, norepinephrine, and epinephrine
Carcinoid	Flushing, wheezing, and right-sided cardiac valvular disease	Serotonin and kinins
Somatostatinoma	Nonketotic diabetes mellitus, steatorrhea, diabetes, and gallstones	Somatostatin
Glucagonoma	Skin rash (migratory necrotizing erythema) and mild diabetes	Glucagon
Mastocytosis	Flushing, dermatographism, nausea, vomiting, and abdominal pain	Histamine and tryptase

VIPoma, Vasoactive intestinal polypeptide tumor.

bile acid excretion is high in a patient with steatorrhea, reduced duodenal bile acid concentration can be inferred. Mucosal disease can be evaluated with a small bowel biopsy and bacterial overgrowth can be assessed by breath hydrogen testing after an oral glucose load or by quantitative culture of intestinal contents (Fig. 55.6).

22. How does one make a diagnosis of celiac disease?

Celiac disease is a common cause of chronic fatty diarrhea, but it may present without diarrhea. The population prevalence in the United States is estimated to be just less than 1%. Serologic testing for immunoglobulin A (IgA) antibodies against tissue transglutaminase is the preferred noninvasive test, and small bowel mucosal biopsy is the definitive test. If serologic testing is done, total IgA levels should be measured because 10% of patients with celiac disease may have IgA deficiency, which would produce a false-negative test serologic result (see Chapter 40).

23. What other conditions can produce villous atrophy or blunting?

The differential diagnosis of villous changes on biopsy includes conditions other than the celiac disease: drug-induced enteropathy (e.g., olmesartan and nonsteroidal anti-inflammatory drugs), hypogammaglobulinemia and common variable immunodeficiency, autoimmune enteropathy, small bowel bacterial overgrowth, giardiasis, collagenous sprue, tropical sprue, Crohn disease, ulcerative jejunoileitis, and enteropathy-associated T cell lymphoma.

24. Describe the further evaluation of chronic inflammatory diarrhea.

Inflammatory diarrheas can be due to idiopathic inflammatory bowel diseases, such as ulcerative colitis or Crohn disease; invasive chronic infectious diseases, such as tuberculosis or yersiniosis; ischemic colitis; radiation colitis; and some tumors. To sort through these diagnoses, the most appropriate tests include colonoscopy to inspect the colonic mucosa visually, colonic biopsy to look for microscopic evidence of inflammation, small bowel radiography or CT scanning of the abdomen, and special cultures for chronic infections, such as tuberculosis or yersiniosis. In most cases the diagnosis will be apparent after these tests are completed (Fig. 55.7).

25. How does one distinguish irritable bowel syndrome from chronic diarrhea?

The diagnosis of irritable bowel syndrome should be based on the presence of abdominal pain that is associated with defecation and abnormal bowel habits. Chronic continuous diarrhea in the absence of pain is not irritable bowel syndrome, although it may be functional in nature. Symptom criteria (Rome IV criteria) have been published for clinical and research purposes and include the onset of symptoms at least 6 months ago and the presence of

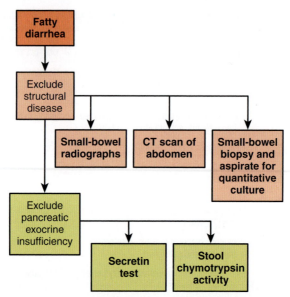

Fig. 55.6 Evaluation of chronic fatty diarrhea is designed to determine whether malabsorption or maldigestion is the cause of the excess fecal fat excretion. *CT*, Computed tomography. (From Fine KD, Schiller LR. AGA technical review on the evaluation and management of chronic diarrhea. Gastroenterology.1999;116:1464-1486.)

at least 1 day per week of abdominal pain or discomfort in the last 3 months that is associated with at least two of the following three features:

1. Relieved by defecation.
2. Onset associated with a change in stool frequency.
3. Onset associated with a change in stool form or appearance. Symptom onset must be at least 6 months prior to diagnosis.

Three causes account for symptoms in most patients with IBS-D and should be considered in designing treatments:

- Dietary intolerances (~40%)
- Bile acid diarrhea (~30%)
- Small intestinal bacterial overgrowth or dysbiosis (~15%–20%)

26. What causes of chronic diarrhea may be difficult to diagnose?

These conditions are seen in referral centers after routine evaluation has failed to disclose a diagnosis. In general, the tests necessary to make these diagnoses are not difficult but have not been done because physicians have not considered these diagnoses in the differential diagnosis of chronic diarrhea.

- Fecal incontinence
- Iatrogenic diarrhea (drugs, surgery, and radiation)
- Surreptitious laxative ingestion
- Microscopic colitis syndrome
- Bile acid–induced diarrhea
- Small bowel bacterial overgrowth
- Pancreatic exocrine insufficiency
- Carbohydrate malabsorption
- Peptide-secreting tumors
- Chronic idiopathic secretory diarrhea

27. What are common causes of iatrogenic diarrhea?

Most iatrogenic diarrheas are due to ingestion of drugs, some of which may not be considered as common causes of diarrhea. Approximately two-thirds of the drugs listed in the *Physician's Desk Reference* mention diarrhea as a possible side effect. Therefore the physician should obtain a history of all ingested drugs, including prescription medications, over-the-counter drugs, and herbal remedies (Box 55.1). Other causes of

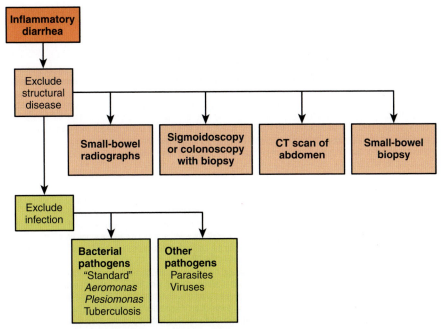

Fig. 55.7 Chronic inflammatory diarrhea has a diverse differential diagnosis. Structural evaluation with endoscopic or radiographic techniques often yields a diagnosis. Mucosal biopsy may be needed to confirm the diagnosis. *CT*, Computed tomography. (From Fine KD, Schiller LR. AGA technical review on the evaluation and management of chronic diarrhea. Gastroenterology. 1999;116:1464-1486.)

Box 55.1 Drugs Associated With Diarrhea

- Acarbose
- Antibiotics (most)
- Antineoplastic agents (many, especially immune checkpoint inhibitors)
- Anti-inflammatory agents (e.g., NSAIDs, gold, and 5-aminosalicylates)
- Antiarrhythmics (e.g., quinidine)
- Antihypertensives (e.g., β-receptor–blocking drugs and olmesartan)
- Antacids (e.g., those containing magnesium)
- Acid-reducing agents (e.g., H_2-receptor antagonists, and proton pump inhibitors)
- Prostaglandin (e.g., misoprostol)
- Vitamin and mineral supplements
- Herbal products

H2, Histamine-2; *NSAIDs*, nonsteroidal anti-inflammatory drugs.

---

iatrogenic diarrhea include surgical operations, such as vagotomy, gastrectomy, and cholecystectomy, and radiation therapy, during which the intestine is exposed to high doses of ionizing radiation.

28. **What features should suggest surreptitious laxative ingestion?**
    Some patients who present with chronic diarrhea have diarrhea due to laxative abuse. Laxatives can be detected by chemical testing of stool or urine. The diagnosis should be confirmed before confronting the patient, and psychiatric consultation should be available to help with further management. In general, four groups of patients have this diagnosis:
    - Patients with bulimia: usually adolescent or young adult females concerned about body weight or with overt eating disorders
    - Patients seeking a secondary gain: disability payments, concern, or caring behavior by others
    - Munchausen syndrome: peripatetic patients who relish being diagnostic challenges and may undergo extensive testing repeatedly

- Polle syndrome (Munchausen syndrome by proxy): dependent child or adult given laxatives by caregiver to show effectiveness as a caregiver or to gain sympathy from others and may have a history of a sibling who died with chronic diarrhea

29. What is microscopic colitis syndrome?

Microscopic colitis is a syndrome characterized by chronic secretory diarrhea, a normal gross appearance of the colonic mucosa, and a typical pattern of inflammation in colon biopsy specimens. This pattern includes changes in the surface epithelium (flattening and irregularity), intraepithelial lymphocytosis, and an increased density of inflammatory cells in the lamina propria. There are two varieties. The first type is collagenous colitis in which the subepithelial collagen layer is thickened, and the second type is lymphocytic colitis in which the subepithelial collagen layer is of normal thickness. Microscopic colitis is as common as Crohn disease in the general population. It occurs frequently in older patients and may be associated with fecal incontinence. In many cases, a rheumatologic or autoimmune disorder may be present. Treatment is variably effective: budesonide has the most evidence for efficacy; bile acid–binding drugs and bismuth subsalicylate have some efficacy.

30. Define bile acid diarrhea.

In patients with ileal resection or disease, the part of the small intestine with high-affinity bile acid transporters has been removed or is dysfunctional. Thus, excessive bile acid finds its way into the colon. If the bile acid concentration in colonic contents reaches a critical level of approximately 3–5 mmol/L, salt and water absorption by the colonic mucosa is inhibited in diarrhea results. Patients who have had extensive small bowel resections (more than 100 cm) often have so much fluid entering the colon that this critical bile acid level is not reached, even though bile acid malabsorption may be extensive (Fig. 55.8).

In addition to this classic form of diarrhea caused by bile acid malabsorption, some investigators have shown that bile acid malabsorption causes chronic diarrhea in some patients with IBS-D. These patients have defective feedback inhibition of hepatic bile acid synthesis by fibroblast growth factor–19 (FGF19). This results in excessive synthesis of bile acids, reflected by high circulating levels of an intermediary metabolite of bile acid synthesis, C4, and overflow of bile acid into the colon. Treatment with bile acid–sequestering resins, such as cholestyramine, may be effective in this group of patients.

31. What is the best nonspecific therapy for chronic diarrhea?

Because the evaluation of chronic diarrhea may extend over several weeks and because the diagnosis is not always forthcoming, patients may need symptomatic therapy. The most effective agents are opiates. Traditional antidiarrheal agents, such as diphenoxylate and loperamide, work well in many patients but should be given on a routine schedule in patients with chronic diarrhea rather than on an as-needed basis. Typical doses of one or two tablets or capsules of these agents before meals and at bedtime will improve symptoms in most people.

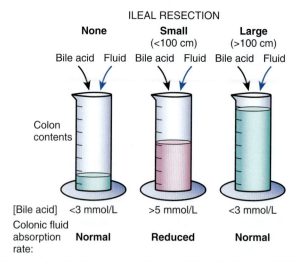

Fig. 55.8 Bile acid diarrhea occurs when bile acid malabsorption in the ileum is linked with relatively low fluid flows into the colon. As a result, the concentration of bile acid in the colon contents is greater than the cathartic threshold of 3–5 mmol/L. If fluid flows are high (as with substantial small bowel resection), bile acid malabsorption may be just as severe, but bile acid concentrations are not high enough to impair absorption by the colon.

Table 55.4 Nonspecific Therapy for Chronic Diarrhea.

DRUG CLASS	AGENT	DOSAGE
Opiates (μ-opiate receptor selective)	• Diphenoxylate • Loperamide • Codeine • Morphine • Opium tincture	2.5–5 mg qid 2–4 mg qid 15–60 mg qid 2–20 mg qid 2–20 drops qid
Adrenergic agonist	• Clonidine	0.1–0.3 mg tid
Somatostatin analog	• Octreotide	50–250 mcg tid sc
Bile acid–binding resin	• Cholestyramine	4 g qd to qid

qid, Four times daily; *qd*, every day; *tid*, three times daily; *sc*, subcutaneously.

When this therapy is ineffective, more potent opiates, such as codeine, opium, or morphine, can be used. With the stronger agents, doses should be low at first and increased gradually, so that tolerance to the central nervous system effects can develop. Fortunately, the gut does not become tolerant to these agents; thus one can usually find a dose that will control symptoms without producing severe side effects. Other agents that are sometimes used to manage chronic diarrhea include clonidine, octreotide, and cholestyramine, but they tend to be less effective than opiates and are often less well tolerated by patients, making them second-line agents in most circumstances (Table 55.4).

CLINICAL VIGNETTE

Available Online

BIBLIOGRAPHY

Available Online

WEBSITES

Available Online

CHAPTER 56

ACQUIRED IMMUNE DEFICIENCY SYNDROME AND THE GASTROINTESTINAL TRACT

C. Mel Wilcox, MD, MSPH and Michael Saag, MD

 Additional content available online

1. **Describe the time course of opportunistic diseases in patients with human immunodeficiency virus (HIV) infection and acquired immune deficiency syndrome (AIDS).**
   There is a stereotypical time course for the development of opportunistic processes in patients with HIV (PWH) infection. The risk for these disorders increases when the CD4 count falls to less than 200 cells/mL. For some processes, such as lymphoma and tuberculosis, presentation may occur at a CD4 count of more than 200. Cytomegalovirus (CMV) infection, cryptosporidia, microsporidia, and *Mycobacterium avium* complex (MAC) occur when the CD4 count is less than 100 and often less than 50.

2. **Is there a role for barium esophagogram in PWH and esophageal symptoms?**
   Barium esophagogram has a limited role in patients with AIDS. Given that infections and neoplasms are the most common cause of disease in patients with significant immunodeficiency (CD4 count <100 cells/mL), endoscopic inspection with tissue acquisition with biopsy or brushings is mandatory for a specific diagnosis. In addition, some of these disorders have a similar appearance radiographically, and toxicity can be associated with treatments directed at these infections. Thus a specific diagnosis is mandatory before empiric therapy is given. Motility disorders and reflux may be important to exclude in patients infected with HIV without immunodeficiency.

3. **What are the implications of odynophagia in a PWH?**
   Odynophagia, or painful swallowing, is an uncommon symptom. In patients with AIDS, this almost always represents an esophageal ulcer. In such patients, associated chest pain may be a concomitant complaint. Upper endoscopy is mandatory for a specific diagnosis. Rarely, *Candida* esophagitis may result in severe odynophagia, but more typically is milder and dysphagia is prominent.

4. **What is the role of endoscopy in PWH with upper gastrointestinal (GI) symptoms?**
   Patients with AIDS (CD4 count <200) are at risk for opportunistic infections and neoplasms, particularly when the CD4 lymphocyte count falls to less than 100 cells/mL. Given the broad differential diagnosis of upper GI symptoms in these patients, generally upper endoscopy should be performed so all lesions can be biopsied for a definitive diagnosis.

5. **How has antiretroviral therapy (ART) altered the incidence of opportunistic GI disorders?**
   Since the introduction of protease inhibitors and ART in 1995, there has been a constant and dramatic decline in all GI opportunistic disorders (ODs) in patients with AIDS. In addition, highly active ART (HAART) has also been shown to indirectly treat many GI ODs. Once the immune status of the patient improves, the OD generally resolves. However, careful follow-up of patients receiving ART early on is mandatory as their condition can decompensate as a result of immune reconstitution inflammatory syndrome (IRIS).

6. **What is the role of empiric therapy for new-onset esophageal symptoms in PWH infection?**
   Candida esophagitis is the most common cause of esophageal disease in patients with AIDS presenting with dysphagia or odynophagia (Fig. 56.1). Because of this high prevalence, an empiric approach to new-onset esophageal symptoms with potent antifungal therapy is commonly undertaken and accepted. A fluconazole loading dose of 200 mg followed by 100 mg/day for 10 days should be instituted. Because *Candida* esophagitis responds rapidly to fluconazole, patients who do not symptomatically improve within the first few days of treatment should undergo endoscopic evaluation to exclude other causes of disease (viral esophagitis). This is the only condition for which enough data exist to document empiric therapy. Empiric therapy for suspected viral, fungal, and parasitic diseases is not indicated.

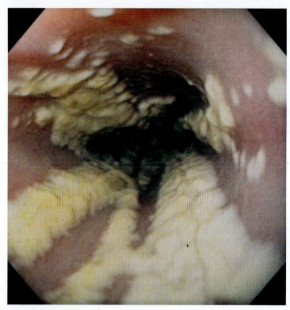

Fig. 56.1 Candidal esophagitis. Yellow plaques coating the esophageal wall are typical for *Candida*. Note that on one portion of the wall, the material has been removed and the underlying mucosa is normal.

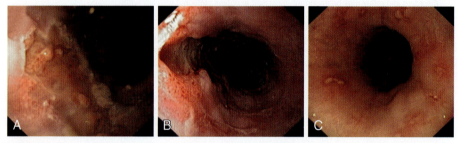

Fig. 56.2 Ulcerative esophagitis in acquired immune deficiency syndrome. Cytomegalovirus (A), idiopathic esophageal ulcer (B), and herpes simplex virus (C).

7. What is the role of empiric therapy for upper GI symptoms in PWH?

With improving ART, patients commonly have CD4 counts higher than 200 cells/mL. In these patients, an empiric trial of a proton pump inhibitor is reasonable for symptoms consistent with gastroesophageal reflux disease (GERD) or other dyspeptic complaints. If symptoms do not improve within 1–2 weeks, endoscopic evaluation to exclude other causes of disease is mandatory.

8. What are the most common causes of esophageal ulceration in patients infected with HIV?

The most common causes are CMV and idiopathic esophageal ulcer (IEU). On endoscopy, CMV and IEU appear most often as multiple, large, well-circumscribed solitary ulcerations, with normal-appearing surrounding mucosa (Fig. 56.2).

Herpes simplex virus (HSV) is usually associated with multiple small, shallow esophageal ulcerations, often raised with a volcano crater appearance. GERD can also present with ulcerations of the distal esophagus generally involving the gastroesophageal junction; these lesions are generally linear and superficial. Neoplasms (e.g., lymphoma), parasites (e.g., leishmaniasis), and fungal infections (e.g., histoplasmosis and *Candida* spp.) are rare causes of esophageal ulcers (Table 56.1).

Table 56.1 Reported Causes of Esophageal Ulcers in Acquired Immune Deficiency Syndrome.

Viruses	Cytomegalovirus, herpes simplex virus type II, Epstein-Barr virus, papovavirus, and human herpesvirus-6
Fungi	*Candida* spp., *Histoplasma capsulatum*, *Cryptococcus neoformans*, mucormycosis, aspergillosis, *Penicillium chrysogenum*, and *Exophiala jeanselmei*
Bacteria	*Mycobacterium avium* complex, *Mycobacterium tuberculosis*, *Bartonella henselae*, *Nocardia asteroides*, and *Actinomyces israelii*
Protozoa	*Cryptosporidia, Leishmania donovani*, and *Pneumocystis carinii*
Tumors	Non-Hodgkin lymphoma and Kaposi sarcoma, cancer (squamous cell and adenocarcinoma), and lymphoma
Pill induced	Zalcitabine, zidovudine, and other
Gastroesophageal disease and idiopathic	Idiopathic esophageal ulcer

9. **What biopsy technique should be used to sample an esophageal ulcer?**
   The exact number of biopsies required for maximal sensitivity and specificity is not clearly established, but several studies suggest the range of 8–10. It is important to obtain biopsy samples from the ulcer margin and from the ulcer base. This is because biopsy of the ulcer edge reveals a cytopathic effect that is present in squamous epithelium associated with HSV; conversely, CMV resides in granulation tissue in the ulcer base. The role of culture and cytologic examination for esophageal ulcers is not settled. If all biopsies are negative for viral, bacterial, fungal, and parasitic infections, a diagnosis of IEU can be made.

10. **What is AIDS cholangiopathy? How do patients present?**
    AIDS cholangiopathy is a spectrum of biliary tract abnormalities resembling sclerosing cholangitis that can be caused by a wide array of microorganisms (*Cryptosporidium, Microsproidium*, and CMV) and neoplasms (non-Hodgkin lymphoma), usually in patients with advanced immunodeficiency (CD4 count <100 cells/mL). Patients generally present with epigastric or right upper quadrant pain, fever, and malaise. Although AIDS cholangiopathy is a cholestatic disease, jaundice and pruritus are uncommon.

11. **How is AIDS cholangiopathy best diagnosed?**
    The most common laboratory finding in this syndrome is a markedly elevated alkaline phosphatase, usually more than three times the upper limit of normal. Typically, bilirubin is not elevated and rarely exceeds 3 mg/dL, and transaminases are only mildly elevated. Generally, these patients have a dilated bile duct that is identifiable on abdominal ultrasonography.
    The diagnosis of AIDS cholangiopathy is best established by endoscopic retrograde cholangiopancreatography. The diagnosis is usually established by obtaining biopsy specimens of the ampulla or duodenal mucosa, bile duct biopsy, aspirated bile specimens, or biliary epithelial brush cytologic examination. Several cholangiographic patterns have been described, including papillary stenosis, sclerosing cholangitis, combined papillary stenosis and sclerosing cholangitis, isolated intrahepatic disease, and long extrahepatic bile duct strictures. The most common pattern is papillary stenosis with intrahepatic sclerosing cholangitis. Endoscopic sphincterotomy is appropriate for the relief of pain in patients with papillary stenosis and dilated ducts.

12. **What are the most common causes of pancreatitis in patients infected with HIV?**
    Several studies have documented chronic and recurrent elevations of serum amylase and lipase in up to 50% of patients with AIDS. The most common medications associated with pancreatitis in AIDS are pentamidine, didanosine, and zalcitabine, the latter two are not currently used. Protease inhibitors frequently cause hyperlipidemia. Ritonavir is associated with the most dramatic increases in serum triglycerides, with 10% of patients developing severe hypertriglyceridemia. Pancreatitis is well described in patients with elevations in triglycerides from protease inhibitors. Reported infectious causes of pancreatitis include CMV, HSV, MAC, and tuberculosis. An infectious cause of pancreatitis is difficult to establish and requires pancreatic biopsy.

Table 56.2 Studies and Laboratory Tests Used in the Evaluation of Diarrhea in Acquired Immune Deficiency Syndrome.

Stool	Cultures (*Salmonella*, *Shigella*, and *Campylobacter* spp.) Toxin (*Clostridium difficile*) Ova and parasites (*Giardia lamblia*, *Entamoeba histolytica*, and *Cryptosporidium* spp.) Modified Kinyoun acid-fast (*Cryptosporidium* spp. and *Isospora belli*) Concentrated stool (zinc sulfate and Sheather's sucrose flotation) (microsporidia)
Blood	Cultures (*Mycobacterium avium* complex, *Salmonella*, and *Campylobacter* spp.) Antibodies (*Entamoeba histolytica* and CMV)
Gastrointestinal fluids	Duodenal aspirate (*Giardia lamblia* and microsporidia) Electron microscopy (*Cryptosporidium* spp. and adenovirus)
Biopsy stains	Hematoxylin-eosin GMS or methenamine silver (fungi) Methylene blue-azure II-basic fuchsin (microsporidia) Fite (mycobacteria)
Immunohistochemical stains (CMV) and immunologic methods	In situ hybridization (CMV) DNA amplification (CMV) Culture of tissue CMV Herpes simplex virus Mycobacteria

CMV, Cytomegalovirus.

13. What is the clinical presentation of diarrhea in AIDS?

When evaluating a PWH with diarrhea, careful attention should be directed to the history and physical examination. Enteritis (small bowel diarrhea) is associated with voluminous, watery bowel movements, abdominal bloating, cramping, borborygmi, and nausea. Abdominal pain, if present, tends to be periumbilical or diffuse. Abdominal examination reveals an increase in number and frequency of bowel sounds, which may be high-pitched. Conversely, colitis (large bowel diarrhea) is characterized by frequent, small bowel movements, with the presence of mucus, pus, or blood (dysentery). Patients with prominent involvement of the distal colon also have proctitis symptoms, such as tenesmus, dyschezia (pain on defecation), and proctalgia (rectal pain).

14. What is the approach to diarrhea in PWH?

It is important to consider patient exposures. A history of new medications or an alteration in a current regimen, such as antiretrovirals or antibacterials, is important because many protease inhibitors are associated with diarrhea and antibacterials are associated with *Clostridium difficile* colitis. In febrile patients, blood cultures should be obtained for common bacteria are mandatory. If stool and blood culture studies are negative, the next step is an endoscopic evaluation with biopsy. In the presence of colitis symptoms, flexible sigmoidoscopy or colonoscopy is recommended. Table 56.2 summarizes the studies and laboratory tests used in the evaluation of diarrhea in AIDS.

Table 56.3 lists the most common infectious causes of diarrhea in AIDS. Table 56.4 lists common associations between exposures and infections.

15. Describe the clinical features of HSV proctitis in AIDS.

HSV proctitis is the most common cause of nongonococcal proctitis in sexually active homosexual males. HSV proctitis classically presents with tenesmus, purulent rectal discharge, severe proctalgia, fever, constipation, and anorectal bleeding. Painful inguinal lymphadenopathy is an almost universal finding. The pain tends to distribute in the region of the sacral roots (i.e., buttocks, perineal region, and posterior thigh). Because of the neural involvement by HSV and the presence of severe pain, patients may complain of impotence and difficulty in initiating micturition. Visual inspection and anoscopy commonly reveal the following lesions: vesicles, pustular rectal lesions, or diffuse ulcerations. HSV is a pathogen of the squamous mucosa; therefore diffuse proctitis involving the entire rectum is rare. In severe cases, the columnar rectal and sigmoid mucosa has been involved. The differential diagnoses of HSV proctitis include lymphogranuloma venereum (*Chlamydia trachomatis*), *Entamoeba histolytica*, *Salmonella* spp., and *Campylobacter jejuni*.

Table 56.3 Infectious Causes of Diarrhea in Acquired Immune Deficiency Syndrome.

VIRUSES	BACTERIA	PARASITES	FUNGI
Cytomegalovirus	*Salmonella* spp.	*Giardia lamblia*	Histo-
Astrovirus	*Shigella* spp.	*Entamoeba histolytica*	plasma
Picornavirus	*Campylobacter jejuni*	*Microsporidia*	capsula-
Coronavirus	*Clostridium difficile*	*Enterocytozoon bieneusi*	tum
Rotavirus	*Mycobacterium avium* complex	*Encephalitozoon intestinalis*	Candida
Herpesvirus	*Treponema pallidum*	(formerly *Septata*)	albicans
Adenovirus	*Spirochetes*	*Cyclospora cayetanensis*	
Small round virus	*Neisseria gonorrhoeae*	*Cryptosporidium* spp.	
HIV	*Vibrio cholera*	*Isospora belli*	
	Aeromonas spp.	*Blastocystis hominis* (?)	
	Pseudomonas spp. (?)		
	Staphylococcus aureus		

HIV, Human immunodeficiency virus.

Table 56.4 Sources of Infectious Diarrhea.

INFECTIOUS AGENT	ASSOCIATION
Clostridium difficile	Recent antibiotics, nursing home, or hospital exposures
Cryptosporidiosis *Microsporidiosis*	Recent visit to a farm, contact with farm animals, and use of a public swimming pool
Giardia	Camping and stream water
Mycobacterium avium	CD4 count less than 50 cells/mL
Cyclospora cayetanensis	Common cause of diarrhea in South America
Microsporidiosis	Uncommon in the Southern United States
Rotavirus	Common cause of diarrhea in Australia

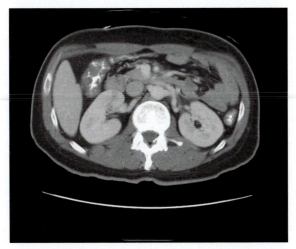

Fig. 56.3 Cytomegalovirus colitis. Abdominal computed tomography scan shows colonic wall thickening most pronounced in the right colon.

16. **What is the preferred endoscopic procedure for the evaluation of diarrhea in AIDS?**

    The advantage of endoscopy is that it permits direct visualization of the mucosa and retrieval of tissue for histologic examination. The diagnostic yield of colonoscopy in patients infected with HIV with chronic diarrhea and negative stool studies ranges from 27% to 37%; in patients with AIDS, CMV is the most common etiologic factor identified (Fig. 56.3). CMV colitis is usually present in the distal colon; however, isolated, right-sided CMV colitis has been reported. Therefore, if CMV is suspected as the cause of diarrhea, a full colonoscopy is warranted, especially if sigmoidoscopy is negative. However, it is still not clear whether colonoscopy has a higher yield than flexible sigmoidoscopy for the detection of organisms other than CMV. Evaluation with colonoscopy is prudent if right-sided abdominal complaints are also reported. The value of upper endoscopy and small bowel biopsy in the evaluation of chronic diarrhea has also been demonstrated, although specific treatment options for most small bowel pathogens are limited. Some would obtain ileal biopsy at the time of colonoscopy rather than proceed with upper endoscopy and biopsy. The most commonly detected organisms involving the small bowel are cryptosporidia and microsporidia.

17. **What is the most common cause of viral diarrhea in AIDS?**

    CMV is one of the most common opportunistic infections in patients with AIDS, occurring late in the course of HIV infection when immunodeficiency is severe (CD4 lymphocyte count <100 cells/mL). CMV has been identified in mucosal biopsy samples in as many as 45% of patients with AIDS and diarrhea, especially in those patients with negative stool studies. CMV causes both enteritis and colitis. A number of other viral pathogens—adenovirus, rotavirus, astrovirus, picobirnavirus, and coronavirus—have been reported to involve the GI tract in patients with AIDS, but their clinical importance remains to be determined. HSV can cause proctitis that mimics diarrhea because of the rectal mucous discharge. However, HSV does not cause enterocolitis because it invades the squamous mucosa, not the columnar epithelium, such as the one lining the colonic and small bowel mucosa.

18. **What are the treatment options for CMV enterocolitis?**

    The natural history of CMV colitis is variable. In untreated patients, it usually has a chronic course characterized by progressive diarrhea and weight loss, although occasionally symptoms and histologic abnormalities remit spontaneously. Unlike CMV retinitis, for which strong evidence supports induction therapy followed by lifelong maintenance therapy, the optimal duration of therapy and the need for maintenance therapy in CMV colitis are undefined. Consensus guidelines recommend 3–6 weeks of induction therapy, typically ganciclovir, followed by maintenance therapy if there is a history of relapses. Valganciclovir can be given orally and achieves serum concentrations similar to intravenous ganciclovir. Studies for GI disease are limited. Funduscopic examination at the time of diagnosis of CMV enterocolitis is mandatory because the duration of therapy is considerably longer for disseminated diseases than for diseases limited to the GI tract.

19. **Name the common parasites that cause diarrhea in AIDS.**

    Among the protozoa, *Cryptosporidium parvum* is the most common parasite causing diarrhea in AIDS and has been identified in up to 11% of symptomatic patients. Although a cause of acute diarrhea, cryptosporidiosis is found most commonly in patients infected with HIV with chronic diarrhea. In some studies of HIV-infected patients with chronic diarrhea, microsporidia (*Enterocytozoon bieneusi* and *Encephalitozoon intestinalis*) are the most commonly identified pathogens. *Giardia* is also a consideration in patients with diarrhea, especially when chronic and associated with the upper GI symptoms of nausea and bloating. *Isospora belli* is a rare GI pathogen in patients infected with HIV in North America, whereas it is endemic in many developing countries, such as Haiti.

20. **Is strongyloidiasis more prevalent in HIV infection?**

    Strongyloides stercoralis is an endemic parasite in the subtropical areas worldwide, including the southeastern United States. There is no clear evidence that HIV infection predisposes to strongyloidiasis. However, PWH may be more prone to develop the *Strongyloides* hyperinfection syndrome. In addition, during therapy with HAART an IRIS with hyperinfection syndrome has been reported. Therefore it is important to keep this potentially life-threatening infection in mind when evaluating PWH and GI symptoms such as diarrhea, abdominal pain, and dyspepsia. In PWH with eosinophilia, empiric therapy with ivermectin is warranted while the workup of eosinophilia is in progress. *Strongyloides* can infect any part of the GI tract. However, the classic finding is a *catarrhal* duodenitis, with edema of the villi and massive amounts of yellow exudate covering the mucosa (Fig. 56.4).

21. **Compare the clinical features and therapies for cryptosporidiosis and microsporidiosis.**

    GI microsporidial infection is generally attributed to two species: *E. bieneusi* and *E. intestinalis*. In general, intestinal disease is relatively mild in contrast to the severe diarrhea typical for cryptosporidiosis. Loose stools and mild weight loss are common, with colonic symptoms typically absent. GI bleeding suggests another diagnosis as this infection does not cause mucosal ulceration. Although stool studies can establish the diagnosis, small bowel biopsies, of either the duodenum or ileum, with special stains are more sensitive. Although there is no effective antimicrobial therapy for *E. bieneusi*, albendazole is highly effective for *E. intestinalis*. As with all opportunistic infections in AIDS, ART may result in clinical remission.

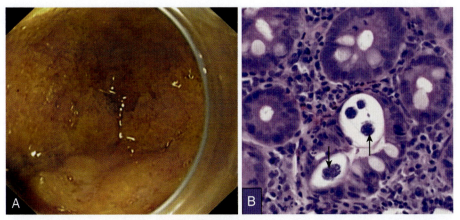

Fig. 56.4 *Strongyloides stercoralis* duodenitis in a patient infected with human immunodeficiency virus with hyperinfection syndrome. The classic duodenal finding is a *catarrhal* duodenitis (A). Histologic examination is mandatory in the evaluation of strongyloidiasis (B). The preferred biopsy site is always the duodenum.

Cryptosporidia are a common cause of chronic diarrhea in patients with HIV infection with severe immunodeficiency. There are at least 40 species of *Cryptosporidia*, but the most common cause of human disease is *Cryptosporidium muri*. The diarrhea is generally voluminous and watery. Dehydration and weight loss are common in patients with advanced immunodeficiency. Disease severity correlates with immune function. The disease may wax and wane, but persistent or progressive disease may be manifested by dehydration and electrolyte imbalances. Constitutional symptoms are prominent, including low-grade fever, malaise, anorexia, nausea, and vomiting. Both of these infections improve with reconstitution of the immune system following successful ART.

22. **Which bacteria most commonly cause diarrhea in AIDS?**
    Campylobacter, *Salmonella*, *Shigella* spp., and *C. difficile* are the most common causes of diarrhea in AIDS. *Yersinia enterocolitica*, *Staphylococcus aureus*, and *Aeromonas hydrophila* have also been associated with severe enterocolitis in patients infected with HIV. *C. difficile* colitis has become the most frequent bacterial cause of diarrhea in patients infected with HIV, perhaps because of frequent exposure to antimicrobials and the requirement for hospitalization. MAC is a common pathogen in patients with advanced immunosuppression (i.e., CD4 count <50 cells/mL). An incidence of 39% has been described when the CD4 count remains less than 10 cells/mL. Tuberculosis is most frequent in developing countries, is less likely to present with diarrhea alone, and can present at any level of immune dysfunction.

23. **When do you initiate hepatitis B virus (HBV) therapy in PWH?**
    HBV-HIV coinfection represents a significant problem in HIV care. As ART has improved the prognosis of HIV and AIDS, significant increases in morbidity and mortality resulting from liver disease have been observed. HBV and HIV are acquired by similar mechanisms and thus coinfection is common. Patients with coinfection of HIV and HBV have higher HBV DNA levels and are less likely to convert from hepatitis B e-antigen–positive to hepatitis B e-antibody–positive, indicating a poorer response to HBV therapy. Patients with an HBV DNA greater than 2000 IU and F2 or greater fibrosis on biopsy should receive HBV treatment. If a patient has cirrhosis, he or she should be treated if HBV DNA is greater than 200. For patients with a high CD4 count, HBV monotherapy that is not active against HIV should be the first-line therapy. When initiating HAART, HBV also should be treated with two antiviral agents active against HBV. If CD4 counts are between 350 and 500 cells/mL, one can elect to treat both HIV and HBV. HAART with two agents active against HBV should be used instead of HBV monotherapy in these individuals.

24. **Why is it important to know the HBV treatments that are also active in treating HIV?**
    Initiating HBV monotherapy which is also active in treating HIV can result in HIV resistance, potentially limiting HAART options. Furthermore, if ART is initiated without concurrent HBV treatment, immune reconstitution can result in a potentially life-threatening flare of untreated HBV. Table 56.5 shows treatments active against HBV and HIV or HBV alone.

Table 56.5 Hepatitis B Treatments and Human Immunodeficiency Virus (HIV) Activity.

TREATS HIV AND HBV	TREATS HBV WITHOUT HBV RESISTANCE
Lamivudine	Interferon/PEG-IFN
Tenofovir	Adefovir (at 10-mg dosing)
Emtricitabine	Telbivudine (in vitro)
Entecavir (in vivo)	

HBV, Hepatitis B virus; *PEG-IFN*, pegylated interferon.

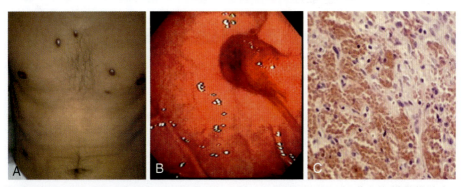

Fig. 56.5 Kaposi sarcoma (KS) usually involves the skin (A). Any part of the gastrointestinal tract may be affected by KS (B). Histologic examination is important to confirm the diagnosis (C).

25. **How is the natural history of hepatitis C virus (HCV) infection altered in patients with AIDS?**
    HCV is common in patients infected with HIV given the similar routes of exposure. In the normal host, progression from infection to cirrhosis takes several decades. A number of studies now suggest that the progression rate is markedly accelerated in patients with AIDS. Indeed, currently HCV infection–related cirrhosis is one of the most common causes of death in these patients. This alteration in natural history suggests that early diagnosis of HCV infection and treatment are important.

26. **What are the GI manifestations of Kaposi sarcoma (KS) in AIDS?**
    KS is a vascular neoplasm caused by HSV-8, seen predominantly in homosexual males with HIV infection. PWH are prone to develop KS at any stage of the disease. GI tract involvement occurs in up to 40% of patients. However, most cases of KS of the GI tract are asymptomatic. AIDS-related KS most frequently manifests with skin disease (Fig. 56.5). However, cutaneous manifestation may be absent in visceral KS. Symptoms of GI KS are dyspepsia, diarrhea, GI bleeding, perforation, and ileus resulting from tumor obstruction (Fig. 56.5).

CLINICAL VIGNETTE

Available Online

BIBLIOGRAPHY

Available Online

CHAPTER 57

ISCHEMIC BOWEL DISEASE

Gina A. Wideroff, MD, Siobhan Proksell, MD and Amar R. Deshpande, MD

 Additional content available online

1. What is ischemic bowel disease?

Ischemic bowel disease is caused by tissue hypoxia and ischemic injury of the small or large intestine as a result of a persistent decrease in mesenteric blood flow, decreased oxygen content of red blood cells, or mesenteric venous stasis. Ischemic bowel disease can manifest in numerous ways, such as acute or chronic midabdominal pain (meal-induced), vomiting, sitophobia (fear of eating), weight loss, diarrhea, ileus, gastrointestinal bleeding, intestinal infarction, peritonitis, or fibrotic strictures.

2. Describe the gross anatomy of the mesenteric vascular system.

Three major arteries and two major veins comprise the majority of the mesenteric circulation.

ARTERIES	VEINS
• Celiac artery	• Superior mesenteric vein (SMV)
• Superior mesenteric artery (SMA)	• Inferior mesenteric vein (IMV)
• Inferior mesenteric artery (IMA)	

The connection of major arteries and veins via capillaries, arterioles, and venules is known as splanchnic circulation, which receives up to 25% of cardiac output under basal conditions and 35% or more postprandially (Fig. 57.1).

The celiac artery provides blood to the stomach, proximal duodenum, part of the pancreas, spleen, liver, gallbladder, and biliary tree. The SMA provides blood to the rest of the duodenum and pancreas, the entire small intestine, and the colon up to the splenic flexure. The IMA supplies the remainder of the colon and rectum, with the latter receiving dual blood supply from the internal iliac arteries of the systemic circulation as well. The IMV drains into the splenic vein, and the SMV and splenic vein anastomose to form the portal vein. Mirroring the arterial blood supply, there is dual venous drainage of the rectum into the systemic system through the inferior vena cava via the internal iliac veins and through the IMV to the portal circulation.

3. What are the protective responses to intestinal ischemia?

Abundant collateralization, autoregulation of blood flow, and the intestine's ability to increase oxygen extraction from the blood.

4. What are the watershed zones and explain their clinical significance.

These are regions between two major arteries that are susceptible to nonocclusive ischemic injury. Griffith point occurs in the region of the splenic flexure and is the anastomosis between ascending left colic artery and the marginal artery of Drummond. Sudeck point is at the rectosigmoid junction and is the anastomosis between the last sigmoid arterial branch of the IMA and a branch of the superior rectal artery.

5. An extensive collateral circulatory system exists between the systemic and splanchnic vascular networks. Describe this system.

The several systemic-splanchnic and intersplanchnic collateral channels that connect the three major mesenteric arteries and their branches become apparent in the event of occlusion of one of the major branches (Fig. 57.2):

• Pancreaticoduodenal arcade provides collateral channels between the celiac axis (via the superior pancreaticoduodenal arteries) and SMA (via the inferior pancreaticoduodenal arteries).
• Marginal artery of Drummond, composed of branches of the SMA and IMA, is a continuous arterial pathway that runs parallel to the entire colon.
• The middle colic branch of the SMA and the left colic branch of the IMA are connected by the arc of Riolan.
• The IMA connects with the systemic circulation via the iliac artery by the ileomesenteric arcade.
• A slowly developing occlusion promotes the opening of these collateral channels; thus, chronic mesenteric arterial insufficiency (e.g., abdominal angina) is unusual unless there is virtually complete occlusion of two of the three major mesenteric arteries, including the SMA.

6. What is meant by autoregulation?

Autoregulation is the concept by which blood flow remains relatively constant via the response of arterioles and venules to changes in perfusion. A steep gradient of pressure exists between the artery and proximal portion of

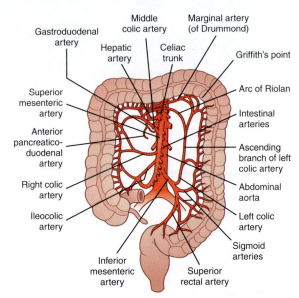

Fig. 57.1 Mesenteric arterial anatomy. Three unpaired arterial branches of the aorta (celiac, superior mesenteric, and inferior mesenteric arteries) provide oxygenated blood to the small and large intestines. In most instances, veins parallel arteries. The superior mesenteric vein joins the splenic vein to form the portal vein, which enters the liver at its hilum. The inferior mesenteric vein joins the splenic vein near the juncture of the superior mesenteric and splenic veins. (Adapted from Rogers AI, Rosen CM. Mesenteric vascular insufficiency. In Schiller, LR, ed. Small Intestine, Current Medicine. Philadelphia, PA: Lange; 1997, with permission.)

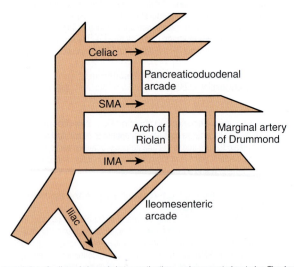

Fig. 57.2 Schematic representation of collateral channels between the three major mesenteric arteries. The development of alternative anastomoses and collateral flow makes it theoretically possible that any single artery could supply all of the abdominal viscera with arterial blood given sufficient time and opportunity, that is, gradual occlusion of one or two of the other major arterial vessels. One major anastomosis exists between the left branch of the middle colic artery (from the superior mesenteric artery [SMA]) and the left colic artery from the inferior mesenteric artery (IMA), forming the meandering mesenteric artery or the arc of Riolan. Its demonstration by angiography indicates occlusion of the SMA or IMA. The marginal artery of Drummond is an arterial connection that provides a continuous channel of collateral flow via the vasa recta to the small and large intestines. The ileomesenteric arcade establishes an important anastomosis between the mesenteric and systemic circulation between the superior hemorrhoidal artery, a branch of the IMA, and the hypogastric artery, a branch of the iliac artery. (Adapted from Rogers AI, Rosen CM. Mesenteric vascular insufficiency. In Schiller, LR, ed. Small Intestine, Current Medicine. Philadelphia, PA: Lange; 1997, with permission.)

the arteriole. If there is a decrease in arterial perfusion or an increase in oxygen demand (as in the postprandial state), arterioles dilate and additional capillaries are recruited to prevent tissue hypoxia. Additionally, adjustments in the resistance of the venous system are employed to maintain adequate cardiac output. For example, an increase in tone occurs in the setting of hypotension to enhance venous blood return to the heart (Fig. 57.3).

7. How can we classify ischemic bowel disease?
- Acute or chronic
- Arterial or venous
- Occlusive or nonocclusive
- Embolic or thrombotic (Fig. 57.4)

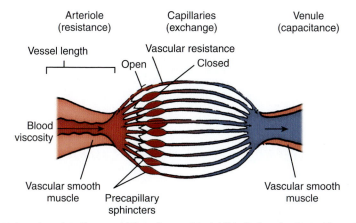

Fig. 57.3 Intramural vascular anatomy. The assured delivery of oxygen-rich arterial blood to the various layers of the small and large intestinal wall during basal, meal-stimulated, and stress states depends on the interplay between various anatomic and physiologic factors, including blood viscosity, red blood cell oxygen saturation, arteriole length and resistance to flow, tone of precapillary sphincters, tone of vascular smooth muscle, and venous capacitance. (Adapted from Rogers AI, Rosen CM. Mesenteric vascular insufficiency. In Schiller, LR, ed. Small Intestine, Current Medicine. Philadelphia, PA: Lange; 1997, with permission.)

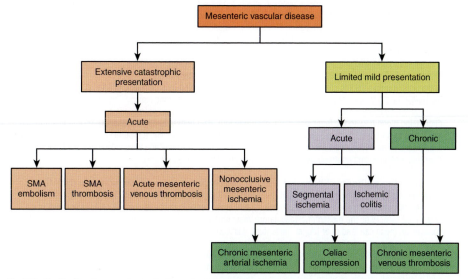

Fig. 57.4 Classification of mesenteric vascular disease based on the extent of resulting ischemia. This particular classification, proposed by Williams, may facilitate more effective evaluation and management by focusing on the extent of gut involvement. *SMA,* Superior mesenteric artery. (From Williams LF. Mesenteric ischemia. Surg Clin North Am. 1988;68:331-353.)

8. What clinical circumstances predispose to ischemic bowel disease?

	ACUTE MESEN-TERIC ARTERIAL EMBOLISM	ACUTE MESENTERIC ARTERIAL THROMBOSIS	NONOCCLUSIVE MESENTERIC ISCHEMIA	MESENTERIC VENOUS THROMBOSIS
Risk factors	Atrial fibrillation, valvular heart disease, myocardial infarction, mural thrombus, atrial myxoma, endocarditis, and trauma	Diffuse atherosclerotic disease, hypercoagulable states (e.g., pregnancy, hyperhomocysteinemia, antiphospholipid syndrome, oral contraceptive pills, neoplasms, polycythemia vera, essential thrombocytosis, and paroxysmal nocturnal hemoglobinuria), vasculitides, vascular aneurysms, and dissections	Cardiac arrhythmias, hypoperfusion (cardiogenic shock, sepsis, and hypovolemia), and vasoconstricting drugs (digoxin and cocaine)	Hypercoagulable states (arterial causes, deficiencies of factor V Leiden, protein C and S, and antithrombin III), congestive heart failure, shock, portal hypertension, hepatic vein thrombosis (Budd-Chiari syndrome), malignancy, trauma, sclerotherapy, peritonitis, diverticulitis, pancreatitis, inflammatory bowel disease, intestinal obstruction, postoperative states, and trauma

9. **Describe the pathophysiologic findings of occlusive acute mesenteric ischemia (AMI).**
Intestinal ischemia results from tissue hypoxia, which can be secondary to a decrease in blood volume, red blood cell mass, flow rate, or oxygen content. As the radius of an artery decreases, the resistance to flow increases by a power of 4. Autoregulation (Question 6) results in vasodilation to maintain flow up to a finite point, beyond which flow decreases. Examples of such instances are acute or chronic arterial thrombi, an embolus, or transient vasoconstriction.

10. **What is abdominal angina? What is its clinical significance?**
Abdominal angina refers to chronic, recurrent abdominal pain caused by a decrease in arterial blood flow through the mesenteric arteries, usually resulting from stenosis from atherosclerotic lesions. The postprandial state can be regarded as an exercise stimulus; food entering the stomach causes an increase in oxygen demand, thereby decreasing blood flow to the intestines (steal phenomenon). Pain begins to occur within 30–90 minutes and can last for up to 4 hours. Initially, abdominal angina is usually minimal; however, it progressively increases in severity over weeks to months. Long-term hypoxia of the small intestinal mucosa can cause villous atrophy leading to diarrhea, protein-losing enteropathy, steatorrhea, weight loss, and malnutrition.

11. **Describe the pathophysiologic findings of nonocclusive mesenteric ischemia (NOMI).**
NOMI occurs, as the name implies, without the presence of an embolus or thrombus. The risk of intestinal hypoperfusion can increase with shock, severe hypovolemia, decreased cardiac output, and major thoracic or abdominal surgery as the mesenteric vasculature vasoconstricts. It can also be seen in patients taking digoxin or cocaine, as these can lead to or trigger mesenteric vasoconstriction.

12. **What is focal segmental (short segment) ischemia?**
Focal segmental ischemia refers to ischemia that is confined to a short segment of the bowel because it involves only a few small arteries or veins. This occurs by the same pathophysiologic processes that cause extensive bowel ischemia.

13. **What are the common symptoms of occlusive mesenteric ischemia?**
    The common presenting symptoms of occlusive mesenteric ischemia vary by the cause of ischemia.
    - Patients with mesenteric ischemia caused by an acute embolus of the SMA usually present with the abrupt onset of severe, colicky, midabdominal pain. These patients may also become incontinent of bowel function because of tonic contractions of smooth muscle provoked by ischemia. These contractions cause severe pain but produce few abdominal physical examination findings. It is important to note that late findings of abdominal distension and blood in the stool may be the only presenting signs in patients who are unable to communicate (e.g., those who are sedated, demented, or with altered mental status).
    - Patients with mesenteric ischemia caused by a thrombotic occlusion tend to present with a history consistent with mesenteric angina—recurrent postprandial mid or diffuse abdominal pain, weight loss due to sitophobia, diarrhea, steatorrhea, or protein-losing enteropathy, which can further complicate the chronically ischemic-induced atrophy of the small intestine.
    - Patients with venous occlusive disease generally describe a more nonspecific, insidious onset of severe midabdominal pain out of proportion to abdominal physical examination findings, diarrhea, and emesis. Pain may be acute or subacute, occurring over weeks to months. This occurs when a massive influx of fluid into the bowel wall and lumen causes systemic hypotension and an eventual decrease in arterial flow.

14. **What are the common symptoms of NOMI?**
    These patients have less dramatic complaints with pain that is generally more diffuse and episodic associated with poor cardiac performance. A small proportion of patients do not have abdominal pain.

15. **What are the physical findings in a patient with mesenteric ischemia?**
    Again, the physical findings associated with mesenteric ischemia vary based on etiologic factors and duration of ischemia.
    - The classic finding of a patient with an acute occlusion of the SMA is abdominal pain out of proportion to physical examination findings. Early in the course of the disease process, the abdominal examination usually consists only of mild abdominal distension and normal or hypoactive bowel sounds. With the progression of ischemic injury, bowel sounds decrease, ileus develops, and abdominal distension worsens. Stool becomes heme-positive, and sometimes grossly bloody stool may develop. Volume sequestration is manifested by hypotension and tachycardia, whereas fever and peritoneal signs are indications of transmural injury and likely infarction.
    - Patients with venous occlusive disease present with physical examination findings based on the severity and etiology of ischemia: congestive heart failure, abdominal mass, stigmata of chronic liver disease and portal hypertension, or hypercoagulability.
    - NOMI should be suspected in the correct clinical setting as physical examination findings vary with the duration of ischemia. Patients usually describe chronic, recurrent abdominal pain secondary to compromised flow through the SMA. There are no specific physical examination findings. Of note, most patients have evidence of peripheral vascular disease and may also have weight loss.

16. **Do laboratory findings help at all?**
    In the early stages of mesenteric ischemia, there are no specific abnormal laboratory values, only those that are associated with the underlying condition from which the ischemia developed. Nonspecific laboratory abnormalities that develop over the course of the disease process are a result of the consequences of ischemia (i.e., tissue hypoxia, inflammation, necrosis, and volume sequestration) and include hemoconcentration, leukocytosis, and lactic acidosis.

17. **What imaging modality should be considered first? What is the role of a plain film?**
    The recommended first-line imaging study for AMI is computed tomography angiography (CTA) or biphasic multidetector computed tomography of the abdomen and pelvis with intravenous (IV) contrast. CTA is not only rapid, noninvasive, easily available, and highly accurate in diagnosing mesenteric ischemia, but it is also helpful in detecting the underlying etiology of ischemia. CTA may show bowel wall thickening, bowel wall hypoenhancement, intramural hemorrhage, fluid-filled dilated bowel loops, arterial or venous thrombus, decreased filling, narrowing, irregularity, spasm or engorgement of mesenteric vessels, pneumatosis intestinalis, portomesenteric venous gas, or infarction of other viscera. Considering the serious and lethal consequences of a missed diagnosis of AMI, CTA should be done as soon as possible in patients with suspected AMI, even considering it with impaired renal function.
    Plain radiograph has a limited role in diagnosing mesenteric ischemia but may show free intraperitoneal air if bowel infarction and perforation occur.

18. **What is the role of magnetic resonance angiography (MRA) in patients with suspected abdominal angina?**
    MRA is an excellent radiation-free, noninvasive test with high sensitivity and specificity. However, it is not considered a practical test in diagnosing AMI considering the longer duration of the study, potential lack of

availability in urgent situations, and high cost. This study may be helpful in patients with suspected abdominal angina or in those with severe iodine allergy.

19. **Describe the role of duplex ultrasound studies in diagnosis.**

Duplex ultrasound (that includes Doppler technology) is a noninvasive test that evaluates the patency of blood flow through the major mesenteric vessels. It should be performed while the patient is fasting and subsequently when meal-stimulated. It is most helpful in diagnosing multivessel stenosis in suspected mesenteric angina by demonstrating narrowing or occlusion at a vessel origin and excessively turbulent flow.

Of note, duplex ultrasound has limited capabilities in obese patients, as ultrasound waves must pass through body tissue prior to producing a diagnostic image.

20. **What is the diagnostic role of endoscopy and laparoscopy?**

Endoscopy has a limited role in AMI since it does not visualize much of the small bowel, which is the organ most frequently involved. Additionally, endoscopy may not have adequate sensitivity and specificity in detecting ischemic changes (rather than infarction). Also, endoscopy can be dangerous because of the high risk of bowel perforation in the setting of ischemia. Colonoscopy, however, has been shown to be relatively safe and can aid in determining the diagnosis of a patient with suspected ischemic colitis.

Laparoscopy, although invasive, has also been shown to be a relatively safe technique in assisting with diagnosis and assessing the degree of injury to the intestines, and it allows for same-time therapeutic intervention (e.g., bowel resection for infarction). It can easily detect full-thickness mesenteric injury; however, it is limited in the fact that it will miss the earlier stages of potentially reversible ischemia because injury starts at the mucosal surface and then progresses to involve the serosa to become transmural. Additionally, when intraperitoneal pressure exceeds 20 mm Hg, a level often attained after insufflation during laparoscopy, splanchnic blood flow decreases.

21. **Why should you undertake invasive mesenteric angiographic studies?**

Traditional angiography was previously the gold standard for diagnosis of mesenteric arterial occlusion. However, with advances in technology, CTA has largely taken over as the first-line diagnostic technique. Angiography is now reserved for treatment, with the aim of rapid restoration of blood flow to the intestines. Angiography can be used therapeutically to selectively infuse vasodilating drugs or thrombolytics and aid in the completion of angioplasty, balloon embolectomy, or stent placement. Therapeutic choice depends on the patient's clinical stability (evidence of sepsis or peritonitis), surgical candidacy, degree of bowel necrosis, type of occlusion, and response to initial treatment. In stable patients with AMI without peritonitis, endovascular therapy can be attempted before laparotomy as the primary revascularization method, with low threshold for laparotomy if symptoms do not resolve quickly thereafter. In the case of chronic mesenteric ischemia, endovascular therapy has become the primary treatment option, allowing for safe revascularization with stent placement. Additionally, patients with mesenteric venous thrombosis who do not respond to anticoagulation may be treated endovascularly to remove the thrombus.

As with all procedures, angiography has associated risks. Atherosclerosis commonly involves the femoral artery, which is usually the site of entry for the angiographic catheter. This makes it harder to access the mesenteric system and can also cause emboli to distant arteries. Furthermore, iodinated contrast can increase the risk of worsening renal function.

22. **When the diagnosis of AMI is made, what management should be initiated immediately?**

The focus is to correct the underlying cause to improve mesenteric perfusion. Concurrently, hemodynamic monitoring as well as urine output and frequent mental status checks should be initiated. Fluid resuscitation with isotonic crystalloid infusion is essential to enhance visceral perfusion; the fluid volume requirement may be high due to extensive capillary leakage. Vasopressors should be used with caution, as they decrease splanchnic blood flow via mesenteric vasoconstriction. If necessary, vasopressor agents like dobutamine, low-dose dopamine, or milrinone can be used to maintain blood pressure. Broad-spectrum antibiotics should be administered immediately due to the risk of bacterial translocation. Supplemental oxygen should be provided and electrolyte and acid-base abnormalities should be corrected. Unless contraindicated, patients should be anticoagulated with IV unfractionated heparin. Nasogastric tube insertion can be considered for decompression.

23. **What is the role of angioplasty and stenting in the management of ischemic bowel disease?**

Endovascular treatment is less invasive with less intensive care unit requirement in elderly patients with multiple comorbidities compared to open surgical procedures. The endovascular interventions include endovascular embolectomy by transcutaneous mechanical aspiration, percutaneous aspiration thrombectomy, intra-arterial pharmacological thrombolysis infusion, and percutaneous transluminal angioplasty with or without stenting.

24. **When should a patient with ischemic bowel disease undergo laparotomy?**

Prompt laparotomy should be performed on patients with signs of peritonitis, as bowel infarction has already occurred and the chance of survival is dramatically reduced. The goals of surgical intervention include assessment of the extent of injury, reestablishment of blood supply to the ischemic bowel, resection of all nonviable regions, and preservation of all viable bowel.

25. What is meant by a second-look operation?
During initial surgery (whether or not revascularization has been attempted), some affected bowel may be left intentionally in place, as the status of its viability may not be clear. Patients may undergo a second operation 24–48 hours later to identify and resect necrotic bowel and preserve viable bowel.

26. Can ischemia be isolated to the colon?
Ischemic colitis is the most common form of nonocclusive intestinal ischemia, oftentimes occurring in older patients with impaired cardiac output. In younger patients, however, the cause can be occlusive (sickle cell disease and hypercoagulable states) or nonocclusive (cocaine use, vasculitis, and long-distance running).

27. How does ischemic colitis present clinically?
Ischemic colitis most commonly presents with the sudden onset of cramping, mild left lower quadrant abdominal pain, and the urge to defecate. Additionally, patients may present with bright red blood per rectum or hematochezia. Palpation of the abdomen over the affected segment of bowel elicits tenderness. Differential diagnoses include infectious colitis, diverticulitis, and inflammatory bowel disease.

28. How do you confirm a suspected diagnosis of ischemic colitis?
Abdominal plain films may demonstrate thumbprinting along the affected segment of the colon wall, often at the splenic flexure, secondary to subepithelial edema and hemorrhage.

If ischemic colitis is suspected and there are no signs of peritoneal irritation, the patient should undergo colonoscopy within 48 hours for diagnostic confirmation. Any region of the colon may be involved but the key feature is segmental distribution, classically at watershed areas between the SMA and IMA. The rectosigmoid colon (20%), descending colon (20%), splenic flexure (11%), and all three in combination (14%) are affected most commonly. A sigmoidoscopy may be nondiagnostic in those with more proximal disease. The rectum is almost always spared because of its dual blood supply from the IMA and internal iliac artery branches.

Barium enema may reveal thumbprinting but is rarely used for diagnostic purposes due to low sensitivity in comparison to colonoscopy. Angiography is not generally indicated, as the common predisposing factors are nonocclusive in nature and have often resolved by the time ischemia has occurred.

29. What are the sequelae of ischemic colitis? Can anything be done to modify the course of the disease?
Optimizing cardiac function is imperative; impaired cardiac output and cardiac arrhythmias should be corrected. Factors predisposing to vasoconstriction, digoxin therapy, vasopressor agents, and hypovolemia should be avoided when possible. Vasodilating agents are ineffective because low colonic blood flow has often already returned to normal by the time the ischemia is evident. Patients should receive IV isotonic crystalloid fluids and bowel rest. A distended colon should be decompressed by placing a rectal tube or by rolling the patient from a supine position to right and left lateral decubitus positions. If the precipitating event is occlusive in nature, the underlying cause should be corrected, possibly including prolonged anticoagulation. There are no strong supporting data demonstrating the effectiveness of antibiotics.

Ischemic colitis is reversible in up to 70% of patients whose symptoms abate within 24–48 hours; in these patients, healing occurs without stricture in 1–2 weeks while those with severe injury require 1–6 months to heal completely. Irreversible damage occurs in less than 50% of cases and can lead to toxic megacolon, gangrene, perforation, fulminant colitis, and ischemic strictures. Unfortunately, the course cannot be predicted at the time of initial presentation.

Isolated right colon ischemia has a higher mortality and need for surgery, as its pathophysiologic findings are closely related to AMI. Early diagnosis and aggressive management are critical and mirror that of AMI.

30. When is surgery indicated in patients with ischemic colitis?
Surgery is indicated in patients who present with or develop peritoneal signs, massive bleeding, gangrene, perforation, toxic megacolon, or fulminant colitis. It should be considered even with apparent healing in patients who have recurrent bouts of sepsis and in patients who fail to respond to conservative measures over 2–3 weeks. Symptomatic colon strictures may also warrant surgical or endoscopic correction (e.g., balloon dilation or stent placement).

BIBLIOGRAPHY

Available Online

CHAPTER 58

NUTRITION, MALNUTRITION, AND PROBIOTICS

Peter R. McNally, DO, MSRF, MACG

 Additional content available online

1. What is meant by nutritional status?

Nutritional status reflects how well nutrient intake contributes to body composition and function in the face of the existing metabolic needs. The four major body compartments are water, protein, mineral, and fat. The first three compose the lean body mass (LBM); functional capacity resides in a portion of the LBM called the body-cell mass. Registered dietitians or registered dietitian nutritionists concentrate their efforts on the preservation or restoration of this vital component.

2. Define malnutrition.

Malnutrition refers to states of overnutrition (obesity) or undernutrition relative to body requirements, resulting in dysfunction.

3. How do different types of malnutrition affect function and outcome?

- Marasmus is protein-calorie undernutrition associated with significant physical wasting of energy stores (adipose tissue and somatic muscle protein) but preservation of visceral and serum proteins. Patients are not edematous and may have mild immune dysfunction.
- Hypoalbuminemic malnutrition occurs with stressed metabolism and is common in hospitalized patients. They may have adequate energy stores and body weight but have expanded extracellular space, depleted intracellular mass, edema, altered serum protein levels, and immune dysfunction.
- A similar state of relative protein deficiency occurs in classic *kwashiorkor*, in which caloric provision is adequate but quantity and quality of protein are not.

4. How is a simple nutritional assessment performed?

Simple bedside assessment may be as valuable for predicting nutrition-associated outcomes as sophisticated composition and function tests. Two popular methods, the Subjective Global Assessment and the Mini Nutritional Assessment, are simple-to-use validated nutritional assessment tools. Each incorporates basic questions about weight history, intake, gastrointestinal (GI) symptoms, disease state, functional level, and a physical examination to classify patients as well-nourished, mildly to moderately malnourished, or severely malnourished (Fig. 58.1).

A weight history, estimate of recent intake, brief physical examination, consideration of disease stress and medications, and assessments of functional status and wound healing allow a good estimate of nutritional status. They predict the risk for malnutrition-associated complications as well as or better than laboratory data. Poor intake for longer than 1–2 weeks, a weight loss of more than 10%, or a weight less than 80% of desirable warrants closer nutritional assessment and follow-up.

5. Serum proteins are a marker of overall nutritional health. Which plasma proteins will have the most sensitive turnover rate?

Ferritin: 30 hours
Retinol-binding protein: 2 days
Prealbumin: 2–3 days
Transferrin: 8 days
Albumin: 18 days

6. What simple blood tests offer an instant nutritional assessment?

- Serum albumin <3.5 g% is abnormal.
- Total lymphocyte count <1500/mm³ is abnormal.

7. List desirable weights for males and females.

Body mass index (BMI) is calculated from a person's weight and height and is a reliable indicator of body fatness. It is used to determine categories of disease risk based on weight status.

NESTLÉ NUTRITION SERVICES

Nestlé

Mini Nutritional Assessment
MNA®

Last name:	First name:	Sex:	Date:
Age:	Weight, kg:	Height, cm:	I.D. Number:

Complete the screen by filling in the boxes with the appropriate numbers.
Add the numbers for the screen. If score is 11 or less, continue with the assessment to gain a Malnutrition Indicator Score.

Screening

A Has food intake declined over the past 3 months due to loss of appetite, digestive problems, chewing or swallowing difficulties?
0 = severe loss of appetite
1 = moderate loss of appetite
2 = no loss of appetite ☐

B Weight loss during the last 3 months
0 = weight loss greater than 3 kg (6.6 lbs)
1 = does not know
2 = weight loss between 1 and 3 kg (2.2 and 6.6 lbs)
3 = no weight loss ☐

C Mobility
0 = bed or chair bound
1 = able to get out of bed/chair but does not go out
2 = goes out ☐

D Has suffered psychological stress or acute disease in the past 3 months
0 = yes   2 = no ☐

E Neuropsychological problems
0 = severe dementia or depression
1 = mild dementia
2 = no psychological problems ☐

F Body Mass Index (BMI) (weight in kg) / (height in m)^2
0 = BMI less than 19
1 = BMI 19 to less than 21
2 = BMI 21 to less than 23
3 = BMI 23 or greater ☐

Screening score (subtotal max. 14 points) ☐ ☐
12 points or greater   Normal – not at risk – no need to complete assessment
11 points or below   Possible malnutrition – continue assessment

Assessment

G Lives independently (not in a nursing home or hospital)
0 = no   1 = yes ☐

H Takes more than 3 prescription drugs per day
0 = yes   1 = no ☐

I Pressure sores or skin ulcers
0 = yes   1 = no ☐

Ref.: Guigoz Y, Vellas B and Garry P.J. 1994. Mini Nutritional Assessment: A practical assessment tool for grading the nutritional state of elderly patients. *Facts and Research in Gerontology.* Supplement #2:15-59.
Rubenstein LZ, Harker J, Guigoz Y and Vellas B. Comprehensive Geriatric Assessment (CGA) and the MNA: An Overview of CGA, Nutritional Assessment, and Development of a Shortened Version of the MNA. In: "Mini Nutritional Assessment (MNA): Research and Practice in the Elderly". Vellas B, Garry PJ and Guigoz Y , editors. Nestlé Nutrition Workshop Series. Clinical & Performance Programme, vol. 1. Karger, Bâle, in press.

© Nestlé, 1994, Revision 1998. N67200 12/99 10M

J How many full meals does the patient eat daily?
0 = 1 meal
1 = 2 meals
2 = 3 meals ☐

K Selected consumption markers for protein intake
• At least one serving of dairy products
  (milk, cheese, yogurt) per day?   yes ☐   no ☐
• Two or more servings of legumes
  or eggs per week?   yes ☐   no ☐
• Meat, fish or poultry every day   yes ☐   no ☐
0.0 = if 0 or 1 yes
0.5 = if 2 yes
1.0 = if 2 yes   ☐ . ☐

L Consumes two or more servings
of fruits or vegetables per day?
0 = no   1 = yes ☐

M How much fluid (water, juice, coffee, tea, milk…) is consumed per day?
0.0 = less than 3 cups
0.5 = 3 to 5 cups
1.0 = more than 5 cups   ☐ . ☐

N Mode of feeding
0 = unable to eat without assistance
1 = self-fed with some difficulty
2 = self-fed without any problem ☐

O Self view of nutritional status
0 = views self as being malnourished
1 = is uncertain of nutritional state
2 = views self as having no nutritional problem ☐

P In comparison with other people of the same age, how does the patient consider his/her health status?
0.0 = not as good
0.5 = does not know
1.0 = as good
2.0 = better   ☐ . ☐

Q Mid-arm circumference (MAC) in cm
0.0 = MAC less than 21
0.5 = MAC 21 to 22
1.0 = MAC 22 or greater   ☐ . ☐

R Calf circumference (CC) in cm
0 = CC less than 31   1 = CC 31 or greater ☐

Assessment (max. 16 points) ☐ ☐ . ☐

Screening score ☐ ☐

Total Assessment (max. 30 points) ☐ ☐ . ☐

Malnutrition Indicator Score

17 to 23.5 points	at risk of malnutrition	☐
Less than 17 points	malnourished	☐

Fig. 58.1 Mini Nutritional Assessment.

Calculation of BMI.

BMI is calculated the same way for both adults and children. The calculation is based on the formulas given in Table 58.1.

The standard weight status categories associated with BMI ranges for adults are shown in Table 58.2.

BMI can be easily determined by using a BMI calculator (https://www.cdc.gov/widgets/healthyliving/index.html#bmicalculator) or by referring to a BMI chart (Fig. 58.2).

Table 58.1 Calculation of Body Mass Index (BMI).

MEASUREMENT UNITS	FORMULA AND CALCULATION
Kilograms and meters (or centimeters)	Formula: weight (kg) ÷ [height (m)]^2 With the metric system, the formula for BMI is weight in kilograms divided by height in meters squared. Because height is commonly measured in centimeters, divide height in centimeters by 100 to obtain height in meters Example: Weight = 68 kg, Height = 165 cm (1.65 m) Calculation: $68 \div (1.65)^2 = 24.98$
Pounds and inches	Formula: weight (lb.) ÷ [height (in.)]^2 × 703 Calculate BMI by dividing weight in pounds (lb.) by height in inches (in) squared and multiplying by a conversion factor of 703 Example: Weight = 150 lb., Height = 5′5″ (65″) Calculation: $[150 \div (65)^2] \times 703 = 24.96$

Table 58.2 Body Mass Index (BMI) Ranges for Adults.

BMI (KG/M^2)	WEIGHT STATUS
Below 18.5	Underweight
18.5–24.9	Normal
25.0–29.9	Overweight
30.0 and above	Obese

From Centers for Disease Control and Prevention. How is BMI calculated and interpreted?

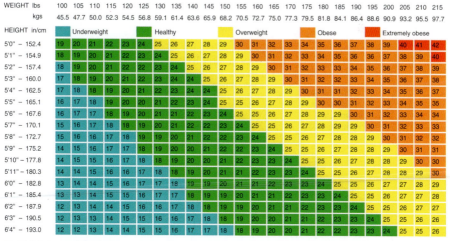

Fig. 58.2 Body mass index chart.

Basal energy expenditure (BEE) in calories can be derived from the Harris-Benedict equation:

$$♀BEE = 655.1 + [9.6 \times weight(kg)] + [1.8 \times height(cm)] - [4.7 \times age(yr)] = kcal/day$$

$$♂BEE = 66.5 + [13.7 \times weight(kg)] + [5.0 \times height(cm)] - [6.8 \times age(yr)] = kcal/day$$

BEE × stress factor = daily caloric need
Stress factor (multiplier)
Mild stress: (× 1–1.3)
Moderate stress: (× 1.3–1.4)
Severe stress: (× 1.5)

See Table 58.3.

8. **What is sarcopenia and is it important in persons with hepatic and digestive diseases?**
   - Sarcopenia often refers to an age-related process of involuntary loss of skeletal muscle mass and strength. This typically begins in the fourth decade with a steady decline in muscle mass and strength, with up to 50% decline by the eighth decade. Resistance exercises, protein supplementation, and vitamin D have been established as the basic treatments.
   - Sarcopenia is commonly seen in persons with hepatic and digestive diseases that cause nutrient maldigestion, malabsorption, and catabolic states. The administration of corticosteroids to treat conditions such as inflammatory bowel disease (IBD) and autoimmune hepatitis are often underappreciated accelerators of sarcopenia. The combination of carbohydrate excess and sedentary lifestyle is a counterintuitive cause of sarcopenia among obese persons with fatty liver and nonalcoholic steatohepatitis. While insulin resistance promotes weight gain and appearance of *health*, it promotes a deceptive loss of muscle mass. The breadth of disorders with sarcopenia that can be seen by GI/hepatology is illustrated in Fig. 58.3.

Table 58.3 Quick Formulas for Calculation of Protein and Caloric Requirements.

ILLNESS SEVERITY	PROTEIN (G/KG/DAY)	CALORIES (KCAL/KG/DAY)
Minimal	0.8	20–25
Moderate	1–1.5	25–30
Severe	1.5–2.5	30–35

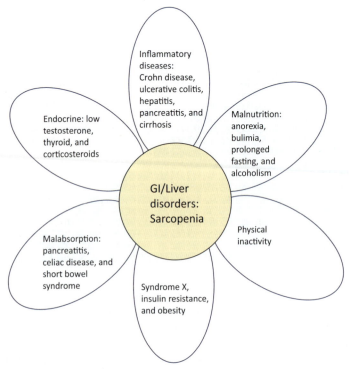

Fig. 58.3 Gastrointestinal (GI)/liver disorders associated with sarcopenia.

9. **Can sarcopenia be quantified or measured?**

Yes. Standardized measures of muscle mass, muscle function, and muscle strength have been developed and are more commonly used in physical therapy, geriatrics, rehabilitative medicine, and nutrition. Hepatology and liver transplant teams employ these measurements to determine waitlist mortality and candidacy for transplant. Routine measurements of sarcopenia include computed tomography at the L3 vertebra level, midarm muscle circumference, muscle strength, and function (hand grip strength and chair stands). Other common muscle function tests include:

- Liver Frailty Index (LFI): composed of three performance-based tests (grip strength, chair stands, and balance). LFI is a tool specifically developed for patients with cirrhosis to objectively measure physical function, a critical determinant of health outcomes.
- Six-minute walk distance.
- Thirty-second sit-to-stand test.

Health care providers need a heightened awareness of medications and diseases that can accelerate sarcopenia. Weight resistance exercise, increased protein intake, and vitamin D have all been shown to be beneficial in slowing sarcopenia. Early intervention with formal nutrition and physical therapy support, along with avoidance of catabolic medications (corticosteroids) are important countermeasures for patients at risk for accelerated sarcopenia.

10. **Describe the types of commonly prescribed oral diets.**

The clear liquid diet supplies fluid and calories in a form that requires minimal digestion, assimilation, and elimination by the GI tract. It provides approximately 600 calories and 150 g of carbohydrates per day but inadequate protein, vitamins, and minerals. Clear liquids are hyperosmolar; diluting the beverages and eating slower may minimize bloating and diarrhea-like GI symptoms. If clear liquids are needed for longer than 3 days, a dietitian can assist with supplementation.

The full liquid diet is used often in progressing from clear liquids to solid foods. It also may be used in patients with chewing problems, gastric stasis, or partial ileus. Typically, the diet provides more than 2000 calories and 70 g of protein per day. It may be adequate in all nutrients (except fiber), especially if a high-protein supplement is added. Patients with lactose intolerance need special substitutions. Progression to solid foods should be accomplished with modifications or supplementation, as needed.

11. **What is a *hidden* source of calories in the intensive care unit?**

Watch out for significant amounts of lipid calories from propofol, a sedative in 10% lipid emulsion (1.1 kcal/mL).

12. **Summarize the typical findings in deficiency or excess of various micronutrients.**

For the typical findings in deficiency or excess of various micronutrients, see Table 58.4.

Table 58.4 Vitamin and Mineral Deficiencies and Toxicities.

MICRONUTRIENT	DEFICIENCY	TOXICITY
Vitamin A	Follicular hyperkeratosis, night blindness, corneal drying, and keratomalacia	Dermatitis, xerosis, hair loss, joint pain, hyperostosis, edema, hypercalcemia, hepatomegaly, and pseudotumor
Vitamin D	Rickets, osteomalacia, hypophosphatemia, and muscle weakness	Fatigue, headache, hypercalcemia, and bone decalcification
Vitamin E	Hemolytic anemia, myopathy, ataxia, ophthalmoplegia, retinopathy, and areflexia	Rare: possible interference with vitamin K, arachidonic acid metabolism, headache, and myopathy
Vitamin K	Bruisability and prolonged prothrombin time	Rapid intravenous infusion: possible flushing and cardiovascular collapse
Vitamin C	Scurvy: poor wound healing, perifollicular hemorrhage, gingivitis, dental defects, anemia, and joint pain	Diarrhea; possible hyperoxaluria and uricosuria; interference with glucose and occult blood tests; and dry mouth and dental erosion

Continued

Table 58.4 Vitamin and Mineral Deficiencies and Toxicities.—cont'd

MICRONUTRIENT	DEFICIENCY	TOXICITY
Vitamin B_1 (thiamine)	Dry beriberi (polyneuropathy): anorexia and low temperature Wet beriberi (high-output congestive heart failure): lactic acidosis Wernicke-Korsakoff syndrome: ataxia, nystagmus, memory loss, confabulation, and ophthalmoplegia	Large-dose intravenous: anorexia, ataxia, ileus, headache, and irritability
Vitamin B_2 (riboflavin)	Seborrheic dermatitis, stomatitis, cheilosis, geographic tongue, burning eyes, and anemia	None
Vitamin B_3 (niacin)	Anorexia, lethargy, burning sensations, glossitis, headache, stupor, and seizures Pellagra: diarrhea, pigmented dermatitis, and dementia	Hyperglycemia, hyperuricemia, GI symptoms, peptic ulcer, flushing, and liver dysfunction
Vitamin B_6 (pyridoxine)	Peripheral neuritis, seborrhea, glossitis, stomatitis, anemia, CNS/EEG changes, and seizures	Metabolic dependency and sensory neuropathy
Vitamin B_{12}	Glossitis, paresthesias, CNS changes, megaloblastic anemia, depression, and diarrhea	None
Folic acid	Glossitis, intestinal mucosal dysfunction, and megaloblastic anemia	Antagonizes antiepileptic drugs and decreases zinc absorption
Biotin	Scaly dermatitis, hair loss, papillae atrophy, myalgia, paresthesias, and hypercholesterolemia	None
Pantothenic acid	Malaise, GI symptoms, cramps, and paresthesias	Diarrhea
Calcium	Paresthesias, tetany, seizures, osteopenia, and arrhythmia	Hypercalciuria, GI symptoms, and lethargy
Phosphorus	Hemolysis, muscle weakness, ophthalmoplegia, and osteomalacia	Diarrhea
Magnesium	Paresthesias, tetany, seizures, and arrhythmia	Diarrhea, muscle weakness, and arrhythmia
Iron	Fatigue, dyspnea, glossitis, anemia, and koilonychia	Iron overload (hepatic and cardiac) and possible oxidation damage
Iodine	Goiter and hypothyroidism	Goiter and hypo-/hyperthyroidism
Zinc	Lethargy, anorexia, loss of taste/smell, rash, hypogonadism, poor wound healing, and immunosuppression	Impaired copper, iron metabolism, reduced HDL, and immunosuppression
Copper	Anemia, neutropenia, lethargy, depigmentation, and connective tissue weakness	GI symptoms and hepatic damage
Chromium	Glucose intolerance, neuropathy, and hyperlipidemia	None
Selenium	Keshan cardiomyopathy and muscle weakness	GI symptoms
Manganese	Possible weight loss, dermatitis, and hair disturbances	Inhalation injury only
Molybdenum	Possible headache, vomiting, and CNS changes	Interferes with copper metabolism and possible gout
Fluorine	Increased dental caries	Teeth mottling and possible bone integrity/fluorosis

CNS, Central nervous system; *EEG*, electroencephalography; *GI*, gastrointestinal; *HDL*, high-density lipoprotein.

13. **What are the nutritional concerns in patients with short bowel syndrome (SBS)?**
Loss of bowel surface puts the patient at great risk for dehydration and malnutrition. The small bowel averages 600 cm in length and absorbs approximately 10 L/day of ingested and secreted fluids. A patient may tolerate substantial loss of small bowel, although preservation of less than 2 feet with an intact colon and ileocecal valve or less than 5 feet in the absence of the colon and ileocecal valve may make survival impossible when just the enteral route of nutrition is used. In addition, the loss of the distal ileum precludes absorption of bile acids and vitamin B_{12}. The remaining bowel, especially the ileum, may adapt its absorptive ability over several years, but the underlying disease may hamper this process.

14. **Describe the management of nutritional problems in patients with SBS.**
Therapy in the acute postsurgical phase is aimed at intravenous fluid and electrolyte restoration. Parenteral nutrition may be required while the remaining gut function is assessed and adaptation takes place. Attempts at oral feeding should include frequent, small meals with initial limitations in fluid and fat consumption. Osmolar sugars (e.g., sorbitol), lactose, and high-oxalate foods are best avoided. In patients with small bowel-colon continuity, increased use of complex carbohydrates may allow the salvage of a few hundred calories from colonic production and absorption of short-chain fatty acids (SCFAs). Antimotility drugs and gastric acid suppression should be used if stool output remains high. Oral rehydration with glucose- and sodium-containing fluids (e.g., sports drinks) may help prevent dehydration. Pancreatic enzymes, bile acid–binding resins (if bile acids are irritating the colon), and octreotide injections may play a role in selected cases. If oral diets fail, the use of elemental feedings may enhance absorption and nutritional state. Teduglutide is a glucagon-like peptide 2 analog that has been approved for the treatment of adult and pediatric SBS-associated intestinal failure. Intestinal or combined intestinal-liver transplantation is available at selected centers.

15. **Describe the approach to nutritional support in patients with acute pancreatitis (AP).**
Historical management of AP allowed the patient to take little by mouth in order to avoid a theoretical risk of further stimulating an inflamed pancreas. The idea of *pancreatic rest* in severe AP is an old paradigm that should be abandoned. Over the last decade further evidence has accrued to suggest early feeding does not exacerbate pancreatic parenchymal inflammation, and is actually beneficial in AP. This rationale stems from the understanding that enteral nutrition likely serves to protect the mucosal barrier of the gut and reduce bacterial translocation. This in turn may reduce the risk of developing infected pancreatic and peripancreatic necrosis. Delayed feeding (generally defined as >24 hours) is associated with higher rates of infected peripancreatic necrosis, multiple organ failure, and total necrotizing pancreatitis. Success of early feeding has been demonstrated with low-fat, normal fat, and soft or solid consistency, and thus it is not necessary to start patients with AP on a clear liquid diet before advancement to a solid diet. Patients who cannot tolerate an oral diet may require enteral tube placement for nutritional support; however, the risk of aspiration should be considered in patients with severe AP. There does not appear to be an advantage to postpyloric tube placement over gastric tube placement. Pancreatitis is considered a high-stress condition requiring high caloric and protein replacement (25 kcal/kg/day up to a maximum of 30 kcal/kg/day with 1.2–1.5 g/kg of protein/day). Carbohydrates and lipid intake should be ~3–6 and up to 2 g/kg/day, with careful monitoring and adjustments for hyperglycemia and hypertriglyceridemia.

16. **What adverse GI effects may be encountered in a patient using herbal supplements?**
It is estimated that one-third to one-half of the US population uses herbal products in supplementary form and that 60%–75% do not inform health care providers. Because herbal products are not regulated and their composition is not standardized, toxicity data are less clear than with regulated pharmaceuticals. However, popular products that may cause adverse GI effects include saw palmetto, *Ginkgo biloba* (nonspecific GI upset), garlic (nausea and diarrhea), ginseng (nausea and diarrhea), aloe (diarrhea and abdominal pain), and guar gum (obstruction). In addition, hepatotoxicity (ranging from asymptomatic enzyme elevation to fulminant necrosis) has been documented with germander, chaparral, senna, *Atractylis*, and *Callilepis*. Hepatotoxicity associated with the use of valerian, mistletoe, skullcap, and various Chinese herbal mixtures has been noted but awaits a cause-and-effect confirmation. The pyrrolizidine alkaloids in *Crotalaria*, *Senecio*, *Heliotropium*, and comfrey have long been implicated in cases of veno-occlusive liver disease.

17. **How is *obesity* defined, and how common is it among US residents?**
BMI has become the standard of measurement for obesity.

$$BMI = weight(kg) \div body\ surface\ area(m^2)$$

A BMI higher than 30 kg/m² is defined as obese.
In 1999–2000 the prevalence of obesity and severe obesity in the United States was 30.5% and 4.7%, respectively. An even more frightening statistic is the rise in the prevalence of obesity (41.9%) and severe obesity (9.2%) from 2017 to March 2020. All states and territories had more than 20% of adults with obesity. Only the District of Columbia, Colorado, Hawaii, and Massachusetts have obesity rates of less than 25% of adults (http://www.cdc.gov/obesity/data/adult.html).

18. **Does obesity carry a significant risk for death?**
Yes. In the United States, 300,000 persons die annually from obesity-related diseases.

19. **What are the medical therapies for obesity?**
Dietary restriction of calories, while maintaining adequate protein, fluid electrolyte, mineral, and vitamin intake, is the key. A sensible weight reduction program targets gradual weight reduction by behavior modification, including dietary and activity changes. Numerous fad diets claim success, but key to the weight loss is patient commitment and total lifestyle modification. The US Preventive Services Task Force 2019 recommendations include screening all adults for obesity. Clinicians should offer or refer patients with a BMI of $30 \, kg/m^2$ or higher to intensive, multicomponent behavioral interventions.

20. **What are the surgical options for obesity?**
Bariatric surgery dates back to the 1950s when intestinal bypass was first performed. The total weight lost correlates with the total length of bowel bypassed. Gastric bypass (GBP) is the most common weight loss surgery performed in the United States (see Chapter 77). The laparoscopic adjustable gastric banding procedure is the most common bariatric surgery in Australia and Europe. A recent systematic review concluded that weight loss outcomes strongly favored Roux-en-Y GBP over laparoscopic adjustable gastric banding.

21. **What are the National Institutes of Health consensus criteria thought to be appropriate indications for bariatric surgery?**
Failure of a major weight-loss program + excessive obesity BMI of more than $40 \, kg/m^2$
    or
Failure of a major weight-loss program + BMI of more than $35 \, kg/m^2$
    and
Obesity-related comorbidities

22. **What is the operative mortality of GBP surgery?**
Operative mortality ranges from 0.3% to 1.6%, and perioperative complications occur in up to 10% of patients, see Chapter 77.

23. **What are the medical benefits of bariatric surgery?**
- Diabetes: 83% of patients with type 2 diabetes and 99% of those with glucose intolerance maintained normal levels of plasma glucose, glycosylated hemoglobin, and insulin; 88% of diabetics no longer required medication.
- Cardiovascular: 15% of patients experienced a decrease in cholesterol, 50%, a decrease in triglycerides, and prescription-treated hypertension was decreased from 58% to 14%.
- Pulmonary: 14% of patients have preoperative obstructive or hypoventilation syndrome, with most improved postoperatively.

24. **What nutritional deficiencies are seen with bariatric surgery?**
Water-soluble vitamins B_{12}, B_1 (thiamine), folate, and C; fat-soluble vitamins A, D, E, and K; and minerals iron, zinc, calcium, and copper. Deficiencies in B_{12} and iron are most commonly observed, with iron deficiency seen in 30% by 5 years.
Deficiencies in vitamin B_1 may cause "bariatric beriberi" and with vitamin A night blindness and corneal Bitot spots.

Recommended postbariatric surgery supplements.
- Iron 325 mg twice daily.
- Vitamin B_{12} as part of a multivitamin.
- Folate as part of a multivitamin.
- 1200–1500 mg calcium in divided doses over the day. Calcium citrate is better absorbed in low acid environment.

25. **Is there a benefit to instituting an anti-inflammatory diet (AID) for patients with immune-mediated inflammatory diseases (IMIDs) to include IBD, rheumatoid arthritis (RA), psoriasis, and psoriatic arthritis?**
Maybe to a qualified Yes. See Table 58.5 for a list and description of some AIDs.
    Mediterranean diet (MD): The MD seems to have promise across all IMIDs based on larger cohort and survey-based studies primarily conducted in patients with RA. It has been studied to a lesser extent in IBD. Without apparent harm from the MD and potential life longevity data shown to occur with the consumption of MD, it would seem reasonable for patients with IBD to consider MD.

Table 58.5 Antiinflammatory Diets.

DIET	INCLUDE	AVOID
Mediterranean diet	Vegetables, fruits, whole grain, nuts, and olive oil	High red meat intake, sweets, sugar, and processed meats
Specific carbohydrate	Fruits, meat, and most vegetables	Grains, potatoes, yams, corn, processed/smoked meat, and dairy
Gluten free	All nongluten-containing foods: including potatoes, maze soy, and rice	Gluten dash containing grains: wheat, rye, barley, oats, etc.
Vegetarian/vegan	Vegetables, fruits, whole grains, nuts, and vegetable oils	Vegetarian: meat plus or minus fish/seafood, and eggs Vegan: meat, fish/seafood, eggs, and other animal-based products
Low FODMAP	Certain fruits: berries, blueberries, grapes, oranges, carrots, cucumbers, and olives	Short-chain carbohydrates, polyols, certain vegetables, fruits, grains, animal-based products—for example, garlic, onions, apples, wheat, and dairy
Calorie restriction/ fasting	Reduced calorie intake or intermittent fasting	

FOODMAP, Fermentable oligosaccharides, disaccharides, monosaccharides, and polyols.

Vegetarian and vegan diet: Vegetarian diets vary considerably but generally eliminate meat products, while vegan diets are void of all animal-based food products, including eggs, dairy, and seafood. These diets gained popularity as a potential therapeutic tool for inflammatory diseases after multiple clinical trials with patients with RA demonstrated positive results.

Calorie restriction/fasting: Diets that restrict total calories or include periods of fasting have gained attention as a potential treatment for IMIDs based on animal and clinical studies showing anti-inflammatory effects. These studies have focused on this type of diet as a treatment for RA and psoriasis. However, a study of 60 patients with IBD in remission analyzed the effects of Ramadan fasting. No adverse effects of fasting on the patients were noted. Additionally, a significant decrease in the clinical colitis activity index was evident.

26. **Is the number of bacteria populating the human intestine greater than the total number of cells in the human body?**
Yes. The average human body consists of approximately 10 trillion cells, whereas there are approximately 10 times that number of microorganisms in the gut.

27. **What value is gut microbiotica to human existence?**
There are estimated to be 200–300 colonic species of bacteria in the gut, each with a unique function (Table 58.6).

28. **Is there a link between gut microbiotica and obesity?**
Yes. Intestinal microbiotica of obese (*ob/ob*) mice were examined and compared with wild-type (*WT/WT*) mice; it was found that *ob/ob* animals have a 50% reduction in the abundance of *Bacteroidetes* and a proportional increase in *Firmicutes* species that are more efficient in extracting calories from otherwise nondigestible polysaccharides in our diet and ultimately generating SCFAs.

29. **What is the definition of a probiotic?**
Probiotic refers to live microbial food supplements that beneficially affect the host by improving intestinal microbial balance and fulfill the following criteria:
- When ingested, they survive and colonize the gut, but rapidly disappear when discontinued.
- They are of human origin.
- They do not produce plasmids.

30. **What are some of the common probiotics?**
Probiotics are generally derived from four bacterial species: *Lactobacillus*, *Bifidobacter*, *Streptococcus*, and *Escherichia coli* (Table 58.7).

Table 58.6 Commensal Effects of Gut Microbiotica on Humans.

ACTION	EFFECT
Carbohydrate fermentation	Reduction of intraluminal colonic pH
Protein fermentation	Production of NH_4 and sympathetic amines
Synthesis of short-chain free fatty acids	Main source of energy and nutrition for the colon
Synthesis of vitamins K, B_1, B6, and B_{12}, folic acid, and pantothenic acid	Essential components for biologic processes
Deconjugation of bile salts, bilirubin, drugs, and steroid hormones	Biotransformation and absorption
Fat malabsorption	Regulation of plasma levels of cholesterol and triglycerides

Table 58.7 Common Probiotics.

LACTOBACILLUS (LAB)	BIFIDOBACTERIA	STREPTOCOCCUS	ESCHERICHIA COLI
L. acidophilus	B. bifidum	S. thermophilus	Nissle 1917
L. casei GG	B. infantis	S. lactis	Serotype
L. rhamnosus	B. longum	S. salivarius	06:K5:H1
L. salivarius	B. thermophilum		
L. delbrueckii	B. adolescentis		
L. reuteri			
L. brevis			
L. plantarium			

31. **Have probiotics been shown to benefit the treatment of GI disorders?**

    Yes.

DISEASE STATE	PROBIOTIC
Irritable bowel disease	Bifidobacter, VSL#3[a]
Ulcerative colitis	VSL#3[a]
Traveler diarrhea	Lactobacillus, VSL#3[a]
Antibiotic-related diarrhea	Lactobacillus, Bifidobacterium, and Saccharomyces boulardii
Relapsing Clostridium difficile diarrhea	Saccharomyces boulardii
Recurrent pouchitis	VSL#3[a]

    [a]VSL#3 is a concentration of eight strains of bacteria.

32. **How are probiotics and prebiotics believed to exert a beneficial effect on the gut?**

    Gut dysbiosis has been identified as a contributor to the errant immune response in a variety of IMIDs, such as IBD, RA, and psoriatic disease (psoriasis and psoriatic arthritis). Probiotics and prebiotics have been investigated as therapeutic options in these disease states. However, the American Gastroenterology Association practice guidelines on the role of probiotics in the management of GI disorders currently do not recommend their use outside of a clinical trial.

    Types of prebiotics, including fructans and galacto-oligosaccharides (a type of oligosaccharide that is not hydrolyzed by humans but rather fermented by gut bacteria), are found naturally in foods, such as asparagus, beets, garlic, and lentils to name a few. Omega-3 fatty acids from sources, such as fish oils, have been used to treat chronic inflammatory disorders, such as IBD. There has been considerable evidence associating low vitamin D levels and inflammation. Providing supplemental vitamin D when a deficiency exists is appropriate. Curcumin, a strong antioxidant derived from the turmeric root, has been used in many cultures for millennia for its antioxidative and anti-inflammatory properties. Green tea is a form of the *Camellia sinensis* plant that contains caffeine and antioxidants and may have anti-inflammatory benefits.

Proposed mechanisms by which probiotics and prebiotics work in IMID:

- Toll-like receptors
- Antimicrobial activity
- Enhanced barrier integrity
- ↓↓ Tumor necrosis factor and interferon
- Induce T regulatory cells
- Induce T cell apoptosis
- Dendritic cell modulation
- Limited adhesion
- ↑↑ Immunoglobulin A
- ↓↓ Chloride secretion
- ↑↑ Mucus secretion
- ↑↑ Interleukins 10 and 12
- •Enhance tight junctions

ACKNOWLEDGMENT

The author would like to acknowledge the contribution of Bonnie Jortberg, PhD, RD, CDE, who was a coauthor of this chapter in the previous edition.

CLINICAL VIGNETTE

Available Online

BIBLIOGRAPHY

Available Online

WEBSITES

Available Online

CHAPTER 59

SMALL BOWEL AND COLON PATHOLOGY

Shalini Tayal, MD

 Additional content available online

SMALL INTESTINE

1. **What are the morphologic features of celiac disease?**

   The normal duodenal mucosa has numerous finger-like projections, or villi, as shown in Fig. 59.1A, whereas in celiac disease the normal villous architecture is lost (blunted villi and crypt hyperplasia) and intraepithelial lymphocytes (IELs) are increased, as shown in Fig. 59.1B. Increased IELs are seen more toward the tips of the villi. These are T lymphocytes that can be highlighted by CD3 immunohistochemical stain.

   The Marsh criteria represent a morphologic classification that defines the many histologic features of this entity. The modified classification (Marsh-Oberhuber) subdivides Marsh 3 into A, B, and C as partial, subtotal, or total villous atrophy, respectively. The Corazza classification simplifies it further into Grade A, B1, and B2, representing Marsh type 1, 3a, and 3c, respectively. The comparison and summary of histologic classifications are depicted in Table 59.1.

   Treated celiac disease may show normal villous architecture but the IELs are still increased.

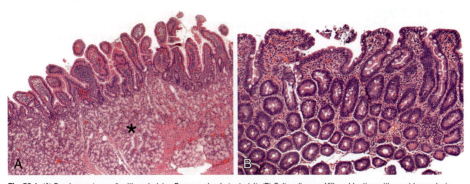

Fig. 59.1 (A) Duodenum (normal) with underlying Brunner glands (*asterisk*). (B) Celiac disease. Villous blunting with crypt hyperplasia and increased intraepithelial lymphocytes (tip heavy pattern). Hematoxylin and eosin stain.

2. **What is the differential diagnosis of the biopsy showing villous blunting?**
   - Allergy to other proteins (e.g., cow's milk in the pediatric population)
   - Dermatitis herpetiformis
   - Nonsteroidal anti-inflammatory drugs (NSAIDs)
   - Peptic duodenitis
   - Giardiasis
   - Tropical sprue
   - Crohn's disease
   - Severe malnutrition
   - Bacterial overgrowth
   - Common variable immunodeficiency
   - Autoimmune enteropathy
   - Graft-versus-host disease (GVHD)
   - Zollinger-Ellison syndrome
   - Chemotherapy effect

Table 59.1 Histologic Classifications of Celiac Disease.

MARSH MODIFIED (OBERHUBER)	HISTOLOGIC CRITERIA			CORAZZA
	IEL[a]	Crypt hyperplasia	Villous atrophy	
Type 0	No	No	No	None
Type 1	Yes	No	No	Grade A
Type 2	Yes	Yes	No	
Type 3a	Yes	Yes	Yes (partial)	Grade B1
Type 3b	Yes	Yes	Yes (subtotal)	
Type 3c	Yes	Yes	Yes (total)	Grade B2

IEL, Intraepithelial lymphocytes.
[a]*More than 40 IEL per 100 enterocytes for Marsh modified (Oberhuber); >25 IEL per 100 enterocytes for Corazza.*
Adapted from Rubio-Tapia A, Hill ID, Kelly CP, Calderwood AH, Murray JA, American College of Gastroenterology. ACG clinical guidelines: diagnosis and management of celiac disease. Am J Gastroenterol. 2013;108(5):656-676.

3. What are the complications of celiac sprue?
   - Collagenous sprue: Some cases of long-standing sprue, unresponsive to gluten-free diet, exhibit a thickened subepithelial collagen table greater than 10 μm along with marked villous blunting.
   - Ulcerative jejunoileitis is characterized by multiple transverse ulcers in the small intestine, predominantly in the jejunum.
   - Enteropathy-associated T cell lymphoma is mostly seen in older adult patients with celiac disease.
   - Carcinoma: Increased incidence of small bowel adenocarcinoma and carcinoma at other gastrointestinal (GI) tract sites has been reported. Also reported are carcinomas of the oropharynx, lung, breast, and ovary.

4. Discuss a few causes of infectious enteritis.
   - Giardiasis: *Giardia lamblia* is seen as a pear-shaped organism that resides in the upper small intestine (duodenum and jejunum) (Fig. 59.2) and exists in two forms—trophozoite and cyst. The trophozoite form (7 μm wide, 14 μm long) shows two symmetrical nuclei with nucleoli and four pairs of flagella. On longitudinal sections, it appears as a long, curved organism.
   - *Mycobacterium avium* intracellulare infection: This opportunistic infection affects both the small and large bowel in immunocompromised hosts in a patchy distribution. Histologic examination shows numerous histiocytes in the lamina propria (Fig. 59.3A) that contain numerous acid-fast bacilli highlighted by Kinyoun stain (Fig. 59.3B). Granulomas may not be identified.
   - Whipple disease: *Tropheryma whippelii* infects the small intestine, cardiac valves, nervous system, and lymph nodes. Histologic examination shows the expansion of lamina propria by positive periodic acid-Schiff (diastase resistant) Whipple bacilli that are negative with acid-fast bacilli stain. The other feature that points to Whipple infection is the dilated lymphatics in the lamina propria caused by obstruction of the lymphatic ducts by bacilli. Other tests include polymerase chain reaction (PCR) assay and electron microscopy.
   - Other infections include *cryptosporidium*, disseminated *histoplasmosis*, *Isospora belli*, *Microsporidium* spp. (*Enterocytozoon bieneusi* and *E. intestinalis*), *Strongyloides*, and *Yersinia* spp.

Miscellaneous Conditions
   - Lymphangiectasia: Primary lymphangiectasia presents in the pediatric age group generally before 3 years. The biopsy sample shows dilated lymphatics in the superficial lamina propria (Fig. 59.4). Secondary causes will show similar histologic findings and include local inflammatory or a neoplastic process.
   - Ischemic enteritis: This is often the result of mechanical obstruction and, histologically, shows hemorrhage in the lamina propria or transmural hemorrhage with mucosal sloughing.
   - GVHD: Histologic findings are graded as follows:
     - Grade 1—Apoptosis (single-cell necrosis) of the crypt epithelium
     - Grade 2—Apoptosis with crypt abscesses
     - Grade 3—Individual crypt necrosis or crypt dropout
     - Grade 4—Total surface denudation of areas of bowel
   - Eosinophilic gastroenteritis: The biopsy shows villous blunting with numerous eosinophils in the lamina propria forming clusters or sheets. The etiologic factors include food allergies, parasites, drugs, hypereosinophilic syndrome, and idiopathic disease.

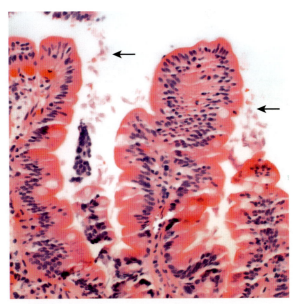

Fig. 59.2 Photomicrograph of *giardiasis*. Small bowel biopsy shows pear-shaped trophozoite forms (*arrows*) on the luminal surface. Hematoxylin and eosin stain. (Courtesy Dr. Loretta Gaido, Denver Health Medical Center, Denver, CO.)

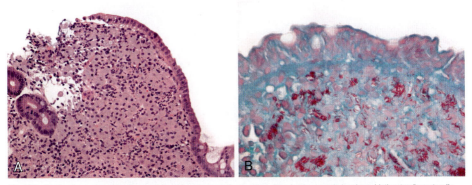

Fig. 59.3 (A) *Mycobacterium avium intracellulare*. There is marked expansion of the lamina propria by plump histiocytes (hematoxylin and eosin stain). (B) *Mycobacterium avium intracellulare*. Acid-fast bacilli (magenta staining rods within histiocytes) highlighted by the Kinyoun stain. *Tropheryma whippelii* organisms are not acid-fast.

Small Intestinal Neoplasms

- Peutz-Jeghers polyps: The small intestine is the most common site for polyps in Peutz-Jeghers syndrome. Histologic examination shows arborizing smooth muscle bundles in the lamina propria without much expansion of lamina propria by inflammatory infiltrate (Fig. 59.5). The overlying epithelium is that of small intestinal type and may show hyperplasia. Dysplasia can occasionally be seen in these polyps.
- Adenomas: Duodenum is the most common upper GI site for an adenoma. The morphologic characteristics are similar to those in the colon: tubular, tubulovillous, or villous patterns are seen. Ampullary adenomas arise in the ampulla or periampullary region and are indistinguishable from each other based on morphologic examination.
- Adenocarcinomas: The primary adenocarcinoma of the small intestine is uncommon (2% of GI tract tumors), and the duodenum is the most common site. Usually, these arise from a sporadic adenoma. Histologic examination resembles colonic adenocarcinoma. Other predispositions include familial adenomatous polyposis (FAP), hereditary nonpolyposis colorectal cancer (HNPCC), or hamartomatous polyp syndromes. Risk factors include chronic inflammatory conditions such as celiac disease, Crohn's disease, ileostomy, and protein-losing enteropathy.

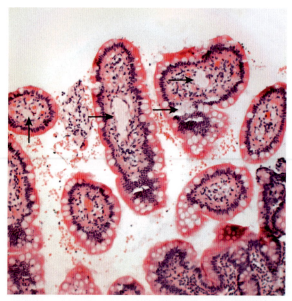

Fig. 59.4 Photomicrograph of lymphangiectasia (secondary). Small bowel biopsy showing villi with dilated lacteals (*arrows*). Hematoxylin and eosin stain.

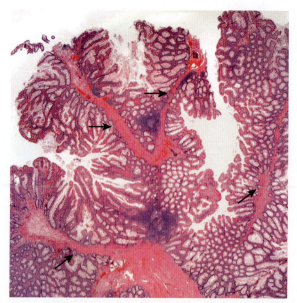

Fig. 59.5 Photomicrograph of Peutz-Jeghers polyp. Note the arborizing smooth muscle bundles (*arrows*) traversing the lamina propria. Hematoxylin and eosin stain.

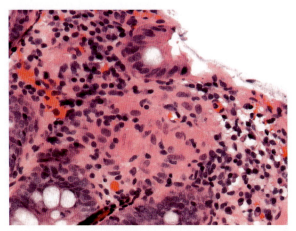

Fig. 59.6 Photomicrograph of Crohn's disease. A microgranuloma is seen in the lamina propria in this biopsy from the transverse colon. Note the epithelioid histiocytes with ample eosinophilic cytoplasm and ovoid nuclei. Hematoxylin and eosin stain.

LARGE INTESTINE

5. **What are the histologic features of idiopathic inflammatory bowel disease (IBD)?**
   - Chronic ulcerative colitis (UC): Grossly, there is diffuse involvement of rectosigmoid and left-sided colon, and proximal extent of the disease varies. Infections such as *Cytomegalovirus*, *Salmonella*, *Shigella*, and *Clostridium difficile* can complicate UC. Toxic megacolon is a fulminant acute complication of the disease. Histologically, the features of acute disease include cryptitis (neutrophilic infiltration in the crypt epithelium), crypt abscesses (neutrophils in the crypt lumens), and mucosal erosions and ulcers. The features of chronicity include architectural distortion of crypts (crypt dropout, bifid crypts, and crypt branching), mucin depletion (loss of goblet cells), Paneth cell metaplasia, basal plasmacytosis, increased eosinophils, and prominent lymphoid aggregates. These changes are diffuse except in the resolving phase, in which these may be focal (they should not be confused with Crohn's disease). Fibrosis is unusual in UC, in contrast to Crohn's disease. The differential diagnosis, especially in the acute disease process, includes infection, ischemic colitis, and Crohn's disease.
   - Quiescent colitis: Histologically, mucosal atrophy (short crypts, loss of crypts, and crypt distortion), thickened muscularis mucosae, and normal inflammatory component in the lamina propria appear. Inflammatory pseudopolyps can be seen in long-standing cases.
   - Backwash ileitis: Some patients with pancolitis demonstrate backwash ileitis, and the biopsy sample shows acute disease without features of chronicity.
   - Crohn's disease: Colon biopsy samples show variable morphologic findings. Some foci may appear normal and the others show aphthous ulcers, cryptitis, glandular distortion and loss, and occasionally granulomas (Fig. 59.6). Transmural inflammation is characteristic of Crohn's disease and distinguishes Crohn's disease from UC. The rectum is usually spared. The resection (done in complicated cases) specimen shows segmental involvement with skip areas, linear ulcers, cobblestoning, strictures, fissures and fistulas, inflammatory pseudopolyps, serosa with creeping fat, and a firm pipe-like bowel resulting from fibrosis. Involvement of the terminal ileum shows villous blunting and increased inflammation in the lamina propria.

6. **Discuss colitis-associated dysplasia in IBD.**
   The Surveillance for Colorectal Endoscopic Neoplasia Detection and Management in Inflammatory Bowel Disease Patients International Consensus Recommendations (SCENIC) Development Panel published a consensus statement in 2015. Per the recommendations, dysplastic lesions in IBD are classified as (endoscopically) visible (polypoid or nonpolypoid) or invisible dysplasia (seen on random biopsy). The visible lesions could be polypoid (pedunculated or sessile) or nonpolypoid (superficially elevated, flat, or depressed).
   The old term dysplasia-associated lesion or malignancy is avoided and no longer in use.

7. **What is the differential diagnosis of focal active colitis?**
   - Infectious colitis
   - Crohn's disease
   - UC early or resolving
   - Bowel preparation artifact

8. **Histologically, which findings help differentiate infectious colitis and NSAID-associated colitis?**
   - Infectious colitis on histologic examination shows acute inflammation in the lamina propria with cryptitis, crypt abscesses, and lack of prominent chronic inflammatory infiltrate or basal plasmacytosis (as seen in IBD). Chronic architectural changes may not be pronounced. Causative organisms include *Escherichia coli* O157:H7, *Salmonella*, *Shigella*, *Clostridium*, *Campylobacter*, *Yersinia*, cytomegalovirus colitis (Fig. 59.7), amebic colitis, and histoplasmosis. Granulomas can be seen in tuberculosis, *Yersinia pseudotuberculosis*, and *Chlamydia* infections.
   - Intestinal spirochetosis (Fig. 59.8) shows organisms on the luminal surface that may not cause an active inflammatory response or injury in the mucosa. These anaerobic organisms belong to *Brachyspira* spp.
   - NSAID-associated colitis changes are patchy, may involve any part of the colon, and histologically include focal active colitis, erosions and ulcers, increased apoptosis in crypts, and diaphragm strictures. Diaphragm-like strictures are formed as a result of repeated injury and repair and are seen microscopically as mucosal and submucosal fibrosis. These may cause luminal narrowing and occasionally serosal strictures. Thickened subepithelial collagen layer in long-standing cases has been associated with NSAIDs that can be confused with collagenous colitis and requires correlation with clinical history and endoscopic findings.

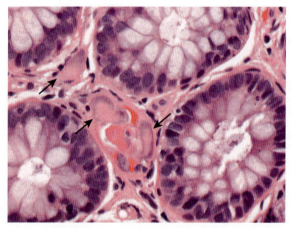

Fig. 59.7 Photomicrograph of cytomegalovirus colitis. Note the large eosinophilic intranuclear viral inclusions (*arrows*). Hematoxylin and eosin stain.

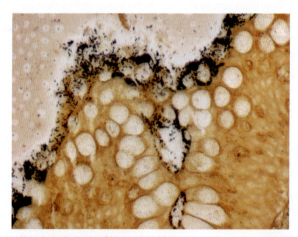

Fig. 59.8 Photomicrograph of intestinal spirochetosis. Steiner stain highlights the spirochetes obscuring the luminal border. No significant inflammation was seen within crypts or lamina propria.

9. **What is the differential diagnosis of polypoid lesions that can mimic adenoma?**
   - Mucosal prolapse, solitary rectal ulcer syndrome, colitis cystica profunda, and eroded polypoid hyperplasia: These are seen in rectosigmoid colon as an ulcerated or a polypoid lesion in patients with the history of constipation or straining during defecation. The histologic examination shows surface erosion, epithelial hyperplasia with distorted and dilated crypts, vertical stranding of muscle fibers in the lamina propria, fibrosis, and lymphoplasmacytic infiltrate. Inflammatory cloacogenic polyps are present at the anorectal junction and show similar histologic characteristics with both squamous and colonic epithelia.
   - Lymphoid polyps: These are benign reactive lymphoid aggregates in the mucosa.
   - Inflammatory polyps: Generally associated with IBD or diverticulitis and consist of marked inflammation in the lamina propria with granulation tissue and fibrosis. The mucosal lining may show regenerative change or erosions.

POLYPS AND NEOPLASMS

10. **What are the histologic features of conventional adenomas?**
    Tubular adenomas (Fig. 59.9) have a tubular architecture with the surface epithelium showing low-grade dysplasia that extends downward in the base. These can show focal areas of high-grade dysplasia with architectural complexity and marked cytologic atypia. Focal high-grade dysplasia does not have a metastatic potential. The tubulovillous adenomas (Fig. 59.10) show a combination of tubular and villous architecture (villous component greater than 25%). Villous adenoma displays a predominant villous architecture (greater than 75%)

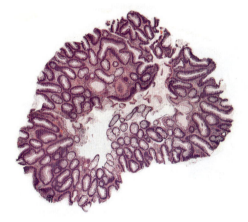

Fig. 59.9 Photomicrograph of tubular adenoma. Polyp showing tubular architecture lined by cells with nuclear stratification and hyperchromasia. Hematoxylin and eosin stain.

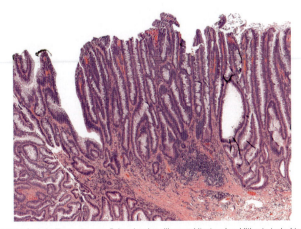

Fig. 59.10 Photomicrograph of tubulovillous adenoma. Polyp showing villous architecture in addition to typical tubular areas. Hematoxylin and eosin stain.

and has a greater propensity for malignant transformation. All of these can have focal areas of pseudoinvasion that should not be interpreted as intramucosal carcinoma. The conventional adenomas show *KRAS* mutations (*BRAF* negative).

11. **What is meant by *intramucosal carcinoma* in an adenoma?**
Invasion of dysplastic glands into the lamina propria is intramucosal carcinoma. In the colon, it is equivalent to high-grade dysplasia, because it is not associated with metastatic potential and a polypectomy with negative margins should suffice.

12. **What is meant by the term *depressed* or *flat* adenoma?**
Endoscopically (Fig. 59.11A), the adenoma shows subtle depression in the mucosa or may be flat. Histologically (Fig. 59.11B), the adenomatous glands show long, tubular architecture with a narrow opening at the surface and are lined by dysplastic epithelium. These tend to have high-grade dysplasia more often than tubular adenomas and are more aggressive.

13. **What is the difference between hyperplastic polyp (HP), traditional serrated adenoma (TSA), and sessile serrated adenoma (SSA)?**
   - HPs are characterized by serrated crypt lumens that are lined by colonic epithelial cells that lack dysplasia (Fig. 59.12).
   - TSAs are polyps that show serrated crypt lumens with stratified pencil-like nuclei at the base of crypts (Fig. 59.13) that resemble the ones seen in tubular adenoma. Some authors have described ectopic crypt formation in TSA. These are short crypts away from muscularis mucosae and are considered as precursors to colorectal cancer (CRC).

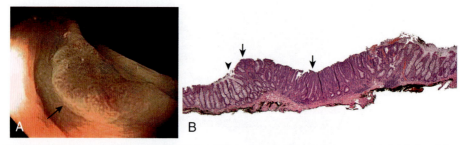

Fig. 59.11 (A) Depressed adenoma (*arrow*), endoscopic view. (B) Photomicrograph of depressed adenoma, morphologic findings. Note the abrupt junction between normal (*arrowhead*) and abnormal (*arrow*) and the depression with tubular glands showing narrow openings at the surface (*central arrow*). Hematoxylin and eosin stain. (A, Courtesy Dr. Norio Fukami, University of Colorado Denver Health Sciences Center.)

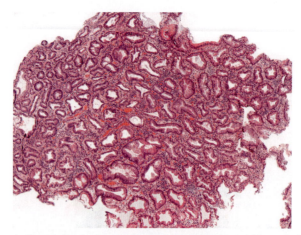

Fig. 59.12 Photomicrograph of hyperplastic polyp. Polyp with hyperplastic glands showing serrated lumens lined by epithelial cells without dysplasia. Hematoxylin and eosin stain.

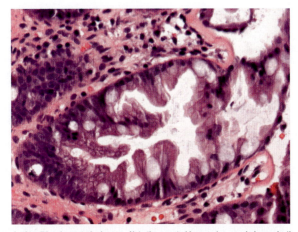

Fig. 59.13 Photomicrograph of traditional serrated adenoma. Note the serrated lumens (as seen in hyperplastic polyps) lined by cells that show pencillate nuclei and stratification (as seen in tubular adenomas). Hematoxylin and eosin stain.

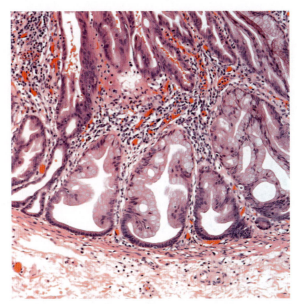

Fig. 59.14 Photomicrograph of sessile serrated adenoma. Note the serrated lumens and broad (boat-shaped) base of the crypts in this polyp resected from the cecum. Hematoxylin and eosin stain.

- SSAs are seen more on the right side of the colon in older adult women and are always sessile. A few (10%) may occur in the left colon. In various studies, these account for 4%–15% of serrated polyps. Architecturally, it differs and shows serrated lumens with a horizontal, broad, or boat-shaped base (Fig. 59.14). The lining epithelium is variable and shows goblet or mucinous cells or may be mucin depleted and may show nuclear stratification. A subset of these polyps may show focal conventional dysplasia; however, architecture is the key finding. This adenoma has been associated with microsatellite instability-high (MSI-H)–related sporadic CRCs (hypermethylation of promoter gene). The majority of these show *BRAF* mutation, and approximately 1 in 25 (4%) of these may progress to cancer.
- Mixed polyps are HPs with typical adenoma foci.

14. What are the genetic abnormalities in conventional CRCs?

- Colorectal adenocarcinomas usually arise from adenomas and can be sporadic (85%) or syndromic. These are graded as well, moderately, or poorly differentiated based on the glandular differentiation (Fig. 59.15). The variants include mucinous (greater than 50% mucinous morphologic characteristics) (Fig. 59.16) and signet ring cell carcinomas (greater than 50% signet ring cell morphologic characteristics). Histologically, neoplastic glands with necrotic debris show invasion through the muscularis mucosa into the submucosa or beyond. On immunohistochemistry (IHC), these usually show staining with cytokeratin 20 (*CK20*) and *CDX2* and are usually negative for staining with *CK7*. The most common genetic alteration (somatic) in sporadic CRCs is the inactivation of *APC/beta-catenin* pathway which can have multiple consequences. Clonal accumulation of additional genetic alterations then occurs, including activation of proto-oncogenes such as *c-myc* and *ras* and inactivation of additional tumor suppressor genes (*TP53* on chromosome 17). These tumors are microsatellite stable (MSS). *BRAF* mutation is not common and is seen in a few (less than 10%) conventional CRCs.
- Small cell carcinoma is a rare variant of CRC with poor prognosis, which shows small cell morphologic characteristics and positive immunostaining with neuroendocrine markers such as chromogranin, synaptophysin, and neural cell adhesion molecule (*CD56*). These are not associated with carcinoid tumors (well-differentiated neuroendocrine tumors) and may be seen with conventional CRC.

15. What genetic abnormalities point to HNPCC?

HNPCC presents in a younger age group and has an autosomal dominant pattern of inheritance. Revised Bethesda criteria are set to screen the patients for MSI. DNA mismatch repair (*MMR*) gene defect is tested for *hMLH1* (50%), *hMSH2* (39%), *hMSH6* (8%), and *hPMS2* (1%) genes. These defects result in the insertion or deletion

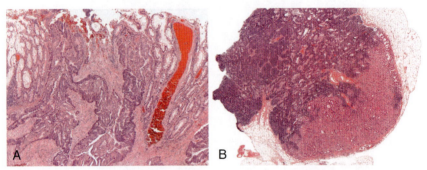

Fig. 59.15 (A) Colon adenocarcinoma, moderately differentiated. Note the infiltrating neoplastic glands with surface involvement in the center of the image and the nonneoplastic epithelium adjacent to it (for comparison). (B) Lymph node with metastasis from colon adenocarcinoma (*right*). Hematoxylin and eosin stain.

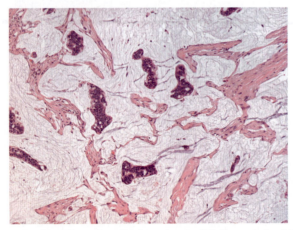

Fig. 59.16 Photomicrograph of mucinous adenocarcinoma. Note the mucin pools with floating neoplastic cell clusters. Hematoxylin and eosin stain.

of nucleotides in the microsatellite sequences, which are tested using PCR and reported as high (MSI-H), low (MSI-L), or stable (MSS). At least five microsatellite sequences are tested and MSI-H is defined as instability in 30%–40% of markers (two of five at least).
- Loss of *hMSH2* indicates HNPCC.
- Loss of *hMLH1* indicates HNPCC or sporadic CRC (loss caused by hypermethylation of *hMLH1* promoter in sporadic CRC).
- The IHC on paraffin sections (of normal and tumor) to test for mismatch repair is also done, which shows loss of staining in the tumor (caused by mutated gene) compared with the normal. Loss of *hMSH2* and/or *hMSH6* is highly associated with Lynch syndrome. Direct gene sequencing can be done in highly susceptible cases and to confirm the results of MSI and IHC. A negative test in an at-risk patient does not rule out other hereditary causes of CRC.

16. **What histologic features seen in CRCs can predict MSI-H?**
These tumors are usually right-sided, show a medullary or syncytial growth pattern, have mucinous or signet ring cell features, are poorly differentiated, and show lymphocytic infiltration. Also, a Crohn-like reaction (nodular lymphoid aggregates) is seen beyond the advancing edge of the tumor. These features, along with the age at diagnosis, are used to determine the MSI by pathology score.

17. **What is the abnormality in MSI-unstable sporadic CRCs?**
These constitute approximately 12%–15% of CRCs. The MSI-H is caused by somatic inactivation of the *hMLH1* mismatch repair gene due to hypermethylation of the promoter region preceding the gene sequence, whereas in HNPCC, the instability is due to germline mutation in the *MMR* genes. Most of the sporadic ones show *BRAF* mutations (*V600E* mutation of *BRAF* oncogene). The histologic findings are similar to those seen in HNPCC.

POLYPOSIS SYNDROMES

18. **Name the hamartomatous polyp syndromes.**
- Hamartomatous polyps include juvenile hamartomatous polyp and the hamartomatous polyp of Peutz-Jeghers type.
- Peutz-Jeghers syndrome involves the entire GI tract (small intestine most common); there is a 93% lifetime risk of cancer. Sporadic Peutz-Jeghers polyps can occur but are extremely rare. Follow-up of these patients is warranted. Histologically, these typically show arborizing smooth muscle bundles in the lamina propria lined by normal or hyperplastic epithelium, occasionally with dysplastic foci.
- Juvenile polyposis syndrome involves the colon or the entire GI tract (pedunculated polyps); the risk of CRC is approximately 30%–40% and is less (10%–15%) for upper GI cancer. This is the most common polyp in the juvenile population. Germline mutation in the *SMAD4/DPC4* tumor suppressor gene accounts for half the cases. Histologically, these are lobulated polyps with cystically dilated crypt (mucus retention cysts) with inflamed edematous lamina propria and occasionally with superficial erosions. Other than juvenile polyp syndromes, juvenile polyps are seen in Cowden syndrome and Bannayan-Riley-Ruvalcaba syndrome.
- Cowden syndrome involves the entire GI tract from esophagus to rectum; the risk of developing CRC is generally not increased. The most commonly recognized cancer is breast, followed by thyroid. It arises from *PTEN* germline mutation. Histologically, juvenile polyps are common; also seen are HPs, adenomas, lipomas, and, rarely, ganglioneuromas.
- Bannayan-Riley-Ruvalcaba syndrome is a variant of Cowden syndrome with similar histologic features.
- Cronkhite-Canada syndrome occurs in any portion of the GI tract (sessile polyps); the risk of developing cancer is not well described. Histologically, the polyps seen are similar to juvenile-type (retention) polyps with marked edema in the lamina propria; the intervening mucosa shows similar changes in the lamina propria. Differential diagnosis includes Ménétrier disease and juvenile polyposis syndrome.
- Hyperplastic polyposis is a rare syndrome with an increased risk for CRC. It is characterized by the presence of HPs predominantly (adenomas—tubular or serrated also can be seen) in the colon proximal to the sigmoid colon. The number of polyps ranges from 5 to 100. Most of these are nonfamilial and the genetic abnormalities include *BRAF* and *KRAS* mutations.
- All are hereditary except Cronkhite-Canada syndrome and hyperplastic polyposis.

19. **Name the adenomatous polyp syndromes.**
- FAP affects the entire colon and rectum; there is 100% risk of cancer. Histologically, tubular adenomas and occasionally tubulovillous and villous adenomas are identified.
- The variants include attenuated FAP, Gardner syndrome, Turcot syndrome, hereditary flat adenoma syndrome, and Muir-Torre syndrome.
- All are hereditary syndromes.

20. **How are neuroendocrine tumors classified?**
The spectrum ranges from well-differentiated neuroendocrine tumors (carcinoid tumors) to poorly differentiated (small cell carcinomas) and large cell neuroendocrine carcinomas. The common site of involvement is the rectum, followed by the cecum and sigmoid colon. The histologic characteristics are similar to those described in the small intestine section (available online). These are sporadic tumors. A malignancy rate of 11%–14% has been calculated for rectal carcinoids. The malignancy criteria include size greater than 2 cm, invasion into the muscularis propria, and increased mitoses.

21. **What are the most common primary tumor sites that can show colon metastases?**
These include the lung, stomach, breast, ovary, endometrium, and melanoma. These tumor cells creep under the surface epithelium or form submucosal nodules of varying sizes. More than one focus is generally seen. The surface epithelium lacks dysplasia (expected with primary colon adenocarcinomas). IHC may be helpful in poorly differentiated neoplasms. Usually, primary colonic adenocarcinomas show immunoreactivity with *CK20* (95%) and *CDX2* (intestinal epithelium marker). Difficulty arises in some poorly differentiated tumors that have lost antigenicity or show lineage infidelity.

DISEASES OF THE APPENDIX

22. **What is the effect of IBD on the appendix?**
The appendix is involved in 50% of cases with ileal Crohn's disease and UC with cecal involvement. Isolated involvement is rare.

23. **Describe the mucinous lesions of the appendix.**
- Mucocele is a cystically dilated appendiceal lumen containing mucus. It can be nonneoplastic or neoplastic. Any obstruction of the lumen can give rise to mucocele.
- In low-grade mucinous adenocarcinomas, with pseudomyxoma peritonei, the mucin/tumor cells dissect through the wall of the appendix into the peritoneum. Most cases of synchronous tumors in the ovary and appendix are now considered metastases from the appendiceal tumor. Acellular pools of mucin pose a diagnostic problem. A diagnosis of adenoma (or cystadenoma) should be rendered only if the entire muscularis mucosae is intact. A diagnosis of *low-grade appendiceal mucinous neoplasm or LAMN* previously known as *uncertain malignant potential* is favored in the cases in which intact muscularis mucosae cannot be seen.
- Mucinous adenocarcinomas with mucinous carcinomatosis include signet ring cell carcinomas, invasive well-differentiated carcinomas, and cystadenocarcinoma.

24. **What is the incidence of carcinoid tumors in appendectomy specimens (performed for appendicitis)?**
Appendiceal carcinoid has been reported in 0.3%–0.9% of appendectomy specimens. It is the most common appendiceal neoplasm. The functioning tumors are commonly serotonin-producing neoplasms. The risk factors for malignancy include size greater than 2 cm and the invasion of mesoappendix.

25. **What are the histologic types of mixed endocrine-exocrine neoplasms?**
These include goblet cell carcinoid, tubular carcinoid, and mixed carcinoid-adenocarcinoma. Mixed carcinoid-adenocarcinoma carries the worst prognosis.

DISEASES OF THE ANAL CANAL

26. **The typical findings of Hirschsprung disease include absence of ganglion cells. What other stain can help support the diagnosis, and what is the ideal site of biopsy?**
Acetylcholinesterase stain highlights the proliferation of thickened nerve fibers in the lamina propria and muscularis mucosae. This stain is done on the frozen tissue. So, ideally, two biopsy samples are sent—one in formalin and another fresh for freezing. The site of biopsy is at least 2 cm above the dentate line. The lower rectum (adjacent to the dentate line) is physiologically hypoganglionic. Also, the submucosa should be included in the biopsy samples to assess the nerves in both the lamina propria and muscularis mucosae.

27. **How is anal intraepithelial neoplasia (AIN) graded, and what is the risk of progression to squamous cell carcinoma (SCC)?**
AIN is graded as low grade (AIN I or mild dysplasia) and high grade (encompasses AIN II and AIN III or moderate and severe dysplasia or carcinoma in situ, respectively). The term Bowen disease (Fig. 59.17A) is used for lesions with severe dysplasia (carcinoma in situ) seen at the anal verge or perianal skin. The high-grade lesions are associated with high-risk human papillomavirus 16 and 18, among others. These lesions are known to recur after local treatment. The risk of progression to SCC (Fig. 59.17B) is low (approximately 5%).

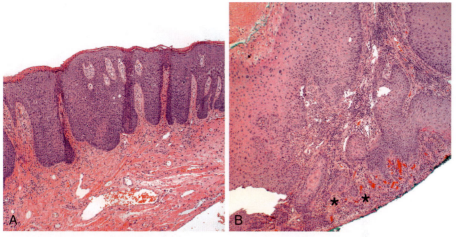

Fig. 59.17 (A) Bowen disease. Note the thickened squamous epithelium showing severe full-thickness dysplasia. (B) Squamous cell carcinoma (*asterisks*) at another focus within the same specimen. Hematoxylin and eosin stain.

28. **What are the cells of origin and the immunohistochemical profile of perianal Paget disease?**

    The Paget cells (intraepithelial large cells with pale pink cytoplasm and large nuclei) are believed to be of apocrine lineage and show immunoreactivity with low-molecular-weight keratins *Cam 5.2, CK7*, and carcinoembryonic antigen. Mucin stain may be positive. The differential diagnosis includes pagetoid spread from adjacent CRC and melanoma in situ. The immunoprofile helps to distinguish between these types of cancer.

BIBLIOGRAPHY

Available Online

WEBSITES

Available Online

CHAPTER 60

FOREIGN BODIES AND THE GASTROINTESTINAL TRACT

Trevor Dunbar, DO, Kenneth Leung, MD and George Saffouri, MD

 Additional content available online

1. **How common are foreign body ingestions in the gastrointestinal (GI) tract?**
   An estimated 90,000 cases of foreign body ingestion occur every year in the United States, of which 75% are seen in children. Up to 90% of foreign bodies may pass spontaneously without intervention. However, with intentional ingestion, the need for endoscopic and surgical intervention may be much higher.

2. **Who is at risk of foreign body ingestion?**
   Most foreign body ingestions involve children aged 5 years or younger and are usually unintentional. Among adults, accidental ingestions often involve alcohol use, while intentional ingestions often involve cognitive or mental health disorders, incarceration, and drug smuggling. Food impactions occur more frequently around holidays and athletic events.

3. **What underlying GI pathologies are often seen in cases of esophageal food impaction?**
   Underlying structural, inflammatory, or motility disorders are often encountered at the time of endoscopy. Structural findings include strictures, rings, Zenker diverticulae, and malignancies. Nearly 50% of esophageal biopsies performed in food impaction cases reveal underlying eosinophilic esophagitis. Of the motility disorders, achalasia is the most salient.

4. **What foreign bodies are commonly ingested?**
   Among children, household items such as coins, small toys, marbles, erasers, and magnets are frequently ingested. Common foreign bodies encountered in adults include meat and fish bones, jewelry, toothpicks, and dental prostheses. In contrast, among incarcerated individuals or those with mental health disorders, sharp and other potentially dangerous items such as razor blades, shanks, metal hardware, pencils, and drug packets are frequently encountered. Occasionally, endoscopic video capsules may be retained (Fig. 60.1).

5. **What are common presentations of foreign body ingestions?**
   Esophageal foreign bodies are typically symptomatic and may present with dysphagia, odynophagia, or retrosternal discomfort. In severe cases, there may be difficulty managing secretions. While patients with food

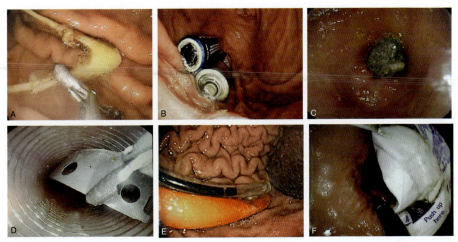

Fig. 60.1 Examples of foreign bodies in the gastrointestinal tract. (A) Fish bone being grasped. (B) Two AA batteries. (C) Rock. (D) Razor blade being extracted within an overtube. (E) Ballpoint pen (*black*) and straw (*orange*). (F) Milk carton seen in retroflexion.

impactions can often localize a particular area of discomfort, the perceived location does not correlate well with the true location of the obstruction.

6. What is the general approach to management?

Whenever possible, a careful history regarding the ingested material, timing of ingestion, history of dysphagia or similar episodes, allergies, previous endoscopies, and previous GI surgeries is essential.

Medical decision-making in cases of foreign body ingestion and food impactions is guided by clinical presentation, patient characteristics, as well as the type, quantity, and location of foreign material within the GI tract (Fig. 60.2). In every case, consideration must be made regarding airway protection, need for early surgical consultation, urgency of endoscopy, need/type of procedural sedation, and necessary management equipment.

7. What are the *red flag* signs or symptoms?

Careful examination should assess for airway compromise, luminal perforation, or bowel obstruction. Coughing, choking, stridor, or respiratory distress may result from aspiration or compression of the trachea from the foreign

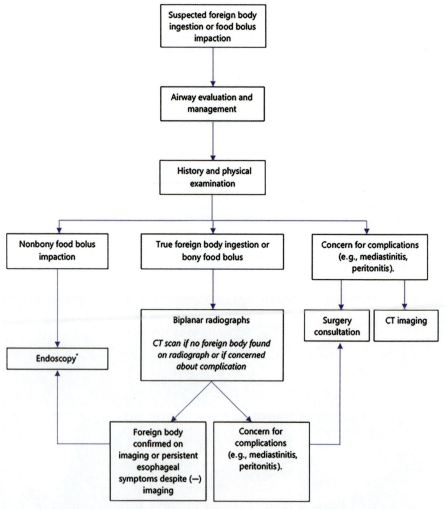

*If food bolus impaction is at or above the cricopharyngeus, consider otolaryngology consultation for laryngoscopy

Fig. 60.2 Management algorithm for adults with suspected foreign body ingestion or food bolus impaction. *CT,* Computed tomography.

body. Excessive salivation and inability to swallow secretions suggest the presence of complete esophageal obstruction. A neck and chest examination to look for swelling, erythema, tenderness, or crepitus should be performed, the presence of which should raise suspicion for oropharyngeal or esophageal perforation. Abdominal examination should be thorough to evaluate for peritonitis from perforation or distension from obstruction.

8. **What are the high-risk locations for obstruction within the GI tract?**
   The most frequent site of obstruction is the esophagus. This is due to both structural and functional features of the esophagus as well as underlying pathology. Within the esophagus, normal anatomy consists of areas of acute narrowing which are vulnerable to obstruction, including the upper esophageal sphincter, aortic arch impression, and lower esophageal sphincter. Other high-risk locations along the GI tract include the pylorus, duodenal sweep, ileocecal valve, and anal canal.

9. **What is the role of imaging in the initial evaluation of foreign body ingestion?**
   Diagnostic imaging can locate and characterize the foreign body and evaluate for related complications. Most foreign bodies are radiopaque. Common radiolucent objects include fish and chicken bones, wood, and plastic. Biplanar radiographs of the neck, chest, and abdomen can identify and clarify the number, size, location, and configuration of the foreign body. However, uncomplicated nonbony food impactions may reasonably proceed to endoscopy without imaging. Whenever clinical suspicion for foreign body ingestion is high or if there is evidence of esophageal obstruction, endoscopy should be performed even with negative imaging.

   Computed tomography (CT) has higher sensitivity for detecting foreign bodies. CT may be considered when the location of a foreign body is uncertain based on radiographs or if evaluating for complications, such as abscess, peritonitis, perforation, or fistulae. Oral contrast should be avoided due to aspiration risk—particularly if there is concern for esophageal obstruction—as well as potentially coating and obscuring the foreign body during endoscopy.

10. **What is the optimal timing for endoscopy?**
    Timing is determined by the perceived risks of aspiration, perforation, and obstruction associated with the foreign body. Emergent endoscopy within 2–6 hours should be performed in individuals unable to manage secretions, or those with disk batteries or sharp, long objects in the esophagus. Otherwise, objects in the esophagus should be removed within 24 hours to maximize the chance of successful removal and minimize complications. Asymptomatic patients with objects in the stomach do not always require endoscopy. However, objects in the stomach that are wider than 2.5 cm should be removed as these are less likely to pass the pylorus. Similarly, objects longer than 6 cm, such as pencils, pens, or toothbrushes, should be removed due to difficulty passing the duodenal sweep. Sharp objects also carry an increased risk of perforation, and therefore removal is suggested. Ingested objects identified in the colon on initial imaging can often be monitored with serial imaging and will likely pass without intervention.

11. **How should foreign bodies be endoscopically removed?**
    Over 95% of foreign bodies in the upper GI tract can be removed safely and effectively with flexible endoscopes. Esophageal food impactions are often successfully managed using the push technique, in which the endoscopist uses air insufflation and the endoscope to gently push the food bolus into the stomach. However, if pushing demonstrates resistance, alternative strategies include fragmenting the bolus into smaller pieces to facilitate passage, piecemeal extraction, or cap-assisted suction.

    Endoscopic accessories are chosen based on the size, shape, and nature of the foreign body as well as endoscopist preference. Retrieval devices are used to either capture foreign bodies whole or to grasp objects securely for removal. These include forceps, graspers, snares, baskets, and nets. Protective devices, such as overtubes or rubber hoods, can be utilized to minimize the risks of mucosal laceration and aspiration of the foreign body in an unprotected airway.

12. **What objects should not be removed endoscopically?**
    Body stuffing and packing involve the smuggling of illicit drugs through the concealment of the drug in the GI tract. Drugs may be packed in a protective covering such as a condom or balloon and swallowed or inserted into the rectum. Rupture of these packets can lead to overdose and fatal intoxication. Endoscopy should not be attempted. Rather, patients should be monitored in the hospital until passage. Individuals who develop signs or symptoms of intoxication or bowel obstruction should promptly undergo surgery.

13. **When should endotracheal intubation be considered?**
    While most procedures can be performed under conscious sedation or with monitored anesthesia care, endotracheal intubation should be considered in cases with high risk for aspiration, such as obstruction at the level of the upper esophageal sphincter and anticipated prolonged or riskier procedures (e.g., multiple ingested objects and large or sharp objects).

14. **Are pharmacologic therapies beneficial in the management of esophageal foreign body impactions?**

Pharmacologic therapy to facilitate the passage of esophageal foreign bodies that have been studied include glucagon and papain. While glucagon is frequently given in the emergency department, it is often unsuccessful and is associated with nausea and vomiting, potentially increasing the risk of aspiration. Papain can cause mucosal erosion and perforation and should be avoided.

15. **When should foreign body ingestions be referred for surgery?**

While endoscopy can successfully remove most foreign bodies in the upper GI tract, at times, early surgical consultation is warranted. Due to limited, difficult working space, otolaryngology consultation for laryngoscopy should be considered in obstruction at or above the cricopharyngeus. Signs/symptoms of perforation or complete luminal obstruction require urgent surgery consultation. Rarely, if a foreign body cannot be retrieved endoscopically and the item does not pass spontaneously, surgical removal may be needed.

16. **When should diet be resumed?**

For successful uncomplicated foreign body removals, a regular diet can be resumed immediately following recovery from the procedure. Additional postprocedural monitoring while NPO (*nil per os*) or on a liquid diet may be warranted for technically difficult procedures.

17. **What is a common rectal foreign body presentation and the recommended management?**

Anorectal foreign body cases are primarily seen in young males involving a wide range of objects. In rare pediatric cases, a thorough investigation for potential child abuse is warranted. Many anorectal foreign body presentations are delayed as individuals choose to reveal symptoms rather than the actions that preceded them. Colorectal surgery consultation is typically warranted. Imaging should be obtained to assess for sharp objects, and careful rectal examination should be performed to evaluate the retained object before attempted extraction. Strategies for removal include transanal extraction, endoscopic extraction with rigid or flexible scopes, or operative management. General anesthesia may be utilized to help relax the anal sphincter.

BIBLIOGRAPHY

Available Online

CHAPTER 61

FUNCTIONAL GASTROINTESTINAL DISORDERS AND IRRITABLE BOWEL

Vikram Rangan, MD and Anthony Lembo, MD

 Additional content available online

1. What is irritable bowel syndrome (IBS)?

IBS is a disorder of gut-brain interactions characterized by chronic or recurrent abdominal pain, usually in the lower abdomen, that is associated with altered bowel habits (diarrhea, constipation, or a combination of diarrhea and constipation). Bloating, distention, and disordered defecation are commonly associated features. IBS is characterized by abnormalities in gastrointestinal (GI) motility, visceral sensation, altered intestinal microbiome, and immune cell activation. The diagnosis of IBS is generally made based on the Rome IV criteria which are shown below:

Recurrent abdominal pain on average at least 1 day/week in the last 3 months, associated with two or more of the following criteria:
1. Related to defecation
2. Associated with a change in frequency of stool
3. Associated with a change in the form (appearance) of stool
Criteria must be fulfilled for 3 months, with symptom onset at least 6 months prior to diagnosis.

2. How common is IBS?

A recent worldwide prevalence study that included 24 countries involving over 50,000 individuals using internet surveys found the prevalence of IBS using the Rome IV criteria ranging from 1.3% to 5.9% of the population, with an average of 4.1%. Younger individuals (less than age 50) are more likely to report IBS symptoms as compared with older individuals, although IBS can occur at any age. In some cases, symptoms of IBS date back to childhood. IBS symptoms are more prevalent in female patients rather than male patients.

The female-to-male ratio of IBS is 2:1, though this ratio is significantly higher for IBS constipation (IBS-C), while the ratio is nearly 1:1 for IBS diarrhea (IBS-D). Not only do females have symptoms more frequently than males, but they are also more likely to seek medical attention for their symptoms.

3. What is the effect of IBS on quality of life?

IBS can have a significant negative effect on Health-Related Quality of Life (HR-QOL). However, because IBS is not a life-threatening illness, many clinicians underestimate its effect on individuals, family, and friends. Using the standard health-related questionnaire 36-Item short form survey (SF-36), individuals with IBS symptoms report lower scores on all scales compared with the general population. Compared with other illnesses such as diabetes and depression, patients with IBS have similar or significantly worse HR-QOL scores.

4. What is the economic burden of IBS?

Only approximately 25%–50% of individuals with IBS symptoms ever seek health care. Nevertheless, given the prevalence of symptoms, IBS has a significant economic burden. IBS is one of the top 10 reasons for consultation with a primary care physician, and the most common reason for consulting a gastroenterologist. Nearly one-third of all consultations by gastroenterologists are for IBS symptoms. In the United States alone, there were an estimated 2.7 million visits per year for IBS between 2007 and 2015. In addition, patients with IBS undergo a multitude of diagnostic and therapeutic procedures, which are often unnecessary and sometimes dangerous. IBS is also thought to have a significant effect on work productivity. Between absences and periods of impaired productivity due to IBS symptoms, it was estimated in one study that patients with IBS have the equivalent of 14 hours of lost productivity per 40-hour work week.

CAUSES OF AND DIAGNOSIS OF IRRITABLE BOWEL SYNDROME

5. What is the current belief about the causes and risk factors for IBS?

IBS is the result of a complex interaction between psychosocial and physiologic factors via the gut-brain axis. The pathogenesis of IBS appears to be multifactorial. Factors believed to play a role in the pathogenesis of IBS include heritability and genetics, environment and social learning, diet, intestinal microbiota, intestinal immune activation, central processing of visceral sensations, and gut dysmotility. Early life factors, such as family attitudes toward

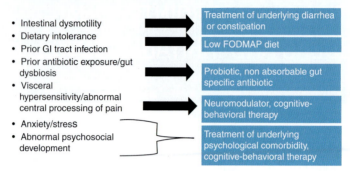

- Intestinal dysmotility
- Dietary intolerance
- Prior GI tract infection
- Prior antibiotic exposure/gut dysbiosis
- Visceral hypersensitivity/abnormal central processing of pain
- Anxiety/stress
- Abnormal psychosocial development

Treatment of underlying diarrhea or constipation

Low FODMAP diet

Probiotic, non absorbable gut specific antibiotic

Neuromodulator, cognitive-behavioral therapy

Treatment of underlying psychological comorbidity, cognitive-behavioral therapy

Fig. 61.1 Irritable bowel syndrome causes and possible treatments. *FODMAP*, Fermentable oligo-, di-, and monosaccharides and polyols; *GI*, gastrointestinal.

illness, major loss, or abuse history, or, possibly, genetic predisposition, may influence a person's psychosocial development (e.g., psychologic state, coping skills, social support, or susceptibility to life stress) or gut dysfunction (e.g., gut dysmotility or hypersensitivity). Although closely interrelated, the importance of any one factor in the generation of IBS symptoms varies greatly between individuals (Fig. 61.1).

6. **What is the role of intestinal dysmotility in IBS?**
Patients with IBS have both a reduction and an increase in the number of colonic contractions per minute compared with healthy individuals. However, these abnormal motility patterns rarely correlate with IBS symptoms, nor do they explain many of the symptoms associated with IBS.

7. **What is the role of abnormal central processing of pain?**
Abnormal central processing, such as downregulation of incoming visceral sensations, has also been found in patients with IBS. In patients with IBS, rectal distention fails to activate the perigenual anterior cingulated cortex (ACC), the area containing large amounts of B-endorphin activity, which may serve to downregulate pain but instead shows increased activation of the rostral ACC, an area associated with unpleasantness and attention. Also, patients with IBS and a history of abuse reported greater activation of the middle and posterior dorsal cingulate regions, reduced activity of the supragenual anterior cingulate, which are implicated in pain inhibition and arousal. Therefore, patients with IBS may have an alteration of the pain modulatory system, as well as upregulation of afferent signals at the primary splanchnic afferent or its spinal connections.

8. **What is the role of the intestinal microbiota in IBS?**
Several studies have suggested that some differences exist in the intestinal microflora of patients with IBS compared with healthy individuals including a decrease in microbial diversity. Using conventional microbiologic techniques, fecal microflora of patients with IBS have been shown to have higher numbers of facultative organisms, such as *Klebsiella* species and enterococci, and lower numbers of Enterobacteriaceae, lactobacilli, and bifidobacteria. Using more sophisticated DNA techniques, investigators have shown significant differences between patients with IBS and controls for several bacterial genera, including *Coprococcus*, *Collinsella*, and *Coprobacillus*. In addition, IBS-D and IBS-C also appear to have distinct microbial populations.

9. **What is the significance of visceral hypersensitivity in IBS?**
Visceral hypersensitivity as demonstrated by lower pain thresholds to balloon-distention volumes in the GI tract of patients with IBS in comparison with healthy individuals is a cause of pain symptoms in IBS. The cause of visceral hypersensitivity in IBS is not completely understood. However, researchers now believe that noxious stimuli can change the synaptic efficiency of peripheral and central neurons. This may occur through altered release of serotonin (5-HT) from the enteroenteric cells in the myenteric plexus or the release of inflammatory cytokines from activated immune or inflammatory cells in response to infection or injury. Through a process known as the windup, neurons can develop a pain memory that can persist long after the noxious stimulus is removed. Patients with IBS may also be prone to developing sensitization. Repetitive sigmoid contractions, such as those that may occur during intense stress, could induce sensitization in a person predisposed to developing IBS, thereby causing rectosigmoid hypersensitivity.

10. **What is postinfectious IBS (PI-IBS)?**
IBS symptoms develop in approximately 10% of healthy individuals after an infectious gastroenteritis. PI-IBS is most commonly reported after a bacterial infection such as *Campylobacter*, *Salmonella*, and *Shigella* but has

also been reported after viral, bacterial, protozoa, and nematode infections. Even after clearing the infection, there remains an increase in inflammatory (including CD3 lymphocytes, CD8 intraepithelial lymphocytes, and calprotectin-positive macrophages) and neuroendocrine cells that can release cytokines, serotonin, and other molecules that are capable of stimulating motor and sensory neurons in the GI tract. Risk factors for developing PI-IBS in persons who have had gastroenteritis are (1) female sex, (2) age younger than 60 years, (3) absence of vomiting, and (4) prolonged diarrhea with the infection. Additionally, anxiety, neurosis, somatization, and stressful life events before or during the infection also appear to be risk factors for determining who will develop IBS.

Two novel biomarkers, cytolethal distending toxin B (CdtB) antibody and antivinculin antibody, have been proposed to be a biomarker for postinfectious IBS. Studies have shown that patients with IBS-D are more likely to have elevated antibody levels compared to patients with inflammatory bowel disease and celiac disease.

11. What is the role of stress in IBS?
Although most people have experienced the effect of anxiety and stress on their GI tract with urgency, cramps, constipation, or diarrhea, patients with IBS appear to have exaggerated GI response to stress. Additional, major stressful life events, such as a death of a loved one, divorce, and physical, mental, or sexual trauma, are frequently associated with the onset of IBS symptoms.

12. What are the common comorbid symptoms associated with IBS?
Individuals with IBS often have other GI and non-GI symptoms. Common upper GI symptoms include dyspepsia, heartburn, early satiety, and nausea. Common extraintestinal symptoms include urinary frequency and urgency (especially in females), sexual dysfunction, muscle discomfort and other rheumatologic conditions, dyspareunia, poor sleep, low back pain, headaches, chronic fatigue, loss of concentration, and insomnia. The number of these symptoms tends to increase with the severity of IBS. The presence of one or more of these intestinal or extraintestinal symptoms does not discriminate between IBS and organic intestinal diseases.

13. How is IBS diagnosed?
IBS can be confidently diagnosed in the vast majority of patients based on identifying typical symptoms and evaluating for alarm features, performing general physical examinations and routine laboratory studies. While IBS has historically been thought of as a diagnosis of exclusion, studies have confirmed the accuracy of making a positive diagnosis of IBS without performing extensive testing, which shortens the time to appropriate therapy and reduces the amount of expensive and sometimes invasive testing that patients with suspected IBS ultimately undergo.

14. What are the typical symptoms of IBS?
The key defining symptom of IBS is abdominal pain, which is typically localized to the lower abdomen but can be noted throughout the abdomen. Symptoms are often intermittent and are associated with changes in stool frequency and/or consistency. Although the Rome IV criteria require abdominal pain to be present only one day per week over the prior 3 months, they often occur more frequently, particularly in individuals who seek medical care. Other symptoms that are common but not essential for the diagnosis include bloating or feeling of abdominal distention, rectal urgency, and incomplete evacuation.

15. What testing is necessary for patients with suspected IBS?
CBC should be checked in all patients with suspected IBS without alarm symptoms. In patients with suspected IBS-D, it is also recommended that serologic testing to rule out celiac disease, as there is a significantly higher prevalence of this condition in patients meeting symptom criteria for IBS. Fecal calprotectin and serum C-reactive protein be checked as well. In patients with suspected IBS-C, a thyroid-stimulating hormone if clinically appropriate could be considered. Current guidelines recommend against stool testing for enteric pathogens, food allergy testing, and routine colonoscopy in those under the age of 45, unless there is a specific clinical rationale for doing so. It should be noted that if a colonoscopy is performed on a patient with suspected IBS-D, random biopsies should be obtained to exclude microscopic colitis, as a recent study found microscopic colitis present in 2.5% of patients older than the age of 35.

16. What alarm features warrant further testing in diagnosing IBS?
Alarm features such as rectal bleeding, unintended weight loss, fever, older age of onset of symptoms, nocturnal awakening from sleep, or a family history of colon cancer or inflammatory bowel disease may suggest the presence of an organic disease and generally warrant further testing.

17. What is the role of fructose intolerance?
Fructose is the sweetest of sugars and therefore is commonly used as a sweetener in soft drinks, chocolate, syrups, and jams. Fructose is also naturally present in many fruits and vegetables and in honey. Up to one-half of healthy adults have evidence of malabsorption after ingesting 25 g of fructose (10% concentration). Fructose

Carbohydrate Breath Testing for SIBO

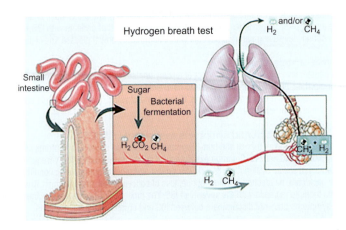

Fig. 61.2 Carbohydrate breath testing for small intestinal bacterial overgrowth (SIBO).

intolerance can cause symptoms similar to those found in IBS; therefore patients ingesting large amounts of fructose should be advised to reduce their intake. The prevalence of fructose malabsorption in IBS is similar to that in healthy individuals and therefore it is unlikely to be the cause of IBS in most patients.

18. What is the role of lactose intolerance?

The prevalence of lactose intolerance is slightly higher in adults with IBS; however, even though the symptoms due to lactose intolerance can be similar to IBS, lactose intolerance is not the cause of IBS in most patients. Nevertheless, an empiric trial of a lactose-free diet or testing with a lactose hydrogen breath test, which measures the exhaled hydrogen produced from colonic bacterial degradation of lactose, should be considered. Patients who respond to a lactose-free diet should be encouraged to gradually reintroduce lactose into their diet to determine if and when symptoms recur. Most people with lactose intolerance can consume up to 1.25 cups (280 mL) of milk per day without significant symptoms. Avoidance of lactose can lead to a significant reduction in calcium intake, which may increase the risk of osteoporosis. Therefore patients on a restricted lactose diet should be advised to increase their calcium intake from other sources. Live-culture yogurt is another alternative source of calcium that is well tolerated by many patients with lactose intolerance.

19. What is the role of small intestinal bacterial overgrowth (SIBO) in IBS?

SIBO is a condition in which the small bowel is colonized by microbes normally found in the large intestine. SIBO appears to be more common in IBS, although the reported incidence of SIBO varies according to the detection method employed. SIBO can be evaluated by breath testing, which assesses end-expiratory breath concentration of hydrogen and methane, and in some cases hydrogen sulfide, after ingestion of a fermentable carbohydrate (either glucose 50–75 g or lactulose 10 g). In those with SIBO, microbial anaerobic fermentation of glucose/lactulose leads to increased production of these gases, which then diffuse into a patient's systemic circulation and are subsequently expired from the lungs (Fig. 61.2).

NONPHARMACOLOGIC IRRITABLE BOWEL SYNDROME APPROACHES

20. What is the role of food in IBS?

Most patients with IBS report worsening symptoms following ingestion of foods. The most commonly implicated foods are milk and dairy products, wheat products, onions, peas and beans, hot spices, cabbage, certain meats, smoked products, fried food, and caffeine. However, the dietary composition of patients with IBS is similar to that of the general community. There is no documented evidence showing that a food allergy mediated by immunoglobulin E plays a role in IBS symptoms.

Many patients adopt an inappropriately restrictive diet in the setting of IBS symptoms. Dietary history can help to determine if a significant correlation exists between a particular food and IBS symptoms. If a correlation exists, the offending food should be eliminated from the diet to discover if symptoms resolve. Resolution of symptoms suggests, but does not confirm, a diagnosis of a causal relationship between the food and IBS.

Diets deficient in fiber (e.g., fruits, vegetables, and grains) may help to explain constipation. Diets with excessive amounts of gas-producing foods (e.g., beans, cabbage, legumes, cauliflower, broccoli, lentils, and Brussels sprouts), poorly absorbed carbohydrates (e.g., fructose or sorbitol), or lactose in patients who are lactose intolerant, may explain excessive flatus, bloating, or diarrhea. Excessive air swallowing, which commonly occurs in people who smoke, chew gum, or eat rapidly, may help explain excessive flatulence. Diets consisting of large fatty meals or caffeine may help explain postprandial rectal urgency and bowel frequency.

The low fermentable oligo-, di-, and monosaccharides and polyols (FODMAP) diet (discussed below) is the most evidence-based dietary intervention for IBS. While many other dietary interventions have been proposed, caution should be exercised before recommending dietary restriction, as it has been estimated that up to 20% of individuals with IBS may screen positive for avoidant restrictive food intake disorder, which can be exacerbated by the recommendation for a restricted diet.

21. What are FODMAPs?

FODMAPs are fermentable oligosaccharides, disaccharides, monosaccharides, and polyols. They include fructose, lactose, fructans, galactans, and sugar alcohols, such as sorbitol, maltitol, mannitol, xylitol, and isomalt. Fructose and lactose are present in apples, pears, watermelon, honey, fruit juices, dried fruits, milk, and dairy products. Polyols are used as a sugar replacement in low-calorie food products. Galactans and fructans are present in common dietary constituents, such as wheat, rye, garlic, onions, legumes, cabbage, artichokes, leeks, asparagus, lentils, inulin, soy, Brussels sprouts, and broccoli. Recent studies suggest many patients with IBS have improvement in symptoms on a low FODMAP diet, although further studies are needed to determine which patients are most likely to improve.

22. What is the FODMAP diet?

As previously noted, FODMAPs are poorly absorbed in the small intestine. A diet high in FODMAPs has been associated with higher levels of hydrogen produced in the breath in both patients with IBS and healthy individuals as well as GI symptoms and lethargy primarily in patients with IBS. It is likely that a low FODMAP diet reduces the fermentation of these carbohydrates and subsequent hydrogen production, therefore reducing IBS symptoms such as bloating, abdominal pain, and flatulence (Table 61.1).

The low FODMAP diet is a significantly restrictive diet and thus may not be the best option for patients with a history of eating disorder or for whom there is concern over malnutrition or weight loss. Additionally, it may not be the best treatment option for those individuals who do not consume a large quantity of FODMAP-containing foods at baseline. Nonetheless, it does represent an attractive nonpharmacologic option for treating IBS for many individuals when done correctly. The low FODMAP diet starts with a 4–6 week elimination phase, in which all high FODMAP foods are significantly reduced from a given patient's diet. If no symptom improvement is noted, the trial of a low FODMAP diet is abandoned. If significant improvement is noted; however, the patient then goes through

Table 61.1 The Fermentable Oligosaccharides, Disaccharides, Monosaccharides, and Polyols (FODMAP) Diet.

HIGH FODMAP FOODS	LOW FODMAP FOODS
High-fructose-containing fruit: apples, pears, and watermelon	Low-fructose-containing fruit: bananas, grapes, and strawberries
Fructan-containing vegetables: onions, asparagus, and artichokes	Low-fructan-containing vegetables: spinach, carrots, and eggplant
High-galactan-containing foods: legumes, lentils, and soy	Low-galactan-containing foods: tofu and peanuts
Wheat-based products: bread, pasta, and cereals	Wheat-free grains: oats, quinoa, and corn
Sorbitol-containing foods	Sucrose, glucose, and pure maple syrup
Lactose-containing foods: milk, ice cream, and soft and fresh cheeses	Lactose-free foods: lactose-free milk, rice milk, and hard cheese

a reintroduction phase, where various classes of FODMAP-containing foods are individually reintroduced (usually over 3 days, with increasing quantity over this 3-day period) to better identify specific FODMAP-containing foods that a given patient is intolerant to. The goal by the end of this reintroduction phase is to arrive at a personalized diet that eliminates obvious trigger foods but is also not unnecessarily restrictive. It has been estimated that 76% of patients following the low FODMAP diet are able to liberalize their diet after completion of the reintroduction phase. This is often best accomplished with the assistance of a registered dietician though many web and app-based tools are available to assist patients.

23. What is the role of gluten-free diet in IBS?
Although many patients with IBS empirically report an improvement in symptoms on a gluten-free diet, rigorous evidence from controlled trials is lacking. Gluten elimination is a significant component of the previously discussed low FODMAP diet. However, a recent study suggested that even among those with self-reported gluten sensitivity, fructans rather than gluten was the major trigger of symptoms.

24. What is the role of fiber in IBS?
Recent guidelines suggest the use of soluble fiber supplementation in patients with IBS, as it has been shown to improve global IBS symptoms with only minor side effects. However, insoluble fiber has not been shown to significantly improve global IBS symptoms and is more commonly associated with bloating and abdominal pain. Fiber is frequently associated with increased gas production, abdominal cramps, and bloating, many patients are reluctant to follow a high-fiber diet.

Therefore a prudent approach in patients with IBS with mild to moderate IBS is to initially instruct them to gradually increase dietary fiber intake to approximately 20–25 g per day over several weeks. If adding fiber to the diet fails to relieve symptoms, psyllium should be tried next because of its ability to absorb water. If psyllium is not tolerated, then a trial with the semisynthetic fiber methylcellulose or the synthetic fiber polycarbophil should be considered.

25. What is the role of cognitive-behavioral therapy (CBT) in IBS?
CBT is the best-studied psychologic treatment for IBS. Cognitive techniques (typically administered over 4–15 sessions) are aimed at changing catastrophic or maladaptive thinking patterns underlying the perception of somatic symptoms. Behavioral techniques aim to modify dysfunctional behaviors through relaxation techniques, contingency management (rewarding healthy behaviors), or assertion training. Randomized controlled trials have also shown reductions in IBS symptoms with CBT versus control therapy (including waiting list, symptom monitoring, and usual medical treatment). A home-based CBT (with minimal therapist contact) has also demonstrated significant symptom improvement compared to those receiving standard IBS education. App-based CBT without any direct therapist contact has recently received Food and Drug Administration (FDA) clearance.

Other psychologic treatments may also play a role in improving IBS symptoms, though further study is needed for all of these psychologic interventions, including gut-directed hypnosis, which involves relaxation, change in beliefs, and self-management.

26. Can exercise improve IBS symptoms?
Physical activity has a number of positive physiologic and psychologic effects. In the GI tract, exercise can increase overall gut motility, including colonic motility and colon transit time. In a recent study, 12 weeks of moderate to rigorous exercise (20–60 minutes three times per week) resulted in significant improvement in IBS symptoms, although there were no differences in stool quality or characteristics, or in symptoms like bloating.

PHARMACOLOGIC APPROACHES TO IRRITABLE BOWEL SYNDROME

27. What is the pharmacologic approach in treating IBS?
Pharmacologic treatment is usually aimed at treating and preventing the predominant symptoms, such as diarrhea, constipation, and abdominal pain. Pharmacologic treatment options for patients who report diarrhea as their predominant symptom include antidiarrheals, such as loperamide, cholestyramine, eluxadoline, or alosetron. For patients who report constipation as their predominant symptom, treatment options include fiber, osmotic laxatives (i.e., polyethylene glycol), secretagogues (lubiprostone, linaclotide, plecanatide, and tenapanor), or prokinetic agents (prucalopride and tegaserod). For patients who report pain as the predominant symptom, treatment options include antispasmodics (peppermint oil, dicyclomine, and hyoscyamine) and neuromodulators (most often a tricyclic antidepressant [TCA] such as amitriptyline or desipramine) (Fig. 61.3).

28. What is the role of antidepressants in IBS?
Antidepressants are commonly used for moderate to severe abdominal symptoms associated with IBS. TCA medications are the most commonly used antidepressants for IBS symptoms. Typically, the TCAs are administered in low doses (e.g., between 10 and 50 mg), though guidelines do allow for dose escalation past this level. The exact mechanism of action is not clear but includes visceral analgesia, improvement in sleep, and slowing of

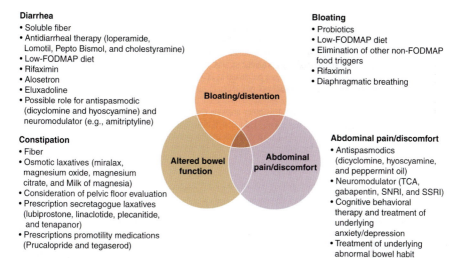

Diarrhea
- Soluble fiber
- Antidiarrheal therapy (loperamide, Lomotil, Pepto Bismol, and cholestyramine)
- Low-FODMAP diet
- Rifaximin
- Alosetron
- Eluxadoline
- Possible role for antispasmodic (dicyclomine and hyoscyamine) and neuromodulator (e.g., amitriptyline)

Constipation
- Fiber
- Osmotic laxatives (miralax, magnesium oxide, magnesium citrate, and Milk of magnesia)
- Consideration of pelvic floor evaluation
- Prescription secretagogue laxatives (lubiprostone, linaclotide, plecanitide, and tenapanor)
- Prescriptions promotility medications (Prucalopride and tegaserod)

Bloating
- Probiotics
- Low-FODMAP diet
- Elimination of other non-FODMAP food triggers
- Rifaximin
- Diaphragmatic breathing

Abdominal pain/discomfort
- Antispasmodics (dicyclomine, hyoscyamine, and peppermint oil)
- Neuromodulator (TCA, gabapentin, SNRI, and SSRI)
- Cognitive behavioral therapy and treatment of underlying anxiety/depression
- Treatment of underlying abnormal bowel habit

Bloating/distention

Altered bowel function

Abdominal pain/discomfort

Fig. 61.3 Pharmacologic treatments of irritable bowel syndrome. *SNRI*, Serotonin and norepinephrine reuptake inhibitor; *SSRI*, selective serotonin reuptake inhibitor; *TCA*, tricyclic antidepressant.

the GI transit. Their effects on IBS appear to be independent of the effect on depression or other psychologic parameters. In clinical practice, these medications are often used in patients in whom pain is a predominant symptom. A recent meta-analysis noted 12 randomized controlled trials comparing TCAs to placebo and noted that TCAs were significantly associated with improvement in IBS symptoms, with a number needed to treat of 4.5. Notably though, this class of medication is also associated with adverse effects like dry mouth, constipation, and drowsiness, which can be of particular concern in older individuals.

Selective serotonin reuptake inhibitors (SSRIs) are a very commonly utilized class of medication for anxiety and depression symptoms. Though anxiety and depression often coexist with IBS, there is a lack of clear evidence that these medications improve IBS symptoms and current guidelines suggest against the use of SSRIs in patients with IBS. Nonetheless, there are some patients who do experience clear improvement in their IBS symptoms with this class of medications. Because serotonin is associated with diarrhea, SSRIs may be better tolerated in IBS-C. Other psychiatric medications like buspirone, mirtazapine, and serotonin-norepinephrine reuptake inhibitors (SNRIs) like duloxetine are often utilized in IBS. However, large-scale clinical trials for these classes of antidepressants in IBS are lacking, and there is currently no guideline recommendation for or against their use in IBS.

29. What is the role of antispasmodics in IBS?
Antispasmodics decrease contractions or spasms in the GI tract and thereby reduce abdominal cramps. Patients with IBS have exaggerated sigmoid contractions in response to meals and to stress, which may explain the postprandial discomfort and urgency in some patients. There are three antispasmodics currently available in the United States: hyoscyamine, dicyclomine, and peppermint oil (there are multiple different formulations of the latter).

Hyoscyamine and dicyclomine work by blocking the acetylcholine-mediated depolarization of intestinal smooth muscles, while peppermint oil blocks the entry of calcium into smooth muscle cells and resulting in smooth muscle contraction. Antispasmodics can be taken at regular intervals (up to four times daily) or intermittently for more episodic symptoms. For patients with postprandial symptoms, the medications can be taken 30–45 minutes before a meal. For patients with less predictable and more intermittent symptoms, hyoscyamine is often preferable because it also comes in an easily dissolvable tablet, which can be taken sublingually and acts within minutes. Current guidelines suggest the use of antispasmodics in patients with IBS, as they have been shown to help with both abdominal pain and global IBS symptoms (though their impact on global IBS symptoms has not been consistently shown in studies). Though they can be used in patients with different underlying stool consistency, they are more often utilized in those with IBS-D, as the anticholinergic effects of hyoscyamine and dicyclomine can further slow gut transit.

30. What is the role of probiotics in IBS?
Given the postulated role of gut microbiota in IBS, probiotic medications have also been commonly utilized in their treatment. Probiotics are live organisms (bacteria) that are thought to exert a health benefit on the host through

multiple proposed mechanisms including modulation of bacterial flora, improvement of the barrier function of the epithelium, modulation of expression of pain receptors, and alteration of the immune activity of the host. However, mechanistic evidence for these hypotheses in IBS is still very limited.

Additionally, the large number of probiotic products that are available has made it difficult to draw definitive conclusions about the efficacy of individual probiotic strains. Well-conducted large multicenter dose-ranging studies are generally lacking. A meta-analysis published in 2018 included 53 randomized controlled trials evaluating the efficacy, safety, and tolerability of probiotics in patients with IBS and found some evidence of beneficial effects on global IBS symptoms and abdominal pain, though noting that it was unclear which particular strain or species was of maximal benefit. This meta-analysis did note that adverse events were not significantly increased in those taking probiotics compared to placebo. It also noted that there were insufficient data to support the use of prebiotics or symbiotics in IBS. Due to the lack of strong evidence for their efficacy, current guidelines do not recommend probiotics for the treatment of global IBS symptoms.

DIARRHEA

31. What is the role of loperamide in IBS?

Loperamide is a synthetic peripheral opioid agonist that reduces gut transit, as well as reducing the secretion of water into the gut. Loperamide has long been a mainstay in the treatment of IBS. Loperamide reduces gut motility, which allows for greater fluid absorption and improved stool consistency. Loperamide does not cross the blood-brain barrier at standard doses and therefore does not have central nervous system effects. While older studies of it did not demonstrate improvement in global IBS symptoms, most patients with IBS-D do experience a reduction in diarrhea and frequency with it, as well as improvement in stool consistency. Loperamide 2–4 mg each morning after the initial bowel movement and before social events can reduce undesirable urges to defecate and increase confidence and willingness to engage in social activities. Current guidelines suggest using loperamide in patients with IBS-D.

32. What is the role of antibiotics in IBS?

Rifaximin is a minimally absorbed oral antibiotic with a broad spectrum of activity and a favorable tolerability profile that has been extensively studied in IBS-D. Rifaximin has been shown to improve global IBS symptoms and is approved by the US FDA for the treatment of IBS-D. The recommended dose is 550 mg three times daily for 2 weeks. Patients taking rifaximin are more likely to achieve adequate relief of their global IBS symptoms, IBS-related bloating, and IBS-related pain compared with placebo-treated patients, although its efficacy declines over time in some patients (one study showed that in those with recurrence of abdominal pain symptoms following initial treatment, the median time to recurrence was 3.5 months). Notably, it has also been shown that two additional courses of treatment with rifaximin after loss of initial response can be effective.

Other antibiotics have also been utilized in the treatment of IBS, although they are less studied than rifaximin. One example is the antibiotic neomycin, which is sometimes used in combination with rifaximin for treatment of a phenomenon called intestinal methanogen overgrowth (IMO), which results from colonization with a nonbacterial organism called *Methanobrevibacter smithii*, and is often associated with both bloating and constipation. While it has been shown to improve symptoms in the subset of patients with IBS-C and IMO, neomycin also has the potential to cause adverse reactions, including ototoxicity, nephrotoxicity, and neuromuscular blockade and respiratory paralysis, especially when given soon after anesthesia or muscle relaxants. Therefore it should be used cautiously for the treatment of IBS. Other antibiotics like metronidazole and augmentin have been utilized by some providers for treating IBS, though large-scale trials evaluating their effectiveness are lacking.

33. What is the role of alosetron in IBS?

Alosetron is a selective serotonin receptor antagonist used to treat diarrhea symptoms. Although alosetron was approved in 2000 by the FDA for adult females with IBS-D, it was removed from the market later that year because of concerns about its safety, particularly severe constipation, and ischemic colitis. However, as a result of public demand, the FDA in June 2002 reinstated Alosetron for females with chronic, severe IBS-D unresponsive to conventional therapy. This required adherence to the manufacturer's prescribing program starting at a lower dose of 0.5 mg twice daily (with instruction for further dose reduction if constipation occurs on this dose). This prescribing program was effective in achieving global improvement in bowel symptoms for females with severe IBS-D and produced much fewer complications of constipation. The risk of ischemic colitis remained similar though relatively low (approximately one case per 1000 patient-years). Current American Gastroenterological Association guidelines suggest its use in patients with IBS-D who have failed more conventional therapies.

34. What is the role of eluxadoline in IBS?

Eluxadoline was FDA-approved treatment for the management of IBS-D in 2015. It is classified as a mixed opioid receptor agonist and antagonist; it acts as an agonist on μ and κ receptors and as an antagonist on δ receptors. It has been shown to improve stool consistency, fecal urgency, and to a lesser extent abdominal pain, though its effect on the latter symptom may be comparatively less pronounced. It is contraindicated in those with a history of cholecystectomy, as there is an increased risk of pancreatitis in these patients. There is also thought to be an increased risk of sphincter of Oddi spasm in those with a history of excessive alcohol use (i.e., those who drink more than three alcoholic beverages per day) or known sphincter of Oddi disease.

CONSTIPATION

35. What is the role of laxatives in IBS?

When constipation associated with IBS does not improve with fiber, osmotic laxatives should be tried first as they tend to be gentler and cause fewer side effects such as cramps and diarrhea than other laxatives. Osmotic laxatives such as polyethylene glycol have not been proven to improve abdominal pain, though on an individual level, many patients do not show improvement in pain symptoms with regular usage of osmotic laxatives.

It should be remembered that patients with constipation should be evaluated for pelvic floor dyssynergia, because many of these patients may respond to biofeedback therapy, a technique that retrains patients to relax their pelvic floor muscles when attempting defecation.

36. What is the role of guanylate cyclase activators in IBS?

Linaclotide and plecanatide are two guanylate cyclase-C agonists that are FDA approved for the treatment of IBS-C. Both medications work by increasing intestinal fluid secretion. In two large, randomized trials, linaclotide resulted in improvement in abdominal pain, bowel function, and global outcomes in patients with IBS-C. This, combined with a good safety and tolerability profile, suggests that linaclotide is an effective treatment for IBS-C. There was similar evidence for the efficacy of plecanatide in phase 3 trials.

Diarrhea is a common side effect with both medications, though may be less frequent with plecanatide. Linaclotide is available in three different dosages (72, 145, and 290 mcg), which may allow for easier dose titration for individual patients.

37. What is the role of lubiprostone in IBS?

Lubiprostone is a chloride channel activator that increases secretions in the intestines, thereby increasing bowel transit. It acts locally on the epithelial cells that line the intestines and is rapidly metabolized, which leads to low systemic bioavailability. This medication is typically administered twice daily, at a dose of 8 mcg, though 24 mcg is also available for patients with chronic constipation. It is approved by the FDA for females with IBS-C; however, for chronic constipation, lubiprostone is approved for males and females.

38. What is the role of 5-HT4 agonists in IBS?

Stimulating serotonin type 4 (5-HT4) receptors has a promotility effect in the GI tract. Tegaserod is a 5-HT4 agonist that can be used for the treatment of IBS-C. It has been shown in multiple large placebo-controlled clinical trials to improve both global IBS symptoms, and may also improve additional symptoms like abdominal pain, stool consistency, stool frequency, and bloating. It was previously approved in 2002 but was withdrawn from the US market in 2007 due to concern over excessive cardiovascular events with it. This medication was more recently reapproved in 2019 specifically for females less than 65 years of age, with one or fewer cardiovascular risk factors.

Prucalopride is another high-affinity 5-HT4 agonist that was approved by the FDA in 2018 for the treatment of chronic idiopathic constipation. In clinical trials in patients with chronic idiopathic constipation, prucalopride improves constipation symptoms as well as HR-QOL. It is also thought to have a promotility effect on the stomach and small bowel as well and may thus be utilized as a treatment option in individuals with concomitant delayed gastric emptying.

39. What is the role of tenapanor in IBS?

Tenapanor is an inhibitor of sodium/hydrogen exchanger isoform 3 in the small intestine and colon. It reduces absorption of sodium and phosphate and thus increases water secretion in the intestine. It has been shown in clinical trials to improve both abdominal pain and bowel frequency in those with IBS-C. As is the case with other prescription medications utilized for constipation, its main associated side effect is diarrhea. This medication was approved by the FDA for the treatment of IBS-C in 2019, and current guidelines suggest its use in patients with IBS-C.

BIBLIOGRAPHY

Available Online

CHAPTER 62

ENDOSCOPIC CANCER SCREENING AND SURVEILLANCE

Zachary Johnston, MD and Jeffrey Laczek, MD, FACP, FACG

 Additional content available online

1. **What is endoscopic cancer screening and surveillance?**
   Endoscopic screening is the use of endoscopy (i.e., upper endoscopy, colonoscopy, endoscopic ultrasound [EUS], or wireless capsule endoscopy) in apparently healthy individuals to detect cancer or precancerous conditions.
   Endoscopic surveillance is the use of endoscopy in patients with known malignant or premalignant conditions to detect cancer or identify changes that need additional treatment or evaluation.

2. **Why is endoscopic cancer screening and surveillance performed for gastrointestinal (GI) cancers?**
   Colorectal cancer (CRC) is the third leading cause of cancer death in the United States for both males and females, with an estimated 151,030 new cases and 52,580 deaths in 2022. The lifetime risk of developing CRC is 4.1% based on 2017–19 data. CRC has well-defined premalignant lesions that are easily identifiable on endoscopy; recognition and treatment of these lesions have contributed to the decline in new cases and deaths from colon cancer over the past decades. Other GI conditions have similar premalignant conditions that can also be identified to prevent cancer and cancer-related deaths.

ESOPHAGUS

3. **Endoscopic cancer screening of the esophagus is primarily undertaken for what two types of esophageal cancers? What risk factors are associated with these two types of cancers?**
   Esophageal adenocarcinoma (EAC) and esophageal squamous cell carcinoma (SCC) are the two major types of esophageal cancer. Esophageal cancer is much more common in males than females, with a relative risk of 3.4.
   - EAC is the most common type of esophageal cancer in the United States; it is increasing in prevalence and is highly associated with Barrett esophagus (BE), gastroesophageal reflux disease (GERD), and obesity. EAC is more common in White Americans than Black Americans.
   - SCC is the most common type of esophageal cancer worldwide but less common than EAC in the United States. Esophageal SCC is more common in Black Americans than White Americans. The major risk factors for esophageal SCC include alcohol use, tobacco use, and human papillomavirus infection. Achalasia, caustic injury to the esophagus, tylosis, and Plummer-Vinson syndrome, while uncommon, are also associated with esophageal SCC.

4. **What is BE? Is endoscopic screening and surveillance for BE necessary?**
   BE is intestinal metaplasia in the tubular esophagus (i.e., replacement of the normal esophageal squamous epithelium with specialized columnar epithelium containing goblet cells). For the diagnosis of BE, there must be at least 1 cm of columnar epithelium within the esophagus. Screening for, and subsequent surveillance of, BE is important because BE is the only known precursor lesion to EAC.

5. **Which patients should undergo endoscopic screening for BE?**
   Patients with chronic GERD (at least weekly symptoms for 5 or more years) should undergo screening for BE if they have three or more of the following risk factors:
   - Male sex
   - Age >50 years
   - White race
   - Tobacco smoking
   - Obesity
   - First-degree relative (FDR) with BE or EAC
     After a negative screening examination, repeat screening is not recommended unless significant esophagitis (Los Angeles grade B or worse) was noted on the index examination.

6. What techniques are used to perform endoscopic screening in BE?

During upper endoscopy, all salmon-colored mucosa within the esophagus should be evaluated with a careful high-definition white light examination plus electronic chromoendoscopy or acetic acid chromoendoscopy. Electronic chromoendoscopy, typically achieved using narrow wavelengths of light, highlights mucosal and vascular patterns. Nondysplastic BE (NDBE) has a cerebriform mucosal pattern (resembling the gyri of the brain) and elongated pit patterns. Disordered or crowded pit patterns suggest dysplasia or early neoplasia. Dilute (1.5%–3%) acetic acid causes a white change in the mucosa, highlighting mucosa patterns; premature loss of this white color may indicate early neoplasia.

7. How is BE histologically graded?

BE is histologically graded as follows:
- Nondysplastic.
- Low-grade dysplasia (LGD).
- High-grade dysplasia (HGD).
- Indeterminant for dysplasia (IND) indicates that the pathologist is unable to determine if dysplasia is truly present or if the histology represents inflammatory changes. BE IND should be confirmed by a second pathologist with GI experience. Studies of patients with BE IND have shown similar rates of progression to HGD and/or EAC as patients with BE with LGD, leading to the management recommendations below.

8. What is the rationale for endoscopic surveillance in BE?

The incidence of EAC in patients with BE is approximately 5 per 1000 patient-years. Given the dismal prognosis of EAC, surveillance of BE offers the opportunity to detect and treat precursor lesions (LGD or HGD) or very early EAC that is curable with endoscopic treatment.

9. How often should patients with BE undergo endoscopic surveillance?

The American Society for Gastrointestinal Endoscopy recommends an upper endoscopy every 3–5 years for surveillance of NDBE. The American College of Gastroenterology recommends an upper endoscopy every 3 years for NDBE 3 cm or greater in length and every 5 years for NDBE less than 3 cm in length. BE with LGD or IND should undergo more frequent surveillance (Table 62.1).

10. How is LGD managed in patients with BE?

LGD should be confirmed by an expert GI pathologist. If LGD is confirmed, the overall annual risk of progression to HGD/EAC is 4.6 per 100 patient-years, with the rate being significantly higher (8.8 per 100 patient-years) in the first year after diagnosis. Endoscopic eradication therapy (EET) and intensive surveillance, as outlined in Table 62.1, are both options for managing LGD; the risks and benefits of these options should be discussed with the patient.

11. How do you manage HGD in patients with BE?

BE with HGD is associated with a 6% per year risk of progression to EAC. HGD should be confirmed by an expert pathologist. Given the high risk of progression to EAC and the significant morbidity and mortality associated with

Table 62.1 2022 American College of Gastroenterology Guidelines: Recommended Endoscopic Surveillance Intervals for Barrett Esophagus Based on the Degree of Dysplasia and Segment Length.

BASELINE ENDOSCOPIC FINDING	SUGGESTED ENDOSCOPIC SURVEILLANCE
Nondysplastic BE of <3 cm in length	EGD every 5 years
Nondysplastic BE of ≥3 cm in length	EGD every 3 years
BE indefinite for dysplasia, any length (confirmed by a second pathologist)	Repeat EGD within 6 months after increasing PPI to twice-daily dosing, if not already on high-dose PPI If repeat EGD yields a diagnosis of NDBE or LGD, treat using that algorithm If repeat EGD demonstrates BE indefinite for dysplasia, EGD annually
BE with LGD (confirmed by a second pathologist and opting for endoscopic surveillance)	EGD at 6 months from diagnosis EGD 12 months from diagnosis EGD annually thereafter

BE, Barrett esophagus; *EGD*, esophagogastroduodenoscopy; *LGD*, low-grade dysplasia; *NDBE*, nondysplastic BE; *PPI*, proton pump inhibitor.

Adapted from Shaheen N, Falk GW, Iyer PG, Souza RF, Yadlapti RH, Sauer BG, et al. Diagnosis and management of Barrett's esophagus: an updated ACG guideline. Am J Gastroenterol. 2022;117:559-587.

esophagectomy, EET is the recommended treatment for BE with HGD. Intramucosal EAC (T1a), which is usually diagnosed on a specimen from endoscopic mucosal resection (EMR), is treated similar to BE with HGD. More advanced EAC (i.e., T1b) is generally treated with esophagectomy due to the unacceptably high risk of lymph node metastases, but EET may be an option for patients with superficial submucosal invasion (sm1—invasion into the upper third of the submucosa to a depth <500 μm) and low-risk features such as a negative deep margin, well to moderate differentiation and no lymphovascular invasion.

12. **What is the role of endoscopic resection (ER) of visible lesions in BE?**
    All visible lesions in BE (i.e., nodules within Barrett mucosa) should undergo ER using either EMR or endoscopic submucosal dissection (ESD). The specimens obtained by ER are larger and deeper (usually including the muscularis mucosa and submucosa) than forceps biopsies, helping to more accurately stage early EAC. ER is particularly important prior to EET.

13. **What EET options are available?**
    Radiofrequency ablation (RFA) and cryotherapy are the two EET methods currently in widespread use. The goal of EET is the complete elimination of intestinal mucosa (CEIM). Patients undergoing EET should be treated at high-volume centers, and intensive surveillance is recommended following CEIM. EUSs are often performed prior to EET to evaluate for evidence of occult cancer, such as lymphadenopathy.

14. **Describe the workup once EAC is identified while performing endoscopic surveillance for BE.**
    Patients in whom EAC is identified during surveillance of BE should undergo a computed tomography (CT) scan of the chest and abdomen. If no evidence of metastatic disease is detected on CT scan, further evaluation should be performed with EUS and positron emission tomography–CT scan. When technically feasible, ER should be performed for early-stage cancers for the most accurate T staging. After the completion of the workup, patients should undergo multidisciplinary evaluation prior to determining a treatment course.

15. **Do patients with achalasia have an increased risk of esophageal cancer?**
    Yes. Individuals with achalasia have an increased risk of developing esophageal SCC compared with the general population. Estimates of this risk range from 16 to 28 times the risk of age- and sex-matched controls. Overall, cancer tends to occur when patients are in their 70s, following decades of symptoms.

16. **What is the role of endoscopic cancer surveillance in patients with achalasia?**
    Surveillance for SCC in patients with achalasia is not routinely recommended but may be considered 15 years after the onset of symptoms. All surface abnormalities of the esophagus identified during the examination should undergo biopsy. The frequency of surveillance endoscopy has not been defined.

17. **Is there a link between caustic ingestion and the development of esophageal cancer?**
    Yes. A caustic injury to the esophagus, most commonly after lye ingestion, is associated with an increased risk of developing SCC of the esophagus. A history of caustic ingestion is present in 1%–4% of patients with esophageal cancer and surveillance is recommended starting 20 years after the ingestion.

18. **What is tylosis and what endoscopic surveillance is recommended for it?**
    Tylosis is an uncommon autosomal dominant disorder that is distinguished by the thickening of the skin (hyperkeratosis) on the palms and soles. The syndrome is associated with a 27% incidence of esophageal SCC. The average age of onset of esophageal cancer is 45 years with mortality from esophageal cancer occurring in patients as young as 30 years. Patients with tylosis should be under surveillance for SCC with an upper endoscopy every 1–3 years starting at the age of 30 years. Most cases of esophageal cancer in these patients have been noted in the distal esophagus; attention should be focused on this area during the examination.

19. **What type of endoscopic surveillance is recommended in patients with tylosis?**
    Patients with tylosis should begin endoscopic surveillance at the age of 30 years. Most cases of esophageal cancer in these patients have been noted in the distal esophagus, so attention should be focused on this area during the examination. Repeat endoscopy should not be conducted more frequently than every 1–3 years in these patients.

STOMACH AND SMALL BOWEL

20. **What is the malignant potential of gastric polyps?**
    Gastric polyps are often found incidentally during endoscopy and most can be histologically classified as hyperplastic, fundic gland, or adenomatous polyps.
    - Hyperplastic polyps occur in response to chronic inflammation in the stomach (i.e., *Helicobacter pylori* infection or chronic atrophic gastritis). In areas of the world where *H. pylori* infection is common, hyperplastic polyps

are the most common type of gastric polyps. Hyperplastic polyps may have malignant potential, but the risk appears low. The risk of malignancy is higher in large (>1 cm) polyps or pedunculated polyps.

- Fundic gland polyps are associated with proton pump inhibitor use, familial adenomatous polyposis (FAP), and MUTYH-associated polyposis (MAP). Sporadic and proton pump inhibitor—associated fundic gland polyps have essentially no malignant potential. In a study of 75 patients undergoing surveillance of FAP, fundic gland polyps were found in 88% of patients and were dysplastic in 41%. The dysplasia in FAP-associated fundic gland polyps is typically low grade and, interestingly, the dysplasia in FAP-associated fundic gland polyps rarely progresses to cancer.
- Adenomatous polyps have definite malignant potential, which correlates with the size of the polyp and the age of the patient.

21. **How are gastric polyps managed when encountered radiographically or endoscopically?**
Endoscopic evaluation is warranted for polyps of any size that are detected radiographically. Endoscopically, fundic gland polyps appear similar in color to the surrounding mucosa and are shiny, often with tiny surface blood vessels. Other types of gastric polyps cannot reliably be distinguished by their endoscopic appearance, so a biopsy or polypectomy should be performed when such polyps are detected. When multiple polyps are encountered, the largest polyp(s) should be biopsied or removed as well as any atypical appearing polyps. If the polyps all appear similar, a representative polyp or polyps should be biopsied or removed.

22. **Is endoscopic surveillance required after the removal of a gastric polyp?**
After complete removal of an adenomatous gastric polyp, repeat endoscopy is recommended in 1 year, followed by a surveillance endoscopy every 3–5 years. HGD or other aggressive features necessitate closer surveillance. Fundic gland polyps generally do not need surveillance. The surveillance necessary for small hyperplastic polyps remains unclear but *H. pylori* infection, if present, should be treated. Large hyperplastic polyps tend to be recalcitrant and need close follow-up after removal.

23. **What is gastric intestinal metaplasia (GIM)?**
GIM, intestinal mucosa occurring in the stomach, is part of the Correa cascade, whereby there is a progression from normal gastric mucosa to chronic gastritis, atrophic gastritis, intestinal metaplasia, dysplasia, and ultimately to gastric cancer. *H. pylori* infection, tobacco use, and dietary factors (i.e., nitroso compounds and a high salt diet) have been implicated as causative factors, as has autoimmune metaplasia.

24. **How common is GIM? What is its malignant potential?**
GIM is common in the United States. Based on a 2020 study encompassing over 36,000 upper endoscopies performed during a 15-year period, the point prevalence of GIM was 12%. Non-White race, increasing age, and *H. pylori* infection were associated with GIM. The overall risk of gastric cancer in US patients with GIM is 0.16% per year, although patient and disease characteristics have been identified that portend a higher risk (see Question 25).

25. **What role does endoscopic surveillance have in GIM?**
In its 2020 guideline, the American Gastroenterological Association recommends against the routine use of endoscopic surveillance for GIM but does note that surveillance may be reasonable in patients at increased risk of gastric cancer, such as:
- Incomplete versus complete GIM (histology showing at least partial colonic type, compared with small intestinal type)
- Extensive versus limited GIM (intestinal metaplasia involving the gastric body plus antrum and/or incisura compared with involving the antrum and/or incisura only)
- Patients with a family history of gastric cancer
- Racial/ethnic minorities
- Immigrants from high-incidence regions

If endoscopic surveillance is performed, an upper endoscopy every 3–5 years is a reasonable strategy. During upper endoscopy, biopsies should be taken of the antrum, body (5 biopsy site or Sydney protocol), and any focal lesions. *H. pylori* infection should be treated in any patient with GIM.

GIM with dysplasia is associated with a significantly higher risk of gastric cancer and needs close surveillance, in addition to endoscopic treatment or ablation if the dysplastic focus is visible.

26. **Are patients with pernicious anemia at an increased risk for gastric cancer? Is endoscopic screening or surveillance required?**
Yes. Individuals with pernicious anemia have an estimated two- to threefold increased risk of developing gastric cancer. The risk of developing gastric cancer in patients with pernicious anemia is highest within the first year of diagnosis, so an upper endoscopy is recommended within 6 months of diagnosis. There are insufficient data to support subsequent endoscopic surveillance.

27. **Is partial gastrectomy a risk factor for the development of gastric cancer?**
   Partial gastrectomy for benign gastric or duodenal ulcers has become increasingly uncommon. There are conflicting results from studies evaluating the risk of gastric cancer following partial gastrectomy for benign disease. In studies suggesting an association, the risk of gastric cancer begins to increase 15–20 years after the initial surgery. Periodic upper endoscopy after this point may be reasonable.

28. **Who is at risk for ampullary and nonampullary duodenal adenomas?**
   Ampullary and nonampullary duodenal adenomas can occur sporadically or in association with FAP or MAP. Both ampullary and nonampullary duodenal adenomas have the potential for malignant transformation and should be removed, ideally endoscopically.

29. **How should endoscopic surveillance be performed for sporadic duodenal adenomas?**
   Sporadic nonampullary duodenal adenomas should be completely removed, which can generally be accomplished using standard endoscopic techniques, such as snare polypectomy or lift-assisted endoscopic mucosa resection. The surveillance interval for duodenal adenomas is not well-defined, but a repeat EGD in 5 years seems reasonable for small (i.e., <10 mm) polyps without advanced histology. Large (i.e., >20 mm) duodenal adenomas have been shown to have a high recurrence risk, requiring close follow-up.

30. **What is the upper GI tract endoscopic surveillance strategy for patients with FAP or MAP?**
   Individuals with FAP should undergo endoscopic surveillance for duodenal adenomas starting between the ages of 20 and 25 or before undergoing colectomy for colonic disease. In MAP, duodenal polyposis is less frequent and occurs at a later age, so surveillance can begin between the ages of 30 and 35 years. Surveillance should consist of an EGD with the use of a duodenoscope or a cap-assisted gastroscope (to adequately examine the ampulla). Duodenal polyposis can be staged using the modified Spiegelman staging system and surveillance intervals are guided by the resulting stage. The modified Spiegelman staging system does not specifically account for ampullary adenomas, and endoscopic treatment or closer surveillance may be required based on ampullary findings.

31. **How often is surveillance endoscopy performed on patients who have undergone ER of ampullary adenomas?**
   Multiple surveillance protocols exist for follow-up after an endoscopic ampullectomy. One such protocol is a repeat endoscopy in 3 months. If there is no recurrent polyp tissue, surveillance should be performed in 1 year, then every 3–5 years.

PANCREAS

32. **Who should undergo endoscopic screening and surveillance for pancreatic cancer?**
   Screening for pancreatic cancer is indicated for patients with:
   - Hereditary pancreatitis
   - A strong family history of pancreatic cancer (at least one FDR and one second-degree relative with pancreatic cancer)
   - Peutz-Jeghers syndrome (PJS), regardless of family history
   - Familial atypical multiple mole melanoma (FAMMM), regardless of family history, if there is a CDKN2A mutation leading to changes in the p16 protein
   - *BRCA2* mutations and at least one affected FDR or two affected relatives of any degree
   - *BRCA1*, *MLH1*, *MSH2*, *MSH6*, *PALB2*, or *ATM* gene mutations and at least one FDR with pancreatic cancer

33. **When should endoscopic screening begin for patients at increased risk for pancreatic neoplasia?**
   Screening or surveillance for pancreatic cancer in high-risk individuals should generally begin at the age of 50 years, with the following exceptions:
   - Patients with *PRSS1* gene mutations (associated with hereditary pancreatitis) or FAMMM should begin surveillance at the age of 40 years.
   - Patients with PJS should begin surveillance between the ages of 30 and 40 years.
   - If there is a family history of pancreatic cancer, screening should begin 10 years earlier than the youngest relative with pancreatic cancer or at the ages noted above, whichever comes earlier.
   - New-onset diabetes in a high-risk individual should prompt evaluation for pancreatic cancer.

34. **What is the recommended endoscopic surveillance interval for patients at high risk for pancreatic cancer?**
   Pancreatic cancer screening should be repeated at a 1-year interval following a negative examination.

COLON

35. At what age is CRC screening recommended for average-risk patients? What are the preferred testing modalities for CRC screening?

CRC screening should be offered to average-risk individuals beginning at the age of 45 years. There is growing evidence that heavy cigarette smoking and obesity may be linked to an increased risk of CRC and to the development of CRC at an earlier age; however, there are no formal recommendations for earlier screening in these patients. The risks and benefits of CRC screening options should be discussed with the individual patient. Colonoscopy and fecal immunochemical testing (FIT) are considered first-tier methods while CT colonography, FIT-fecal DNA testing, and flexible sigmoidoscopy should be reserved for those who decline a first-tier option. Colon capsule endoscopy has significant limitations, which minimize its utility for CRC screening (Table 62.2).

36. When should endoscopic screening begin for individuals with a family history of CRC? How often should endoscopic surveillance be performed in these individuals?

Patients with an FDR with CRC (or an advanced adenoma) before the age of 60 years or multiple FDRs with colon cancer (or an advanced adenoma) at any age should undergo screening colonoscopy every 5 years starting at the age of 40 or 10 years younger than the youngest affected relative. Individuals with a single FDR diagnosed with CRC (or an advanced adenoma) after age 60 can be offered average-risk screening options starting at the age of 40 years.

37. What are the endoscopic surveillance guidelines for individuals with a personal history of colon cancer?

If a complete endoscopic examination was not performed at the time of colon cancer diagnosis, a colonoscopy should be performed within 6 months after surgical resection. Endoscopic surveillance should be performed 1 year after surgery, then be repeated in 3 years, and then every 5 years. Shorter intervals may be recommended due to genetic conditions or for surveillance of polyps removed during colonoscopy.

38. Outline the endoscopic surveillance guidelines for individuals with a personal history of rectal cancer.

For patients with full surgical staging, a surveillance colonoscopy should be performed 1 year after surgery, repeated in 3 years, then every 5 years. Patients treated with transanal excision alone should also get proctoscopy with EUS or contrast-enhanced magnetic resonance (MR) imaging (MRI) every 3–6 months for the first 2 years, then every 6 months for a total of 5 years.

39. Do individuals with an FDR diagnosed with adenomatous polyps require earlier screening for CRC? Do they have an increased risk for CRC?

Persons with an FDR with a documented advanced adenoma (an adenoma ≥1 cm in size, with HGD, or with a villous component) before the age of 60 years, or with two FDRs diagnosed with advanced adenomas at any age, should begin CRC screening at the age of 40 or 10 years younger than the youngest affected relative. Without documentation of an advanced adenoma, family members' polyps should be presumed to be nonadvanced. An FDR with adenomatous polyps increases an individual's risk for CRC by twofold but screening for patients with family members that had nonadvanced adenomas can be conducted for patients at average risk for CRC.

40. What are sessile serrated polyps (SSPs) and are they premalignant?

SSPs, also referred to as sessile serrated lesions or sessile serrated adenomas, are premalignant lesions. They are flat or sessile lesions, often with a mucus cap, predominantly occurring in the cecum and ascending colon.

Table 62.2 2017 Multi-Society Task Force Ranking of Current Colorectal Cancer Screening Tests.

Tier 1	Colonoscopy every 10 years Annual fecal immunochemical test (FIT)
Tier 2	CT Colonography every 5 years FIT-fecal DNA every 3 years Flexible sigmoidoscopy every 10 years (or every 5 years)
Tier 3	Capsule colonoscopy every 5 years

Adapted from Rex DK, Boland CR, Dominitz JA, Giardiello FM, Johnson DA, Kaltenbach T. Colorectal cancer screening: recommendations for physicians and patients from the U.S. Multi-Society Task Force on Colorectal Cancer. Gastroenterology. 2017;153(1):307-323.

SSPs are thought to lead to CRC through a different pathway than adenomatous polyps (with early KRAS or BRAF mutations and CpG island methylation occurring in SSPs).

41. What are the surveillance recommendations after the removal of adenomatous colon polyps or SSPs?

After the removal of adenomatous colon polyps or SSPs, a colonoscopy should be performed for surveillance with the interval dependent on the number and histology of the polyps removed (Table 62.3).

42. What endoscopic surveillance should be performed following piecemeal resection of an adenoma or SSP ≥20 mm?

Intensive surveillance is recommended following piecemeal resection of an adenoma or SSP ≥20 mm. The first surveillance examination should be performed 6 months after the resection with the second examination 1 year thereafter and the third examination 3 years later. Careful examination of the postmucosectomy scar should be performed, including the use of image enhancement techniques (i.e., dye-spray chromoendoscopy or electronic chromoendoscopy). Biopsies of the scar site should be performed, even if no visible polyp tissue is seen, because the combination of normal endoscopic and histologic findings is most highly predictive of long-term eradication.

43. When should screening colonoscopy not be offered or surveillance stopped?

The benefits of colon cancer screening decrease and the risks of colonoscopy increase as patients get older. The US Preventive Services Task Force recommends that colon cancer screening not be continued after age 85 years and that the decision to continue colon cancer screening be individualized for patients 75–85 years old based on comorbidities and findings of any prior colonoscopy (i.e., previous advanced adenomas).

44. How is serrated polyposis syndrome diagnosed?

To diagnose serrated polyposis syndrome, the World Health Organization requires at least one of the following:
- At least five serrated polyps proximal to the sigmoid colon, two or more of which being 10 mm or larger
- Serrated polyp(s) proximal to the sigmoid colon in a patient with a family history of serrated polyposis syndrome
- More than 20 serrated polyps of any size were found throughout the colon

Table 62.3 2020 US Multi-Society Task Force Recommendations for Postcolonoscopy Follow-Up in Average-Risk Adults With a Normal Colonoscopy, Adenomas, or Serrated Polyps.

BASELINE COLONOSCOPY FINDING	RECOMMENDED INTERVAL FOR SURVEILLANCE COLONOSCOPY
Normal colonoscopy ≤20 hyperplastic polyps <10 mm	10 years
1–2 tubular adenomas <10 mm	7–10 years
1–2 SSPs <10 mm	5–10 years
3–4 tubular adenomas <10 mm 3–4 SSPs <10 mm Hyperplastic polyp ≥10 mm	3–5 years
5–10 tubular adenomas <10 mm 5–10 SSPs <10 mm Adenomas or SSPs ≥10 mm Adenomas with villous or tubulovillous histology Adenoma with HGD SSP with dysplasia Traditional serrated adenoma	3 years
>10 adenomas on a single examination	1 year
Piecemeal resection of adenoma or SSP ≥20 mm	6 months

HGD, High-grade dysplasia; *SSP*, sessile serrated polyp.
Adapted from Gupta S, Lieberman D, Anderson JC, Burke CA, Dominitz JA, Kaltenbach T, et al. Recommendations for follow-up after colonoscopy and polypectomy: a consensus update by the US Multi-Society Task Force on Colorectal Cancer. Gastroenterology. 2020;158(4):1131-1153.e5. https://doi.org/10.1053/j.gastro.2019.10.026. Epub February 7, 2020. PMID: 32044092; PMCID: PMC7672705.

45. **What is FAP? What is the risk of developing in patients with FAP?**
    FAP is an autosomal dominant disease caused by mutations in the APC gene. The syndrome presents as an extensive number of adenomas throughout the colon (the colon may appear carpeted with polyps) and is associated with a near 100% risk of cancer by the age of 40–50 years. Attenuated FAP (AFAP) presents with lesser numbers of colon polyps (i.e., 20–100), and patients with AFAP typically develop colon cancer at a later age than patients with classical FAP.

46. **When should endoscopic surveillance begin in patients with FAP?**
    Genetic testing should be offered to all at-risk family members of patients with FAP. Family members found to carry a pathogenic variant of the APC gene, who decline genetic testing, or for whom genetic testing is not feasible, should begin screening with an annual colonoscopy at the age of 10–15 years. While colonoscopy is the preferred screening modality, flexible sigmoidoscopy can be considered based on patient/family preferences.

47. **Do patients with PJS require endoscopic surveillance for CRC?**
    CRC surveillance endoscopy is offered to patients with PJS syndrome because the lifetime risk of CRC is 39%. The lifetime risk of gastric cancer (29%) and small bowel cancer (13%) are also significantly increased in patients with PJS. Colonoscopy, upper endoscopy, and small bowel screening (wireless capsule endoscopy or CT/MR enterography) should start at age 8–10 years. If normal, they should be repeated at age 18, then every 2–3 years thereafter. Annual pancreas imaging (EUS or MRI) should be performed starting at the age of 30–35 years.

48. **What is Lynch syndrome?**
    Lynch syndrome, previously known as hereditary nonpolyposis colorectal cancer syndrome, is an autosomal dominant disorder characterized by the early development of CRC (average age 44 years), endometrial cancer, and/or cancer of the stomach, ovary, small bowel, and urothelium; cancers also occur at other sites at a lower frequency. Lynch syndrome is caused by defects in the mismatch-repair genes (*MLH1*, *MSH2*, *MSH6*, and *PMS2*) or the epithelial cell adhesion molecule gene (*EPCAM*). Lynch syndrome is frequently diagnosed based on immunohistochemical testing for mismatch-repair proteins in CRCs, endometrial cancers, and other Lynch syndrome-related tumors.

49. **What are the endoscopic surveillance guidelines for Lynch syndrome?**
    For patients with *MLH1*, *MSH2*, or *EPCAM* mutations, colonoscopy surveillance should begin at the age of 20–25 years (or 2–5 years younger than the earliest cancer diagnosis in an affected relative). For patients with MSH6 or PMS2 mutations, colonoscopy surveillance should begin at the age of 30–35 years (or 2–5 years younger than the earliest cancer diagnosis in an affected relative). For all patients with Lynch syndrome, colonoscopy surveillance should be repeated every 1–2 years. For all patients with Lynch syndrome, upper endoscopy should be performed every 2–4 years starting at the age of 30–40 years, with random biopsies of the proximal and distal stomach taken at least on the initial upper endoscopy. These biopsies will allow for the diagnosis of *H. pylori* infection, GIM, or autoimmune gastritis, which may further increase the risk for gastric cancer. Upper endoscopy should preferably be performed in conjunction with a colonoscopy.

50. **Do patients with ulcerative colitis (UC) and Crohn disease require endoscopic surveillance?**
    Yes. Long-standing colonic inflammatory bowel disease (IBD) increases an individual's risk for the development of dysplasia and CRC. Ulcerative proctitis is not associated with an increased risk of CRC.

51. **Which clinical characteristics increase the risk of CRC in patients with UC and Crohn disease?**
    The most significant risk factors for the development of CRC in patients with IBD are as follows:
    - Longer duration of disease
    - Extent of colitis
      Other risk factors include as follows:
    - History of dysplasia
    - Family history of CRC
    - Young age at onset of disease
    - Personal history of primary sclerosing cholangitis (PSC)

52. **How should endoscopic surveillance be performed in patients with UC and Crohn disease?**
    Dysplasia surveillance should begin 8–10 years after diagnosis in patients with colonic IBD (UC or Crohn disease) or immediately after the diagnosis of PSC. Surveillance consists of colonoscopy using a high-definition endoscope with dye-spray chromoendoscopy or electronic chromoendoscopy (narrow wavelength spectrum, filters, or postimage processing to enhance the vascular and mucosal detail). Any concerning lesions should be biopsied (targeted biopsies), and nontargeted biopsies should also be obtained during the initial surveillance examination and if white light endoscopy is used without dye-spray or virtual chromoendoscopy. After a negative examination,

a surveillance colonoscopy should be repeated in 1–5 years (based on factors such as the presence of PSC, previous dysplasia, the burden of prior colonic inflammation, and family history of CRC).

53. What is the treatment strategy for dysplasia in patients with UC or Crohn disease?

Small (<2 cm) lesions *without* features of invasive cancer or submucosal invasion (i.e., mucosal depression, irregular surface architecture, or failure to symmetrically lift following the injection of saline or a lifting agent) can be removed using standard endoscopic removal techniques. Large lesions may need removal by a highly experienced endoscopist or surgical techniques. Surveillance is imperative following the removal of dysplastic lesions in patients with IBD, with the interval dependent upon the size of the dysplastic lesions and the degree of dysplasia (i.e., LGD or HGD).

When dysplasia without a visible lesion (invisible dysplasia) is encountered, the patient should undergo dye-chromoendoscopy to identify subtle lesions. Persistent HGD or multifocal dysplasia should be managed with surgery, while persistent unifocal LGD can be managed with intensive surveillance.

54. How are adenomatous-appearing polyps managed in patients with UC and Crohn disease?

Adenomatous-appearing polyps occurring within an area of the colon previously affected by colitis should be removed as above. Some guidelines recommend that biopsies be obtained from the adjacent flat mucosa, but recent evidence suggests visual inspection by a trained endoscopist is sufficient. For the lowest risk lesions (i.e., subcentimeter low-grade adenomas), surveillance colonoscopy should occur in no more than 2 years. Polyps occurring in areas not previously affected by colitis can be removed and followed with less-intensive surveillance.

ACKNOWLEDGMENT

The authors would like to acknowledge the contributions of Dr. David Jones who was the author of this chapter in the previous edition.

CLINICAL VIGNETTE

Available Online

BIBLIOGRAPHY

Available Online

WEBSITES

Available Online

RHEUMATOLOGIC MANIFESTATIONS OF GASTROINTESTINAL DISEASES

Kristine A. Kuhn, MD, PhD, FACR

 Additional content available online

IBD-ASSOCIATED SPONDYLOARTHRITIS

1. **How often does an inflammatory peripheral or spinal arthritis occur in patients with inflammatory bowel disease (IBD)?**
   Over 50% of patients with IBD develop joint pain (arthralgia), and 25% have evidence of joint inflammation on exam or imaging. Spondyloarthritis (SpA) is the most common extraintestinal manifestation (EIM) of IBD. SpA in Crohn disease (CD) can be peripheral (15%), localized to the sacroiliac joints (SIJs, 13%), or manifest as ankylosing spondylitis (AS; 4%). For ulcerative colitis (UC) the incidence of peripheral SpA is 12%, sacroiliitis 7%, and spondylitis 2%. While those patients with sacroiliitis are often *HLA-B27* gene negative, those with AS are often B27 positive.

2. **What are the most common joints involved in patients with UC and CD with an inflammatory peripheral arthritis?**
   Although ankles and knees are most common, any peripheral joint can be affected (Fig. 63.1).

3. **Describe the clinical characteristics of the inflammatory peripheral SpA associated with idiopathic IBD.**
   Type I (acute, pauciarticular, parallels IBD activity) occurs in ~5% of patients with IBD, sometimes prior to (30% of cases) or early in the course of IBD. It is strongly associated with flares of IBD in 80% of those affected and

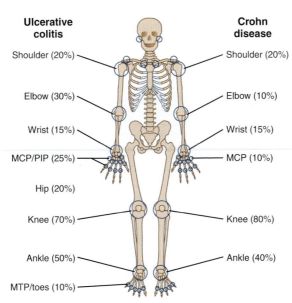

Ulcerative colitis		Crohn disease
Shoulder (20%)		Shoulder (20%)
Elbow (30%)		Elbow (10%)
Wrist (15%)		Wrist (15%)
MCP/PIP (25%)		MCP (10%)
Hip (20%)		
Knee (70%)		Knee (80%)
Ankle (50%)		Ankle (40%)
MTP/toes (10%)		

Fig. 63.1 Joints commonly involved as an extraintestinal manifestation of ulcerative colitis and Crohn disease. *MCP*, Metacarpophalangeal; *MTP*, metatarsophalangeal; *PIP*, proximal interphalangeal.

co-occurs with other EIMs like erythema nodosum and uveitis. Synovial fluid analysis reveals an inflammatory fluid with up to 50,000 white blood cells (WBC)/mm³ (predominantly neutrophils) and negative findings on crystal examination and cultures. Most arthritic episodes are self-limited with 90% resolving within 3–6 months. This type of arthritis does not result in radiographic changes or deformities. There is an increased prevalence of *HLA-B27, HLA-B35*, and *HLA-DRB1*0103* in this type of arthritis.

Type 2 (chronic, polyarticular, independent of IBD activity) also occurs in ~5% of patients. Arthritis tends to be symmetric (80%), polyarticular (metacarpophalangeal joints > knees and ankles > other joints), runs a course independent of the activity of IBD, and does not coincide with extra-articular manifestations (except uveitis). Active arthritis is chronic (90%) and episodes of exacerbations and remissions may continue for years. Because of its chronicity, this type of arthritis can cause erosions and deformities. There is an association of this arthritis with *HLA-B44* but not with *HLA-B27*.

4. What other EIMs commonly occur in patients with idiopathic IBD and inflammatory peripheral arthritis?

By 30 years following IBD diagnosis, approximately 50% of patients with IBD will have developed EIMs, with 25% of individuals having an EIM preceding IBD diagnosis. The development of one manifestation increases the risk of developing another. The most common nonarthritic EIMs can be remembered with the following mnemonic:

P = Pyoderma gangrenosum (<2%)
A = Aphthous stomatitis (<10%)
I = Inflammatory eye disease (acute anterior uveitis) (2%–5%); more common with CD
N = Nodosum (erythema) (~15%)

5. Does the extent and activity of IBD correlate with the activity of the peripheral SpA?

Patients with UC and CD are more likely to develop a peripheral SpA if the colon is extensively involved. In patients with type 1 arthritis, most arthritic attacks occur during the first few years following the onset of the bowel disease, but late occurrences also occur. The episodes coincide with flares of bowel disease in 60%–80% of patients. The arthritis may precede symptoms of IBD in up to 30% of cases, especially in children with CD. Consequently, lack of gastrointestinal (GI) symptoms and even a negative stool guaiac test does not exclude the possibility of occult CD in a patient who presents with characteristic arthritis.

6. Which points in the history and physical examination are helpful in separating axial SpA from mechanical low back pain in a patient with IBD?

On the basis of history and physical examination, 90% of patients with axial SpA can be differentiated from patients with mechanical low back pain (Table 63.1).

7. Does the activity of axial SpA correlate with the activity of the IBD?

No. The onset of sacroiliitis or spondylitis can precede the onset of IBD by years, occur concurrently, or follow onset by years. Furthermore, the course of spinal arthritis is completely independent of the course of IBD.

Table 63.1 Clinical Differentiation of Inflammatory Spinal Arthritis and Mechanical Low Back Pain.

	INFLAMMATORY BACK PAIN	MECHANICAL LOW BACK PAIN
Onset of pain	Insidious	Acute
Duration of morning stiffness	>60 min	<30 min
Nighttime pain	Yes	Infrequent
Movement effect on pain	Improvement	Worsen
Sacroiliac joint tenderness	Usually	No
Range of back motion	Global loss of motion	Abnormal flexion
Reduced chest expansion	Sometimes	No
Neurologic deficits	No	Possible
Duration of symptoms	>3 mo	<4 wk

8. **What HLA occurs more commonly than expected in patients with axial SpA associated with IBD?**
   HLA-B27 is found in 8% of the normal, healthy, white population and is enriched in a population of individuals with AS (~80%) with and without IBD. A patient with IBD who possesses the *HLA-B27* gene has 7–10 times increased risk of developing AS compared with patients with IBD who are *HLA-B27* negative. However, the development of sacroiliitis is not associated with *HLA-B27*.

9. **What serologic abnormalities are seen in patients with IBD?**
   - Erythrocyte sedimentation rate (ESR) and C-reactive protein are elevated, whereas rheumatoid factor and antinuclear antibody are negative.
   - Perinuclear antineutrophil cytoplasmic antibody is seen in more than 55%–70% of patients with UC and fewer than 20% of patients with colon-predominant CD. It is usually directed against lactoferrin and less commonly bactericidal permeability increasing protein, cathepsin G, lysozyme, or elastase. It is never directed against myeloperoxidase.
   - Anti–*Saccharomyces cerevisiae* is present in 40%–70% of patients with CD and rarely (<15%) in patients with UC. Antibodies to *Escherichia coli* outer membrane protein C (OmpC) and flagellin (CBir1, Af-Fla2, and Fla-X) are found in 50%–60% of patients with CD and 5%–10% in patients with UC.

10. **Describe the typical radiographic features of axial SpA in patients with IBD.**
    Patients with early inflammatory sacroiliitis frequently have normal radiographs of the SIJs. In these patients, magnetic resonance imaging (MRI) of the SIJs should be pursued. Sacroiliitis on MRI manifests as bone marrow edema on STIR and T2 fat-suppressed sequences, indicating inflammation (Fig. 63.2A). Over several months to years, patients develop sclerosis and erosions in the lower two-thirds of the SIJ (Fig. 63.2B). In some patients, these joints may completely fuse. Later, radiographs may show shiny corners at the insertion of the annulus fibrosis, anterior squaring of the vertebrae, and syndesmophyte formation (Fig. 63.3A). Syndesmophytes (calcification of annulus fibrosis) are thin, marginal, and bilateral. A *bamboo spine* (bilateral syndesmophytes traversing the entire spine from lumbar to cervical) (Fig. 63.3B) is the end stage of AS even in the setting of IBD.

11. **What other rheumatic problems occur with increased frequency in patients with IBD?**
    - Achilles tendon and plantar fascia enthesitis
    - Clubbing of fingernails (5%, mostly CD)
    - Hypertrophic osteoarthropathy (periostitis)
    - Psoas abscess or septic hip from fistula formation (CD)
    - Osteoporosis secondary to medications (i.e., prednisone)
    - Granulomatous lesions of bone and joints (CD)
    - Vasculitis (<5%)
    - Amyloidosis

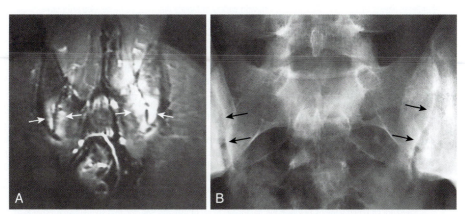

Fig. 63.2 (A) Magnetic resonance image of the sacroiliac joints showing inflammation (*arrows*) (T2-weighted image, TE50, TR2500). (B) Radiograph showing early bilateral sacroiliitis (*arrows*).

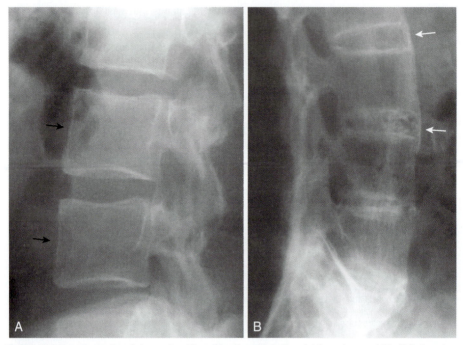

Fig. 63.3 (A) Radiographs showing anterior squaring of the vertebrae in a patient with early inflammatory spondylitis. (B) Radiograph showing thin, marginal syndesmophytes (*arrows*) causing bamboo spine in a patient with Crohn disease with advanced inflammatory spondylitis.

12. Can treatment alleviate the symptoms of peripheral or axial SpA in patients with IBD?

See Table 63.2. Comment: Nonsteroidal anti-inflammatory drugs (NSAIDs) may exacerbate IBD. Cyclooxygenase 2 (cox-2) selective NSAIDs may be safer.

13. What rheumatic disorders are associated with pouchitis, lymphocytic colitis (LC), and collagenous colitis (CC)?

Pouchitis is inflammation of the ileal pouch created following colectomy for UC. It occurs in up to 40%–60% of patients having this surgery. Patients present with watery or bloody diarrhea. Some develop arthritic manifestations (Table 63.3) treatment includes metronidazole and ciprofloxacin, but some patients will develop antibiotic-refractory disease requiring immunosuppression. Surgical revision may be necessary in treatment-resistant cases.

Microscopic colitis includes both LC and CC. Patients present with watery diarrhea and may develop arthritic manifestations (10%–20%) or autoimmune thyroiditis (Table 63.3). Patients older than 65 years (80%) and females (60%) are most commonly affected. The diagnosis can only be made by tissue histologic examination obtained by colonoscopy. Budesonide is effective for inducing and maintaining clinical and histologic remission for CC and LC, and loperamide may ameliorate diarrhea. Evidence for benefit of bismuth subsalicylate and mesalamine with or without cholestyramine for the treatment of CC or LC is weak.

14. Why are patients with IBD more prone to develop an inflammatory arthritis?

The precise pathogenesis of IBD-associated SpA is unknown. However, there is ample clinical evidence supporting that IBD and SpA are along a continuum between pure bowel disease and pure SpA. As noted, ~25% of patients with IBD develop a form of SpA. Conversely, up to 50% of patients with AS have inflammation of the bowel identified on endoscopy. While many of these are asymptomatic, over time, 6%–10% of these patients will develop overt symptomatic CD.

There are common findings between the pathophysiology of IBD and SpA, too that suggest an overlap in the two disease entities. Shared genetic polymorphisms are associated with IBD and AS such as IL-23R as is

Table 63.2 Alleviation of Arthritic Symptoms in Inflammatory Bowel Disease.

DRUG	PERIPHERAL SPA	AXIAL SPA
NSAIDs[a]	Yes	Yes
Corticosteroids		
Systemic	Yes	No
Intra-articular	Yes	Only for sacroiliitis
Sulfasalazine	Yes	No
Mesalamine	No	No
Methotrexate	Yes	No
Azathioprine/6MP	No	No
TNF inhibitors[b]	Yes	Yes
Other biologics		
Vedolizumab[c]	No	No
Secukinumab[d]	Yes	Yes
Ustekinumab	Yes	No
JAKi	Yes	Yes
Bowel resection		
Crohn disease	No	No
UC	Only for Type 1	No

IBD, Inflammatory bowel disease; *NSAIDs*, nonsteroidal anti-inflammatory drugs; *SpA*, spondyloarthritis; *TNF*, tumor necrosis factor; *UC*, ulcerative colitis.
[a]NSAIDs may exacerbate IBD. Cox-2 selective NSAIDs may be safer.
[b]Anti-TNFα approved and effective include infliximab, adalimumab, golimumab, and certolizumab pegol. Etanercept is ineffective for IBD.
[c]There have been reports of SpA developing in the setting of vedolizumab.
[d]Secukinumab should be used with caution in patients with IBD as new cases were observed to occur in clinical trials as was worsening of established IBD.

Table 63.3 Rheumatic Disorders Associated With Pouchitis, Lymphocytic Colitis, and Collagenous Colitis.

	POUCHITIS	LC	CC
Peripheral SpA	Yes	Yes	Yes (10%)
Axial SpA	No	Yes*	No
Rheumatoid arthritis	No	Yes	Yes
Thyroiditis/other autoimmune disease	No	Yes	Yes

CC, Collagenous colitis; *IBD*, inflammatory bowel disease; *LC*, lymphocytic colitis; *SpA*, spondyloarthritis.
*Up to 60% of patients with axial SpA have asymptomatic Crohn-like lesions on right-sided colon biopsies. However, only 4%–5% will evolve into overt IFD.

microbial dysbiosis (i.e., a substantial alteration of the individual bacterial species compared to controls). In both diseases, there is a Th17-mediated inflammation characterized by increased IL-6, IL-17a, and IL-23. Finally, gut-derived lymphocytes and macrophages have been identified in circulation and synovial fluid of individuals with SpA; these cells express intestinal markers such as invariant T cell receptors (mucosal-associated invariant T cells), IL-23R, IL-17a, $\alpha E\beta 7$, $\alpha 4\beta 7$, and CD163. What triggers circulation of the gut-derived cells, though remains unknown but possibly due to microbial signals in the gut and/or increased intestinal permeability due to local inflammation.

REACTIVE ARTHRITIS

15. **What is reactive arthritis, and what are the most common GI pathogens that cause it?**

A reactive arthritis is a sterile inflammatory arthritis that occurs within 1–3 weeks following an infection by an organism that infects mucosal surfaces, especially the urethra or large bowel.

Approximately 1%–3% of patients who have an infectious gastroenteritis during an epidemic subsequently develop a reactive arthritis. It may be as high as 20% in *Yersinia*-infected individuals. The following GI pathogens are often associated:

- *Yersinia enterocolitica* or *Yersinia pseudotuberculosis*
- *Salmonella enteritidis* or *Salmonella typhimurium*
- *Shigella flexneri*, then *Shigella dysenteriae*, and occasionally *Shigella sonnei*
- *Campylobacter jejuni* or *Campylobacter coli*
- *Clostridium difficile*
- *E. coli*

16. **Which joints are most commonly involved in a reactive arthritis following a bowel infection (i.e., postenteritic reactive arthritis)?**

The joints commonly involved in reactive arthritis after bowel infection can be seen in Fig. 63.4.

17. **Describe the clinical characteristics of postenteritic reactive arthritis.**

- Demographically, males are affected more frequently than females; the average age is 30 years old.
- Onset of arthritis is abrupt and acute.
- Distribution of joints is asymmetric and oligoarticular. A lower extremity is involved in 80%–90%. Sacroiliitis occurs in 20%–30%; enthesitis (Achilles tendon, plantar fascia attachments) and toe dactylitis occur.
- Synovial fluid analysis is notable for inflammatory fluid (usually 10,000–50,000 WBC/mm^3), no crystals, and negative cultures.
- ~80% will resolve in 1–6 months; 20% have chronic arthritis with radiographic changes of peripheral and/or SIs.

18. **What extra-articular manifestations can occur in patients with postenteritic reactive arthritis?**

- Sterile urethritis (15%–70%)
- Conjunctivitis
- Acute anterior uveitis (iritis)

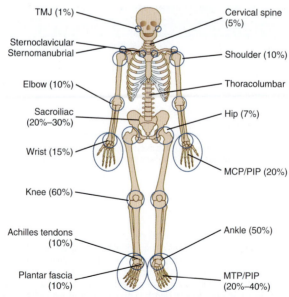

Fig. 63.4 Joints commonly involved in reactive arthritis after bowel infection. *MCP*, Metacarpophalangeal; *MTP*, metatarsophalangeal; *PIP*, proximal interphalangeal; *TMJ*, temporomandibular joint.

- Oral ulcers (painless or painful)
- Erythema nodosum (5% of *Yersinia* infections)
- Circinate balanitis
- Keratoderma blennorrhagicum

19. **How commonly do patients with postenteritic reactive arthritis have the clinical features of reactive arthritis (Reiter syndrome)?**
The triad of inflammatory arthritis, urethritis, conjunctivitis, and uveitis with or without mucocutaneous lesions that characterize reactive arthritis (Reiter syndrome) may develop 2–4 weeks after an acute urethritis or diarrheal illness. The frequency of the triad varies with the causative enteric organism:
- *Shigella*, 85%
- *Yersinia*, 10%
- *Salmonella*, 10%–15%
- *Campylobacter*, 10%

20. **How do the radiographic features of inflammatory sacroiliitis and spondylitis caused by postenteritic reactive arthritis differ from those in patients with IBD?**
See Table 63.4 and Fig. 63.5 for the difference.

21. **Discuss the relationship of *HLA-B27* positivity in patients with postenteritic reactive arthritis compared with a normal healthy population.**
- Patients with reactive arthritis = 60%–80% *HLA-B27* positive; normal healthy controls, 4%–8% *HLA-B27* positive.
- Caucasians and patients with radiographic sacroiliitis or uveitis are more likely to be *HLA-B27* positive.
- A person who is *HLA-B27* positive has 30–50 times increased risk of developing reactive arthritis following an episode of infectious gastroenteritis compared with a person who does not have the *HLA-B27* gene.

Table 63.4 Radiographic Comparison of Spinal Arthritis in Postenteritic Reactive Arthritis Versus Inflammatory Bowel Disease.

	REACTIVE ARTHRITIS	IBD
Sacroiliitis	Unilateral and asymmetric	Bilateral
Spondylitis	Asymmetric, nonmarginal, and jug-handle syndesmophytes	Bilateral, thin, and marginal syndesmophytes

IBD, Inflammatory bowel disease.

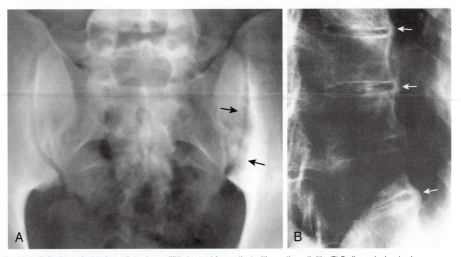

Fig. 63.5 (A) Radiograph showing unilateral sacroiliitis (*arrows*) in a patient with reactive arthritis. (B) Radiograph showing large, nonmarginal syndesmophytes (*arrows*) of the spine in a patient with reactive arthritis.

Table 63.5 Treatment of Postenteritic Reactive Arthritis.

TREATMENT	ACUTE	CHRONIC	SACROILIITIS
NSAIDs	Yes	Yes	Yes
Corticosteroids			
Intra-articular	Yes	Yes	Yes
Oral	Yes*	No	No
Antibiotics			
2-Week course	No	No	No
3-Month course	N/A	No	No
Sulfasalazine	N/A	Yes	No
Methotrexate	N/A	Yes	No
Anti-TNFα[a]	N/A	Yes	Yes

DMARD, Disease-modifying antirheumatic drug; *FDA*, US Food and Drug Administration; *NA*, not applicable; *NSAID*, nonsteroidal anti-inflammatory drug; *TNF*, tumor necrosis factor.
*Approximately 20 mg daily and taper; if >5 mg daily needed or >3 months then consider DMARD.
[a]Anti-TNFα agents include etanercept, infliximab, adalimumab, golimumab, and certolizumab pegol (not FDA-approved).

- Only 20%–25% of all *HLA-B27*–positive individuals who get an infectious gastroenteritis from *Shigella, Salmonella,* or *Yersinia* go on to develop a postenteritic reactive arthritis.

22. **Explain the current theory for the pathogenesis of a postenteritic reactive arthritis.**
Bacterial antigens and nucleic acids as well as phagocytosed bacteria (but not viable organisms) from the pathogens (*Campylobacter, Yersinia, Shigella,* and *Salmonella*) causing the infectious gastroenteritis to have been recovered from joints of patients who develop a postenteritic reactive arthritis. These bacterial components are thought to incite inflammation in the joint. The role that *HLA-B27* plays in the pathogenesis is debated. One possibility is that recirculating *HLA-B27*–restricted T cells present bacteria-derived peptides with arthritogenic properties to the immune system in a unique way, leading to inflammation. Another postulate is that there is molecular mimicry between the *HLA-B27* molecule and the bacterial antigens, causing an aberrant immune response leading to altered or defective intracellular killing by *HLA-B27*–positive cells, resulting in persistence of arthritogenic pathogens. A third hypothesis relates to the tendency for the *HLA-B27* heavy chain to misfold when the cell is under stress. This results in heavy chains accumulating in the endoplasmic reticulum leading to an *unfolded protein response*, causing the release of inflammatory cytokines. The chronic persistence of bacterial antigens may stress the *HLA-B27*–positive cells, leading to *B27* heavy chain misfolding and the unfolded protein response. However, because *HLA-B27* positivity is neither necessary nor sufficient to cause reactive arthritis, additional genetic (endoplasmic reticulum aminopeptidase–1 and IL-23R polymorphisms) and environmental factors likely play a role in the pathogenesis of postenteritic reactive arthritis.

23. **Is any therapy beneficial for postenteritic reactive arthritis?**
See Table 63.5 for the treatment of postenteritic reactive arthritis.

WHIPPLE DISEASE

24. **Who was Whipple?**
George Hoyt Whipple, MD, in 1907 reported the case of a 36-year-old medical missionary with diarrhea, malabsorption with weight loss, mesenteric lymphadenopathy, and migratory polyarthritis. He named this disease *intestinal lipodystrophy*, but it is now known as Whipple disease. Dr. Whipple also became a Nobel laureate in physiology in 1934 and was the founder of the University of Rochester Medical School.

25. **Who gets Whipple disease?**
Only one to six cases worldwide per 10,000,000 persons per year are reported. Whipple disease occurs most commonly in middle-aged (48–54 years old) White males (male/female ratio, 8:1). The HLA alleles DRB*13 and DQB1*06 are associated with Whipple disease. Most (~2/3) have poor personal hygiene and occupational exposure to animals, soil (e.g., farmers), and sewage.

26. **What are the multisystem manifestations of Whipple disease?**
The clinical manifestations of Whipple disease can be remembered using the following mnemonic:

W = Wasting and weight loss	**D** = Diarrhea
H = Hyperpigmentation (skin)	**I** = Interstitial nephritis
I = Intestinal pain	**S** = Skin rashes
P = Pleurisy	**E** = Eye inflammation
P = Pneumonitis	**A** = Arthritis
L = Lymphadenopathy	**S** = Subcutaneous nodules
E = Encephalopathy	**E** = Endocarditis
S = Steatorrhea	

27. **Describe the clinical characteristics of the arthritis associated with Whipple disease.**
Seronegative oligoarthritis or polyarthritis (knees, ankles, and wrists) is the presenting symptom in 60% of patients and may precede the intestinal symptoms by up to 5 years. More than 70% of patients will develop arthritis at some time during their disease course. The arthritis is inflammatory, is often migratory, and does not correlate with intestinal symptoms. Sacroiliitis or spondylitis occurs in 7%–4% of patients, respectively. Synovial fluid analysis shows an inflammatory fluid with 5000–100,000 cells/mm^3 (predominantly neutrophils). Radiographs usually remain unremarkable.

28. **What are the etiologic factors of Whipple disease and how is the diagnosis made?**
Whipple disease is caused by a gram-positive actinomycete called *Tropheryma whipplei*. The diagnosis is made by demonstrating periodic acid–Schiff (PAS)-positive inclusions in macrophages of affected tissues, typically a small bowel or lymph node biopsy sample. These deposits contain the rod-shaped free *T. whipplei* bacilli seen on electron microscopy. The diagnosis can be confirmed by a polymerase chain reaction of the DNA sequence of the 16S-ribosomal RNA gene sequence of *T. whipplei* in the PAS-positive tissue sample.

29. **How is Whipple disease best treated?**
Initial treatment is ceftriaxone (or meropenem) for 2 weeks to ensure therapy of the central nervous system (CNS). Oral trimethoprim (TMP)–sulfamethoxazole (SMX) is subsequently used for more than 1 year. Tetracycline can be used in sulfa-allergic patients. Relapses can occur particularly in patients with CNS involvement (30%). These patients should be treated indefinitely with oral TMP/SMX.

OTHER GASTROINTESTINAL DISEASES

30. **What rheumatic manifestations have been described in patients with celiac disease (gluten-sensitive enteropathy)?**
Celiac disease is an enteropathy resulting from an autoimmune reaction to wheat gluten and gliadin by T and B lymphocytes in the gut of genetically predisposed individuals. It is a relatively common disease affecting 1:70–1:300, most often in individuals of Northern European Ancestry. Celiac disease is associated with *HLA-DQ2* or *HLA-DQ8*, usually in linkage with *HLA-DR3* in 99% of patients. Dietary gluten is partly digested by gastric enzymes to peptides including gliadin that is deaminated by tissue transglutaminase (tTG) increasing its immunogenicity. This immunogenic gliadin peptide is presented in the context of *HLA-DQ2* or *DQ8* to CD4+ T cells, resulting in interferon γ release and inflammation, altered gut permeability, and villous atrophy.

The gold standard diagnostic is duodenal biopsy showing villous atrophy. However, autoantibody testing is very helpful in screening individuals prior to biopsy. On a gluten-rich diet in people who are not immunoglobulin A (IgA) deficient, IgA antibodies against tissue transglutaminase have a high sensitivity (95%) and specificity (90%) for celiac disease. Due to poor specificity, antigliadin antibodies are no longer used to screen for celiac disease.

The most frequent rheumatic manifestations include the following:
- Symmetric polyarthritis (~25%) involving predominantly large joints (knees and ankles > hips and shoulders) occurs. Oligoarthritis and sacroiliitis can also occur. Importantly, the arthritis may precede enteropathic symptoms in 50% of cases. The arthritis responds to a gluten-free diet in 46%–60% of cases.
- Metabolic bone disease occurs in most and can be complicated by secondary hyperparathyroidism and even osteomalacia due to steatorrhea from severe enteropathy causing vitamin D deficiency. Some of these patients are mistakenly diagnosed as fibromyalgia with irritable bowel syndrome.
- Dermatitis herpetiformis is present in 15%–25% of individuals with celiac disease and usually responds to a gluten-free diet. Dapsone can also be used.

31. **Describe the bowel-associated dermatosis-arthritis syndrome (BADAS).**

In the past, this syndrome occurred in 20% of patients who underwent intestinal bypass (jejunoileal or jejunocolic) surgery for morbid obesity, but newer techniques of bariatric surgery have drastically reduced the incidence. BADAS can also occur in patients with IBD, diverticular disease, other bowel surgeries, and as a rare consequence of bacterial overgrowth in patients with poor intestinal peristalsis.

The arthritis is intensely painful, inflammatory, oligoarticular, and frequently migratory, affecting both upper and lower extremity small and large joints. Radiographic findings usually remain normal, despite 25% of patients having chronic recurring episodes of arthritis. Up to 80% develop dermatologic abnormalities, the most characteristic of which is a maculopapular or vesiculopustular rash.

The pathogenesis involves bacterial overgrowth in the blind loop, resulting in antigenic stimulation that purportedly causes immune complex formation (frequently cryoprecipitates containing secretory IgA and bacterial antigens) in the serum that deposits in the joints and skin. Treatment includes NSAIDs and oral antibiotics, which usually improve symptoms. Only surgical reanastomosis of the blind loop or improvement in peristalsis can result in the complete elimination of symptoms.

32. **What types of arthritis can be associated with carcinomas of the esophagus and colon?**

Carcinomatous polyarthritis can be the presenting feature of an occult malignancy of the GI tract. The arthritis is typically acute in onset, asymmetric, and predominantly involves lower extremity joints while sparing the small joints of the hands and wrists. Patients have an elevated ESR and a negative rheumatoid factor. Another type of arthritis associated with colorectal malignancy is septic arthritis caused by *Streptococcus bovis*.

33. **What are the clinical features of the pancreatitis, panniculitis, and polyarthritis (PPP) syndrome?**

PPP syndrome is a systemic syndrome occurring in some patients with pancreatitis or pancreatic acinar cell carcinoma due to the release of trypsin, lipase, and amylase from the disease pancreas causing fat necrosis. Its clinical manifestations can be remembered by the following mnemonic:

P = Pancreatitis

A = Arthritis (60%) and arthralgias, usually of the ankles and knees (synovial fluid is typically noninflammatory and creamy in color as a result of lipid droplets that stain with Sudan black or oil red O)

N = Nodules that are tender, red, and usually on extremities (frequently misdiagnosed as erythema nodosum but really are areas of lobular panniculitis with fat necrosis)

C = Cancer of the pancreas (a more common cause than pancreatitis)

R = Radiologic abnormalities caused by osteolytic bone lesions from bone marrow necrosis (10%)

E = Eosinophilia

A = Amylase, lipase, and trypsin released by the diseased pancreas (causes fat necrosis in skin, synovium, and bone marrow)

S = Serositis, including pleuropericarditis, frequently with fever

34. **What musculoskeletal problem can occur with pancreatic insufficiency?**

Osteomalacia is caused by fat-soluble vitamin D malabsorption.

CLINICAL VIGNETTE

Available Online

BIBLIOGRAPHY

Available Online

DERMATOLOGIC MANIFESTATIONS OF GASTROINTESTINAL DISEASE

CHAPTER 64

David Cleaver, DO, FAOCD, FAAD and Peter R. McNally, DO, MSRF, MACG

 Additional content available online

1. **What are and how often are cutaneous, extraintestinal manifestations (EIMs) seen in patients with inflammatory bowel disease (IBD)?**
   Cutaneous EIMs have been reported to occur in 5%–15% of patients with IBD. Erythema nodosum (EN) and pyoderma gangrenosum (PG) are the most frequent cutaneous EIMs seen. Other less common cutaneous EIMs include Sweet syndrome, metastatic Crohn disease, hidradenitis suppurativa, and psoriasis (Table 64.1 and Fig. 64.1).

2. **Are there cutaneous disorders that can be caused by IBD medications?**
   Yes, melanoma, NMSC (nonmelanoma skin cancer—basal cell and squamous cell carcinoma), and EN.
   - ↑ melanoma with anti–tumor necrosis factor alpha treatment
   - ↑ NMSC with azathioprine and 6-mercaptopurine
   - ↑ EN with azathioprine and 6-mercaptopurine

3. **What gastrointestinal disorders are associated with xanthomas and xanthelasmas?**
   These skin manifestations are a classic feature of primary biliary cirrhosis and familial hyperlipidemia that can be associated with pancreatitis.
   - Xanthelasma is a type of plain xanthoma often localized to the periorbital area, while xanthomas are yellow-to-red plaques found in skin folds of the neck and trunk (Fig. 64.2A).

4. **A 60-year-old farmer, seen by primary care for *fragility of skin over the back of his hands* Fig. 64.2B). He has a medical history of intermittent atrial fibrillation and mild type II diabetes mellitus. Liver enzymes are mildly elevated: alanine transaminase (ALT) = 60 U/L and aspartate aminotransferase (AST) = 45 U/L. What is your diagnosis?**
   Porphyria cutanea tarda (PCT).
   PCT clinically manifests with increased skin fragility and blistering skin lesions on sun-exposed areas. The common age of presentation is the fifth to sixth decade and occurs slightly more commonly in males. PCT is the most common human porphyria, due to hepatic deficiency of uroporphyrinogen decarboxylase (UROD), which is acquired in the presence of iron overload and various susceptibility factors, such as alcohol abuse, smoking, hepatitis C virus (HCV) infection, human immunodeficiency virus (HIV) infection, iron overload with hemochromatosis (HFE) gene mutations, use of estrogens, and UROD mutation.
   This patient's serum was ferritin of >1000 ng/mL and HFE genetic testing was homozygous for C282Y. Persons with cirrhosis and PCT and/or hemochromatosis require serial phlebotomy and monitoring for hepatocellular carcinoma with periodic alpha fetal protein and hepatic ultrasound.

5. **Development of a purpuric rash (Fig. 64.2C) over the lower extremities in a previous intravenous drug user, with mild elevation in ALT and AST liver enzyme tests should suggest what disorder?**
   Mixed cryoglobulinemia.
   - About 70%–90% cryoglobulinemia cases are linked to chronic hepatitis C infection. There are three types of cryoglobulinemia:
     - Type I: monoclonal immunoglobulin, most often resulting from an underlying B cell hematologic malignancy (Waldenström's macroglobulinemia or multiple myeloma).
     - Type II: mixed cryoglobulinemia (a mixture of monoclonal immunoglobulin M [IgM] with rheumatoid factor activity directed against polyclonal immunoglobulin G [IgG]). Most often due to chronic HCV infection but also hepatitis B virus and HIV. Also seen in autoimmune disorders, particularly, Sjögren syndrome.
     - Type III: mixed cryoglobulinemia (IgG and IgM are polyclonal) Most commonly seen in HCV infection but also seen in autoimmune disease (e.g., systemic lupus erythematosus and Sjögren syndrome).

Table 64.1 Cutaneous Extraintestinal Manifestations Are Seen in Inflammatory Bowel Disease (IBD) Patients.

CUTANEOUS DISORDER	CUTANEOUS AND CLINICAL FEATURES	PARALLELS IBD ACTIVITY	TREATMENT
PG (Fig. 64.1A)	Erythematous papules evolve into painful ulcerations Anterior tibia and or thigh location Pathergy	Yes: colonic disease activity	Oral steroids, cyclosporin, tacrolimus, and anti-TNFα Avoid skin biopsies and mechanical trauma
EN (Fig. 64.1B)	Painful erythematous nodules and plaques Extensor surfaces of legs Female > male	Yes: bowel activity Other causes: medications (oral contraceptives) infections, sarcoid	Systemic corticosteroids or IBD specific therapy
Sweet syndrome (acute febrile neutrophilic dermatosis) (Fig. 64.1C)	Tender exanthems or nodules Extremities, trunk, or face Female (80%) >> male	Yes: bowel activity Other causes: infection and cancer	Topical or oral prednisone, or immunomodulators
MCD	Great *mimicker* Found anywhere Biopsy for diagnosis: PAS stain (−) granulomas	No	Topical or systemic prednisone, and anti-TNFα surgery, and hyperbaric oxygen
HS (Fig. 64.1D)	Abscesses and nodules with sinus tracts and scarring Intertriginous, mammary, and inguinal regions	No May precede or follow the onset of IBD disease activity	Antibiotics Anti-TNF and/or surgery for refractory cases
Ps	Silvery scales overlying erythematous plaques Scalp, joint flexures Can occur with anti-TNFα	No May precede or follow the onset of disease activity	Topical corticosteroids Apremilast or biologics for refractory case Ustekinumab may treat both PS and IBD

EN, Erythema nodosum; *HS*, hidradenitis suppurativa; *MCD*, metastatic Crohn disease; *PAS*, periodic acid–Schiff; *PG*, pyoderma gangrenosum; *Ps*, psoriasis; *TNFα*, tumor necrosis factor alpha.

6. A patient with chronic and frequent, mushy stools and a body mass index of 20 kg/m², complains of pruritis and the cutaneous lesions seen in Fig. 64.2D/E. What is your diagnosis?

Dermatitis herpetiformis (DH) and celiac disease (CD).

- The characteristic clusters of small vesicles found on an erythematous base are rarely seen in persons with DH, because the lesions are so intensely pruritic that patients will scratch the area and vesicles are replaced by small pustules. People exhibiting DH should undergo serologic antibody testing for CD and small bowel biopsy. Only 10%–15% of people with CD will be affected by DH. People of northern European descent are more likely than those of African or Asian heritage to develop DH. A punch skin biopsy with direct immunofluorescent staining is characterized by granular IgA deposits at the dermal-epidermal junction (Fig. 64.2E). Institution of a gluten-free diet (GFD) is recommended for people with DH and CD or with either disorder alone, as both often respond to GFD. Dapsone can offer dramatic relief in DH symptoms and a diet high in iodine may worsen DH symptoms.

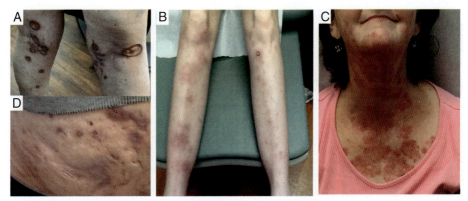

Fig. 64.1 Photographic examples of cutaneous EIMs: (A) pyoderma gangrenosum, rapidly enlarging painful ulcer characterized by blue/purple undermined borders and pathergy; (B) erythema nodosum, tender red to violet nodules; (C) Sweet syndrome, acute painful, febrile neutrophilic dermatosis found over arms, face and back; and (D) hidradenitis suppurativa, also called *acne inversus* manifests as clusters of chronic painful abscesses in the axilla, mammary and inguinal regions—severe scaring deformity is common. (Courtesy David Cleaver, DO.)

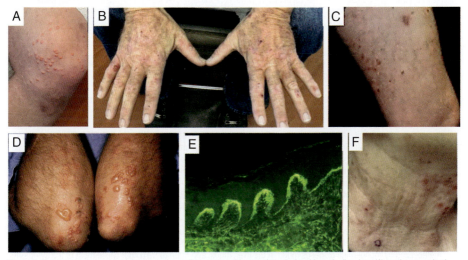

Fig. 64.2 Photographic examples of dermatologic conditions seen with gastrointestinal and hepatic disorders: (A) xanthomas: raised, waxy-appearing, yellowish-colored lesions; (B) porphyria cutanea tarda: painful, blistering skin lesions that develop on sun-exposed skin (photosensitivity); (C) purpura: purplish discoloration of the skin typically seen on the legs and up to the torso; (D–F) dermatitis herpetiformis: intensely itchy blisters filled with a watery fluid, direct immunofluorescence of skin biopsy demonstrates granular IgA deposits along the dermal-epidermal junction. ((A, B, and F) Courtesy David Cleaver, DO. (C) Kartha V, Franco L, Coventry S, McLeish K, Caster DJ, Schadt CR. Hepatitis C mixed cryoglobulinemia with undetectable viral load: a case series. JAAD Case Rep. 2018;4(7):684-687. https://doi.org/10.1016/j.jdcr.2018.04.004. PMID: 30128338; PMCID: PMC6098195. (D and E) From High WA, Prok LD, eds. Dermatitis herpetiformis. In Dermatology Secrets. Philadelphia, PA: Elsevier Ltd; 2021.)

7. **Your local primary care physician evaluated a 30-year-old male patient with chronic severe cracking and fissuring of the hands and feet (Fig. 64.3A). The patient related symptoms of solid food dysphagia and referred the patient for endoscopy. What is your diagnosis?**

Tylosis.

Tylosis is a rare autosomal dominant trait caused by a mutation in RHBDF2 located on the *17q25* gene. It is characterized by focal thickening of the skin of the hands and feet (hyperkeratosis palmaris et plantaris) and esophageal cancer. The lifetime risk for esophageal cancer has been estimated to be as high as 95%. The cutaneous manifestations of tylosis usually arise early in childhood but can present as late as puberty. Esophageal

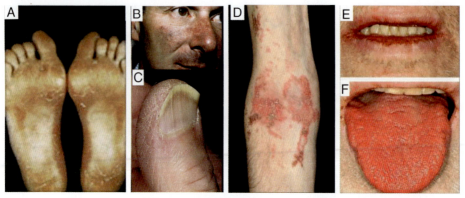

Fig. 64.3 Photographic examples of dermatologic conditions seen with gastrointestinal and hepatic disorders. (A) Howel-Evans syndrome is an extremely rare condition involving thickening of the skin in the palms of the hands and the soles of the feet (palmoplantar keratoderma); (B) carcinoid syndrome: chronic flushing development of thick skin changes with venous telangiectasia and bluish coloration of the malar regions; (C) Koilonychia: spoon-shaped nails; (D–F) Necrolytic migratory erythema: red, blistering rash that spreads across the skin commonly affects the limbs and skin around the mouth, may see a glossy raspberry like tongue. ((A) Courtesy Metze D, Oji V. McKee's Pathology of the Skin. 5th ed. Philadelphia, PA: Elsevier; 2020: 97. (B) Courtesy Fitzsimons Army Medical Center teaching files. (C) From Habif TP, ed. Clinical Dermatology. 4th ed. Philadelphia, PA: Mosby; 2004: 885. (D) Courtesy Boujan N, Géraud C. Neuropsychiatric symptoms, skin disease, and weight loss: necrolytic migratory erythema and a glucagonoma. Lancet. 2020;395(10228):985. https://doi.org/10.1016/S0140-6736(20)30324-X. PMID: 32199485, Copyright © 2020 Elsevier Ltd.)

cancer associated with tylosis usually presents in the fourth to fifth decades. Early endoscopic surveillance, before the onset of dysphagia is recommended.

8. **A 50-year-old male presents to his primary care provider with diarrhea, flushing, rosacea, and malar telangiectasias (Fig. 64.3B). What is your diagnosis?**
Carcinoid syndrome (CS).

CS is a paraneoplastic syndrome caused by the release of serotonin and a variety of other vasoactive hormones from well-differentiated neuroendocrine tumors (NET). Hallmark symptoms of CS are flushing, diarrhea, and wheezing caused by vasoactive hormones: 5-hydroxytryptamine (5-HT), histamine, kallikrein, prostaglandins E and F, and tachykinins. Carcinoid tumors divert tryptophan metabolism toward serotonin production and away from niacin (B3), which can result in pellagra-like symptoms.

CS is most commonly caused by NET arising from the appendix and the midgut (third portion of duodenum to the proximal transverse colon). Foregut carcinoid tumors (arising from the esophagus, stomach, and proximal duodenum) lack aromatic amino acid decarboxylase that converts 5-hydroxytryptophan (5-HTP) to the vasoactive 5-HT; these tumors rarely produce symptoms of CS. Similarly, hindgut carcinoid tumors arising from the rectum and distal colon, rarely secrete 5-HT or other vasoactive hormones. Serotonin released by carcinoid tumors is metabolized by monoamine oxidases found in the liver, lungs, and brain to 5-HT that cause most of the symptoms of CS.

Plasma or 24-hour urinary 5-HIAA tests are used for the diagnosis and monitoring of patients with NET. Computed tomography is poor at detecting primary carcinoids, but helpful in defining the extent of tumor. Somatostatin receptor scintigraphy with indium-111 octreotide and -111 pentetreotide alone or in conjunction with other imaging modalities can be extremely helpful in tumor localization.

9. **Your local primary care physician sees a 25-year-old female patient with symptoms of fatigue, pagophagia, and solid food dysphagia that occurs immediately after swallowing. Physician examination was remarkable for a slender, pale-appearing female with swollen red patches at the corners of the mouth, dry skin, and spooning of the nails (Fig. 64.3C). Laboratory tests have documented iron deficiency anemia. What is your diagnosis?**
Plummer-Vinson syndrome (PVS).

The PVS is characterized by the triad of dysphagia, iron deficiency, and esophageal web. Typically, PVS presents in middle-aged females with weakness, pallor, fatigue, and dysphagia. Cutaneous manifestations include brittle nail koilonychias, angular cheilitis, and pale atrophic mucous membranes. Pagophagia, compulsive eating of

Table 64.2 Hereditary Gastrointestinal Cancers and Associated Dermatologic Manifestations.

SYNDROME	GENES AFFECTED	ASSOCIATED CUTANEOUS FINDINGS	ASSOCIATED CANCER
Adenomatous Polyposis Syndromes			
Lynch syndrome or HNPCC	MLH1, MSH2, MSH6, PMS2, and EPCAM	Sebaceous adenoma, epithelioma, carcinoma, keratoacanthoma	Colon, gastric, endometrium, ovary, and urologic
Muir-Torre syndrome (Fig. 64.4A and B)	MLH1 or MSH2 genes and is inherited in an autosomal dominant manner	Cutaneous sebaceous neoplasms and keratoacanthomas multiple	Colorectal (56%), urogenital (22%), small intestine (4%), and breast (4%)
Familial adenomatous polyposis (Gardner syndrome)	APC	Epidermoid cysts, lipomas, and desmoid tumors Congenital hypertrophy of retinal pigmented epithelium	Colorectal, duodenal, thyroid, adrenal, and hepatoblastoma
Hamartomatous Polyposis Syndromes			
Peutz-Jeghers syndrome (Fig. 64.4C)	STK11	Dark brown to blue macules in the perioral and periocular areas and the buccal mucosa; pigmented macules on the fingers	Duodenal, colon, breast, pancreas, stomach, small bowel, cervix, ovary, testes, and thyroid
Cowden syndrome (Fig. 64.4D and E)	PTEN	Trichilemmomas, papillomatous papules, acral and plantar keratosis, lipomas, and mucocutaneous neuromas	Colon, thyroid, endometrial and breast cancers, and renal carcinoma
Bannayan-Riley-Ruvalcaba syndrome	PTEN	Pigmented macules on glans penis and lipomas	No association with gastrointestinal malignancy, but if PTEN present thyroid, endometrial, breast, and renal cell carcinoma are associated
Juvenile polyposis syndrome	MADH4 and BMPR1A	Digital clubbing	Colon
Neurofibromatosis	RET (protooncogene) (rearranged during transfection)	Café-au-lait spots, cutaneous neurofibromatosis, and axillary freckling Lisch nodules in the iris	Chronic myeloid leukemia of childhood, neurofibrosarcoma, and pheochromocytoma
Cronkhite-Canada syndrome		Nail dystrophy, alopecia, alopecia, diffuse hyperpigmentation on face, palms, soles, and neck	Possible gastrointestinal malignancy

APC, Adenomatosis polyposis coli; HNPCC, hereditary nonpolyposis colorectal cancer; PTEN, phosphate and tension homolog deleted on chromosome 10; RET, protooncogene rearranged during transfection; STK11, serine-threonine kinase.

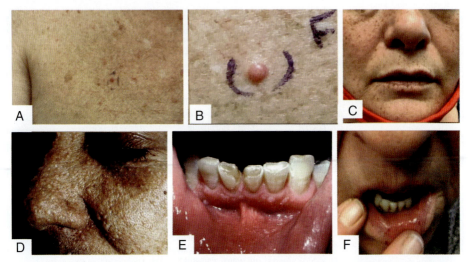

Fig. 64.4 Photographic examples of dermatologic conditions seen with gastrointestinal and hepatic disorders. (A and B) Sebaceous adenoma/adenocarcinoma seen in Muir-Torre syndrome; (C) Peutz-Jeghers syndrome: dark blue or dark brown freckling around the mouth, lips, fingers, or toes; (D and E) Cowden syndrome: trichilemmomas on the face and papillomatous papules on gingiva and mouth; (F) hereditary hemorrhagic telangiectasia: telangiectasias of the lips, fingers and internal organs. ((A–C and E) Courtesy David Cleaver, DO. (D) From High WA, Prok LD. Cowden syndrome. In Dermatology Secrets. Philadelphia, PA: Elsevier Ltd; 2021.)

ice, is a common symptom of iron deficiency. The dysphagia is usually caused by a proximal esophageal web that can be diagnosed with barium swallow radiography or upper endoscopy. Iron supplementation and mechanical esophageal dilation effectively treat PVS.

10. **Your local endocrinologist refers a patient with diabetes mellitus for gastroenterology consultation to evaluate weight loss and oily diarrhea. At the time of your examination the patient points out a recurrent painful erythematous rash over the trunk and lower extremities, blisters around the mouth, and a red tongue (Fig. 64.3D–F). What is your diagnosis?**
The clinical picture of diabetes mellitus, steatorrhea, and migratory painful erythematous rash is very suggestive of glucagonoma syndrome.

Glucagonoma syndrome is caused by a rare glucagon-secreting pancreatic alpha-cell tumor. The cutaneous manifestation of necrolytic migratory erythema (NME) along with elevated glucagon level, abnormal glucose tolerance, weight loss, anemia, diarrhea, steatorrhea, thrombotic disease, and psychiatric disturbances suggest the diagnosis. NME is a painful, annular, and erythematous eruption. NME can occur anywhere and often presents several years before the tumor is identified. Skin biopsies at the edge of the lesion will demonstrate characteristic necrosis and separation of the papillary epidermis with vacuolar degeneration of keratinocytes. Direct immunofluorescent stain reveals apoptosis staining of keratocytes with immunoglobulins, fibrin, and complement 3.

11. **Are there skin characteristic manifestations seen with hereditary polyposis syndromes?**
Yes.

There are a number of characteristic dermatologic manifestations seen with either adenomatous or hamartomatous polyposis syndromes (Table 64.2 and Fig. 64.4).

CLINICAL VIGNETTE

Available Online

BIBLIOGRAPHY

Available Online

CHAPTER 65

DISEASES OF THE APPENDIX

Tomoki Sempokuya, MD and Peter Mannon, MD, MPH

 Additional content available online

1. **Describe the anatomy and functions of the appendix.**

   The appendix is a 5- to 10-cm diverticulum arising from the cecum's posteromedial wall caudal to the ileocecal valve. Its location can vary from retro-cecal ascending (65% of variants) to pelvic (31%) to retro-cecal transverse, para-cecal ascending pre-ileal, and para-cecal ascending post-ileal positions. The appendix is an immunologic organ that is a primary site of immunoglobulin A section whose removal before age 11 may be protective against developing ulcerative colitis. It may also play a role in maintaining a healthy intestinal microbiome.

2. **What is the disease prevalence of appendicitis?**

   A peak incidence of appendicitis is noted between the ages of 10 and 30, and it has a rate of 5.7–50 patients per 100,000 inhabitants per year. In the United States the lifetime risk of appendicitis is estimated to be 9%.

3. **What are the clinical presentations of appendicitis?**

   Acute appendiceal distention initially stimulates visceral afferent pain fibers, producing vague, dull, diffuse pain in the mid-abdomen (periumbilical) or lower epigastrium. Low-grade fever, anorexia, nausea, and vomiting may occur after the onset of pain. The inflammatory process soon involves the serosa of the appendix and, in turn, the parietal peritoneum, producing the characteristic shift in pain to the right lower quadrant.

4. **Describe the pathophysiology of appendicitis.**

   Luminal obstruction, mainly by fecaliths, enteroliths, or hypertrophic lymphoid tissue (children), causes distention of the appendix due to continued mucosal secretion, blocked drainage into the lumen and bacterial overgrowth. Subsequently, distention predisposes to wall infarction and causes bacterial invasion to cause appendicitis. Fecaliths cause approximately 90% of perforated and gangrenous appendicitis.

5. **Where and what is McBurney point?**

   Charles McBurney was an American surgeon (b. 1845) who popularized the physical finding of maximal deep tenderness (McBurney sign) located over an area (McBurney point) at the distal two-thirds along an axis drawn from the umbilicus to the anterior superior iliac spine. Rebound pain at this point is known as Aaron sign. However, due to the variable location of the appendix and other etiologies of tenderness in this area, McBurney sign is not required for nor diagnostic of appendicitis.

6. **What are the psoas and obturator signs?**

   The psoas sign is the finding of pain on right hip extension (elicited by having the patient lie on the left side while the right thigh is flexed backward) and is irritation of the retroperitoneal psoas muscle indicative of a retro-cecal placement of the inflamed appendix. The obturator sign refers to internal obturator muscle (pain on internal rotation of the flexed right hip) by an inflamed retro-cecal appendix.

7. **What is the Rovsing sign?**

   Rovsing sign is the finding of right lower quadrant abdominal pain when the left lower quadrant is palpated. The maneuver stretches the peritoneum only causing pain in the area where the peritoneum is irritating a structure like a muscle, here, right lower quadrant pain in acute appendicitis.

8. **What is the differential diagnosis of appendicitis?**

   Due to nonspecific symptoms, the differential diagnosis of acute appendicitis is broad; acute diverticulitis, Meckel diverticulitis, infectious enterocolitis, inflammatory bowel disease, peptic ulcer disease, cholecystitis, biliary colic, incarcerated hernia, mesenteric lymphadenitis (especially age <15 years), tubo-ovarian abscess, ovarian torsion, ectopic pregnancy, pelvic inflammatory disease, mittelschmerz, and carcinoid tumor. For immunocompromised patients, typhlitis (neutropenic enterocolitis) which can present with necrosis of the intestinal wall, commonly cecum, should be considered.

9. **How do you diagnose appendicitis?**
Diagnosing appendicitis by clinical presentation alone is challenging. To aid diagnosis, several scoring systems have been developed. The Alvarado score was often utilized in the past, but recent studies suggested that the Appendicitis Inflammatory Response (AIR) score (https://www.mdcalc.com/appendicitis-inflammatory-response-air-score) based on vomiting, rebound tenderness, right iliac fossa pain, fever, polymorphonuclear leukocytosis, and elevated C-reactive protein (CRP) performed better for diagnosis of appendicitis. Alternatively, a newer adult appendicitis score (AAS) had been developed. Based on these newer scoring system results, further imaging studies should be considered. Computed tomography (CT) scan is commonly used, but ultrasounds are an alternative option for pediatric or pregnant patients. Performing point-of-care ultrasonography as first-line diagnostic imaging may decrease the need for CT scans with a sensitivity of 76% and a specificity of 95%.

10. **What complications are associated with appendicitis? How do you manage these complications?**
Sixteen to forty percent of patients with appendicitis experience perforation, more commonly at the extremes of age. The estimated mortality rate related to perforation is 5%, compared to 0.6% associated with gangrenous appendicitis. Patients with perforation typically require surgical management. Other infectious complications such as abscess formation, peritonitis, and sepsis may occur. CT-guided drainage should be considered in the presence of an abscess.

11. **What is the treatment modality for appendicitis?**
Patients with appendicitis have been treated with appendectomy for decades. Recently, a randomized clinical trial showed a 10-day course of antibiotics therapy was noninferior to appendectomy for the treatment of uncomplicated appendicitis. However, patients with an appendicolith had a higher risk of complications and underwent appendectomy within 90 days. In select patients with noncomplicated appendicitis without appendicolith, nonoperative management can be considered. However, interval appendectomy is recommended for recurrent disease, children, and young adults (age <40 years) with appendicitis. If the patient requires an appendectomy, laparoscopic appendectomy provides effective treatment with a lower incidence of wound infections and morbidities, shorter hospital stay, and better quality of life.

12. **What are the common postsurgical complications after appendectomy?**
Postsurgical complication rates are estimated to be 11.1% for open appendectomy and 8.7% for laparoscopic appendectomy. The most common postsurgical complication is wound infection, ileus, and abscess formations.

13. **What is the incidence rate for a negative appendectomy?**
Historically, the negative appendectomy rate (NAR, that is the rate of removing a normal appendix) is estimated to be around 15%–25%. However, due to the improvements in imaging modalities, a recent population-based study showed NAR decrease to 4.5% for ultrasonography and 0.6% for CT scan imaging. Surgeons may come across a grossly normal appendix during the surgery, and it often leads to the dilemma of proceeding with appendectomy. Previous studies suggested that 19%–40% of grossly normal appendices had pathologic abnormalities. Early appendicitis may appear grossly normal, and it is recommended to proceed with appendectomy if the suspicion for appendicitis by clinical history and diagnostic imaging is high.

14. **How do you differentiate between pelvic inflammatory disease (PID) and appendicitis?**
Clinical signs such as cervical discharge, cervical motion tenderness (Chandelier sign), dyspareunia, dysmenorrhea, and bilateral pain can help differentiate PID from appendicitis.

15. **How do you manage a pregnant patient with appendicitis?**
Acute appendicitis is the most frequently encountered extrauterine disease requiring surgery during pregnancy. During the increasing size of the gravid uterus, the appendix can move superiorly above the right iliac crest (usually by the fourth month of pregnancy). Ultrasonography should be used as first-line diagnostic imaging. If ultrasound images are inconclusive, magnetic resonance imaging (MRI) images should be considered. Fetal loss increases from 5% in uncomplicated appendicitis to 28% if perforation complicates acute appendicitis; therefore early intervention is the rule if appendicitis is suspected. Laparoscopic appendectomy, rather than an open appendectomy, should be used to improve safety to decrease the risk of fetal loss and preterm delivery.

16. **When do you consider nonoperative management of appendicitis?**
For patients with uncomplicated appendicitis as well as in certain situations of appendicitis with abscess or phlegmon, nonoperative management with antibiotics can be considered. Patients may require percutaneous drain placement if the abscess is present. It was suggested that fever exceeding 38°C and appendiceal diameter $\geq$15 mm are predictors of antibiotic treatment failure. A 5-year follow-up of the APPAC randomized control trial showed a 5-year appendicitis recurrence rate of 39.1% for nonoperative management using antibiotic treatment alone.

17. **What are the emerging management strategies for appendicitis?**
    Endoscopic retrograde appendicitis therapy (ERAT) is an emerging nonoperative treatment for uncomplicated acute appendicitis. Using cap-assisted colonoscopy with fluoroscopy, luminal obstruction is relieved by removing fecalith or drainage of pus by plastic stent placement. This technique is beneficial for patients with high surgical risk and can preserve the physiologic functions of the appendix.

18. **What steps should be taken if an ovarian tumor is discovered during laparoscopic or open exploration?**
    The appendix should be removed after obtaining peritoneal washings, which are studied for cytologic findings of a tumor. The ovarian mass itself should not be touched or biopsied. Ovarian cancer is staged with a strictly performed technique and should be done at a later procedure.

19. **What is the most common tumor of the appendix, and describe the management of the tumor?**
    An appendiceal neoplasm may be found incidentally, and it is estimated to be found in 0.7%–1.7% of appendectomy specimens. However, for patients who are over 40 years old and have complicated appendicitis, the incidence of appendicular neoplasm ranges from 3% to 17%. Neuroendocrine tumors are the most common neoplasm of the appendix, typically accounting for less than 1% of appendectomy specimens. As is seen in the colon, sessile serrated lesions and adenoma can also occur in the appendix. Other appendiceal neoplasms include mucinous neoplasm, adenocarcinoma, goblet cell adenocarcinoma, and mesenchymal neoplasms. In addition, pseudomyxoma peritonei often originates from a primary tumor in the appendix. In general, tumors <1 cm in size and located in the distal appendix can be safely removed by appendectomy. Right hemicolectomy with or without systemic therapy is indicated for larger tumors or invasions into the cecum.

20. **What is stump appendicitis?**
    Stump appendicitis is still a rare but increasingly recognized entity in which patients who have had their appendix removed develop delayed (days to years following surgery) right lower quadrant pain and leukocytosis similar to their initial presentation. The entity relates to a small portion of the appendiceal lumen left in place during surgery. A recent meta-analysis did not show differences in occurrence rates between laparoscopic and open procedures. A high index of suspicion is often needed to make the diagnosis, and treatment ranges from antibiotic therapy to surgical excision.

21. **What is a Meckel diverticulum?**
    A Meckel diverticulum (first described in 1699 and later named by Johann Freidrich Meckel in 1809) is a congenital omphalomesenteric mucosal remnant located on the antimesenteric side of the ileum. Derived from pluripotent cells, it can contain ectopic gastric or, less commonly, pancreatic mucosa. It generally adheres to the rule of 2s: it is found in 2% of the population, within 2 feet of the ileocecal valve, and 2% will develop symptoms.

22. **What is a Mitrofanoff procedure?**
    A Mitrofanoff appendicovesicostomy is a procedure performed to obviate the need for urethral catheterization in those with neurogenic bladder (such as patients with spina bifida). The appendix is removed from its attachments to the cecum while maintaining its blood supply; then, one end is sutured to the urinary bladder, and the other end is sutured to the skin to form a stoma, usually near the umbilicus.

CLINICAL VIGNETTE

Available Online

BIBLIOGRAPHY

Available Online

PLAIN FILM, BARIUM, AND VIRTUAL COLONOGRAPHY

Mike H. Lee, MD and James Latanski, MD

 Additional content available online

1. When requesting an imaging examination, what information should a clinician provide for a radiologist?

By communicating the following information, a clinician helps ensure that an imaging examination will be conducted and interpreted optimally for each patient.

- Provide pertinent or significant medical history and clinical information related to the examination: (1) key findings from history, physical examination, and laboratory tests that suggest the diagnoses in question and (2) any surgical alteration of the anatomy to be examined with imaging.
- Explain the purpose of the examination, including possible diagnoses, potential complications from a recently performed procedure, or an established diagnosis or finding to follow for change. A specific explanation of how the imaging findings may alter management decisions (i.e., follow-up vs. surgery) or confirm a notorious diagnostic dilemma is useful as the radiologist may not be aware of specific treatment algorithms.
- Never hesitate to visit with the radiologist and discuss the case. Effective dialogue and communication between clinicians and radiologists lead to more accurate and diagnostic radiologic imaging.

ABDOMINAL RADIOGRAPHY

2. What is the key radiographic finding of bowel obstruction?

The hallmark of obstruction, whether mechanical or functional, is dilatation of the bowel. The rule of "3s" defines abnormal dilation of the intestine:

- Small bowel 3 cm or larger
- Transverse colon 6 cm or larger
- Cecum 9 cm or larger

It is important to distinguish small bowel from colon when evaluating for bowel obstruction and using the rule of 3s. Small bowel, while typically smaller, is more central in the abdomen and has circumferential dense lines called valvulae conniventes, also known as plicae circulares. Valvulae conniventes form a continuous line around the bowel, whereas the colon has haustral folds that do not form a continuous line around the colon. The colon is also typically found around the periphery of the abdomen.

The differential for dilated air-filled loops of the bowel includes bowel obstruction and paralytic ileus, and it is challenging to differentiate between the two. Several signs favor the diagnosis of small bowel obstruction:

- Prominent abdominal distension, small bowel dilatation, and absence of large bowel dilatation all favor the diagnosis of small bowel obstruction (Fig. 66.1).
- A *stepladder* configuration of dilated small bowel loops extending from the left upper to the right lower quadrants.
- Although less reliable, air-fluid levels in the same loop of small bowel at differing heights.
- String of pearls sign is also known as the string of beads sign.

Compared to bowel obstruction, paralytic ileus could be suggested based on recent surgical history and dilatation of both small bowel and colon.

3. Where in the algorithmic approach for the workup of small bowel obstruction does abdominal radiography lie?

Abdominal radiography is the preferred initial radiologic examination for patients with suspected small bowel obstruction, primarily because of its widespread availability and low cost. However, it is only diagnostic in 50%–60% of cases (Fig. 66.2), so if clinical suspicion for obstruction is high, abdominal computed tomography (CT) should be considered the most definitive test.

4. What are the hallmark features of gallstone ileus?

Although representing an infrequent cause of small bowel obstruction, gallstone ileus has significant associated mortality if the diagnosis is delayed. The characteristic imaging findings are referred to as Rigler triad: pneumobilia, small bowel obstruction, and an ectopic, intra-abdominal, radiodense gallstone (most often lodged at the ileocecal valve).

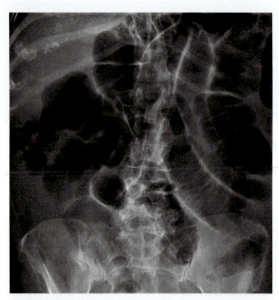

Fig. 66.1 Supine abdomen radiograph. Multiple dilated loops of small bowel are present throughout the abdomen without significant colonic distention. Small bowel mechanical obstruction was found at surgery secondary to a ventral abdominal hernia.

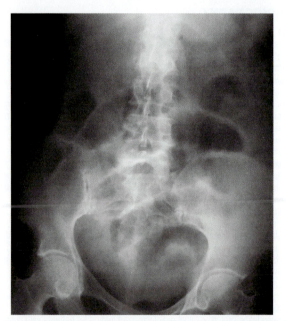

Fig. 66.2 Portable supine abdomen radiograph. Because dilatation of the small bowel does not reach the right lower quadrant, mechanical obstruction of the small bowel substantially upstream of the terminal ileum is probable. This obstruction, however, was functional, as a result of acute pancreatitis.

5. Is ascites detectable on abdominal radiography?

Abdominal radiographs are insensitive for the identification of ascites and should never be used as a diagnostic test for that indication. However, there are several findings that suggest the presence of ascites on supine radiography, such as centrally located, air-filled loops of bowel and lack of visualization of the abdominal contents,

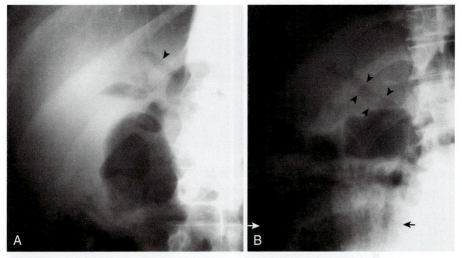

Fig. 66.3 A branching and tapering gas pattern in the liver, if predominantly near the hilum (*arrowheads*), usually is biliary (A) but occasionally is in portal veins. (B) Central hepatic gas pattern which may appear as pneumobilia represents portal venous gas in this case. This is supported by bubbly and linear pneumatosis (*arrow*) below the liver, consistent with bowel ischemia. The large amount of gas and timing of imaging can make the two difficult to distinguish.

to include the liver, spleen, psoas, and urinary bladder outlines. There may also be a hazy density overlying the majority of the abdomen. Ultrasound is the modality of choice for ascites as it can be used diagnostically and for therapeutic paracentesis.

6. **What distinguishes portal venous gas from pneumobilia?**
   Although in both conditions gas is in a branching, tapering pattern, the location within the liver of the gas is usually distinctive. Because portal venous blood normally flows toward the periphery, gas in portal veins tends to accumulate in the periphery of the liver. Because bile normally flows toward the hilum, biliary gas tends to accumulate near the hilum. These rules occasionally fail; however, because at the instant the radiograph is exposed, the location of the constantly moving gas may transiently be atypical (Fig. 66.3). Portal venous gas is an ominous sign, and if suspected, diligent inspection of the radiograph for signs of ischemic bowel, such as pneumatosis intestinalis, is vital. On the other hand, pneumobilia is typically benign and seen after ampullary sphincterotomy or choledocoenterostomy. Gas-producing bacteria is a rare cause of pneumobilia, in such a case the patient will appear septic.

7. **Which types of foreign bodies are encountered on abdominal radiographs?**
   A wide range of foreign bodies is radiopaque and therefore visible at abdominal radiography (Fig. 66.4). On the other hand, radiolucent objects include wood and most fish bones. Aluminum is not entirely radiolucent but can nonetheless be very difficult to appreciate as it is not as radiopaque as other metals. Foreign bodies can be categorized as intraluminal or extraluminal for logistical purposes (Table 66.1).

8. **What are the causes of intra-abdominal calcification?**
   - Renal calculi (80% radiodense) and bladder calculi
   - Cholelithiasis (10%–15% radiodense)
   - Porcelain gallbladder (possible increased risk of cancer)
   - Pancreas (chronic pancreatitis)
   - Calcified lymph nodes (granulomatous disease or chronic inflammation)
   - Vascular calcifications
   - Appendicoliths

CONTRAST MEDIA

9. **What are the roles of barium and water-soluble (iodinated) contrast media for opacification of the lumen of the gastrointestinal (GI) tract?**
   In the setting of fluoroscopy, barium and water-soluble contrast can be used for the evaluation of pathology between the esophagus and the anus. Double-contrast barium studies involve intraluminal gaseous distension

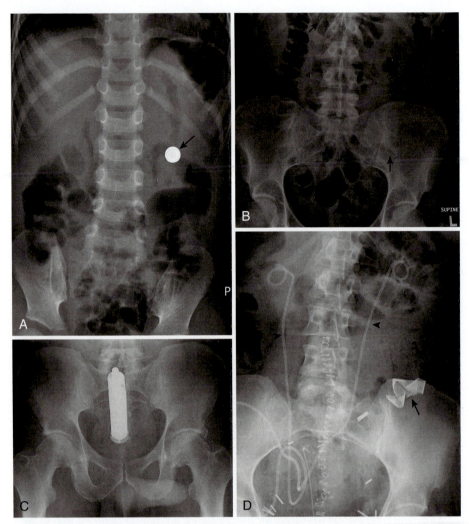

Fig. 66.4 Examples of various abdominal foreign bodies. (A) Round metallic structure (*arrow*) overlies the left hemiabdomen in a 3-year-old girl; in cases of suspected but not witnessed foreign body ingestion, a lateral view can be helpful to confirm the intra-abdominal location. This was confirmed to be button battery ingestion. (B) Three curvilinear radiodense structures (*arrows*) project over the abdomen on this frontal supine view of a 24-year-old woman. The patient initially denied ingestion of foreign bodies but subsequently admitted to swallowing numerous staples. (C) Cylindrical radiopaque structure overlying the midline pelvis represents a vibrator inserted in the rectum. Rectal foreign bodies are typically oriented in the craniocaudal direction. (D) Inadvertent laparotomy sponge (*arrow*) is present within the abdominal cavity following surgery. This portable supine radiograph was obtained after recognition of an incorrect sponge count. The laparotomy sponge itself is radiolucent; however, they are detectable because of an incorporated radiopaque marker. Bilateral ureteral stents are also present (*arrowheads*).

with ingested or rectally inserted barium coating the mucosal surface. The thin layer of barium on the background of gaseous lucency allows detailed mucosal evaluation. Conversely, single-contrast barium studies are without the gaseous background, thus producing a single column of barium. Single-contrast studies are used to evaluate function, stricture position and length, fistulous connections, and for esophageal or postoperative leaks when other imaging modalities are inconclusive. Water-soluble (iodinated) contrast is used as the initial evaluation when an esophageal perforation or a bowel/colonic postoperative leak is suspected. Only after ruling out a large leak is barium appropriate. The reason is that barium can cause significant chemical peritonitis and has a risk of causing pleuritis. On a separate note, aspiration of barium is largely benign as it is not directly toxic to the airways, which

Table 66.1 Common Causes of Radiopaque Foreign Bodies.

INTRALUMINAL	EXTRALUMINAL
Bezoars	Surgical clips (either in expected or migrated position)
Markers for the measurement of colonic transit (Sitz marks)	Migrated intrauterine devices
Packages of illegal narcotics (body packing)	Retained surgical materials (e.g., inadvertent clamp or surgical sponge; the latter typically occurs in the setting of incorrect sponge count)
Dislodged tubes from prior procedures (e.g., feeding tubes and biliary stents)	Intentionally placed surgical materials (e.g., surgical sponge used to control bleeding in traumatic liver laceration—clinical history helps to distinguish from the inadvertent variety)
Ingested or inserted items (coins, batteries, and endoscopic capsules used for workup of small bowel disease)	

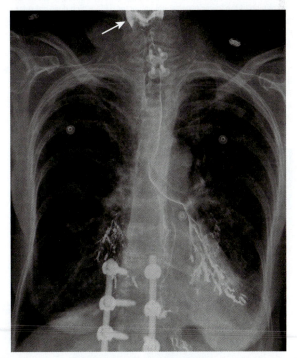

Fig. 66.5 Barium aspiration. Barium contrast is seen coating the trachea, mainstem bronchi, and bilateral lower lobe bronchi following accidental aspiration. A large quantity of contrast is retained with the piriform sinuses (*arrow*), which predisposes to aspiration.

is not the case for hyperosmolar water-soluble contrast media; as a result, hyperosmolar agents are no longer routinely used (Fig. 66.5).

Benefits of barium contrast:
- More radiopaque and more resistant to dilution
- Can be used to evaluate mucosal surface
- Largely benign if aspirated
- Low cost
- Benefits of water-soluble (iodinated) contrast
- Lower risk of chemical peritonitis and pleuritis

SWALLOWING STUDIES

10. What information does a barium swallow provide?

Barium swallow, also referred to as esophagram, is the general term for a fluoroscopic-radiographic examination of oral, pharyngeal, and esophageal swallowing. For the evaluation of dysphagia, a barium swallow study has a few advantages over endoscopy, primarily its ability to diagnose disorders of motility in addition to structural abnormalities. Conversely, endoscopy is superior in detecting milder grades of esophagitis, permits tissue sampling, and does not expose the patient to ionizing radiation. Barium swallow provides the assessment of esophageal motility and emptying, type of hiatal hernia if present, presence of a stricture or mucosal injury, and detection of esophageal reflux.

11. In patients with gastroesophageal reflux disease (GERD), is there a role for barium swallow?

A barium esophagram plays a key role prior to anti-reflux surgery for patients with GERD. This examination allows for the assessment of esophageal emptying, identifies the presence and type of hiatal hernia as well as the presence of a foreshortened esophagus, evaluates esophageal motility, and may detect and qualify the amount of reflux. The caveat with reflux is that its absence at the time of the barium swallow does not exclude this diagnosis; therefore this examination should never be performed solely to detect or exclude reflux.

12. Which esophageal motility disorders are diagnosable by barium swallow?

Achalasia, scleroderma, and esophageal spasm can be diagnosed by barium swallow. Achalasia is typically seen as a severe narrowing of the lower esophageal sphincter (LES) which does not relax (Fig. 66.6 and Table 66.2). Contrast can pool and food material can fill the esophageal lumen, giving the esophagus a more complex appearance. Due to its intermittent nature, esophageal spasm can appear normal but, when active, is diagnosed by multiple nonperistaltic contractions and has been likened to a corkscrew appearance.

13. What findings are suggestive of achalasia secondary to cancer from primary achalasia?

Features suggestive of, but not diagnostic for, secondary achalasia (cancer) are as follows:
- LES *beak* is irregular, eccentric, or abruptly marginated.
- LES *beak* is long, 3.5 cm or longer.
- Esophageal body is relatively narrow, caliber 4 cm or smaller.

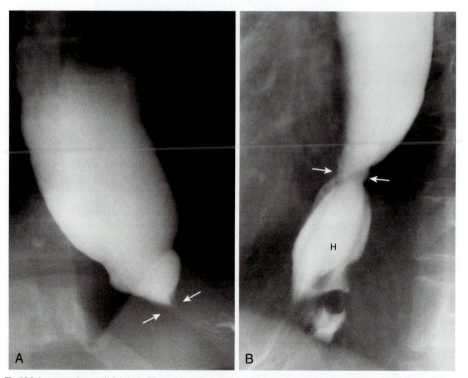

Fig. 66.6 Lower esophagus. (A) Achalasia. Dilatation is marked above a *beak* (*arrows*), formed by the closed lower sphincter. (B) Sclero-derma. Dilatation is moderate above a cylindrical reflux esophagitis stricture (*arrows*), below which is a sliding hiatus hernia (H).

Table 66.2 Achalasia Versus Scleroderma.

	ESOPHAGEAL DILATATION	PERISTALSIS IN PURE SMOOTH MUSCLE PART OF THE ESOPHAGUS	ESOPHAGOGASTRIC JUNCTION
Achalasia	May be marked	Absent	Beak: smooth, concentric, tapered, and flexible No hiatus hernia
Scleroderma	Minimal or moderate	Weak, incomplete, or absent	Stricture from esophagitis: cylindrical, rigid, sometimes irregular, or ulcerated Often a sliding hiatus hernia

Table 66.3 Gastric Ulcers on Upper Gastrointestinal Series: Benign and Malignant Features.

FINDINGS	BENIGN	MALIGNANT
Location in stomach	Other than upstream half of stomach along greater curvature	Upstream half of stomach along greater curvature
Profile view: relationship of ulcer to lumen	Beyond expected lumen	Within expected lumen
Radiating folds	Regular To margin of ulcer or to ulcer mound (of edema)	Nodular, irregular, fused, clubbed, or amputated May not reach ulcer margin
If the ulcer is within a mass	Ulcer location in mass: central Mass: smooth Junction with wall: obtuse angle	Ulcer location in mass: eccentric Mass: irregular Junction with wall: acute angle
Surrounding mucosa	Intact	Distorted or obliterated
Ulcer shape	Round, oval, or linear	Angular
Other	Hampton line	
Healing	Complete	Usually incomplete Occasionally complete, but scar Radiating folds with malignant characteristics

14. **What is the difference between barium swallow, upper GI series, and small bowel follow-through (SBFT)?**

All three refer to a radiographic examination in which the patient ingests a radiopaque contrast medium, typically barium. Unlike a barium swallow, an upper GI series does not evaluate swallowing function but does include evaluation of the stomach and duodenum in addition to the esophagus. An SBFT solely focuses on the duodenum, jejunum, and ileum without evaluation of the esophagus or stomach. Of note, SBFT is not routinely performed, and CT or magnetic resonance (MR) enterography is the modality of choice for the evaluation of the small bowel.

15. **Can benign and malignant gastric ulcers be distinguished?**

While there are features that may suggest benignity or malignancy of gastric ulcers (Table 66.3), they are not sensitive and do not supersede the necessity of endoscopy and biopsy.

16. **What are the indications for either SBFT or enteroclysis?**

In the past, SBFT and enteroclysis (also known as small bowel enema because it involves the injection of contrast medium directly into the small bowel) have been employed in the evaluation of small bowel pathology, including inflammatory bowel disease, neoplasm, and obstruction. CT and MR imaging have largely replaced these imaging modalities. Crohn disease represents one of the few remaining indications for SBFT. Enteroclysis essentially has no role in modern medicine.

COLON AND RECTUM

17. What are the indications for either single- or double-contrast techniques of a barium enema examination?

There has been a substantial decline in the use of double-contrast barium enema as a screening tool for colorectal cancer detection, as it has been largely replaced in favor of optical or virtual colonoscopy. Although once touted as an effective test in this manner because of its relatively low cost, minimal risk, and ability to evaluate the entirety of the colon, double-contrast barium enema has been shown to be less sensitive for polyp detection compared with optical colonoscopy, which has emerged as the accepted gold standard.
- Single contrast: for fistula or sinus tract evaluation, anastomotic integrity prior to ileostomy closure, and obstruction (predominantly colonic volvulus)
- Double contrast: for colorectal cancer

18. What is the role of defecography (evacuation proctography)?

Defecography may identify the cause and help direct therapy if there is anorectal dysfunction. It may also show one or more of the following: rectocele, rectal intussusception (rectorectal or intra-anal), external rectal prolapse, and enterocele. Similar to SBFT and entercolysis, defecography has largely been replaced by MR defecography.

CHOLANGIOPANCREATOGRAPHY

19. What is endoscopic cholangiopancreatography?

Endoscopic cholangiopancreatography is the injection of contrast material through the ampulla to interrogate the pancreatic and biliary ducts. MR cholangiopancreatography (MRCP) is noninvasive and has largely replaced endoscopic retrograde cholangiopancreatography as a primary diagnostic option. Indications for MRCP include congenital abnormalities of hepatobiliary and pancreatic ducts, postsurgical anatomy and complications, choledocholithiasis, and masses of the pancreas or biliary tract (Figs. 66.7 and 66.8).

Percutaneous transhepatic cholangiography (PTC) is an interventional radiology procedure which, as the name suggests, involves inserting a needle into a peripheral hepatic biliary duct and injecting contrast. PTC is typically used when less invasive methods of imaging the biliary ducts are inconclusive. However, it is rarely done alone. In the setting of a known obstruction or infection, PTC can be converted into a percutaneous biliary drainage procedure for both diagnostic and therapeutic benefits.

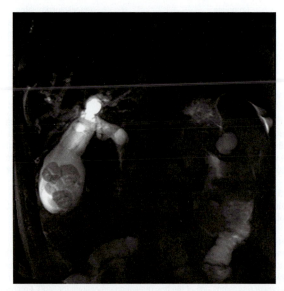

Fig. 66.7 Magnetic resonance cholangiopancreatography image showing multiple nonobstructing cholelithiasis layering at the fundus of the gallbladder. Of note, there is also intrahepatic and extrahepatic biliary dilatation.

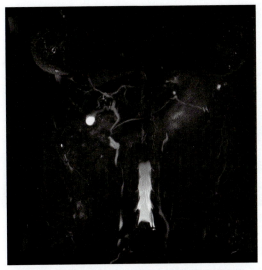

Fig. 66.8 Magnetic resonance cholangiopancreatography image demonstrating pancreatic divisum.

Table 66.4 Virtual Colonoscopy Versus Optical Colonoscopy.

	VIRTUAL COLONOSCOPY (CTC)	OPTICAL COLONOSCOPY
Safety profile	Less complications, including lower rate of bowel perforation	More frequent incidence of bowel perforation Less well tolerated than CTC
Complete colonic wall visualization	Better complete colonic wall visualization (4% for CTC vs. 7% for optical colonoscopy in one large series of direct comparison*)	Higher rate of incomplete examination
Bowel prep	Potential for no bowel prep (laxative-free CTC) with the use of fecal tagging	Required
Radiation exposure	Uses ionizing radiation, although dose to the patient is not significantly different from that of a routine abdominal CT scan	None
Ability to perform procedures	Unable to perform interventions	Able to perform procedure (biopsy or polypectomy) at the same time lesions are identified
Extracolonic findings	Ability to visualize the colon wall, in addition to detecting incidental findings of the abdomen and pelvis	Can only visualize colonic lumen

CT, Computed tomograpy; *CTC*, computed tomographic colonography.
Data from Halligan S, Taylor SA. CT colonography: results and limitations. Eur J Radiol. 2007;61(3):400-408.

VIRTUAL COLONOSCOPY

20. **Describe the primary differences between virtual colonoscopy, also referred to as computed tomographic colonography (CTC), and optical colonoscopy.**
    Technologic advances over the past few years have allowed CTC to evolve into the premiere radiologic method to investigate colonic neoplasia, surpassing double-contrast barium enema. However, optical colonoscopy continues to be the primary tool used for colorectal cancer screening. There are several inherent differences between these two modalities, and each has its own advantages and disadvantages (Table 66.4). Although it is necessary for physicians to be cognizant of the unique features of both CTC and optical colonoscopy, the most important fact is that they are equivalent in their ability to detect colorectal cancer and large polyps (>10 mm).

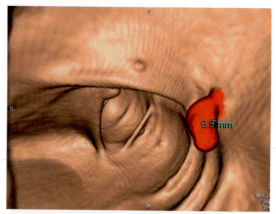

Fig. 66.9 Computed tomography colonography demonstrating a 6.9 mm sessile colon polyp.

21. Do guidelines exist for the appropriate management of CTC findings?

- If a mass is detected, surgical consultation is recommended (Fig. 66.9).
- Strong recommendation, low-quality evidence 9. The European Society of Gastrointestinal Endoscopy/European Society of Gastrointestinal and Abdominal Radiology recommends referral for endoscopic polypectomy in patients with at least one polyp ≥6 mm detected at CTC (Fig. 66.9). Follow-up CTC may be clinically considered for 6- to 9-mm CTC-detected lesions if patients do not undergo polypectomy because of patient choice, comorbidity, and/or low-risk profile for advanced neoplasia.
- For polyps 5 mm or less in size, continued routine screening with CTC is recommended in 5 years.

ACKNOWLEDGMENT

The authors would like to acknowledge the contributions of Dr. Michael Reiter who was the author of this chapter in the previous edition and provided many of the images.

BIBLIOGRAPHY

Available Online

CHAPTER 67

INTERVENTIONAL RADIOLOGY I: CROSS-SECTIONAL IMAGING PROCEDURES

Katherine S. Marchak, MD and Kimi L. Kondo, DO, FSIR

 Additional content available online

IMAGE-GUIDED PERCUTANEOUS BIOPSIES AND FLUID ASPIRATION AND DRAINAGE

1. **What are the indications for image-guided percutaneous needle biopsy (PNB)?**
   - Establish a benign or malignant diagnosis of a lesion. Stage patients with known or suspected malignancy when metastasis is suspected.
   - Molecular analysis for treatment planning.
   - Monitor treatment. Obtain material for microbiological analysis in patients with known or suspected infection. Determine the nature and extent of diffuse parenchymal diseases (e.g., cirrhosis, organ transplant rejection, and glomerulonephritis).

2. **What are the indications for image-guided percutaneous fluid aspiration (PFA) and percutaneous catheter drainage (PCD)?**
   - Obtain a sample for fluid characterization and microbiologic sensitivities.
   - Remove fluid suspected to be infected or the result of an abnormal fistulous connection.
   - Remove fluid collection suspected to be the cause of symptoms sufficient to warrant drainage (e.g., pain).
   - Perform an adjunctive procedure necessary to facilitate the improved outcome of a subsequent intervention (e.g., drainage prior to sclerotherapy).
   - Perform a temporizing maneuver to stabilize the patient's condition before definitive surgery (e.g., drainage of diverticular abscess to allow primary reanastomosis).

3. **Name contraindications (absolute or relative) for image-guided PNB and PFA/PCD.**
   - A competent patient who does not give consent.
   - A patient who is unwilling or unable to cooperate with or to be positioned for the procedure (e.g., a retroperitoneal abscess which is only accessible percutaneously via the back but the patient is unable to lie prone because of pain from an anterior abdominal wound or recent surgical incision). However, general anesthesia could be considered.
   - Uncorrectable coagulopathy.
   - Severely compromised cardiopulmonary function or hemodynamic instability.
   - Lack of a safe percutaneous *window* or pathway to the target (e.g., procedure requires transgression of pleura: risk of pneumothorax, pleural effusion, and empyema).
   - Inability to visualize the target with available imaging modalities.
   - Tumor abscess may require lifelong catheter drainage.
   - Pregnancy in cases in which imaging guidance uses ionizing radiation (the potential risks to the fetus and the clinical benefits of the procedure should be considered before proceeding).

4. **When is an image-guided percutaneous core biopsy required as opposed to a percutaneous fine-needle aspiration (FNA)?**
   When architectural detail is needed for histopathologic diagnosis (e.g., well-differentiated neoplasms) and staging (e.g., staging fibrosis of diffuse liver diseases), a core biopsy is required. FNA specimens are usually obtained using 22- to 27-gauge needles and yield clusters of cells and occasionally small tissue fragments for cytopathologic examination. Core biopsies are performed using disposable, spring-loaded, automated devices (20 gauge or larger) and yield cylinders of tissue 1–3 cm long.

5. **Which imaging modalities are used to guide interventional procedures?**
   Fluoroscopy, ultrasound (US) (Fig. 67.1), computed tomography (CT), and magnetic resonance imaging (MRI) can be used to guide interventions. US and CT are used most often.

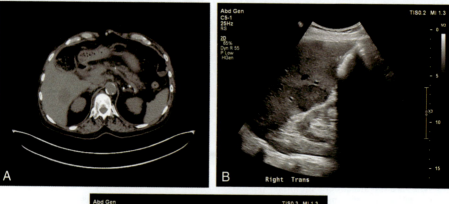

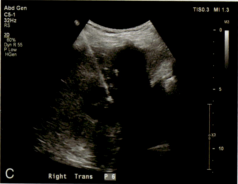

Fig. 67.1 Metastatic urothelial cancer. (A) Noncontrast axial computed tomography scan of the liver demonstrates a 3.3 cm lesion in the liver, which was fluorodeoxyglucose-avid on associated positron emission tomography. (B) Ultrasound of the liver demonstrates the mass to be hypoechoic. (C) The needle is echogenic and well visualized during percutaneous ultrasound-guided biopsy.

6. **What five conditions must be satisfied before a percutaneous procedure can be performed?**
   - The patient or patient's representative must provide written, informed consent for the procedure, intravenous conscious sedation (if applicable), and potential administration of blood or blood products.
   - Code status during the procedure and post-procedural recovery period must be determined if the patient has do-not-attempt-resuscitation order.
   - Depending on the type of procedure (e.g., high risk and low risk), the patient's coagulation profile must be determined and any coagulopathies corrected per the Society of Interventional Radiology Consensus guidelines.
   - The patient must be fasting if conscious sedation will be used during the procedure. Exact times vary depending on the institutional protocols and guidelines. Typical guidelines are fasting for at least 2 hours for *clear* liquids and at least 6 hours for *solids* or food.
   - Appropriate antibiotic coverage must be administered if there is any possibility that the lesion or fluid collection is infected as the percutaneous intervention could cause transient bacteremia.

7. **What coagulation parameters are assessed before a percutaneous procedure?**
   The patient history should be reviewed for bleeding risks, such as anticoagulant (warfarin [Coumadin], low-molecular-weight heparin, and direct-acting oral anticoagulants) or platelet-inhibitor (aspirin, clopidogrel [Plavix], and nonsteroidal anti-inflammatory drugs) agents, uremia, or hepatocellular disease. Routinely assessed parameters include hematocrit, prothrombin time, international normalized ratio (INR), partial thromboplastin time, and platelet count. Additionally, in patients with chronic liver disease, fibrinogen may be assessed.

8. **How and when should coagulopathies be corrected?**
   Coagulopathies should be corrected with appropriate transfusions of packed red blood cells or hemostatic agents such as platelets, fresh-frozen plasma, vitamin K, cryoprecipitate, protamine, and recombinant factor VIIa.

The Society of Interventional Radiology guidelines offer useful coagulation and transfusion parameters for percutaneous procedures based on low or high risk of bleeding. In low-risk procedures, it is not routinely recommended that platelet count or INR be assessed but if they are determined they need to be corrected to $>20 \times 10^9/L$ and <2.0–3.0, respectively. In high-risk procedures, routine assessment of platelet count and INR are recommended with correction to $>50 \times 10^9/L$ and <1.5–1.8, respectively. However, institutional guidelines may vary from this practice.

9. **How and when should anticoagulation and antiplatelet medications be held?**
   The Society of Interventional Radiology Consensus Criteria also offers recommendations for antiplatelet and anticoagulation medications based on low and high risk of bleeding in percutaneous procedures. For low-risk procedures, most medications do not need to be withheld. For high-risk procedures, most medications are recommended to be held and the duration depends on the pharmacologic characteristics of the medication. In patients with coronary stents, atrial fibrillation, or mechanical heart valves, a cardiology consult with a multidisciplinary approach to anticoagulation/antiplatelets may be needed.

10. **What pharmacologic agents can be injected into septated or viscous abdominal fluid collections to improve drainage?**
    Intracavitary fibrinolysis therapy with tissue plasminogen activator (tPA) can be performed through the drainage catheters to shorten treatment time and improve the clinical course of patients treated with percutaneous drainage catheters. Optimal dosing regimens have not been determined. Typical doses of tPA range from 4 to 6 mg of tPA diluted in up to 50 mL normal saline. The total volume of fluid depends on the size of the cavity. The dose is injected into the catheter, which is clamped for 1 hour after the dose is administered. After unclamping, the dose is allowed to drain spontaneously. This is typically performed twice daily for 3 days. Total number of doses varies depending on output response. Caution should be used with hepatic abscesses or in patients who are coagulopathic because of the potential increased risk of bleeding.

11. **What should you suspect if the drainage catheter has persistently elevated outputs and how can this be managed?**
    If a catheter has persistently elevated outputs, a sudden increase in drainage, or a change in the composition of the effluent, a fistula should be suspected. Injection of contrast into the catheter under fluoroscopy often demonstrates the fistula, which can be to the gastrointestinal tract, pancreatic duct, biliary system, or genitourinary tract. Occasionally, an alternative study is necessary such as a small bowel follow-through if the fistula acts as a one-way valve and is not demonstrated by injection of the drainage catheter. Often the fistula will heal but prolonged drainage is required and can last as long as 2–4 weeks or more. The catheter should not be removed until the fistula has healed or has been repaired. To promote healing of the fistula, the drainage catheter should be left to gravity and not placed on suction drainage as this can increase output through the fistula and therefore delay healing. Repair of fistulas can be percutaneous with fibrin glue or laser ablation, or surgical.

12. **When should you remove the drainage catheter?**
    If the catheter output is less than 10–20 mL per 24 hours, there are no other reasons for the decreased outputs (e.g., catheter clogged, kinked, or malpositioned), and the patient has clinically improved, the catheter can be removed. Repeat imaging with US, CT, or contrast injection under fluoroscopy is not necessary unless the patient has a known fistula or is still clinically symptomatic, or unless the overall output is less than expected. An exception to these criteria for catheter removal is percutaneous cholecystostomy and transhepatic catheters. These require an epithelialized tract to form before removal to prevent bile leakage and bile peritonitis. This usually requires a minimum of 3 weeks' time, but if the patient is immunocompromised or in the intensive care unit, the process can take even longer.

13. **What are the major complications of image-guided PNB?**
    Major complications are defined as those that result in an unplanned increase in the level of care, prolonged hospitalization (inpatients), admission to the hospital for therapy (outpatients), permanent adverse sequelae, and death. The complications of PNB can be stratified as general or organ-specific. Major general complications include hemorrhage, infection, solid organ injury, bowel perforation, and pneumothorax. Reported rates of major complications range from 0.1% to 10% with infection as a result of a biopsy being uncommon. Hemorrhage is the most common complication but clinically significant bleeding requiring blood transfusion or intervention is infrequent, and the reported rates increase with larger needle sizes, use of cutting needles, and the vascularity of the organ or lesion biopsied.

14. **Does seeding of the needle tract occur during routine tumor biopsy?**
    Case reports of tumor spread along the needle tract as a result of percutaneous biopsy are described in the medical literature. Overall, seeding of the needle tract is uncommon and the reported rates vary according to the organ biopsied. For masses suspected to be hepatocellular carcinoma (HCC), needle track seeding can be a

potentially devastating complication in transplant candidates in whom immunosuppression may predispose to seeded tumor growth; however, the American Association for the Study of Liver Diseases believes the risk has been overstated in earlier literature. Needle gauge sizes, number of needle passes, traversing normal parenchyma, and coaxial versus single-needle systems are believed to influence the risk of tumor seeding, but robust evidence is still lacking. Although this potential complication should be discussed with the patient prior to the procedure, it should not be considered a contraindication to FNA or core biopsy in patients in whom the diagnosis is in question and when knowledge of a specific diagnosis is likely to alter clinical management.

Cystic lesions like suspected cystadenomas or cystadenocarcinomas of the ovary or pancreas should not be sampled percutaneously, even with small, skinny needles. This is associated with a significant risk of post-procedural needle tract seeding and subsequent pseudomyxoma peritonei or peritoneal carcinomatosis.

IMAGE-GUIDED PERCUTANEOUS PAIN INTERVENTIONS

15. What are the indications for image-guided celiac plexus block (Fig. 67.2)?
    - As a diagnostic maneuver to determine whether abdominal pain is sympathetically mediated.
    - For the palliation of pain in acute pancreatitis and other acute pain syndromes thought to be mediated by the celiac plexus.
    - To alleviate the acute pain associated with embolization of liver malignancies.
    - To treat abdominal *angina* associated with arterial insufficiency to the abdominal viscera.

16. What are the indications for image-guided celiac plexus neurolysis?
    Neurolysis can be performed with either phenol or alcohol to treat pain associated with abdominal and retroperitoneal malignancies (e.g., pancreatic cancer) or for chronic benign pain syndromes (e.g., chronic pancreatitis).

17. What are other image-guided blocks that can be performed?
    - Hypogastric plexus block can be performed for sympathetically mediated pain of the pelvic viscera (e.g., malignancy, proctalgia fugax, and radiation enteritis).
    - Ganglion impar block can be performed for sympathetically mediated pain of the perineum, rectum, and genitalia (e.g., rectal cancer).

HEPATIC INTERVENTIONS

18. Is FNA or core biopsy safe or necessary for all hepatic masses?
    Benign masses such as hemangiomas (Fig. 67.3), focal nodular hyperplasia, and adenomas often have distinguishing characteristics on high-quality cross-sectional imaging modalities. When these masses are present

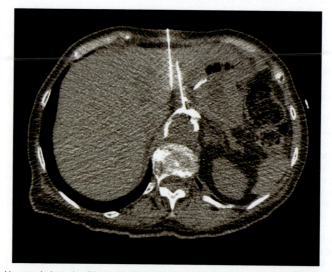

Fig. 67.2 Computed tomography image in a 73-year old with pancreatic cancer with associated chronic abdominal pain. This demonstrates two needles with contrast injection demonstrating good periaortic spread with no retrocrural spread of contrast, prior to injection of anesthetic.

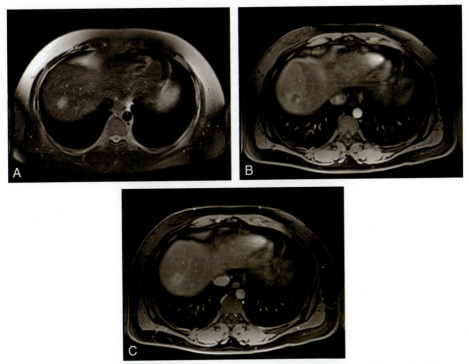

Fig. 67.3 Liver magnetic resonance imaging with hepatic steatosis, fatty sparing near the hepatic dome, and a hemangioma. The hemangioma is T2 hyperintense (A) with nodular peripheral enhancement (B) and gradual fill-in on delayed enhancement images (C).

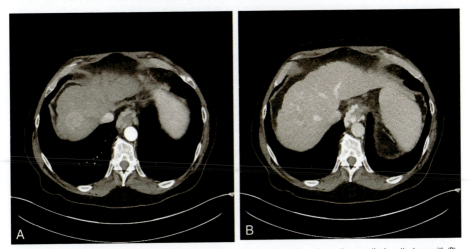

Fig. 67.4 A 68-year old with hepatitis C liver cirrhosis and an (A) arterial enhancing 3.5 cm observation near the hepatic dome with (B) washout on portal venous phase consistent with Liver Imaging Reporting and Data System 5, definitely hepatocellular carcinoma.

in patients with classic corresponding clinical features, obtaining specimens for cytologic or histologic examination is usually not necessary. If any imaging or clinical features are not characteristic, biopsy can be performed safely. Additionally, HCC has specific imaging characteristics. By using the Liver Imaging Reporting and Data System (LI-RADS) criteria, HCC can often be diagnosed without the need for biopsy (Fig. 67.4).

Carcinoid crisis characterized by profound hypotension can be precipitated by FNA of hepatic carcinoid metastases. Patients with carcinoid tumors typically present with characteristic clinical symptoms and can be confirmed biochemically. If biopsy of a suspected hepatic carcinoid metastasis must be performed for diagnosis, appropriate preparatory measures should be taken and resuscitative equipment and medications such as octreotide need to be readily available.

19. How are pyogenic hepatic abscesses treated?

At least 90% of pyogenic hepatic abscesses can be successfully drained percutaneously. Most pyogenic abscesses smaller than 3 cm in diameter are treated with antibiotics either alone or in combination with needle aspiration, with excellent success rates. For pyogenic abscesses larger than 4 cm in diameter, image-guided PCD is required. The size of the self-retaining, pigtail catheter inserted often depends on the viscosity of the fluid encountered.

The possibility of an abscess complicating an underlying hepatic neoplasm should always be considered. Follow-up imaging should be obtained to document eventual complete resolution of the lesion. FNA or core biopsy of any persistent abnormality may be necessary to exclude occult hepatic tumor.

20. When is image-guided PFA/PCD indicated for the treatment of amebic abscesses?

Amebic abscesses respond well to appropriate antibiotic treatment regardless of size, and PCD is usually not required unless response to medical treatment is inadequate. PCD should be considered for large amebic abscesses in a peripheral location or in the left hepatic lobe as these sites are prone to rupture into the peritoneum, pericardium, or pleural space.

21. Is image-guided PFA/PCD indicated for the treatment of hydatid cyst disease?

Cystic echinococcosis is caused by *Echinococcus granulosus*. Echinococcal serology can be considered in suspected cases. Previously, PFA/PCD of a suspected echinococcal cyst or hydatid cyst disease was an absolute contraindication because of fatal anaphylaxis from spillage of the scolices. However, published series describe favorable results with oral albendazole treatment combined with PCD or with the puncture, aspiration, injection, reaspiration (PAIR) technique. The cyst contents are aspirated via the percutaneous puncture. Contrast is injected under fluoroscopic guidance to ensure there is no communication with the bile ducts and then a protoscolicide such as hypertonic saline or ethanol is injected, allowed to sit, and then reaspirated. Modified PAIR uses placement of a catheter, which allows more complete evacuation of the endocyst and repeat injections of protosolicide, and is especially useful for treating large cysts. Oral albendazole treatment must be started at least 4 hours prior to percutaneous intervention. *Caution:* The risk of fatal anaphylaxis is not entirely eliminated and thus appropriate emergency medical treatment and resources must be readily available.

22. Describe the treatment of simple, benign, epithelialized hepatic cysts.

Simple hepatic cysts are often asymptomatic and require no treatment. However, symptomatic epithelialized hepatic cysts (e.g., pain) can be drained successfully and obliterated with sclerotherapy (Fig. 67.5). A self-retaining, pigtail catheter can be used. After catheter placement with US or CT guidance and complete cyst aspiration, samples are sent for culture and cytologic examination. Contrast is injected through the catheter under fluoroscopic guidance to ensure that there is no communication with the biliary tree, vascular structures, or peritoneal cavity. If no connection is demonstrated, then 33%–50% of the original cyst volume is replaced with a sclerosant. Sclerosants used to treat hepatic cysts include ethanol (not to exceed 100 mL), tetracycline, doxycycline, fibrin sealant, and povidone-iodine. The patient is rotated into multiple positions until the entirety of the cyst wall has been in contact with the sclerosing agent for 60 minutes. The entire volume of sclerosant and residual cyst contents are then completely aspirated through the catheter. Large cysts may require repeat treatments. After the final treatment and aspiration, the catheter is removed.

23. Can cysts in patients with polycystic liver disease be treated with sclerotherapy?

Yes, although solitary hepatic cysts are more often successfully sclerosed than cysts in patients with polycystic liver disease. In polycystic liver disease, cysts tend not to collapse, presumably because the surrounding liver is less pliable, making cyst wall apposition and subsequent scarring of the cavity less likely. Surgical or laparoscopic unroofing, fenestration, or removal of cysts may be needed when percutaneous treatment fails.

24. Name the minimally invasive percutaneous ablative therapies for HCC.

Percutaneous ablative techniques for local control of HCC can be divided into three categories: thermal ablation, nonthermal ablation, and chemical ablation. Thermal ablation techniques alter the temperature of the tumor to cause cell death and include heat-based methods (radiofrequency ablation [RFA], microwave ablation [Fig. 67.6], laser ablation, and high-intensity focused US) and cold-based methods (cryoablation). Nonthermal ablation includes irreversible electroporation which uses high-voltage pulses to induce cell death. Chemical ablation involves injecting substances such as ethanol or acetic acid directly into the tumor to produce tissue necrosis.

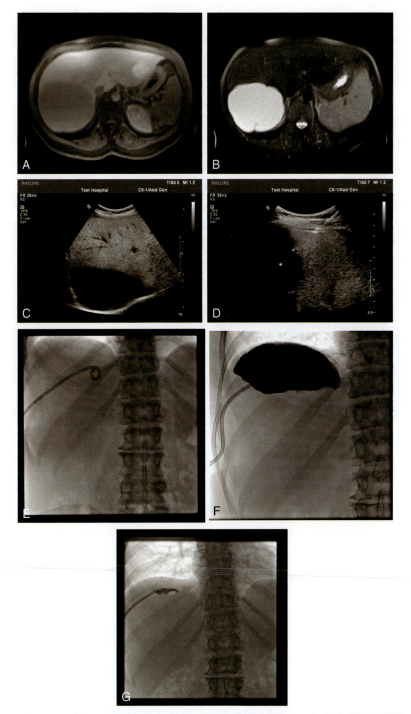

Fig. 67.5 Percutaneous drainage and sclerosis of liver cyst in a 47-year old with right upper quadrant pain. (A) T1 and (B) T2 magnetic resonance imaging of the liver demonstrates a 11 × 9 cm hepatic cyst. (C) Ultrasound (US) demonstrates the cyst and (D) US-guided echogenic needle placement into the cyst. (E) Drain is placed under fluoroscopic guidance and (F) injected to determine the volume for sclerosis. (G) Contrast injection after multiple sessions of alcohol sclerosis demonstrates no significant residual cavity of the cyst.

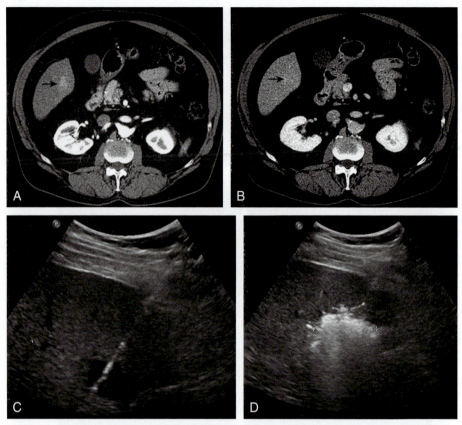

Fig. 67.6 Microwave ablation of hepatocellular carcinoma (HCC). (A) Arterial phase contrast-enhanced computed tomography (CT) scan demonstrates a 2.5-cm hypervascular mass (*arrow*) in the right hepatic lobe of a patient with hepatitis C. (B) There is washout (*arrow*) on the portal venous phase consistent with HCC. (C) Ultrasound image shows the hypoechoic mass with placement of the echogenic microwave probe in the mass. (D) Ultrasound image during microwave ablation depicts the hyperechoic zone of ablation.

25. What temperatures must be achieved to be cytotoxic for tumor destruction?

Irreversible damage with cellular protein denaturation, cell membrane dysfunction, and coagulation necrosis occurs at temperatures between 60° C and 100° C. Above 100° C–110° C, tissue carbonization and charring occur which results in diminished volume of the ablation zone from less effective energy transmission. In cryotherapy, irreversible damage from cellular dehydration, membrane rupture, and ischemic microvascular thrombosis occurs at temperatures between −20°C and −40°C. For adequate tumor destruction, the entire target volume must be subject to cytotoxic temperatures and thus the zone of ablation must be larger than the size of the tumor itself to achieve tumor-free margins.

26. What are the advantages of RFA and other methods of percutaneous thermal ablation?

- Low mortality and complication rates (multicenter surveys report mortality rates ranging from 0.1% to 0.5%, major complication rates ranging from 2.2% to 3.1%, and minor complication rates ranging from 5% to 8.9%).
- Repeatability
- Minimally invasive and shorter recovery times compared with surgery
- Can be used in combination with other treatment therapies
- Less destruction of nonneoplastic tissue than surgery

27. What are the contraindications of RFA or percutaneous thermal ablative techniques?

The only absolute contraindications are uncorrectable coagulopathy or a noncompliant patient. RFA and other percutaneous ablative techniques are local treatments and are usually not performed in patients with vascular invasion or extrahepatic metastases. Patients with colonization of the biliary tract from bilioenteric anastomoses, endoscopic sphincterotomy, or bilioenteric fistula are at increased risk of postablation liver abscess.

28. **Describe the risks of thermal ablation related to the anatomic location of the tumor.**
Superficial tumors adjacent to the gastrointestinal tract are at risk for thermal injury to the bowel wall. The colon appears to be at greater risk for perforation than the stomach and small bowel because of the thinner wall thickness and its lesser mobility. Gas or hydro dissection can be considered. The gallbladder and biliary tract are also at risk for thermal injury. Perforation of the gallbladder is rare, but ablation of tumors adjacent to the gallbladder can be associated with iatrogenic cholecystitis, which is usually self-limited. Tumor location <1 cm from a major biliary duct may result in delayed stenosis. Additionally, bilomas may develop. Lesions in the dome of the liver can result in thermal injury to the diaphragm, pneumothorax, or hemothorax. Vessels in the vicinity or adjacent to lesions are usually protected because of the *heat or cold sink* effect of flowing blood. However, if the vessel is very small or the flow is decreased for any reason, thrombosis can occur. The heat or cold sink effect may also result in incomplete ablation of the neoplastic tissues adjacent to the vessel from temperature loss.

29. **In the treatment of HCC, how do survival outcomes of RFA compare with surgical resection?**
Most studies evaluating surgical resection and RFA show similar long-term outcomes for HCC smaller than 3 cm. In a randomized controlled trial of 112 patients with a solitary HCC less than 5 cm (Cheng et al.), there were no significant differences in local recurrence, overall survival, or disease-free survival between the two groups.

30. **What other liver tumors have been treated with percutaneous thermal ablative techniques?**
Liver metastases from neuroendocrine, gastric, pancreatic, pulmonary, renal, uterine, or ovarian cancer and melanoma have all been successfully treated with RFA. Besides HCC, the majority of percutaneous thermal ablative procedures are performed for the treatment of colorectal liver metastases. Percutaneous RFA has also been used to successfully treat symptomatic giant cavernous hemangiomas in patients choosing not to undergo surgical resection.

SPLENIC INTERVENTIONS

31. **What cross-sectional image-guided interventions are possible in the spleen?**
When clinically indicated, given the increased risk of complications such as bleeding, percutaneous image-guided biopsy, and catheter drainage can be performed safely in the spleen. Focal splenic masses are uncommon, so splenic biopsy is rarely performed. Splenic abscesses also are not common although the incidence is thought to be growing because of the increasing number of immunocompromised patients. If a percutaneous procedure is attempted, the size of the needle or catheter should be conservative because of the risk of hemorrhage. Traversing the least amount of splenic parenchyma en route to the lesion may reduce the risk of bleeding.

PANCREATIC INTERVENTIONS

32. **What procedures are appropriate for solid pancreatic masses?**
Solid masses, usually suspected tumors, can be aspirated percutaneously. Only FNAs should be performed; core biopsies should be avoided because the use of cutting needles can result in severe pancreatitis. As noted previously, percutaneous biopsy of suspected cystadenomas or cystadenocarcinomas should be avoided.

33. **Can FNA be performed for solid pancreatic masses completely surrounded by the bowel?**
If a skinny needle (<20 gauge) is used and the lesion is solid, any organ, including the stomach, small bowel, and colon, can be traversed. Antibiotic coverage is recommended for procedures through the bowel. Major blood vessels should be avoided. The diagnosis of pancreatic adenocarcinoma often can be established by cytopathologic examination alone; a negative result must be interpreted with caution and assumed to be a sampling error until proven otherwise.

34. **What procedures are used for pancreatic and peripancreatic collections?**
Various acute and chronic pancreatic and peripancreatic collections can be percutaneously aspirated and drained using image guidance if clinically indicated. According to the revised Atlanta classification system for acute pancreatitis, collections should be defined as acute peripancreatic fluid collection (APFC), pancreatic pseudocyst, acute necrotic collection (ANC), or walled-off necrosis (WON). The term pancreatic abscess is not used in the current classification. These collections can be aspirated to determine whether they are sterile or infected. In this setting, bowel should not be crossed with the aspiration needle to avoid contaminating and superinfecting otherwise sterile fluid.

35. **Do APFCs require percutaneous image-guided treatment?**
APFCs are adjacent to the pancreas and extra pancreatic only. They occur during the first 4 weeks, have no discernible wall, and do not contain debris or necrosis. Most usually resolve spontaneously without intervention and do not become infected. Percutaneous image-guided drainage is only indicated if infected. The presence of infection can be presumed when there is the presence of extraluminal gas or when percutaneous image-guided FNA is positive for bacteria or fungi on Gram stain and culture.

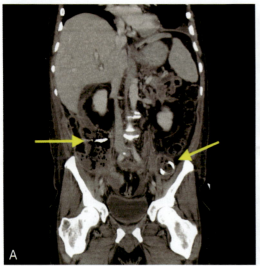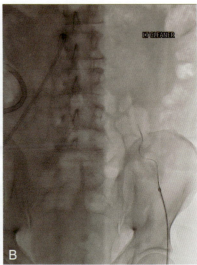

Fig. 67.7 A 47-year-old male with pancreatitis following blunt pancreatic injury. (A) Computed tomography (CT) demonstrates two of three drains within walled-off necrosis. (B) Fluoroscopic image from the sinogram demonstrates a percutaneous necrosectomy.

36. **When is drainage indicated for the treatment of pancreatic pseudocysts?**
    Pancreatic pseudocysts usually occur 4 weeks after the onset of interstitial edematous pancreatitis, have a well-defined wall, and no nonliquid component. Drainage is indicated when pseudocysts are infected, rapidly enlarging, painful, obstructing, or large (>5 cm). Drainage can be achieved via percutaneous image guidance, endoscopic US guidance, or surgically; the optimal technique depends on the clinical situation and location and the decision should be made after multidisciplinary consultation with interventional radiologists, gastroenterologists, and surgeons.

37. **What are the similarities and differences between an ANC and WON?**
    Both collections can be intra pancreatic or extra pancreatic, are associated with necrotizing pancreatitis, and contain variable amounts of fluid and solid necrotic tissue. An ANC occurs within the first 4 weeks and does not have a definable wall encapsulating the collection. WON occurs 4 weeks or more after the onset of necrotizing pancreatitis and is a mature, encapsulated collection with a well-defined inflammatory wall.

38. **What is the role of image-guided PCD in the treatment of infected ANC and WON?**
    The role of PCD in the management of infected ANC and WON is controversial. Open surgical necrosectomy is still considered the gold-standard treatment in infected pancreatic necrosis, because it involves non liquefactive tissue that is difficult to remove with percutaneous drainage catheters. However, open necrosectomy is associated with a high mortality rate and significant morbidity. Image-guided PCD generally has a lower morbidity and mortality rate and can be considered in patients with appropriate percutaneous access either as potential definitive treatment or as a bridge to surgery. It is not uncommon for drains to be left in place for a month or longer. Effective percutaneous drainage also requires vigorous catheter irrigation and frequent catheter upsizing and exchange. Percutaneous necrosectomy is performed with mechanical debridement devices and balloon sweeps of the material (Fig. 67.7).

ADRENAL INTERVENTIONS

39. **When is adrenal gland biopsy indicated?**
    In patients with no history of malignancy, most incidentally discovered adrenal masses less than 4 cm in diameter are benign and should be evaluated with CT scans or MRI. For adrenal masses greater than 4 cm and not typical for adenoma, myelolipoma, hemorrhage, or simple cysts, surgical resection should be considered. In patients with histories of malignancy, an incidental adrenal mass is more often malignant and even small lesions are suspect. In these situations, a biopsy is indicated when noninvasive tests are inconclusive unless the presence of widespread nonadrenal metastases makes the presence or absence of adrenal metastases unlikely to change patient

management. Adrenal biopsies are also indicated when enlarging masses are seen on follow-up imaging and the imaging characteristics are suspicious for malignancy.

40. What adrenal lesions should *not* be biopsied?

Because of the risk of hypertensive crisis, possible pheochromocytomas in any of the above situations should not be needled. Pheochromocytomas do not have specific imaging features and thus must be suspected clinically with confirmation testing for urine or serum catecholamines.

ACKNOWLEDGMENT

The authors would like to acknowledge the contribution of Dr. Paul D. Russ, who was the author of this chapter in the previous edition.

CLINICAL VIGNETTE

Available Online

BIBLIOGRAPHY

Available Online

WEBSITES

Available Online

INTERVENTIONAL RADIOLOGY II: FLUOROSCOPIC AND ANGIOGRAPHIC PROCEDURES

Lisa Walker, MD and Kimi L. Kondo, DO, FSIR

 Additional content available online

1. Name the current radiologic methods of treating hepatic malignancies.
Transarterial chemoembolization (TACE), transarterial embolization (TAE), selective internal radiation therapy (SIRT), percutaneous image-guided chemical ablation, percutaneous image-guided thermal ablation, TACE combined with ablation, and hepatic arterial chemotherapy infusion are the current radiologic methods. Hepatic arterial chemotherapy infusion has been used for the treatment of colorectal cancer metastases to the liver but remains unpopular because of cost, complexity of arterial pump placement, and concerns of liver toxicity.

2. What are the indications for TACE?
Chemoembolization is indicated in patients with liver-dominant hepatic malignancies who are not candidates for curative resection. In patients with hepatocellular carcinoma (HCC), depending on the disease stage, TACE has been used as definitive treatment, palliative treatment, or as a bridge to liver transplantation. It is considered the standard of care for intermediate stages of HCC according to the Barcelona Clinic Liver Cancer staging system. TACE has also been used as a palliative treatment for patients with unresectable cholangiocarcinoma and hepatic metastases from neuroendocrine tumors, colorectal carcinoma, breast carcinoma, as well as soft-tissue sarcomas. The injection of the chemotherapeutic agent (usually doxorubicin) mixed with ethiodized oil followed by embolization with particles is considered conventional TACE as opposed to a more recent refinement of the technique using drug-eluting beads to both deliver the chemotherapy and act as the embolic agent (Fig. 68.1A and B).

3. What is the expected median survival for patients with intermediate HCC after TACE?
For patients with intermediate HCC, the expected median survival is 16 months. After TACE, it is approximately 20 months. This fulfills the standard oncologic criteria for treatment efficacy.

4. Describe exclusion criteria/contraindications for TACE in patients with HCC.
Contraindications for TACE can be categorized based on tumor status, liver disease, patient performance status, Table 68.1 procedural aspects, and chemotherapy characteristics (Table 68.1). Exclusion criteria based on laboratory values are not definitively established. Greater than 50% liver replacement with tumor, bilirubin level

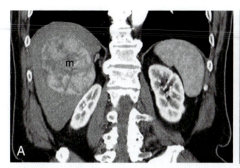
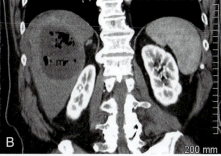

Fig. 68.1 Chemoembolization of a hepatocellular carcinoma (HCC). (A) Coronal arterial phase contrast-enhanced computed tomography (CT) scan demonstrates an 8-cm hypervascular mass (m) in the right lobe of the liver. (B) Coronal arterial phase contrast-enhanced CT scan performed 4 weeks later demonstrates the hypodense, nonenhancing HCC (m) consistent with complete devascularization and response to chemoembolization. The gas bubbles are a result of sterile tumor necrosis from the injection of polyvinyl alcohol particles in addition to the doxorubicin drug-eluting beads.

Table 68.1 Exclusion Criteria and Contraindications for Transarterial Chemoembolization.

CATEGORY	CRITERIA
Tumor status	Single resectable tumor BCLC class D
Liver disease	Child-Pugh class C Active gastrointestinal bleeding
Patient performance status	ECOG >2
Procedural	Renal insufficiency/failure Uncorrectable coagulopathy Intractable systemic infection Severe anaphylactic/anaphylactoid contrast reaction
Doxorubicin related	WBC <3000 cells/mm^3; neutrophils <1500 cells/mm^3 Left ventricular ejection fraction <50%

BCLC, Barcelona Clinic Liver Cancer; *ECOG,* eastern Cooperative Oncology Group; *WBC,* white blood cell.

of more than 2 mg/dL, a lactate dehydrogenase level of more than 425 mg/dL, and an aspartate aminotransferase level of more than 100 IU/L have been reported to be strongly associated with increased postprocedural mortality. However, individual abnormalities of these four parameters have not been shown to predict adverse outcomes from TACE. A total bilirubin cutoff value of more than 3 mg/dL has been described in the literature, although some operators have performed TACE in patients with total bilirubin of more than 3 mg/dL if they are listed for liver transplantation. Portal vein thrombosis is no longer considered an absolute contraindication; however, highly selective embolization and ↓ adjustment of the chemotherapy dose may minimize liver damage.

5. **Describe postembolization syndrome (PES).**
PES is an expected side effect of liver embolization and can occur after TAE, TACE, and SIRT. It is characterized by fever, abdominal pain, anorexia, nausea, vomiting, and fatigue. PES occurs in up to 90% of patients. Symptoms usually arise 24–48 hours after the procedure and last for 1–2 weeks. The severity of symptoms is variable and is usually a self-limited event that is managed supportively. Occasionally, it can require an extended hospital admission. The etiologic factors are not fully understood, but PES is thought to be caused by a combination of liver tissue ischemia, inflammatory response, and tumor necrosis.

6. **How is response to TAE and TACE monitored?**
Post-treatment monitoring is performed with contrast-enhanced multiphase computed tomography (CT) or dynamic magnetic resonance imaging (MRI) 4–6 weeks after all tumor-bearing areas are treated. If treatment of both lobes of the liver are planned, imaging between sessions may be performed based on operator preference. Signs of tumor treatment on CT include uptake of ethiodized oil (conventional TACE only) and absence of arterial phase enhancement when present prior to therapy (Fig. 68.1A and B). The principal determinant of tumor necrosis on MRI is also the absence of arterial enhancement when present prior to treatment.

7. **What is SIRT or yttrium-90 (^{90}Y) radioembolization?**
SIRT, or radioembolization, is a transarterial method for treating hepatic malignancies that involves selective intra-arterial delivery of microspheres loaded with a radioisotope. It is a form of intra-arterial brachytherapy. The primary mode of action is the emission of radiation, and the second mode of action is the embolization of the vasculature. ^{90}Y is the most common radioisotope used for radioembolization. It is a beta emitter, has a mean tissue penetration of 2.5 mm and a maximum penetration of 11 mm, and a half-life of 64 hours (Fig. 68.2A–D).

8. **Name the two US Food and Drug Administration (FDA)–approved and commercially available radioactive microspheres and describe their differences.**
SIR-Spheres are nonbiodegradable resin spheres with a median size of 32 μm and are FDA approved for the treatment of unresectable colorectal liver metastases. TheraSphere therapy consists of nonbiodegradable glass spheres with a median size of 25 μm and is FDA approved for the treatment of unresectable HCC. The activity per particle is higher with TheraSphere, which measures 2500 Bq as opposed to 50 Bq for SIR-Spheres. The number of particles delivered per treatment and the embolization effect with TheraSphere is less compared with SIR-Spheres.

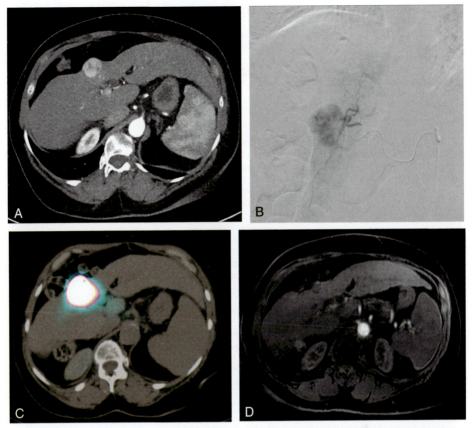

Fig. 68.2 TheraSphere ^{90}Y radioembolization of a hepatocellular carcinoma. (A) Computed tomography (CT) demonstrates an exophytic 2.7 cm Liver Imaging Reporting and Data System 5 mass within segment 4. (B) Macroaggregated albumin mapping angiography demonstrates tumor supply from the middle hepatic artery. (C) Single-photon emission CT/CT with increased radiotracer activity corresponding to the known mass and a lung shunt fraction of 4%. (D) Subsequent ^{90}Y radiation segmentectomy was performed and follow-up magnetic resonance imaging 1 month after treatment showed no residual disease.

9. What are the indications for ^{90}Y radioembolization?

^{90}Y radioembolization is indicated for the treatment of unresectable or medically inoperable primary or secondary liver malignancies. The tumor burden should be liver dominant but does not have to be exclusive to the liver. The Eastern Cooperative Oncology Group performance status should be 0–2, and life expectancy should be at least 3 months.

10. In the pretreatment workup of patients considered for ^{90}Y radioembolization, what imaging procedures besides cross-sectional imaging must occur?

Prior to ^{90}Y radioembolization, mapping visceral arteriography of the celiac, superior mesenteric, left gastric, gastroduodenal, proper hepatic, and right and left hepatic arteries was performed. This is important to determine the areas of possible nontarget embolization and calculate ^{90}Y dosing. At the end of the procedure, injection of technetium-99 macroaggregated albumin into the target artery is performed. Nuclear medicine scanning is then performed to determine pulmonary shunt fraction and areas of nontarget administration. The overall activity of ^{90}Y delivered to the lungs should not exceed >30 Gy per treatment or >50 Gy, as this has been associated with the development of radiation pneumonitis.

11. What are the contraindications of ^{90}Y radioembolization?

- Uncorrectable coagulopathy
- Severe anaphylactic or anaphylactoid contrast reaction
- Severe liver or renal dysfunction
- Lung shunt >20%

- Gastrointestinal (GI) shunts that cannot be corrected
- Untreated varices at high risk of bleeding
- Total bilirubin greater than 2 mg/dL in the absence of a reversible cause
- Greater than 70% tumor replacement of liver unless synthetic function (prothrombin time and albumin) is maintained
- Prior radiation therapy to the liver or upper abdomen that included a significant volume of the liver
- Systemic chemotherapy agents in the preceding 4 weeks not known to be used safely concurrently with radioembolization
- Granulocyte count less than 1.5×10^9/L
- Pregnancy

12. **Discuss the potential advantages of ^{90}Y radioembolization compared with TACE.**
^{90}Y radioembolization has a decreased incidence and severity of PES and thus can be performed as an outpatient procedure without the need for hospitalization. Recent studies suggest better disease control (longer time to progression) with less toxicity with ^{90}Y radioembolization than TACE, although no survival differences between the two treatments have been demonstrated. Additionally, ^{90}Y radioembolization for HCC (TheraSpheres) is a microembolic procedure causing minimal occlusion of the hepatic arteries and may be safely used in the setting of portal vein thrombosis.

13. **Define preoperative portal vein embolization (PVE).**
PVE is an image-guided procedure performed prior to resection of liver malignancies to increase the size of the future liver remnant (FLR) or the liver segments that will remain after surgery. By embolizing the portal vein branches supplying the tumor-bearing segments, flow is redirected to the non-tumor-bearing segments, resulting in hypertrophy of the FLR (Fig. 68.3A and B).

14. **In major hepatic resection candidates with normal liver function, what is the standardized FLR (sFLR) cutoff for PVE?**
The size of the FLR needs to be standardized to patient size as larger patients require a larger liver mass to support their essential functions compared to smaller patients. sFLR is expressed as a percentage of FLR in relation to total functioning liver volume. The cutoff for PVE is an sFLR less than 20% for normal liver, 30% for fibrosis/severe liver injury/prior chemotherapy, and 40% for cirrhosis. Studies have shown significantly higher rates of postoperative liver insufficiency and death from liver failure in patients with sFLR of less than 20% and if the degree of hypertrophy after PVE is less than 5%.

15. **Is PVE indicated for patients with HCC and clinically evident portal hypertension?**
No. Clinically evident portal hypertension is a contraindication to hepatectomy, so these patients are not candidates for major hepatic resection.

16. **When might PVE be indicated in patients with cirrhosis?**
PVE is considered in patients with well-compensated cirrhosis (i.e., Child-Pugh [CP] class A), who are surgical resection candidates, and who have an sFLR of less than 40%. Patients with cirrhosis often demonstrate

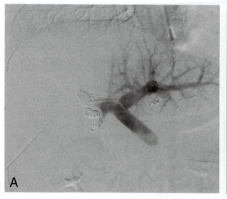
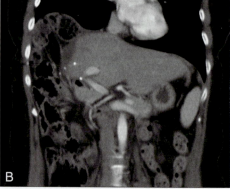

Fig. 68.3 Portal vein embolization (PVE). (A) Patient with hepatic metastases from colon carcinoma with prior chemotherapy in which PVE of segments 5, 6, 7, and 8 was performed to induce hypertrophy of the planned residual hepatic remnant. (B) Initial standardized future liver remnant (sFLR) of 29% and after 1 month after PVE had an sFLR of 39%.

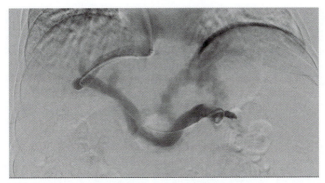

Fig. 68.4 Patient with nonalcoholic fatty liver disease cirrhosis complicated by portal hypertension with gastric varices, portal hypertensive gastropathy, and portosystemic shunt syndrome who had transjugular intrahepatic portosystemic shunt (TIPS) creation. Preprocedure portocaval gradient of 19 mm Hg, which then decreased to 10 mm Hg postprocedure.

attenuated rates and degrees of hypertrophy, so it is not uncommon that PVE might be performed in combination with other techniques, such as TACE. TACE is performed prior to PVE and may prevent disease progression that could result in the patient no longer being eligible for resection.

17. **What are the indications for transjugular intrahepatic portosystemic shunt (TIPS)?**
    - Uncontrollable variceal hemorrhage (Fig. 68.4)
    - Acute or prior variceal bleeding not controlled with initial or continued endoscopic therapy
    - Refractory ascites
    - Prophylaxis against recurrent variceal bleeding in high-risk patients
    - Portal hypertensive gastropathy
    - Hepatic hydrothorax
    - Budd-Chiari syndrome or other veno-occlusive diseases
    - Hepatorenal syndrome
    - Hepatopulmonary syndrome
    - Decompression of portosystemic collaterals prior to abdominal surgeries

18. **What are the contraindications to performing the TIPS procedure?**
    - Elevated right or left heart pressures
    - Heart failure or cardiac valvular insufficiency
    - Marked pulmonary hypertension
    - Rapidly progressing liver failure
    - Clinically significant hepatic encephalopathy
    - Uncontrolled sepsis or systemic infection
    - Unrelieved biliary obstruction
    - Severe, uncorrectable coagulopathy
    - Extensive hepatic malignancy (primary or secondary)

19. **How is TIPS patency followed?**
    TIPS patency can be followed noninvasively by color Doppler ultrasound or venography. Protocols differ among institutions. Two-year primary patency rates with the use of the Viatorr stent graft are 76%–84%, and thus, the need for frequent routine ultrasound surveillance is in question. If an early ultrasound evaluation is performed, it should be done at least 5 days after TIPS creation because air bubbles in the expanded polytetrafluoroethylene fabric create gas artifacts, which do not allow complete visualization and evaluation in the first 2–4 days. TIPS stenosis on ultrasound is suspected when velocities are >190 cm/s, <50 cm/s, or a change in velocity along the stent by 50 cm/s. If the patient becomes symptomatic (e.g., variceal bleeding or ascites) or if significant interval change is demonstrated by ultrasound, venography with therapeutic intervention should be performed to restore normal shunt function.

20. **Define balloon-occluded retrograde transvenous obliteration (BRTO).**
    BRTO is an endovascular technique used as a therapeutic adjunct or alternative to TIPS in the management of gastric varices. It involves the use of occlusion balloons to occlude the outflow veins of a portosystemic shunt and endovascular injection of a sclerosing agent directly into the varix. BRTO is the primary method used in Japan

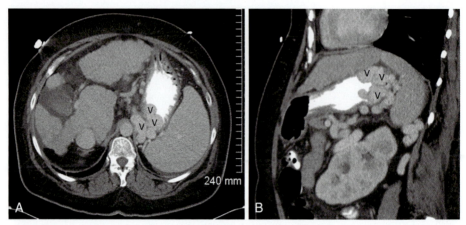

Fig. 68.5 Balloon-occluded retrograde transvenous obliteration treatment of bleeding gastric varices in a 62-year-old male with primary biliary cirrhosis. (A) Axial and sagittal (B) contrast-enhanced computed tomography scan demonstrates large gastric varices (v).

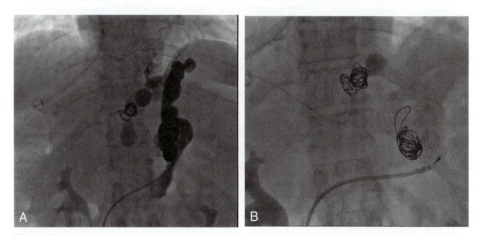

Fig. 68.6 Patient with cirrhosis and portal hypertension with gastric varices with prior transjugular intrahepatic portosystemic shunt who presents for balloon-occluded retrograde obliteration of gastrorenal shunt. Subsequent coil and plug occlusion was performed of the proximal and distal shunt.

and Korea for the management of gastric varices as opposed to the United States and Europe, where the primary management of gastric varices has been portal decompression with TIPS. Its use is growing in the United States. Indications include gastric varices that are actively bleeding or at high risk for bleeding (fundal location, wale sign on endoscopy, >5 mm, or CP class B/C). BRTO may be useful in patients in which TIPS is contraindicated including patients with high Model for End-Stage Liver Disease (MELD), hepatic encephalopathy, or heart failure. Contraindications include portal and/or splenic vein thrombosis due to the risk of occluding portal system outflow, which may result in mesenteric or splenic infarction or lack of a gastrorenal shunt (Figs. 68.5A and B and 68.6).

21. **Name the most common portosystemic shunt occluded during a BRTO procedure.**
    A gastrorenal shunt is the most common type to be occluded during a BRTO procedure because a gastrorenal shunt provides venous outflow in 90% of gastric varices cases with the remaining 10% draining via a gastrocaval shunt.

22. **When might BRTO rather than TIPS be indicated to treat gastric varices?**
    BRTO may be useful in patients in which TIPS is contraindicated, including patients with high MELD >18, hepatic encephalopathy, heart failure, or low portal pressure. With TIPS, portal flow is diverted away from the liver and

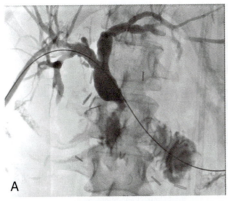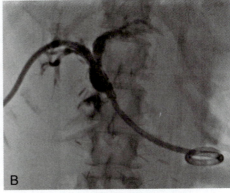

Fig. 68.7 Patient with Roux-en-Y complicated by stricture at the hepaticojejunostomy anastomosis. (A) Cholangiogram demonstrates severe narrowing at the anastomosis site. (B) Subsequent decompression of biliary system after placement of an external-internal biliary stent. Benign biliary stricture protocol was then initiated on the patient.

through the shunt; thus, there is a risk of hepatic encephalopathy and deterioration of hepatic function. With BRTO, the portal flow is often diverted toward the liver, which can potentially reduce hepatic encephalopathy and improve hepatic function. In patients with a decompressive gastrorenal or splenorenal shunt, the portal pressure might already be lower than the traditional hemodynamic endpoint of the TIPS procedure (<12 mm Hg) and there is little gain to further lower the gradient by creating a TIPS.

23. Postprocedurally, what condition can BRTO aggravate?
Portal hypertension can increase after BRTO. As a result of increased portal hypertension, there can be aggravation of nongastric (esophageal or duodenal) varices, development of portal hypertensive gastropathy, ascites, and hydrothorax or pleural effusion.

24. How is the hepatic venous pressure gradient (HVPG) measured?
Access into the hepatic veins can be obtained via the more common transjugular approach or via a transfemoral approach. A balloon occlusion catheter is placed into a hepatic vein 2–3 cm from the hepatic vein ostium, and a free hepatic vein pressure (FHVP) measurement is obtained with the balloon deflated. A wedged hepatic vein pressure (WHVP) measurement is obtained with total occlusion of the hepatic vein on inflation of the balloon. The HVPG is the difference between WHVP and FHVP.

25. Is percutaneous transhepatic biliary drainage (PTBD) the most appropriate initial method to treat biliary obstruction?
The selection of the most appropriate modality (percutaneous, endoscopic, or surgical) to provide biliary drainage depends on the interventional options available, the location and extent of the obstructing lesion, and the expertise of the operator. Currently, endoscopic drainage is the initial procedure of choice for biliary decompression because of its reported lower complications and better patient tolerance compared with the transhepatic approach. However, not all endoscopic drainages are successful, and PTBD continues to play an important role in the management of biliary disease. Biliary disease is best managed by a team that includes an endoscopist, interventional radiologist, and surgeon (Fig. 68.7A and B).

26. What are the indications for PTBD?
- Unsuccessful endoscopic drainage
- Biliary obstruction at or above the level of the porta hepatis
- Biliary obstruction following biliary-enteric anastomosis
- Bile duct injuries after laparoscopic cholecystectomy
    The most common of these indications is failed endoscopic drainage for any reason.

27. Discuss the role of metallic stents for the treatment of biliary obstruction.
The use of permanent metallic stents for the treatment of malignant biliary obstruction is well accepted, especially for inoperable patients whose life expectancies are 6–12 months. In these patients, metallic stents have been shown to be cost-effective and provide a better quality of life than external catheters. Long-term patency of

noncovered metallic stents is poor, with an occlusion rate of 30%–60% by 6 months, and nearly all patients require reintervention within 1 year. The use of metallic stents in benign diseases remains highly controversial.

28. When is percutaneous cholecystostomy indicated?
Two primary indications are as follows:
- Persistent and unexplained sepsis in critically ill patients with acalculous cholecystitis.
- Acute cholecystitis in patients who are poor surgical candidates.

In unstable patients, it can be performed at the bedside if necessary. Less frequent indications include temporary treatment for gallbladder perforation, drainage for distant malignant biliary obstruction, and transcholecystic biliary intervention.

29. What are the indications for angiography in GI bleeding?
For upper GI bleeding, endoscopy is the first line for diagnosis and treatment. However, angiography is indicated if there is an inability to control bleeding, rapid recurrence after bleeding, bleeding too fast to localize the source of bleeding, or anatomic reasons precluding endoscopy. For lower GI bleeding with active bleeding demonstrated on tagged red blood cell (RBC) scan or CT angiography (CTA), angiography is the first line of treatment.

For the interventional radiologist to identify the bleeding site, the following conditions must be met:
- The patient must be actively bleeding at the time of the study unless a structural lesion is the cause of intermittent bleeding.
- The bleeding must be brisk enough to be detectable during the arteriogram, usually more than 0.5 mL/min.
- The bleeding must be arterial or capillary bleeding; venous bleeding is rarely detected on the venous phase of an arteriogram.

Once the bleeding site is identified, transcatheter embolization is a treatment option.

30. How important is localization of the bleeding site before angiography?
Preangiographic localization of the GI bleeding site is extremely helpful. A visceral arteriogram involves evaluation of the celiac, superior mesenteric, and inferior mesenteric arteries; selective catheterization of these vessels and the multiple angiographic projections needed when looking for a bleeding site can make this a tedious and time-consuming procedure, requiring large contrast volumes. Localization of a bleeding vessel or even distinguishing an upper from a lower GI source is helpful, can guide the interventionalist in choosing which vessel should be studied first, and can shorten the procedure.

31. What are the three different modalities to detect GI bleeding and what rate of bleeding is detected?
Tagged RBC can detect bleeding rates of 0.1 mL/min, CTA can detect bleeding rates of 0.3 mL/min, and angiography can detect bleeding rates of 0.5 mL/min.

32. What two types of transcatheter therapy are used for GI bleeding?
Selective embolization with coils or cyanoacrylate glue is used for the treatment of GI bleeding. Modern coaxial systems and microcatheters permit superselective catheterization with accurate deployment of embolic material at the bleeding site (Fig. 68.8A and B). These advances have decreased the risk of bowel infarction, making transcatheter embolization a relatively safe procedure even in the small bowel and colon.

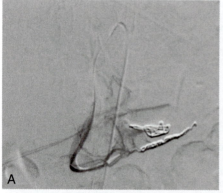
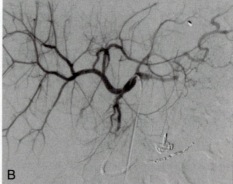

A   B

Fig. 68.8 Patient with upper gastrointestinal bleeding from a duodenal ulcer who failed endoscopic treatment with clipping. (A) Initial arteriogram and coil embolization of the gastroduodenal artery was performed; however, the patient continued to bleed. (B) Repeat angiogram was done and further embolization with glue was performed and subsequent cessation of bleeding.

33. **What is the role of endovascular therapy in patients with acute occlusive mesenteric ischemia?**

The primary goal of any treatment is revascularization of the affected bowel to restore normal function and prevent infarction. Open surgery has traditionally been the standard of care. Endovascular techniques including aspiration embolectomy, thrombolysis, and stenting, have been successfully described in the literature to treat acute occlusive mesenteric ischemia but, most are case reports and small series. If there are no indications of bowel infarction (peritoneal symptoms, pneumoperitoneum, or intramural air on CT), then endovascular treatment may be considered but this should be a multidisciplinary decision based on local expertise with the involvement of a vascular surgeon, interventional radiologist, and intensivist.

34. **Compare open surgical versus percutaneous endovascular treatment for patients with chronic mesenteric ischemia.**

Endovascular treatment with percutaneous angioplasty and stenting is minimally invasive and thus has better short-term morbidity and mortality than open surgical repair. Open surgical repair, however, is more durable and has a decreased reintervention rate compared with endovascular therapy.

ACKNOWLEDGMENT

The authors would like to acknowledge the contribution of Dr. Paul Russ, who was the author of this chapter in the previous edition.

CLINICAL VIGNETTE

Available Online

BIBLIOGRAPHY

Available Online

WEBSITES

Available Online

NONINVASIVE GASTROINTESTINAL IMAGING: ULTRASOUND, COMPUTED TOMOGRAPHY, AND MAGNETIC RESONANCE IMAGING

Michael G. Fox, MD, MBA, Andrew P. Sill, MD and Ryan Kaliney, MD

 Additional content available online

GENERAL

1. **Describe the use of multidetector computed tomography (MDCT) in the evaluation of the liver, pancreas, and biliary system.**
   MDCT uses very thin collimation (0.6 mm) and reconstruction intervals (0.5 mm) to generate true isotropic volumetric data sets and exquisite multiplanar reformations (MPRs) in any imaging plane (Fig. 69.1). Imaging can be performed in the following phases: noncontrast CT (NCCT), early hepatic arterial (HA), late HA, and the portal venous (PV) with the early HA approximately 20 seconds, the late HA phase (HAP) 35–40 seconds, and the PV phase (PVP) 60–70 seconds after injection. The dominant contrast effect in the liver occurs in the PVP. This ability to image rapidly can take advantage of the dual blood supply of the liver—75% from the portal vein and 25% from the hepatic artery.

LIVER IMAGING

2. **How is segmental liver anatomy defined?**
   The liver is divided into four lobes based on the surface configuration and the hepatic veins (HVs). The different hepatic segments are divided by intersegmental fissures, which are traversed or are in the same plane as the HVs.

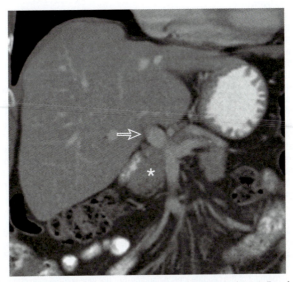

Fig. 69.1 Multiplanar reformats. Coronal reformatted image from axial computed tomography data set allows for multidimensional evaluation. *Open arrow* marks the main portal vein with the pancreatic head (*) inferior.

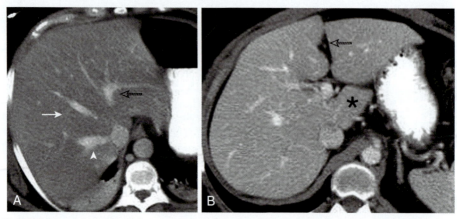

Fig. 69.2 Hepatic vascular anatomy. (A) Computed tomography image depicts the right hepatic vein (*arrowhead*) that divides the anterior and posterior segments of the right lobe of the liver. The middle hepatic vein (*arrow*) divides the right lobe from the left lobe. The left hepatic vein (*open arrow*) divides the medial and lateral segments of the left lobe of the liver. (B) The falciform ligament (*open arrow*) divides the medial and lateral segments of the left lobe of the liver. The caudate lobe is marked by the *.

The main lobar fissure divides the liver into right and left lobes and is represented by a line extending from the gallbladder recess through the inferior vena cava (IVC). It is represented by the middle HV. The right intersegmental fissure divides the right lobe of the liver into anterior and posterior segments and is approximated by the right HV. The left intersegmental fissure divides the left lobe of the liver into medial and lateral segments. It is marked on the external liver margin by the falciform ligament, and it is represented by the left HV. The caudate lobe is the portion of the liver located between the IVC and the fissure of the ligamentum venosum (Fig. 69.2A and B).

Couinaud anatomy further subdivides the liver into eight segments, each with its own blood supply. The eight segments are the caudate lobe (I), the left superior (II) and inferior (III) lateral segments, the left superior (IVa) and inferior (IVb) medial segments, the right anterior (V) and posterior (VI) inferior, and the right posterior (VII) and anterior (VIII) superior segments.

3. **Describe the ultrasound (US), CT, and magnetic resonance imaging (MRI) findings of fatty infiltration of the liver.**
   1. US: Fatty infiltration is seen as areas of focal or diffuse increased echogenicity that do not demonstrate mass effect on the adjacent biliary structures or blood vessels. Fatty infiltration may limit or prevent visualization of intrahepatic vessels, the deeper posterior portion of the liver, and the diaphragm posterior to the liver. Hepatitis or cirrhosis can also present with diffusely increased liver echogenicity.
   2. CT: On NCCT the liver is normally 8 Hounsfield units (HU) greater in density than the spleen. In fatty infiltration, the spleen is 10 HU denser than the liver. In diffuse fatty infiltration, the hepatic vessels are more conspicuous and may appear as if they contain contrast even on an NCCT scan. In focal fatty infiltration, the normal hepatic vessels traverse the area of decreased attenuation, a finding not usually present in malignancy. Focal fatty infiltration tends to be in a lobar distribution (wedge-shaped) with linear margins (Fig. 69.3). Areas where fatty infiltration or sparing typically occur include the gallbladder fossa, subcapsular, left lobe medial segment near the fissure for the ligamentum teres, anterior to the porta hepatis, and around the IVC.
   3. MRI: Signal differences in the liver may be subtle. As with CT, vessels should course normally through the area of signal abnormality without mass effect on adjacent structures. MRI with fat suppression is more sensitive than T1-weighted (T1-w) and T2-weighted (T2-w) imaging for fatty infiltration, with fatty infiltration having decreased signal intensity compared with normal liver. Areas of fatty infiltration will also reliably demonstrate decreased signal on opposed-phase T1-w imaging.

4. **Describe the US, CT, and MRI findings in cirrhosis.**
   1. US: The hepatic parenchyma is typically heterogeneous and hyperechoic with "coarsened" echoes and poorly defined intrahepatic vasculature. Unfortunately, these findings are nonspecific, with increased parenchymal echogenicity also present in fatty infiltration, and parenchymal heterogeneity also present in infiltrating neoplasms. Sonographic features with greater specificity for cirrhosis include nodularity of the liver surface and relative enlargement of the caudate lobe. A caudate-to-right lobe volume ratio of more than 0.65 is highly specific but not sensitive in diagnosing cirrhosis.

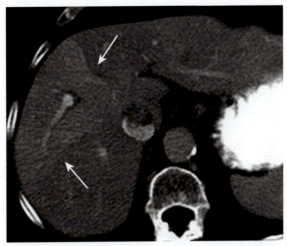

Fig. 69.3 Computed tomography (CT) image of fatty infiltration in a 66-year-old female with lung carcinoma. A large geographic area of focal fatty sparing (*arrows*) extending to the liver capsule with fatty replacement of the remainder of the liver parenchyma is noted on this axial CT image.

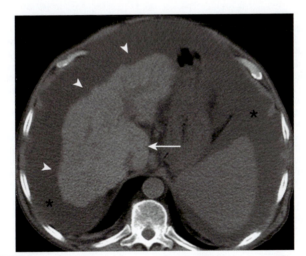

Fig. 69.4 Computed tomography images of cirrhosis in a 67-year-old male with renal failure. The liver margin is nodular in contour (*arrowheads*). The caudate lobe (*arrow*) is hypertrophied as compared with the right and left lobes. Perihepatic and perisplenic ascites (*) are present.

2. MDCT: The caudate lobe and the left-lateral segment typically enlarge, and the right lobe and the left-medial segment typically atrophy, resulting in an enlarged gallbladder fossa. Enlargement of the hilar periportal space, due to left lobe medial segment atrophy, is more than 90% sensitive and specific for early cirrhosis. In advanced cirrhosis, liver volume usually decreases and periportal fibrosis and regenerative nodules can compress the portal and hepatic venous structures, which may result in altered hepatic perfusion and portal hypertension. The presence of isodense regenerating nodules can often only be inferred from the nodular contour of the liver edge. Complications of portal hypertension, especially varices, are exquisitely demonstrated with MDCT; however, unlike sonography, CT cannot determine the direction of vascular flow (Fig. 69.4). Increased attenuation of the mesenteric fat is also noted.
3. MRI: MRI findings in cirrhosis are similar to those on MDCT, with early changes manifesting as enlargement of the hilar periportal space as a result of atrophy of the left lobe medial segment and later findings presenting

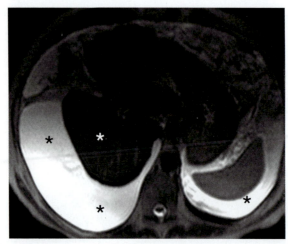

Fig. 69.5 Axial T2-weighted (T2-w) magnetic resonance image of a 53-year-old male with hepatic encephalopathy, preliver transplant demonstrates a small cirrhotic liver having markedly decreased T2-w signal consistent with hemochromatosis (*white* *). Also noted is extensive ascites (*black* *).

as a caudate/right hepatic lobe ratio of more than 0.65 and an expanded gallbladder fossa sign. Regenerative nodules are usually smaller than 1 cm in diameter, have variable T1-w and usually iso to decreased T2-w and gradient-recalled echo (GRE) signal. Regenerative nodules are usually isointense to the liver following contrast.

4. Dysplastic nodules are considered premalignant and are usually larger than regenerative nodules. They often demonstrate increased T1-w and decreased T2-w signal; however, there is overlap with hepatocellular carcinoma (HCC). Imaging findings of portal hypertension are similar to those on MDCT and initially include dilation of the portal and splenic veins with later occlusion and cavernous transformation of the portal vein and development of portosystemic collaterals and ascites.

5. Which is the most sensitive examination for detecting hemochromatosis?

1. MRI is more sensitive and specific than CT in detecting hemochromatosis with the paramagnetic effects caused by iron deposition resulting in decreased T2-w and GRE signal intensity (Fig. 69.5). While less sensitive, liver attenuation on NCCT is typically more than 70 HU in hemochromatosis, compared with a normal level of approximately 45–60 HU. Because many patients with hemochromatosis will develop cirrhosis and 25% will develop HCC, it is important to diagnose early.

6. What are the three growth patterns of HCC?

1. Large solitary mass (50%)
2. Multifocal HCC (40%)
3. Diffuse infiltration (10%)

7. What is the most common benign neoplasm of the liver?

Cavernous hemangioma is the most common benign liver neoplasm.

8. Describe the appearance of focal nodular hyperplasia (FNH) on US, CT, and MRI.

1. General: FNH is the second most common benign hepatic tumor and it is more common in females. FNH contains all of the normal liver elements but in an abnormal arrangement. It is typically smaller than 5 cm in diameter and solitary. The characteristic feature of FNH is the central scar, containing radiating fibrous tissue with vascular and biliary elements. The central scar may be seen with other lesions such as fibrolamellar HCC. Therefore although a characteristic feature of FNH, it is not specific for FNH.
2. US: Often subtle; therefore minimal contour abnormalities or vascular displacement should raise the possibility of FNH. A well-demarcated hypo- to isoechoic mass, possibly demonstrating a central scar, may be identified. Doppler images, especially if a stellate arterial pattern is present, are suggestive of FNH.
3. MDCT: FNH is hypo- to isodense on NCCT and without calcifications. FNH is hyperdense on HAP images because it is supplied by the hepatic artery. On PVP images, it is isodense to normal liver with a hyperdense pseudocapsule. The central scar is present in 35% of lesions smaller than 3 cm and 65% of lesions larger than 3 cm. The scar has lower attenuation than the normal liver on HAP and PVP images but becomes hyperdense

on 5- to 10-minute delayed images. Enlarged feeding arteries and draining veins may be seen, especially with the use of MPRs.

4. MRI: FNH is T1-w hypo- to isointense and T2-w iso- to hyperintense to liver. The central scar is T1-w hypointense and T2-w hyperintense, unlike HCC in which the central scar is T2-w hypointense. The lesion demonstrates diffuse enhancement in the HAP except for the central scar, which demonstrates delayed enhancement similar to CT. Unlike HCC and hepatocellular adenomas (HCAs), capsular enhancement is not identified in FNH. FNH has delayed enhancement with gadoxetic acid.

9. **How does HCA appear on US, CT, and MRI?**
    1. General: HCAs are more common in females and are associated with oral contraceptive use. HCAs can cause morbidity and mortality because of their propensity for hemorrhage and rare malignant degeneration to HCC. HCAs are often 8–15 cm in diameter when diagnosed. HCAs contain few, if any, bile ducts or Kupffer cells, but they are more likely to demonstrate calcification or fat than FNH.
    2. US: Typically shows a heterogeneous, hyperechoic mass caused by internal hemorrhage and high lipid content.
    3. MDCT: A hypodense mass is typically seen on NCCT resulting from intratumoral fat. Internal areas of higher attenuation may be present as a result of recent hemorrhage, a key distinguishing feature from FNH. Contrast-enhanced CT (CECT) may show centripetal enhancement similar to a hemangioma. In contrast to hemangiomas, the enhancement is transient.
    4. MRI: HCA is commonly heterogeneous as a result of necrosis and internal hemorrhage. HCA is usually T2-w iso- to slightly hyperintense. The T1-w signal is variable, but often hyperintense because of fat or hemorrhage, although similar findings may be seen in HCC. HCA can demonstrate decreased signal on opposed-phase T1-w imaging because of the high lipid content. Enhancement is most pronounced in the HAP with rapid washout in the PVP. The presence of hemorrhage helps differentiate HCA from HCC.

10. **Describe the appearance of a hepatic abscess on US, CT, and MRI.**
    1. General: Hepatic abscesses can develop from (1) biliary, (2) PV, (3) arterial, (4) local extension, and (5) traumatic etiologic factors.
    2. US: A hepatic abscess appears as a complex fluid collection, typically with septations, an irregular wall, and internal debris or air. Air is seen as a focal area of echogenicity with posterior shadowing. An abscess can also appear as a simple fluid collection, similar to a cyst.
    3. MDCT: CT is the most sensitive imaging modality; however, the CT findings vary with the size and age of the abscess. Generally, an abscess is a well-defined, low-attenuating uni- or multilocular mass with a well-defined enhancing wall that may contain internal septations. Air bubbles within the abscess cavity, although present in a minority of cases, are the most specific sign of an abscess (Fig. 69.6).
    4. MRI: An abscess appears as a well-defined homogeneous or heterogeneous lesion with decreased T1-w and increased T2-w signal. The cavity may contain septations and is surrounded by a low-signal enhancing capsule. Other complex cystic lesions, such as necrotic or hemorrhagic neoplasms, may have a similar appearance.

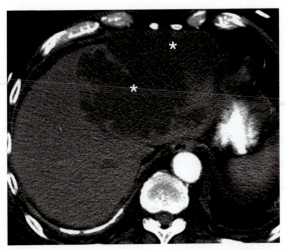

Fig. 69.6 A 74-year-old male with abnormal liver function tests and a large hepatic abscess. Axial contrast-enhanced computed tomography image demonstrates a large nonenhancing liver mass (*) with minimal peripheral enhancement. Subsequent percutaneous drainage confirmed a hepatic abscess.

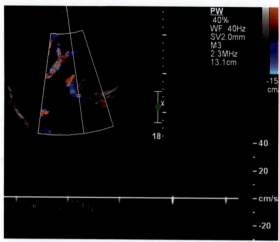

Fig. 69.7 Hepatofugal flow. Color Doppler ultrasound image of the portal vein in the setting of cirrhosis and portal hypertension demonstrates flow away from the transducer (hepatofugal flow) manifested by blue color in the main portal vein and a waveform below the baseline or away from the periphery of the liver.

DOPPLER LIVER IMAGING

11. Describe the sonographic findings of portal hypertension.

Portal hypertension can be suggested when (1) the portal vein diameter is larger than 13 mm, (2) there is less than 20% increase in the portal vein diameter with deep inspiration, (3) a monophasic waveform is present, and (4) flow velocity is decreased. Specific measurements may be unreliable given the portal vein diameter variability and the formation of portosystemic collaterals, which often develop in response to portal hypertension, reducing the portal vein diameter. Common collaterals include (1) a recanalized paraumbilical vein, which runs in the falciform ligament to the abdominal wall and drains the left PV; (2) splenorenal shunts; (3) retroperitoneal veins; (4) hemorrhoidal veins; and (5) the coronary vein, which connects with the portosplenic confluence and ascends to the gastroesophageal junction, producing esophageal varices. A coronary vein diameter larger than 7 mm is highly associated with severe portal hypertension. Retrograde (hepatofugal) PV flow indicates advanced disease and is a useful but late finding (Fig. 69.7).

12. How are Doppler waveforms altered in PV thrombosis?

In acute portal vein thrombosis, PV flow is markedly diminished or absent, with no Doppler waveform or color flow. Cavernous transformation of the portal vein, manifested by multiple tubular channels in the porta hepatis demonstrating Doppler and color flow with nonvisualization of the native portal vein, may develop within 12 months. Echogenic material representing thrombus is usually seen in the portal vein. An arterial waveform within the thrombus is highly specific for malignancy.

13. How does Budd-Chiari syndrome affect Doppler waveforms?

Budd-Chiari syndrome refers to obstruction of hepatic venous outflow. It can occur anywhere from the small hepatic venules to the IVC. It is diagnosed when echogenic thrombus or absent flow is present in one or more of the HVs or the suprahepatic IVC. Intrahepatic collaterals extending from the HVs to the liver surface are common, and the liver parenchyma is usually diffusely heterogeneous. Associated portal vein thrombosis is present in 20% and ascites is often present. The caudate lobe is frequently spared as it has separate drainage to the IVC.

BILIARY TRACT IMAGING

14. Describe the CT findings in acute cholecystitis.

Wall thickening, pericholecystic fluid, and gallstones are seen. CT is better than US at detecting stranding in the adjacent tissues. CECT can also demonstrate enhancement in the adjacent liver. CT can depict intramural gas in emphysematous cholecystitis.

15. What other conditions can result in gallbladder wall thickening?

Numerous conditions including (1) congestive heart failure, (2) constrictive pericarditis, (3) hypoalbuminemia, (4) renal failure, (5) PV congestion or portal hypertension, (6) hepatic venoocclusive disease, (7) chronic cholecystitis,

(8) acquired immune deficiency syndrome–related cholangitis, (9) adenomyomatosis, (10) primary sclerosing cholangitis, (11) leukemic infiltration, and (12) inflammation from hepatitis, pancreatitis, and colitis.

Gallbladder carcinoma also causes wall thickening but is usually differentiated from other causes by a mass-like appearance, adenopathy, and liver metastases.

16. **Describe the differential imaging features seen in the common causes of biliary obstruction.**
    1. Intrahepatic ductal dilatation (>2 mm) with a normal common bile duct (CBD) suggests an intrahepatic mass or abnormality. Dilatation of the pancreatic duct typically localizes the obstruction to the pancreatic or ampullary level.
    2. An abrupt transition from a dilated to a narrowed or obliterated CBD is more characteristic of a neoplasm or stone. Gradual tapering of the CBD at the pancreatic head is more typical of fibrosis associated with chronic pancreatitis, but chronic pancreatitis also can present as a focal mass, and biopsy may be required for differentiation.
    3. Cholangiocarcinoma often arises around the liver hilum (Klatskin tumor). It should be suspected when an abrupt biliary obstruction is present, but no mass or stone is identified.
       a. US: The primary mass is difficult to identify.
       b. MDCT: Low-attenuating mass with mild delayed (10–20 minutes postinjection) peripheral enhancement is typical. Unlike HCC, cholangiocarcinoma usually encases but does not invade the adjacent vessels.
       c. MRI: Usually has low T1-w and high T2-w signal and progressive delayed enhancement caused by fibrous tissue. This can help determine the area to biopsy.

17. **What is magnetic resonance cholangiopancreatography (MRCP) and how does it compare to endoscopic retrograde cholangiopancreatography (ERCP)?**
    MRCP is a noninvasive way to evaluate the hepatobiliary tract using heavily T2-w images. MRCP can reliably demonstrate the CBD, the pancreatic duct, the cystic duct, and aberrant hepatic ducts, and can differentiate dilated from normal ducts. MRCP exceeds the accuracy of CT and US in detecting choledocholithiasis, because CBD stones do not always exhibit acoustic shadowing. This is one reason why US is only 60%–70% accurate in detecting CBD stones (Fig. 69.8).

    MRCP is comparable to ERCP in detecting choledocholithiasis and extrahepatic strictures and in diagnosing extrahepatic biliary and pancreatic duct abnormalities (Fig. 69.9A and B).

18. **Describe the radiologic workup of suspected biliary tree obstruction.**
    1. US: US is the screening examination of choice for suspected biliary ductal disease. Doppler can readily differentiate biliary ducts from vasculature in the portal triad. A CBD diameter larger than 6 mm is more sensitive than dilated intrahepatic ducts in assessing early or partial biliary obstruction; however, the extrahepatic ductal diameter may increase with age, following cholecystectomy or previously resolved obstruction. Normal intrahepatic ducts are smaller than 2 mm in diameter and less than 40% of the diameter of the adjacent portal vein. With intrahepatic ductal dilatation (>2 mm), tubular, low-echogenicity structures are seen to parallel the portal veins, producing the too-many-tubes sign (Fig. 69.10A).

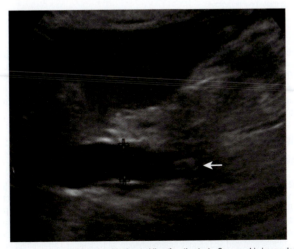

Fig. 69.8 Choledocholithiasis in an 81-year-old female with elevated liver function tests. Sonographic image demonstrates markedly dilated common bile duct (calipers) with obstructing echogenic stone *(arrow)*.

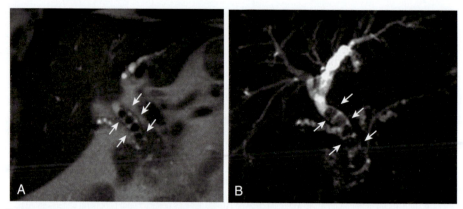

Fig. 69.9 Choledocholithiasis in an 83-year-old female with fever, elevated white blood cell count, elevated total bilirubin, and prior cholecystectomy. (A) Coronal T2-weighted magnetic resonance image demonstrates numerous gallstones (*arrows*) within the common bile duct. (B) Magnetic resonance cholangiopancreatography depicts choledocholithiasis (*arrows*) in same patient.

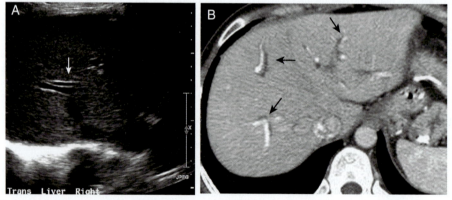

Fig. 69.10 Intrahepatic ductal dilatation. (A) Sonographic image demonstrates the double-duct sign (*arrow*) consistent with intrahepatic ductal dilatation. (B) Contrast-enhanced axial computed tomography image in a 41-year-old female with a gastrointestinal bleed demonstrates nonenhancing dilated ducts (*arrows*).

2. MDCT and MRI/MRCP: Once biliary disease is detected, MDCT or MRI are more efficacious in depicting the degree, site, and cause of obstruction because bowel gas commonly obscures US visualization of the distal CBD (Fig. 69.10B). MDCT and MRI/MRCP also provide more complete delineation of the entire CBD, especially with the use of coronal imaging.
3. ERCP or percutaneous transhepatic cholangiography: These imaging methods provide a more detailed evaluation than US, MDCT, or MRI/MRCP, but both modalities are invasive.

PANCREATIC IMAGING

19. **How can acute pancreatitis be distinguished from chronic pancreatitis on imaging?**
    Acute:
    1. US: US may be limited in the initial evaluation of acute pancreatitis because of overlying bowel gas, resulting in incomplete visualization of the pancreas and underestimation of the extent of peripancreatic fluid collections compared with CT. If pancreatic visualization is not impeded by bowel gas, early or mild pancreatitis often appears normal. In more severe cases of pancreatis, the pancreas may appear enlarged and hypoechoic.
    2. MDCT: CT is not performed to diagnose early or mild pancreatitis as it may be normal. Occasionally, the pancreas may appear enlarged and slightly heterogeneous, with increased attenuation in the peripancreatic fat (dirty fat) caused by inflammation. CT with MPR is the preferred study for patients with clinically severe

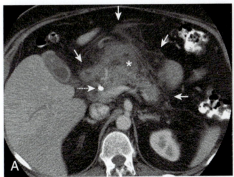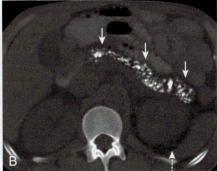

Fig. 69.11 Pancreatitis. (A) Contrast-enhanced computed tomography (CT) image in patients with acute pancreatitis caused by obstruction from pancreatic carcinoma. Extensive stranding in the peripancreatic fat (*arrows*), a nonenhancing pseudocyst anterior to the pancreatic body (*), and a common bile duct stent (*dotted arrow*) are noted. (B) Noncontrast CT image demonstrates numerous calcifications (*arrows*) within the pancreas consistent with chronic pancreatitis. Left perinephric fat stranding (*dotted arrow*) caused by pyelonephritis.

pancreatitis, especially to evaluate for necrosis or other complications. NCCT is initially performed to detect pancreatic ductal or parenchymal calcifications and hemorrhage and to provide a baseline HU for any masses. Imaging in the late HAP and the PVP is then performed. In more severe diseases, intraglandular intravasation of pancreatic fluid causes intrapancreatic fluid collection. Extravasation of fluid results in peripancreatic inflammation, thickened fascial planes, and peripancreatic fluid collection, most commonly in the anterior pararenal space (left greater than right) and the lesser sac (Fig. 69.11A). Fluid extending into the pararenal space can result in the Grey Turner sign (flank ecchymosis) and fluid extending into the gastrohepatic and falciform ligaments can result in the Cullen sign (periumbilical ecchymosis). Posterior leakage of fluid can present with a pleural effusion, classically on the left.

Chronic:
1. US: Calcifications, ductal dilatation, heterogeneous hyperechoic echotexture, focal mass lesions, and pseudocysts may be present. The gland usually atrophies with focally enlarged areas.
2. MDCT: Intraductal calcifications are the most reliable CT indicator of chronic pancreatitis (Fig. 69.11B). The gland size is variable, but focal enlargement caused by a chronic inflammatory mass may necessitate biopsy to exclude carcinoma. The pancreatic duct can be dilated (>3 mm) to the level of the papilla and may appear beaded, irregular, or smooth. Pseudocysts may be seen within or adjacent to the gland.

20. **Describe the role of CT and US in assessing the delayed complications of pancreatitis.**
    1. Ten to twenty percent of patients with acute pancreatitis and fluid collections develop pseudocysts after 4–6 weeks. Most pseudocysts smaller than 5 cm in diameter regress spontaneously. Drainage may be indicated for pseudocysts (1) failing to resolve after 6 weeks, (2) remaining larger than 5 cm in diameter, or (3) causing pain, infection, hemorrhage, bowel obstruction, or fistula.
       US: Pseudocysts appear as anechoic fluid collections with or without internal debris surrounded by a thin wall. May appear complex or even solid because of the debris.
       CECT: Pseudocysts appear as well-defined fluid collections with a uniformly thin, enhancing wall. Gas bubbles inside a pseudocyst relate to infection or enteric fistula formation.
    2. Acute peritonitis may occur if a pseudocyst ruptures into the peritoneal cavity.
    3. Necrosis is diagnosed by a lack of contrast enhancement within the pancreatic tissue. It is best demonstrated by MDCT in the PVP with an accuracy of 85%. CT evidence of necrosis correlated to morbidity/mortality is as follows:
       a. No necrosis: mortality rate (0%) and morbidity rate (6%)
       b. Mild (<30% of the total gland) necrosis: mortality rate (0%) and morbidity rate (≈50%)
       c. Severe (>50% of the total gland) necrosis: mortality rate (11%–25%) and morbidity rate (75%–100%)
       If secondarily infected, gas may be present in the area of necrosis (i.e., emphysematous pancreatitis). Infected areas usually do not contain gas, and a percutaneous aspirate is needed to confirm the diagnosis and identify the organism.
    4. Abscesses result from liquefactive necrosis with subsequent infection and usually occur 4 weeks after the onset of acute pancreatitis. Rate of abscess formation varies with the amount of necrosis.
       US: Abscesses appear as a hypo- to anechoic masses, sometimes containing hyperechoic gas, surrounded by a thickened wall.

MDCT: Abscesses appear as focal low-attenuation fluid collections with thick enhancing walls. If gas is present, an abscess needs to be excluded. The distinction between abscess and infected necrosis is difficult, but important because a pancreatic abscess often requires more aggressive treatment.

5. Enzymatic breakdown of the arterial wall can result in a pseudoaneurysm, most commonly in the (1) splenic, (2) gastroduodenal, or (3) pancreaticoduodenal arteries. Up to 10% of pseudoaneurysms rupture, usually into a pseudocyst, but occasionally into the retroperitoneum, peritoneum, pancreatic duct, or bowel. This results in massive hemorrhage.

   US: Color Doppler US is sensitive in detecting pseudoaneurysms and their complications.

   MDCT: MDCT is best at identifying pseudoaneurysms, which usually present as densely enhancing structures in close proximity to a pseudocyst.

6. Splenic vein thrombosis increases the risk of bleeding gastric varices. It is detected by the absence of enhancement in the expected region of the splenic vein on MDCT in the PVP. It is present in up to 45% of cases of chronic pancreatitis. Color Doppler can also make the diagnosis.

21. What are the imaging findings of pancreatic ductal adenocarcinoma?

1. Pancreatic enlargement is usually focal and best appreciated in the pancreatic body and tail. Diffuse enlargement is often secondary to pancreatitis caused by the neoplasm.
2. Enlargement and distortion of the pancreatic contour or shape are the most frequent findings of pancreatic cancer.
3. Difference in density or echogenicity is present.
   a. US: US usually detects a hypoechoic mass, compared with a normal pancreas, with ill-defined borders.
   b. CT: Pancreatic ductal adenocarcinoma usually appears hypodense compared with a normal pancreas, especially on CECT.
4. Pancreatic duct dilatation (>2–3 mm in diameter) may be the only indirect evidence of a small neoplasm. Dilatation is more common when the neoplasm is located in the pancreatic head and can result in both CBD and pancreatic duct dilatation (double-duct sign). This sign may also be present in chronic pancreatitis.
5. Biliary tract dilatation is more commonly seen with neoplasms in the head of the pancreas. Isolated intrahepatic biliary ductal dilatation may be seen with pancreatic cancer that has spread to the porta hepatis.
6. Local invasion is most commonly into the peripancreatic fat, but occasionally into the porta hepatis, stomach, spleen, and adjacent bowel loops.
7. Regional lymph node enlargement occurs, including nodes in the porta hepatis, para-aortic region, and area around the celiac and superior mesenteric artery (SMA) axis.
8. Liver metastasis occurs as pancreatic metastases that usually are low-density lesions.

22. What are the characteristic features of the four major cystic pancreatic neoplasms?

1. Serous cyst adenoma (SCA) is more common in females older than 60, is overwhelmingly benign, and is often in the pancreatic head. SCA is composed of numerous cysts smaller than 2 cm. It calcifies more commonly than other pancreatic tumors.
2. Mucinous cystic neoplasms are most common in females between 40 and 60 years of age. They are primarily in the pancreatic body or tail and are malignant or potentially malignant.
3. Intraductal papillary mucinous tumors (IPMTs) are rare but are most prevalent in males older than 60 years of age. They produce large amounts of mucin, which can result in ductal dilatation caused by mucin plugs. ERCP is best for diagnosis. IPMTs are usually (40%–80%) malignant. Findings associated with malignancy include (1) ductal dilatation larger than 10 mm, (2) large mural nodules, (3) intraductal calcifications, (4) bulging duodenal papilla, and (5) diffuse or multifocal involvement. Intraductal papillary nodules and a prominent duodenal papilla can distinguish this tumor from chronic pancreatitis.
4. Solid pseudopapillary tumor of the pancreas is most often seen in younger (≈25-year-old) Black or Asian females and is characteristically present in the pancreatic tail. They are often large (9 cm) at presentation and have a low malignant potential. On CT, fluid-debris levels can be present because of hemorrhage.
   a. US: Often appears solid and hyperechoic because of multiple small cysts that may not be individually resolved. A hyperechoic central stellate scar and calcifications suggest the diagnosis.
   b. MDCT: Innumerable minute cysts may appear solid, whereas multiple small but visible cysts may have a honeycomb or "Swiss-cheese" appearance. A central stellate scar and calcifications suggest the diagnosis.
      i. Female predominance (9:1)
      ii. Patients 40–60 years old
      iii. Strong predilection for the pancreatic tail (85%)
      iv. Peripherally calcify in 10%–25% of cases
      v. Considered malignant
      vi. Larger than 5 cm in diameter
      vii. Composed of unilocular or multilocular cysts larger than 2 cm
1. US: Better depicts solid excrescences and internal septations of variable number and thickness, usually thicker than septations in SCA tumors.
2. MDCT: Better demonstrates tumor wall and organ of origin.

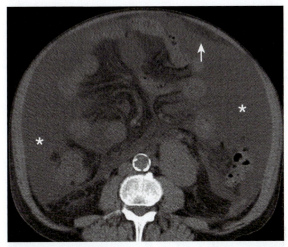

Fig. 69.12 Ascites in a 67-year-old male with renal failure and cirrhosis. Noncontrast computed tomography image demonstrates marked ascites *(*)* with elevation of the omental fat *(arrow)*.

PERITONEAL IMAGING

23. **How is simple ascites distinguished from complicated ascites?**
    Simple ascites:
    1. Watery transudate is usually caused by major organ failure (e.g., hepatic, renal, or cardiac).
    2. CT density is similar to water (0–20 HU); HU is higher as the fluid protein content increases.
    US: Simple ascites is anechoic, with increased through transmission and no internal septations. Ascites is "free-flowing" and located in the dependent portions of the abdomen and pelvis (i.e., Morison pouch, paracolic gutters, and pelvis). US demonstrates a sharp, smooth interface with other intra-abdominal contents (Fig. 69.12). Bowel seems to *float* within the fluid, usually in the center of the abdomen, if large amounts of ascites are present.

    Loculated ascites: Loculated ascites is formed by adhesions, either benign (i.e., prior surgery), infectious, or malignant in etiologic origin. Loculated ascites is typically (1) nondependent, (2) stable when patient changes position, and (3) may displace adjacent bowel loops.

    Complex ascites: Complex ascites is usually secondary to an infectious, hemorrhagic, or neoplastic process. Findings include internal debris or septations, a thick or nodular border or capsule, and HU of more than 20. Aspiration may be required to determine whether a collection is simple or complex.

24. **How is ascites differentiated from pleural effusion on CT?**
    1. Ascites is located anterior and pleural fluid posterior to the diaphragmatic crus.
    2. Pleural effusion can appear to contact the spine.
    3. Ascites has a sharper interface with intra-abdominal organs than pleural fluid.
    4. Unlike pleural fluid, ascites spares the bare area of the liver, which lies along the posterior border of the right hepatic lobe.

25. **Discuss the role of imaging in the assessment of intra-abdominal abscess.**
    US: US is best suited for evaluating pelvic and right and left upper quadrant abscesses, where the bladder, liver, and spleen provide acoustic windows for sound transmission. Abscesses vary in appearance but commonly are irregularly marginated and hypoechoic, with internal areas of increased echogenicity.
    MDCT: CT is the first choice for detecting abscess in acutely ill patients. The CT appearance of an abscess depends on its maturity. Initially, an abscess may appear as a soft-tissue density mass. As it matures and undergoes liquefactive necrosis, the central region develops a near-water attenuation, possibly with internal air bubbles or an air-fluid level (Fig. 69.13). The abscess wall typically enhances, increased density in the adjacent fat is common, and mass effect on the surrounding structures may be seen.

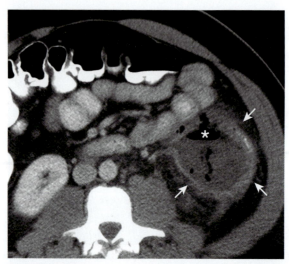

Fig. 69.13 A 23-year-old male with left pericolonic abscess. Axial computed tomography image demonstrates an abscess (*arrows*) likely resulting from diverticulitis. Gas (*) is present within the abscess cavity.

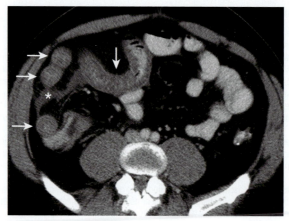

Fig. 69.14 Crohn disease. Computed tomography image depicts small bowel wall thickening (*arrows*) in this patient with Crohn disease. Adjacent fluid within the mesentery is noted (*).

BOWEL IMAGING

26. **What are the causes of small bowel wall thickening (>3 mm) on MDCT?**

Smooth and concentric bowel wall thickening is typical for nonmalignant disease (e.g., Crohn disease, ulcerative colitis, and ischemic, infectious, or radiation enteritis). Extraintestinal findings are important. In acute Crohn disease, MDCT is the best initial examination to evaluate for associated abscesses, fibrofatty proliferation, fistulas, mesenteric inflammation, and engorged vasa recta (comb sign) (Fig. 69.14). However, small bowel follow-through remains more sensitive for subtle mucosal changes and should be performed if suspicion for Crohn disease remains after a normal MDCT. MRI is excellent at diagnosing perianal disease, including fistulas.

Eccentric and irregular bowel wall thickening of more than 2 cm, especially if confined to a short segment, is suspicious for malignancy. Carcinoid is the most common primary malignant small bowel tumor. Carcinoid is typically located in the ileum; however, the actual tumor is often small and not visible on CT. A surrounding desmoplastic reaction with spiculated, often calcified mesenteric lymph nodes suggests the diagnosis. Adenocarcinoma is the most common primary malignant proximal small bowel tumor. It often presents as a mass or annular stricture that may obstruct. B cell lymphoma occurs in the distal small bowel (two-thirds) and T cell

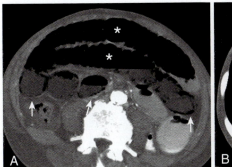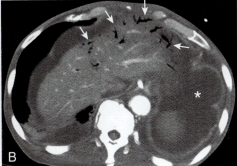

Fig. 69.15 Ischemia. (A) Computed tomography (CT) image demonstrates dilated air and fluid-filled small bowel loops (*). Air is present in the nondependent walls of multiple small bowel loops (*arrows*). (B) CT image demonstrates intrahepatic air within multiple branches of the portal vein (*arrows*). Ascites is also noted (*).

lymphoma in the proximal small bowel (one-third). Massive mesenteric or retroperitoneal adenopathy is often present. Lipomas are easily recognized by their low attenuation (≈−100 HU). The most common metastatic tumors to the small bowel include lung and melanoma.

27. How does MDCT assist in diagnosing small bowel obstruction?

MDCT is useful for evaluating small bowel obstruction; however, supine and erect abdominal radiographs should remain the initial diagnostic examination. MDCT with MPRs can determine the cause and level of obstruction, especially when high-grade. CT enteroclysis is the best imaging modality for low-grade obstruction. The site of obstruction or *transition zone* is the location in which the bowel proximal is dilated and bowel distal is decompressed. MDCT has a high specificity and negative predictive value, but low specificity for detecting ischemia. Bowel ischemia should be considered when wall thickening, mesenteric stranding, and mesenteric fluid are present. Pneumatosis, PV gas, and intramural hemorrhage are present in severe cases (Fig. 69.15A and B). MDCT can also diagnose closed-loop obstructions.

28. How is MDCT used to evaluate the large bowel?

Optimal evaluation of the colon requires bowel preparation and luminal distention with rectal contrast or air to evaluate the true wall thickness. Normal wall thickness of a distended colon is smaller than 4 mm. The addition of intravenous (IV) contrast facilitates the evaluation of the bowel wall and improves the evaluation of solid organs and vascular structures.

29. What are the causes of large bowel wall thickening on MDCT?

Wall thickening is present in numerous conditions, including Crohn disease, ischemic colitis, pseudomembranous colitis, radiation colitis, neutropenic colitis, and infectious (cytomegalovirus or *Campylobacter*) colitis (Fig. 69.16). On CECT, wall thickening can present either as homogeneous enhancing soft-tissue density or as concentric rings of high attenuation from hyperemic enhancement of the mucosa and serosa surrounding the low attenuation of the nonenhancing submucosa, termed the *halo* or *target sign*.

The cause of wall thickening sometimes can be determined by location or associated findings. For example, wall thickening in the splenic flexure region suggests ischemic disease from hypoperfusion in the SMA and inferior mesenteric artery watershed area. Inflammation from a ruptured appendix can produce wall thickening mimicking a primary cecal process, and severe pancreatitis can cause transverse colon wall thickening if inflammatory changes spread through the transverse mesocolon.

Adenocarcinoma can present with an annular narrowing, an intraluminal polypoid mass, or eccentric lobulated wall thickening. Findings of regional or retroperitoneal adenopathy or liver or lung metastases help confirm the diagnosis of carcinoma. Signs of extracolonic extension include strands of soft tissue extending into the pericolonic fat, loss of fat planes between the colon and surrounding structures, and a mass-like appearance. CT is useful in evaluating anastomotic recurrence from colorectal carcinoma, which occurs in the serosa, beyond the reach of the endoscope.

30. What are the CT and US findings of acute appendicitis?

1. US: A distended (>6 mm), noncompressible appendix with or without an adjacent fluid collection, an appendicolith, peritoneal fluid, abnormal flow in the wall of the appendix, and a focal mass representing a phlegmon or abscess.
2. MDCT: The hallmark findings are a distended (>6 mm), thick-walled appendix with abnormal enhancement and inflammatory changes in the periappendiceal fat. An appendicolith may be seen in 25% of cases. Additional

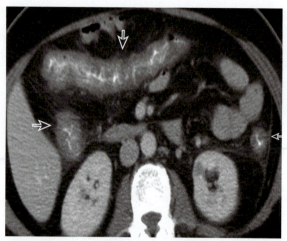

Fig. 69.16 Pseudomembranous colitis in a male who presented with diarrhea and fever. Computed tomography image demonstrates marked circumferential colon wall thickening (*open arrows*) in patient with pseudomembranous colitis.

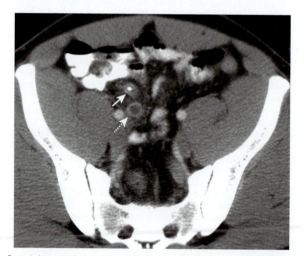

Fig. 69.17 Appendicitis. Computed tomography image demonstrates dilated fluid-filled appendix (*dotted arrow*) with minimal surrounding fat stranding and an appendicolith (*arrow*).

signs of inflammation include focal thickening of the adjacent fascia, focal fluid collections, and adjacent phlegmon or abscess (Fig. 69.17). Findings that suggest perforation include (1) abscess, (2) extraluminal air, (3) extraluminal appendicolith, (4) phlegmon, and (5) focal defect in the enhancing wall. If all findings are present, perforation can be diagnosed with 95% sensitivity and specificity.

31. Which examination is better for diagnosing acute appendicitis?

The sensitivity and specificity of CT are slightly superior to that of US, and CT is better at demonstrating both a normal appendix and the extent of adjacent inflammatory changes. The disadvantages of CT are higher cost and the use of ionizing radiation and contrast material. US is highly operator-dependent but is usually a good first choice for children, pregnant females, and thin people. CT should be used for all other types of patients and is more effective in obese patients.

NEWER TECHNIQUES

32. **What is CT or *virtual* colonoscopy?**

    Optimal performance of MDCT colonoscopy (CTC) requires thin-section (2–3 mm) images using a low-dose technique with additional dedicated CT colonography software. Typical CT scan time is 5–7 seconds, and both prone and supine images are obtained. Bowel preparation requires catharsis usually with magnesium citrate or sodium phosphate. The addition of dilute 2% CT barium to tag residual stool and/or diatrizoate (Gastrografin) to opacify luminal fluid helps differentiate stool from polyps. Distension is performed with either room air or automated CO_2 delivery via a small-caliber flexible catheter. Advantages over optical colonoscopy are that sedation is *not* required and other areas of the abdomen can be evaluated; however, CTC exposes the patient to radiation.

33. **How effective is CT or *virtual colonoscopy* in screening for polyps?**

    Most studies suggest that the accuracy of CTC is greater than barium enemas and approaches optical colonoscopy, especially for polyps >10 mm if the colon is properly prepped and distended. However, interpretation of CTC examinations requires the review of both two- (2D) and three-dimensional images and it is recommended that only radiologists with experience evaluating 50 or more CTC examinations should provide the interpretation.

34. **How has contrast-enhanced US (CEUS) improved the diagnostic evaluation of solid organ masses?**

    IV US contrast agents can be added to traditional sonography to visualize perfusion in lesions of the liver, kidneys, spleen, and other visceral organs. The available contrast agents all consist of gas microbubbles of 1–10 μm in size (equal to or smaller than red blood cells) stabilized by a shell. CEUS requires only 1–2 mL of contrast agent as the microbubbles remain contained within the vascular space and allow real-time visualization of both macrovasculature and microvasculature (e.g., arterial, portovenous, and delayed phases) resulting in higher temporal resolution than other imaging modalities. Prompt elimination (approximately 20 minutes) also permits re-examination within short time intervals.

    Compared with CT or MRI, CEUS decreases the time to diagnosis of liver tumors and can also be utilized to detect the most concerning portion of an indeterminate solid organ lesion during US-guided biopsy. CEUS exceeds the sensitivity of CT and probably MRI in detecting internal vascular flow. Limitations to CEUS generally relate to poor visualization of the target lesion secondary to hepatic steatosis, deep location, or sub-5 mm lesions.

35. **Describe MRI and US elastography and the role they play in the care of patients with chronic liver disease.**

    Chronic liver disease results in progressive hepatic fibrosis and eventual cirrhosis with hepatitis C, alcohol-related liver disease, and nonalcoholic fatty liver disease accounting for a majority of patients awaiting liver transplantation in the United States. Early detection and treatment can improve prognosis; however, morphologic changes may not be evident on imaging until later in the disease course. The degree of fibrosis has historically been evaluated using liver biopsy with histopathologic staging ranging from F0 (no fibrosis) to F4 (cirrhosis) (METAVIR scoring system). Patients with higher stage of liver fibrosis (F3–F4) are at risk for portal hypertension, ascites, variceal hemorrhage, and hepatic encephalopathy and may need portal pressure measurements or surveillance imaging for HCC. Both MRI- and US-based elastography provide a noninvasive method to estimate patients' METAVIR fibrosis stage.

    In general, US-based techniques quantify tissue stiffness and elasticity in response to a compression or shear wave. US elastography is particularly advantageous because of wide availability, versatility, and relatively low cost. Depending on the vendor, 5–10 high-quality measurements are obtained and reported in meters per second or in kilopascals. Reports should include the system-derived interquartile ranger-to-median ratio to denote the quality of the examination.

    MRI elastography requires placement of a mechanical vibrator on the patient's right upper quadrant to generate shear waves, acquisition of a 2D GRE MR elastography sequence which maps propagation and velocity of the shear waves (Fig. 69.18A and B) and an inversion algorithm to quantify and map liver stiffness. MRI elastography is more accurate than US elastography, samples larger portions of liver parenchyma reducing sampling bias, and is usually performed in conjunction with a diagnostic MRI including liver fat and iron quantification.

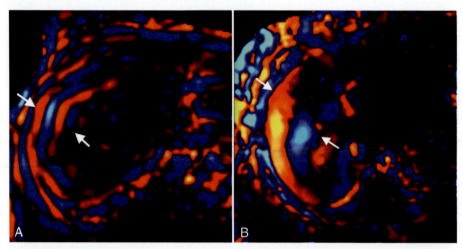

Fig. 69.18 Axial magnetic resonance elastography wave propagation images. (A) A 43-year-old male with normal mean liver stiffness value 1.7 kPa (<2.5–3 kPa is considered normal). (B) A 62-year-old female with mean liver stiffness value 7.9 kPa (>5 kPa indicates stage 4 fibrosis or cirrhosis). Note the visible difference in the wave thickness between these two patients which corresponds with the stiffness of the liver tissue; smaller wavelengths are seen in normal liver whereas larger wavelengths are seen in cirrhotic liver.

ACKNOWLEDGMENT

The authors would like to acknowledge the previous contributions of Dr. David Bean, Dr. Steven H. Peck, and Dr. Kevin Rak to this chapter.

CLINICAL VIGNETTE

Available Online

BIBLIOGRAPHY

Available Online

NUCLEAR IMAGING

Mike H. Lee, MD and James Latanski, MD

CHAPTER 70

🌐 **Additional content available online**

1. **Outline the general advantages of nuclear medicine procedures compared with other imaging modalities.**
   - Provide functional information that is either not available by other modalities or is obtained at greater expense or patient risk.
   - High-contrast resolution (target-to-background ratio) can be achieved in many instances by nuclear medicine techniques, allowing diagnostic studies despite poor spatial resolution.

2. **What are the disadvantages of nuclear medicine procedures compared with other radiographic studies?**
   - Spatial resolution is inferior to that of other imaging modalities.
   - Imaging times can be long, often up to 1 hour or more.
   - Radiation risk is greater than with magnetic resonance imaging (MRI) or ultrasound (US). When compared to radiographs or computed tomography (CT), radiation risk is less straightforward and largely depends on the type of nuclear study. For instance, studies on Gallium 67 and Indium 111 can average two to four times more radiation compared to other nuclear studies. Conversely, for other studies, such as gastric emptying, radiation risk is markedly less compared with traditional imaging methods, such as fluoroscopy.
   - Availability may be limited. Specialized procedures require radiopharmaceuticals or interpretive expertise not available in all centers.

3. **What nuclear medicine tests are most helpful in gastrointestinal (GI) medicine?**
   Nuclear medicine procedures have been used in the evaluation of nearly every GI problem (Table 70.1). Current improvements in and widespread use of endoscopy, manometry, pH monitoring, and diagnostic radiologic imaging techniques (CT, MRI, and US) have limited the use of nuclear medicine to specific clinical problems.

4. **How is cholescintigraphy (hepatobiliary imaging) performed? What is a normal versus an abnormal study?**
   The technique for a basic cholescintigraphic study is the same for nearly all of its clinical indications (see Question 3). The patient is injected with a technetium-99m–labeled iminodiacetic acid derivative, disofenin, and mebrofenin. High bilirubin levels (greater than 5 mg/dL for disofenin and greater than 10 mg/dL for mebrofenin) can cause a competitive inhibition of radiopharmaceutical uptake; however, administering a higher dose can overcome this impediment.
   After injection, sequential images, usually 1 minute in duration, are routinely obtained for 60 minutes. Normally, the liver rapidly clears the radiopharmaceutical. Blood pool activity in the heart is faint or indiscernible by 5 minutes after injection. Persistent blood pool activity and poor liver uptake are indications of hepatocellular dysfunction. Right and left hepatic ducts, the common bile duct, and the small bowel are typically visualized within 30 minutes. The gallbladder usually is seen within 30 minutes but can still be considered normal if visualized within 1 hour. By 1 hour, nearly all the activity is in the bile ducts, gallbladder, and bowel; the liver is seen faintly or not at all. Failure to see an expected structure at 1 hour requires further evaluation with either prolonged images (4 hours for acute cholecystitis, 24 hours for biliary atresia) or various manipulations (Sincalide or Morphine injection) (Fig. 70.1). If the gallbladder is not visualized after 4 hours of Morphine injection, then the findings would be consistent with acute cholecystitis. Overall, the sensitivity for acute calculous cholecystitis is 97% with a specificity of 85%. The sensitivity and specificity are slightly lower in acute acalculous cholecystitis with a sensitivity and specificity of 79% and 87%, respectively. If there is a pericholecystic hepatic activity with a subsequent rim sign, the potential for complicated cholecystitis (i.e., gangrenous or perforated gallbladder) is significantly higher (Fig. 70.2). In adults, absence of activity in the intrahepatic ducts or small bowel can represent a high-grade obstruction (Fig. 70.3).

5. **How should patients be prepared for a cholescintigraphy scan?**
   Patient preparation is vital in ensuring that lack of gallbladder visualization is a true-positive finding.
   Because food is a potent and long-lasting stimulus for endogenous cholecystokinin (CCK) release, the patient should not eat for 4 hours prior to the study. On the other hand, patients who have had a prolonged fast

Table 70.1 Uses of Nuclear Medicine Procedures in Gastrointestinal Diseases.

TEST OR STUDY	USEFUL IN DIAGNOSIS/EVALUATION
Cholescintigraphy (hepatobiliary imaging)	Acute cholecystitis Gallbladder dyskinesis Common duct obstruction Biliary atresia Sphincter of Oddi dysfunction Hepatic mass Biliary leak Cholangioenterostomy patency
Gastric emptying	Quantification of gastric motility
Esophageal motility/transit	Quantification of esophageal transit Evaluation/detection of reflux Detection of pulmonary aspiration
^{14}C-urea breath test	Identification of *Helicobacter pylori* infection
Liver/spleen scan	Hepatic mass lesions Accessory spleen/splenosis
Heat-damaged RBC scan	Accessory spleen/splenosis
^{67}Gallium scan	Staging of abdominal malignancies Abdominal abscess
^{111}In-pentetreotide	Neuroendocrine tumor staging/recurrence
^{111}In WBC scan	Evaluation of abdominal infection/abscess Evaluation of active inflammatory bowel disease
^{99m}Tc-HMPAO WBC scan	Evaluation of active inflammatory bowel disease
^{99m}Tc-RBC scan	GI bleeding localization Hepatic hemangiomas
Pertechnetate (NaTcO4) scanning	Meckel diverticulum
^{99m}Tc-sulfur colloid dynamic imaging	GI bleeding localization
Hepatic arterial perfusion with ^{99m}Tc-MAA	Hepatic intra-arterial catheter perfusion
^{90}Y microspheres	Treatment of unresectable hepatocellular carcinoma Treatment of hepatic metastatic lesions
^{18}F-FDG PET and PET/CT	Evaluation of various malignancies Assessment of inflammatory bowel disease

^{14}C, Carbon-14; *CT*, computed tomography; ^{18}F-FDG, ^{18}F-fluorodeoxyglucose; *GI*, gastrointestinal; *HMPAO*, hexamethyl-propyleneamine-oxime; ^{111}In, indium 111; *MAA*, macroaggregated albumin; *PET*, positron emission tomography; *RBC*, red blood cell; ^{99m}Tc, technetium-99m; *WBC*, white blood cell; ^{90}Y, yttrium-90.

(longer than 24 hours) are receiving intravenous hyperalimentation, or are severely ill can develop viscous bile formation, which may not be adequately emptied out of a normal gallbladder. However, Sincalide can be used to contract the gallbladder and pass the viscous bile. Both scenarios can impair the radiopharmaceutical filling of the gallbladder, which in turn can cause a false-positive study. As previously mentioned, Morphine can be used when the gallbladder is not visualized by 1 hour via increasing sphincter of Oddi contraction and leading to biliary filling. However, if given before the study, Morphine can simulate biliary obstruction. Time from the last Morphine dose is facility dependent and may range from 4 to 8 hours.

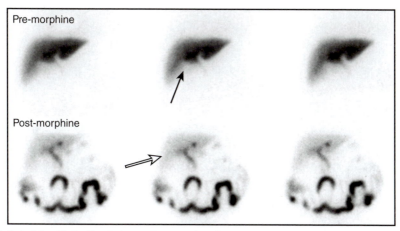

Fig. 70.1 Acute cholecystitis. Pre-Morphine images: After injection with ^{99m}*black arrow*^{99m}Tc mebrofenin, selected 1-min static images during the initial 60-min images demonstrate the absence of radiotracer in the expected location of the gallbladder (*black arrow*). Despite 60 min of imaging, the gallbladder was not visualized. Post-Morphine images: To expedite the examination, Morphine was administered; however, continued imaging for 30 min did not demonstrate gallbladder filling (*white arrow*).

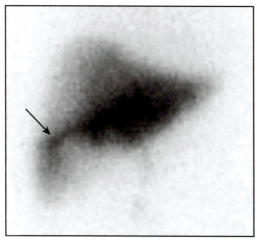

Fig. 70.2 Acute gangrenous cholecystitis. During the initial 60 min of hepatobiliary imaging, pericholecystic hepatic activity (rim sign) is noted without visualization of the gallbladder. The rim sign is thought to be secondary to regional hyperemia, which increases the delivery of the radiopharmaceutical to this area, in addition to localized hepatic dysfunction, which prevents efficient excretion of the radiopharmaceutical. Approximately 40% of patients with this type of activity have a perforated or gangrenous gallbladder.

6. ## How is cholescintigraphy used to diagnose and manage biliary leak?

    Cholescintigraphy is highly sensitive and specific for detecting biliary leak. Non bile fluid collections are common after surgery and can significantly limit the specificity of anatomic studies. In cases of a post-cholecystectomy bile leak, cholescintigraphy can demonstrate the accumulation of activity in the gallbladder fossa with progressive activity in dependent regions, commonly the right paracolic gutter (Fig. 70.4). Additional delayed images up to 24 hours after injection can demonstrate small leaks. Because cholescintigraphy has poor spatial resolution, the exact origin of the leak may not be determined and endoscopic retrograde cholangiopancreatography or percutaneous transhepatic cholangiography may be necessary for further anatomic assessment. Cholescintigraphy can also be used noninvasively to document the resolution of a bile leak. Bilomas can also be detected if there is a focus on increased activity that correlates with a fluid collection noted on previous cross-sectional imaging.

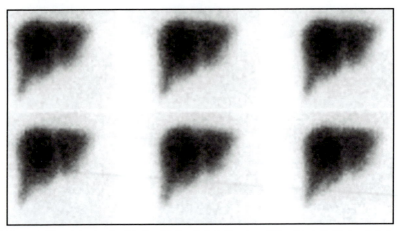

Fig. 70.3 High-grade biliary obstruction. After injection of ^{99m}Tc mebrofenin, there is no visible activity in the intrahepatic ducts or small bowel in the initial 60 min of images. Additional 4- and 24-hr images (not shown) did not demonstrate activity in the small bowel.

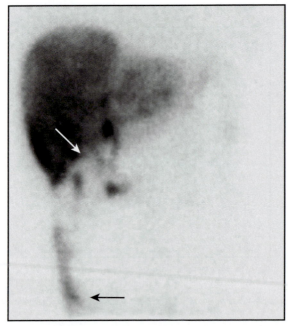

Fig. 70.4 Bile leak. After laparoscopic cholecystectomy, the patient developed severe right upper quadrant pain. Injection of ^{99m}Tc mebrofenin was followed with the acquisition of 1-min sequential images. There is an accumulation of the radiopharmaceutical in the gallbladder fossa (*white arrow*) as well as activity in the right paracolic gutter "tail sign" (*black arrow*) consistent with bile leak.

7. **What is the role of cholescintigraphy in diagnosing biliary atresia?**

If the patient is properly prepared for the examination, cholescintigraphy can be helpful in excluding the diagnosis of biliary atresia. The other primary differential diagnostic possibility in neonates is severe neonatal hepatitis. The role of scintigraphy is not to diagnose biliary atresia but rather to rule out biliary atresia as a possible diagnosis. To improve the sensitivity of the study, premedication of the neonate with oral phenobarbital (5 mg/kg/d in divided doses for 5 days) is imperative, because it stimulates hepatic activity and increases the ability of the liver to extract the radiopharmaceutical. The importance of therapeutic serum levels of phenobarbital cannot be overemphasized because a scan resulting from poor preparation is indistinguishable from a scan consistent with biliary atresia or neonatal hepatitis. If the radiotracer is not seen in the small bowel, delayed images must be obtained and if the small bowel is visualized, biliary atresia is ruled out.

Unfortunately, severe hepatic dysfunction and hepatitis may have a similar appearance to biliary atresia. Additional delayed images should be obtained to assess for activity in the small bowel, which excludes the diagnosis of a high-grade obstruction or biliary atresia.

8. **What is gallbladder dyskinesia? How does cholescintigraphy evaluate the emptying of the gallbladder?**
   A significant number of patients with normal conventional imaging and clinical evaluation have pain referable to the gallbladder, as evidenced by relief of symptoms after cholecystectomy. The poorly understood and heterogeneous entity of gallbladder dyskinesia has been proposed as the cause of this pain. It is thought that poorly coordinated contractions between the gallbladder and cystic duct can cause pain. Gallbladder dyskinesia may be manifested by an abnormally low ejection of bile under the stimulus of CCK (Sincalide).

   After the gallbladder has been filled during cholescintigraphy, gallbladder contraction is stimulated by an infusion of Sincalide, 0.02 mcg/kg in 30 minutes. The amount of gallbladder emptying in 30 minutes reflects the gallbladder ejection fraction (GBEF), normal being greater than 35%. This protocol has demonstrated a correlation of both normal and abnormal GBEF with surgical and medical follow-up.

9. **What is a pulmonary aspiration study? When is it used?**
   Pulmonary aspiration studies are performed by imaging the chest after oral administration of ^{99m}Tc-colloid in water or formula in infants. Activity in the lungs is diagnostic of aspiration. Although sensitivity is low, it is likely higher than that of radiographic contrast studies. The test has the advantage of easy serial imaging to detect intermittent aspiration.

10. **What is the role of nuclear medicine studies in evaluating hepatic mass lesions?**
    The traditional liver and spleen scan using an intravenous injection of ^{99m}Tc-sulfur colloid has largely been replaced by US and dynamic multiphase CT and MRI. In addition to superior resolution with CT and MRI, adjacent structures can also be evaluated. If results are inconclusive, nuclear medicine testing can provide additional information, which can lead to the proper diagnosis.

    Sulfur colloid is composed of small particles (0.3–1 μm) that are phagocytosed by the reticuloendothelial systems, including Kupffer cells in the liver. Lesions that lack Kupffer cells in the liver will not accumulate sulfur colloid. Virtually, all neoplasms, including metastasis, focal inflammatory and infectious diseases of the liver, and vascular malformations, manifest as decreased radionuclide activity (cold) on both liver-spleen and hepatobiliary imaging. However, focal nodular hyperplasia (FNH) can demonstrate a nonspecific appearance on CT, MRI, and US. If a lesion appears isointense (warm) or hyperintense (hot) compared with the rest of the liver, it can be presumed to be FNH because no other hepatic lesion contains a sufficient number of Kupffer cells to concentrate sulfur colloid. Occasionally, FNH can appear cold if there are not enough Kupffer cells to accumulate a sufficient amount of sulfur colloid, which unfortunately does not differentiate it from other hepatic masses. Additional imaging with cholescintigraphy will demonstrate early and prolonged uptake of the radiopharmaceutical because of the presence of hepatocytes in FNH with impaired clearance of the radiopharmaceutical from these lesions.

    The evaluation of hepatic lesions is limited on planar imaging to approximately 1–2 cm. To evaluate smaller lesions, single-photon emission computed tomography (SPECT) imaging, which is produced using rotating gamma camera heads and reconstructing the data into three dimensions, can be used in the evaluation of lesions in the subcentimeter range.

    Using multiphasic imaging with CT or MRI, evaluation for hepatic hemangiomas is excellent. However, if atypical features are noted, imaging using SPECT with ^{99m}Tc-labeled red blood cells (RBCs) can provide additional information for hemangiomas larger than 2 cm and close to the hepatic surface (Fig. 70.5), frequently at lower cost and without intravenous contrast injection. Additional SPECT imaging also improves the ability to evaluate smaller hemangiomas.

11. **How can nuclear medicine procedures assist in detecting ectopic gastric tissue?**
    As a source of pediatric GI bleeding, a Meckel diverticulum invariably contains ectopic gastric mucosal tissue. Because ^{99m}Tc-pertechnetate is concentrated and extracted by gastric tissue, it is an ideal agent to localize sources of GI bleeding caused by a Meckel diverticulum, which can be difficult to detect with traditional radiographic studies.

    The study is performed by injecting pertechnetate intravenously and imaging the abdomen for 60 minutes. Typically, ectopic gastric mucosa appears at the same time as gastric mucosa and does not move during imaging. Sensitivity is 85% for the detection of bleeding from a Meckel diverticulum. Manipulations to increase the sensitivity of the study may include additional pharmaceuticals such as cimetidine (to block pertechnetate release from ectopic mucosa), pentagastrin (to enhance mucosal uptake), and glucagon (to inhibit bowel motility and prevent movement of the radiopharmaceutical).

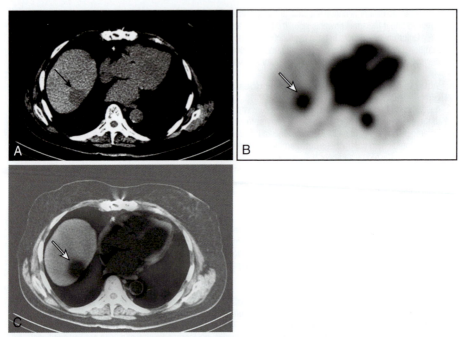

Fig. 70.5 Evaluation of mass lesion. Single-photo emission computed tomography (SPECT)/computed tomography (CT) scan of the liver using in vitro tagged ^{99m}Tc red blood cells (RBCs). (A) Initial CT evaluation of the hepatic mass (*black arrow*) demonstrated findings that were suggestive of an atypical hemangioma. Additional evaluation was suggested. (B) SPECT imaging (using CT attenuation correction from SPECT/CT) demonstrates normal blood pool activity of ^{99m}Tc-RBC with an additional intense focus (*white arrow*) that corresponds to the hepatic mass. (C) Fused images of simultaneously acquired SPECT and CT images reveal the intense focus to be in the exact region of the hepatic mass consistent with hemangioma.

12. Which nuclear medicine procedures are useful in localizing lower GI bleeding?

The difficulty of localizing acute lower GI bleeding is well recognized. Even acute and rapid bleeding can be intermittent and not detected on angiography. Alternatively, the culprit lesion can be obscured by luminal blood during endoscopy. Small bowel bleeding distal to areas accessible by upper endoscopy is notoriously difficult to localize.

Two nuclear procedures have been used to localize GI bleeding sources: short-term imaging with ^{99m}Tc-sulfur colloid injection and extended imaging using ^{99m}Tc-tagged RBC injection. Despite the theoretical advantage of ^{99m}Tc-sulfur colloid in being able to detect smaller bleeds, this technique shares the limitation of angiography: a short intravascular residence time, which mandates the bleed to be active at the exact point of imaging. In addition, the normal biodistribution of sulfur colloid to the liver and spleen limits the evaluation of sources of bleeding around the hepatic and splenic flexures. ^{99m}Tc-RBC imaging has assumed dominance because the long intravascular residence time allows the detection of intraluminal radioactive blood accumulation if extended imaging is necessary.

The first step is performing an in vitro tagging of RBCs with ^{99m}Tc-pertechnetate, which provides the highest RBC tagging efficiency. In vitro tagging of radiolabeled RBCs involves obtaining a small blood sample (1–3 mL) from the patient and using ^{99m}Tc-pertechnetate to label the RBCs in reaction vials. The radiolabeled RBCs are injected back into the patient and dynamic 1- or 2-second flow images are obtained in 60 seconds. In the case of a brisk bleed, the flow images will allow for better localization because delayed images will demonstrate significant radiotracer spread through the bowel (Fig. 70.6). Immediately after dynamic flow images are obtained, sequential 1-minute images are acquired for 90 minutes. The use of dynamic imaging is important because sensitivity for localization is higher when the study is displayed in a cine-loop. If the patient has an intermittent bleed and the initial study is negative, images can be acquired up to 24 hours later if the patient actively bleeds again without reinjecting additional tagged RBCs. Unfortunately, delayed images will have a significant disadvantage in localizing the area of active bleeding because of normal peristaltic activity and the additional time from the beginning of the bleed to the time of imaging.

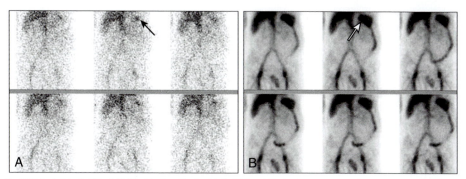

Fig. 70.6 Gastrointestinal bleed. (A) After injection of in vitro-labeled ^{99m}Tc red blood cells, 1-s-per-frame flow images were obtained, which demonstrate a focus of increasing activity (*black arrow*) at the splenic flexure. Because of the brisk nature of this bleed, the flow images were useful in localizing the origin of the bleed. (B) Additional 1-min-per-frame images demonstrate significant radiotracer uptake at the splenic flexure (*white arrow*) and extending activity moving anterograde down the descending colon and into the sigmoid colon. The patient subsequently had a colectomy performed.

13. **Are nuclear medicine procedures clinically useful in localizing GI bleeding, or are simpler techniques adequate?**

    ^{99m}Tc-RBC studies are more sensitive than colonoscopy and angiography in detecting intermittent bleeding. Specifically, tagged RBC studies can detect bleeding rates up to 0.1 mL/min whereas CT angiography detects rates from 0.3 to 0.5 mL/min, and fluoroscopic angiography from 0.5 to 1.0 mL/min. In addition to better visualization, upper endoscopy can also provide therapeutic options. One advantage of the tagged RBC study is that it allows for a survey of both the small and large bowel during a much longer time frame. Once the bleed is localized, therapeutic options with interventional radiology can be facilitated because less time is required to find which vessel to treat. One limitation of tagged RBC studies is the evaluation of gastric bleeds due to physiologic splenic activity.

14. **Are there additional minimally invasive treatments for unresectable malignant liver masses?**

    Use of yttrium-90 (^{90}Y) microspheres is a newer treatment option that delivers concentrated radiation to unresectable hepatocellular carcinoma (HCC) and metastatic disease. ^{90}Y, with a half-life of 64.5 hours, releases beta particles that radiate adjacent soft tissue with an average penetration of 2.5 mm. ^{90}Y microspheres have a diameter of 20–30 μm, which become trapped in the capillary beds of the intended masses and deliver a substantial dose of radiation specifically to these regions without the dangers of systemic radiation.

    To safely deliver the dose of radiation to the targeted disease, hepatic angiography via the femoral artery is performed first. To safely map the perfusion and subsequent delivery area of ^{90}Y microspheres, ^{99m}Tc-MAA is administered directly to the hepatic artery in the same manner that the ^{90}Y microspheres will be delivered. Because ^{99m}Tc-MAA particles are similarly sized compared with ^{90}Y microspheres, the biodistribution of these radiopharmaceuticals should be nearly identical. Using the images from ^{99m}Tc-MAA, the biodistribution is assessed and a shunt fraction is calculated to assess potential unwanted systemic distribution, particularly to the lungs. If these images and calculations demonstrate a safe delivery of ^{99m}Tc-MAA, then treatment with ^{90}Y microspheres is possible.

15. **What is positron emission tomography (PET) and how does it work?**

    PET uses specialized positron-emitting radiopharmaceuticals and equipment to detect areas of increased metabolic activity, a characteristic commonly seen in malignancies. The most commonly used radiopharmaceutical in PET imaging is ^{18}F-fluorodeoxyglucose (^{18}F-FDG), which is a marker for glucose metabolism. Unlike other commonly used radiopharmaceuticals in nuclear medicine, ^{18}F-FDG has a short half-life (110 minutes) and requires a cyclotron for production. Because of the complexity and cost of operating a cyclotron, the vast majority of nuclear medicine clinics do not have an on-site cyclotron and require the use of a separate PET radiopharmacy to provide the PET radiopharmaceutical. In addition, the short half-life of ^{18}F-FDG and the need to transport the ^{18}F-FDG from an outside facility to the imaging site can limit the overall accessibility of PET imaging.

    Tumors demonstrate increased ^{18}F-FDG avidity because of increased expression of glucose transporters and hexokinase, which is responsible for phosphorylating normal glucose and radioactive ^{18}F-FDG. After ^{18}F-FDG is phosphorylated, it is not metabolized any further and becomes effectively trapped intracellularly.

Patient preparation for a study using ^{18}F-FDG entails fasting for 4–6[18] hours prior to the examination to optimize the uptake of ^{18}F-FDG into malignant cells. At the time of the administration of ^{18}F-FDG, blood glucose levels less than 150 mg/dL are optimal, although images obtained in patients with blood glucose levels up to 200 mg/dL can still yield diagnostic results. Use of insulin can interfere with the biodistribution of ^{18}F-FDG, which can complicate the preparation of insulin-dependent diabetics.

ACKNOWLEDGMENT

The authors would like to acknowledge the previous contributions of Dr. Won S. Song to this chapter.

BIBLIOGRAPHY

Available Online

ENDOSCOPIC ULTRASOUND

Linda S. Lee, MD

CHAPTER 71

🌐 **Additional content available online**

1. **How does endoscopic ultrasound (EUS) work?**

   Sound waves used in ultrasonography occur at high frequencies greater than 20,000 Hz, which is beyond the range of human hearing. The ultrasound transducer both generates and receives sound waves to create images through the piezoelectric crystals that convert electrical signals into mechanical vibrations (sound waves) and vice versa. Sound waves occur at a specific frequency, are transmitted through a medium, and can be reflected, absorbed, and refracted as they encounter tissue. Information about the direction from which the sound waves are reflected and the time taken for the sound to return from the object can be used to locate the object. Sound travels readily through liquid, whereas air causes distortion and reverberation of ultrasound waves. The ultrasound transducer at the tip of the echoendoscope should be immersed in a water-filled lumen or covered with a water-filled balloon to transmit and receive defined images.

2. **Define the terminology used to describe EUS findings and name examples of corresponding structures.**

   For definitions of terminology to describe EUS echogenicity and examples of corresponding structures, see Table 71.1.

3. **What is the major difference between radial and linear echoendoscopes?**

   See Fig. 71.1. The major difference between radial and linear echoendoscopes is in the way images are produced. The ultrasound transducer at the tip of the radial echoendoscope acquires images in a 360-degree plane

Table 71.1 Definitions of Terminology to Describe Endoscopic Ultrasound Echogenicity and Examples of Corresponding Structures.

TERMINOLOGY	ECHOGENICITY	EXAMPLES OF STRUCTURES
Anechoic	Black	Fluid (e.g., blood, bile, and pancreatic juice)
Hypoechoic	Gray (darker than surrounding structures)	Lymph node and muscle
Hyperechoic	Bright (light gray to white)	Fat and bone

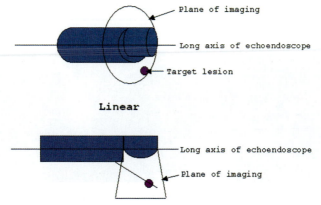

Fig. 71.1 Plane of imaging of radial and linear echoendoscopes.

perpendicular to the long axis of the echoendoscope. A linear echoendoscope provides a 120-degree image parallel to the shaft of the echoendoscope. This enables visualization of a needle passing through the biopsy channel of the echoendoscope into the targeted tissue to allow tissue biopsy and therapeutic maneuvers unlike with a radial echoendoscope.

4. **What are the EUS wall layers of the normal gastrointestinal (GI) tract?**
    See Fig. 71.2. The intestinal wall has five sonographic layers.

5. **Describe generic T staging for luminal GI cancers.**
    See Table 71.2 and Fig. 71.3 for generic T staging for luminal GI cancers.

6. **List the most common indications for diagnostic EUS.**
    -   Staging GI cancers, including esophageal, gastric, pancreatic, ampullary, rectal, and cholangiocarcinoma
    -   Staging lung cancer
    -   Evaluating subepithelial lesions; thick gastric folds; chronic pancreatitis (CP) and idiopathic recurrent pancreatitis; pancreatic lesions, including cysts and masses; and hepatobiliary lesions, including stones, strictures, and masses

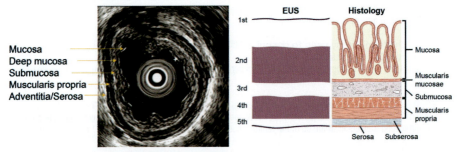

Fig. 71.2 Correlation of endoscopic ultrasound (EUS) image to the histologic composition of the bowel wall and side-by-side correlation of EUS image to the histologic composition of the bowel.

Table 71.2 Generic T Staging for Gastrointestinal Luminal Cancers.

T STAGE	DEFINITION
T1m	Invades mucosa or deep mucosa
T1sm	Invades submucosa
T2	Invades muscularis propria
T3	Invades adventitia or serosa
T4	Invades surrounding structures

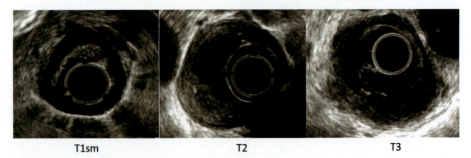

Fig. 71.3 Endoscopic ultrasound for T staging of esophageal cancer.

7. **How does EUS fit into esophageal cancer staging?**
   EUS provides the most accurate method of T and N staging for esophageal cancer with an overall accuracy of 80%–90%. If there is no evidence of distant metastatic disease on radiologic imaging, EUS should be performed to provide locoregional staging.

8. **What lesions are included in TNM staging of esophageal cancers?**
   Staging includes masses at the GE junction and those in the proximal 2 cm of the stomach that extend into the GE junction or esophagus.

9. **How is malignant lymphadenopathy determined in esophageal cancer?**
   See Fig. 71.4. The presence of four EUS criteria (size >1 cm, round, well-defined, and hypoechoic) predicts a malignant LN in nearly 100% of cases. However, only 20%–40% of all malignant LNs have all four EUS criteria. Therefore, when possible, FNA of LN should be performed. The addition of fine-needle aspiration (FNA) to EUS increases sensitivity and specificity to nearly 90% and 100%, respectively.

10. **Discuss regional nodal staging in esophageal cancer.**
    Regional nodes are classified as N0 through N3: N0 with no lymph nodes (LNs), N1 with one or two LNs, N2 with three to six LNs, and N3 with seven or more LNs.
    Regional lymphadenopathy includes LNs in the chest, around the esophagus, and celiac axis.

11. **Discuss some of the limitations of EUS in esophageal cancer staging.**
    The accuracy of T staging by EUS varies with the actual stage of the tumor, with the least accurate being T1 tumors.
    Strictures occur in approximately 30% of esophageal masses. Accuracy for staging is higher for traversable tumors compared with tumors occluding the lumen. Older literature suggested high perforation rates approaching 25% following dilation to allow passage of an echoendoscope, while more recent studies suggested the safety of pre-EUS dilation. Alternatively, a high-frequency ultrasound probe may be carefully advanced through a stricture.
    EUS following chemoradiation is inaccurate with a tendency to overstage; accuracy of EUS for T and N staging ranges from 29% to 60%.

12. **How does EUS affect the management of esophageal cancer?**
    In up to 75% of cases, EUS findings changed the management of esophageal cancer by determining candidates for surgical and endoscopic resection versus neoadjuvant chemoradiation.

13. **What is the role of EUS in gastric cancer staging?**
    Treatment for gastric cancer is stage dependent with endoscopic mucosal resection and submucosal dissection an option for T1N0 cancers and neoadjuvant treatment administered for T3/T4 and nodal positive cancers.

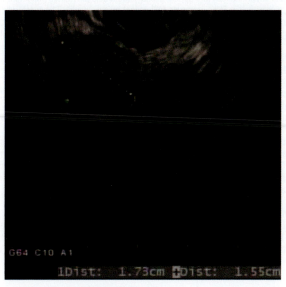

G64 C10 A1
1Dist: 1.73cm Dist: 1.55cm

Fig. 71.4 Endoscopic ultrasound of malignant periesophageal lymph node.

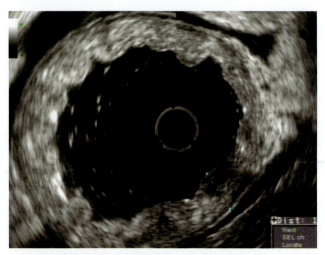

Fig. 71.5 Endoscopic ultrasound of thickened gastric wall caused by submucosal thickening.

Therefore accurate staging is important. If no distant metastatic disease is visible on computed tomography (CT) or positron emission tomography scan, EUS can be the next step for locoregional staging. EUS T staging is highly accurate (86% sensitivity) for distinguishing T1-2 from T3-4 tumors but less accurate for early-stage tumors. For N staging, EUS sensitivity and specificity are 69% and 84%, respectively. CT and magnetic resonance imaging (MRI) appear comparable to EUS for T and N staging.

14. **What EUS findings predict malignancy in thickened gastric folds?**
See Fig. 71.5. Definitive diagnosis of thickened gastric folds is difficult despite the use of EUS. These EUS findings are more predictive of malignancy: thickened submucosa, muscularis propria, or serosa and the presence of ascites or lymphadenopathy. Gastric wall thickening caused by thickened mucosa or deep mucosa can be diagnosed by biopsy or snare resection.

15. **Discuss the accuracy of EUS and endorectal coil MRI in staging rectal cancer.**
Accuracy of EUS and endorectal coil MRI appear overall comparable for T stage (ranging from 65% to 95%) and nodal stage (approximately 75%). However, MRI cannot reliably identify T1 tumors, whereas EUS tends to understage T4 tumors. The addition of FNA may increase the accuracy of N staging. The National Comprehensive Cancer Network guideline suggests staging with MRI although when contraindicated, EUS should be performed.

16. **List some limitations of EUS for rectal cancer staging.**
    • Invasion into the mesorectal fascia cannot be evaluated.
    • Distinguishing peritumoral inflammation from tumor extension may be difficult.
    • Staging stenotic rectal masses may be limited.
    • Post-treatment staging is inaccurate.
    • Endosonographer experience affects the accuracy of staging.

17. **How is EUS used in the diagnosis and staging of pancreatic cancer?**
EUS-guided biopsy is the preferred diagnostic procedure for pancreatic cancer with a sensitivity of 80%–85% and specificity near 100%. This is superior to CT-guided FNA with a sensitivity of 62%–81%. Accuracy of locoregional staging is comparable for CT, MRI, and EUS. EUS is superior for the detection of portal vein invasion, whereas pancreatic protocol CT better visualizes superior mesenteric artery and superior mesenteric vein involvement.

18. **What is the role of EUS in pancreatic neuroendocrine tumors (PNETs)?**
EUS is an integral part of both detecting and diagnosing PNETs with 90% sensitivity for detecting them compared to about 73% for both abdominal CT scan and MRI. In patients with CT negative for PNET, EUS identified PNET in 26% of cases. EUS is superior to CT scan for small (<1 cm) PNETs, detecting 68% of these which were missed by CT.

Table 71.3 Common Subepithelial Lesions and Endoscopic Ultrasound Characteristics.

SUBEPITHELIAL LESION	EUS CHARACTERISTIC
Gastrointestinal stromal tumor	Hypoechoic, second or fourth layer
Lipoma	Hyperechoic, third layer
Neuroendocrine tumor	Mildly hypoechoic, second or third layer
Cyst	Anechoic, second or third layer
Pancreatic rest	Hypoechoic or heterogeneous, second, third, or fourth layer
Granular cell tumor	Hypoechoic, second or third layer
Varices	Anechoic, serpiginous, second or third layer
Inflammatory fibroid polyp	Hypoechoic, second or third layer

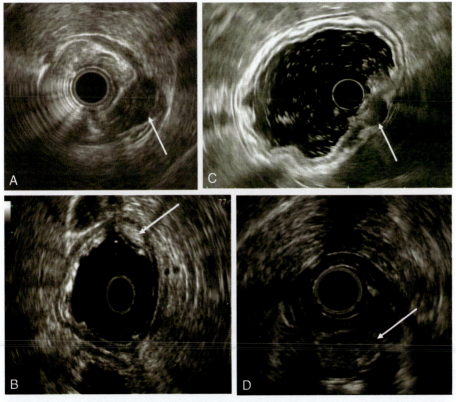

Fig. 71.6 Endoscopic ultrasound of subepithelial lesions. (A) Gastrointestinal stromal tumor. (B) Lipoma. (C) Carcinoid. (D) Pancreatic rest.

19. What are common subepithelial lesions and their EUS characteristics?

For common subepithelial lesions and their EUS characteristics, see Table 71.3 and Fig. 71.6.

20. **Compare EUS with endoscopic retrograde cholangiopancreatography (ERCP), magnetic resonance cholangiopancreatography (MRCP), and abdominal ultrasound for the detection of choledocholithiasis.**
    EUS, ERCP, and MRCP have comparable sensitivity and specificity for detecting choledocholithiasis (85%–95% and 92%–98%, respectively). Although the overall accuracy of EUS is comparable to MRCP, EUS is superior for stones smaller than 5 mm and intrasphincteric stones. All are superior to abdominal ultrasound, which has poor sensitivity of 20%–55% and 83% specificity.

21. **What is the role of EUS in suspected choledocholithiasis?**
    See Fig. 71.7. This depends on the probability of choledocholithiasis being present based on clinical and imaging findings. In patients with a high probability of choledocholithiasis (common bile duct (CBD) stone seen on radiologic imaging, cholangitis, or both dilated CBD with bilirubin >4 mg/dL), ERCP should be performed without further testing, whereas patients with low probability of stones may be managed conservatively. EUS is indicated in patients with intermediate probability of choledocholithiasis (abnormal liver function tests, dilated CBD, age >55 years).

22. **Discuss the accuracy of EUS imaging and cytologic examination in diagnosing pancreatic cystic lesions.**
    EUS imaging differentiates mucinous from nonmucinous cysts with 50% accuracy. Sensitivity of EUS-FNA cytologic examination for distinguishing mucinous from nonmucinous cysts is less than 50%.

23. **How do cyst fluid carcinoembryonic antigen (CEA), glucose, and amylase help differentiate among the common pancreatic cystic lesions?**
    See Table 71.4. Mucinous cysts have elevated CEA >192 ng/mL and low levels of glucose (<50 mg/dL).

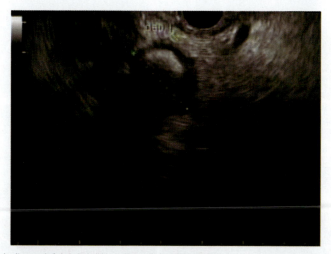

Fig. 71.7 Endoscopic ultrasound of choledocholithiasis (hyperechoic with shadowing).

Table 71.4 Levels of Carcinoembryonic Antigen (CEA), Glucose, and Amylase in Pancreatic Cystic Lesions.

TYPE OF CYST	CEA	GLUCOSE	AMYLASE
Pseudocyst	↓ (<192 ng/mL)	↑ (<50 mg/dL)	↑ (>250 U/L)
Serous cystadenoma	↓	↑	↓
Mucinous cystic neoplasm	↑	↓	↓
Intraductal papillary mucinous neoplasm	↑	↓	↑

Box 71.1 Standard Endoscopic Ultrasound Criteria for Chronic Pancreatitis

Parenchymal Criteria

Hyperechoic foci: small distinct reflectors

Hyperechoic strands: small, stringlike hyperechoic structures

Lobularity: containing lobules—rounded homogeneous areas separated by strands of another echogenicity

Cysts: abnormal anechoic round or oval structure

Calcifications: hyperechoic lesion with acoustic shadowing

Ductal Criteria

Main pancreatic duct dilation: >3.5 mm in body or >1.5 mm in tail

Dilated side branches: at least three anechoic structures, >1 mm in width communicating with main pancreatic duct

Irregular pancreatic duct: uneven outline of duct

Hyperechoic duct wall: at least 50% of the length of main pancreatic duct in body and tail with hyperechoic wall

Adapted from The International Working Group for Minimal Standard Terminology in Gastrointestinal Endosonography. Minimal standard terminology in gastrointestinal endosonography. Dig Endosc. 1998;10:159-184; Catalano MF, Sahai A, Levy M, Romagnuolo J, Wiersema M, Brugge W, et al. EUS-based criteria for the diagnosis of chronic pancreatitis: the Rosemont classification. Gastrointest Endosc. 2009;69:1251-1261.

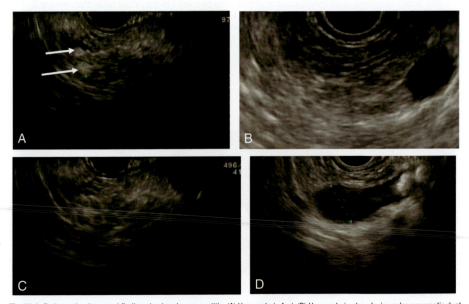

Fig. 71.8 Endoscopic ultrasound findings in chronic pancreatitis. (A) Hyperechoic foci. (B) Hyperechoic strands, irregular pancreatic duct, and hyperechoic duct wall. (C) Lobularity. (D) Calcifications.

24. **What are the standard nine EUS criteria for CP?**

For the standard nine EUS criteria for CP, see Box 71.1 and Fig. 71.8.

25. What are the limitations of EUS in diagnosing CP?

Interobserver agreement for the diagnosis of CP is moderate with kappa of 0.45; for the individual EUS features of CP, there is poor to moderate agreement, with the highest agreement for ductal dilation and lobularity.

Determination of whether EUS findings are pathologic or represent asymptomatic fibrosis, normal age-related changes, or normal variant is not possible. Asymptomatic EUS changes of CP have been reported in alcoholics, patients of advanced age, and patients who smoke without clinical CP.

26. How is EUS helpful in idiopathic recurrent pancreatitis?

EUS can provide an etiologic factor for 40%–80% of idiopathic recurrent pancreatitis cases with negative abdominal ultrasound and CT scan. More than 60% of the EUS findings are biliary pathologic conditions (microlithiasis, sludge, or stone).

27. List common indications of therapeutic EUS.

- Celiac plexus block/neurolysis (Video 71.1)
- Endoscopic cystgastrostomy/necrosectomy (Video 71.2)
- EUS-guided biliary/pancreatic access
- EUS-guided gastrojejunostomy
- EUS-guided gallbladder drainage
- EUS-guided variceal management

28. What are the potential complications of EUS-guided celiac plexus block/neurolysis?

Diarrhea, orthostatic hypotension, transiently worse abdominal pain, infection, and paralysis very rarely.

29. When is endoscopic cystgastrostomy or necrosectomy considered?

In patients with symptoms from their pseudocyst/walled-off necrosis which has a mature wall and is apposed to the stomach or duodenal wall. EUS guidance likely increases the technical success of these procedures.

30. Discuss pros and cons of EUS-guided biliary access compared with percutaneous biliary drainage.

Pros include no external drain needed and can potentially be completed in one setting rather than needing to return for another procedure. Cons include higher risk than standard ERCP although similar overall complication rate as percutaneous biliary drain and technique limited to tertiary care centers with expertise in therapeutic EUS.

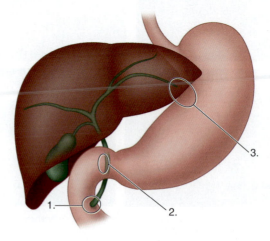

Fig. 71.9 Endoscopic ultrasound (EUS)–guided bile duct access: (1) rendezvous approach after EUS-guided access to extrahepatic or intrahepatic bile duct, (2) choledochoduodenostomy, and (3) hepaticogastrostomy.

31. **What are the different ways to access the bile duct via EUS?**

See Fig. 71.9. EUS-guided access to the intrahepatic or extrahepatic bile duct (depending on where the biliary stricture is) can be performed when ERCP fails. If the ampulla is accessible, either a rendezvous procedure or antegrade stenting following intrahepatic bile duct access can be performed. In a rendezvous procedure, EUS is used to advance the guidewire out of the ampulla into the duodenum, and then ERCP is performed in the usual manner. If the ampulla is inaccessible or rendezvous approach is not feasible, a new fistulous communication between the extrahepatic bile duct and duodenum (choledochoduodenostomy) or intrahepatic bile duct and stomach (hepaticogastrostomy) can be created via EUS using fully covered metal stents.

ACKNOWLEDGMENT

The author would like to acknowledge the contributions of Dr. Peter R. McNally, who was the author of this chapter in a previous edition.

CLINICAL VIGNETTE

Available Online

BIBLIOGRAPHY

Available Online

CHAPTER 72

ESOPHAGEAL SURGERY

Alex D. Michaels, MD and Theodore N. Pappas, MD

 Additional content available online.

ACHALASIA

1. **Define *achalasia*. What are the classic findings of esophageal achalasia?**
   Achalasia is a primary motility disorder of the esophagus characterized by a loss of enteric neurons leading to the absence of peristaltic waveforms in the esophageal body and impaired relaxation of the lower esophageal sphincter (LES) in response to swallowing. The condition is relatively rare, occurring at an incidence of 0.5–1.2 per 100,000 per year, yet it is the most commonly diagnosed primary esophageal motility disorder. Peak incidence is between 20 and 50 years of age, and it typically has an insidious onset.

2. **What are the most common symptoms of achalasia?**
   The nonrelaxing LES causes a functional outflow obstruction to the lower esophagus, resulting in progressive dysphagia, regurgitation, weight loss, and chest pain.

3. **What is pseudoachalasia? How is it diagnosed?**
   Pseudoachalasia, or secondary achalasia, is an esophageal motility disorder caused by a distal esophageal obstruction from an intrinsic tumor at the esophagogastric junction (EGJ) or extrinsic compression of the esophagus from a nonesophageal tumor. Patients exhibit symptoms typical of achalasia, including dysphagia, regurgitation, chest pain, and weight loss. Sometimes, manometry, endoscopy, and two-dimensional radiologic examination cannot distinguish pseudoachalasia from achalasia. Endoscopy helps rule out the possibility of pseudoachalasia but cannot diagnose a mural or extramural tumor. When this is suspected, based on a history of rapidly progressive dysphagia and substantial weight loss, endoscopic ultrasonography or computed tomography is recommended. The main distinguishing feature is the complete reversal of pathologic motor phenomena following successful therapy of the underlying disorder.

4. **What are the nonsurgical options for the treatment of achalasia?**
   - Smooth muscle relaxants (nitrates and calcium channel blockers)
   - Botulinum toxin injection at the LES
   - Pneumatic dilatation of the LES
   - Peroral endoscopic myotomy (POEM)

5. **What are the basic components of laparoscopic Heller myotomy for achalasia?**
   Surgical treatment of achalasia consists of a longitudinal myotomy of the distal esophagus and EGJ. Most myotomies were performed through the chest before the advent of minimally invasive surgery. The transabdominal laparoscopic approach is currently the procedure of choice with good long-term results in 84%–94% of patients.
   The operation starts with an upper endoscopy to evaluate the esophagus and the tightness of the LES. Five trocars are placed in the upper abdomen in an arrangement similar to that of a laparoscopic antireflux operation.
   A myotomy carried down to the level of the mucosa is performed, roughly 6 cm in length along the esophagus and 2–3 cm below the EGJ onto the stomach. Intraoperative manometry, repeat endoscopy, or Endoflip (endoluminal functional lumen imaging probe—an endoscopic device that measures the diameter and distensibility of sphincters within the gastrointestinal tract) is then used to confirm successful ablation of the pathologic high-pressure zone. A partial fundoplication is performed after the completion of the myotomy around a 52-Fr bougie. There is a general consensus that a 360-degree wrap may cause significant obstruction at the distal end of the esophagus and lead to worsening of esophageal function in patients with already impaired peristalsis. A randomized trial compared Heller myotomy and Dor fundoplication (partial anterior wrap) with Heller myotomy and Nissen fundoplication (360-degree wrap); the recurrence rate in the Nissen group was significantly higher than in the Dor group (15% vs. 2.8%, respectively) supporting the addition of Dor fundoplication to the Heller. However, the Toupet fundoplication (partial posterior wrap) and Dor fundoplication are equally effective in preventing reflux with low rates of postoperative dysphagia. Many surgeons prefer the Dor as it only requires an anterior esophageal dissection and provides mucosal protection as all of the exposed mucosa is covered by gastric serosa.

Patients who develop mild-to-moderate reflux after a Heller with a partial fundoplication can be easily managed medically.

6. **Describe the complications of Heller myotomy.**
The most common complication of a surgical myotomy is esophageal perforation, which is reported in up to 4.6% of patients. Previous pneumatic dilatation and botulinum toxin injection increase the technical difficulty in performing a myotomy and may increase the rate of perforation. Mucosal injuries detected during surgery may be repaired primarily. An unrecognized esophageal perforation may present as persistent fever, tachycardia, or left-sided pleural effusion. These patients require close observation and may need reoperation if conservative measures fail.

Early postoperative dysphagia is usually due to incomplete myotomy, whereas causes of late dysphagia also include healing of the myotomy or, more rarely, a reflux-induced stricture. Incomplete myotomy usually responds to extension of the myotomy. However, in patients in whom the first myotomy was complete, a second myotomy is less likely to be successful and such patients may require esophagectomy.

7. **How do long-term results of Heller myotomy compare with mechanical esophageal dilatation?**
Several large retrospective series have compared the two treatments and favor operative myotomy over pneumatic dilatation. With the introduction of the minimally invasive approach, the historical concerns about the morbidity associated with open surgical techniques have essentially disappeared and the morbidity and mortality of both surgical and nonsurgical options are now nearly identical. The long-term success and safety of laparoscopic myotomy have completed the shift in favor of surgery as the primary therapeutic option for patients with achalasia. A randomized controlled trial that compared laparoscopic Heller myotomy with Dor fundoplication versus pneumatic dilatation revealed that the two techniques are equally effective through 2-year follow-up, though patients in the dilation group did receive up to three separate dilations compared to the single operation in the Heller group.

8. **Describe POEM.**
The POEM results in a similar myotomy that is performed in the Heller, but it is performed endoscopically. A high-definition gastroscope with a cautery knife is used to create a mucosal incision to allow the scope access to the submucosal space. A longitudinal submucosal tunnel is then made for 8–10 cm on the esophagus and 3 cm onto the stomach. Selective myotomy of the circular muscle fibers is performed followed by closure of the mucosotomy. The tunnel and myotomy can be performed either anteriorly or posteriorly. Though an anterior tunnel is technically easier to perform, a posterior tunnel is preferred if the patient had previously undergone a Heller myotomy.

9. **How do the results of Heller myotomy compare with POEM?**
As POEM is a newer procedure, there are insufficient long-term studies at this point. A recent meta-analysis showed 92.7% improvement in dysphagia with POEM versus 90.0% with Heller at 2 years. While both procedures had good results for symptomatic improvement of dysphagia, patients who underwent POEM had higher rates of symptomatic gastroesophageal reflux disease (GERD) (odds ratio [OR] 1.69), abnormal pH studies (OR 4.30), and erosive esophagitis (OR 9.31) as there is no antireflux procedure performed with the POEM as there is when a Heller is performed.

10. **Summarize the treatment algorithm for patients with achalasia.**
The treatment options for achalasia are initially medical (nitrates and calcium channel blockers). Endoscopic botulinum toxin injection can be used to temporarily paralyze the LES. Botulinum toxin injection should be reserved for patients who are unable to tolerate surgery because of significant comorbidities, or patients whose clinical presentation is complicated, putting the diagnosis of achalasia in doubt. Endoscopic pneumatic dilation weakens the LES by stretching or tearing the LES muscle fibers. It is effective but often requires repeated procedures. Laparoscopic Heller myotomy with Dor fundoplication is reserved for patients with severe symptoms or younger patients so as to avoid the need for multiple pneumatic dilatations. POEM can either be used as an alternative to a primary Heller or as further treatment of persistent or recurrent dysphagia following a Heller.

11. **What is the association between achalasia and esophageal cancer?**
Patients with achalasia have a 28-fold increased risk of developing squamous cell carcinoma. There is also an increased risk of developing adenocarcinoma, but it is substantially lower than that of squamous cell carcinoma. Even though the relative risk is high, the absolute risk of developing esophageal cancer is still very low. Therefore both the American College of Gastroenterology and the American Society for Gastrointestinal Endoscopy recommend against routine endoscopic surveillance for esophageal cancer in in patients with achalasia.

ESOPHAGEAL CANCER

12. What is the incidence of esophageal cancer?

An estimated 15,310 new cases of carcinomas of the esophagus were diagnosed in men and 3,950 new cases in females in 2021. Approximately 12,410 men and 3120 females will die from the disease. Although it accounts for only 1% of newly diagnosed cancers, it causes 4% of cancer deaths in the United States, making it the seventh leading cause of death from cancer among men. The incidence of esophageal cancer has continued to rise in the last 30 years. Whereas squamous cell carcinoma accounted for most cancers of the esophagus 40 years ago, adenocarcinoma now represents two-thirds of such tumors in the United States. This is primarily caused by the striking increase in the incidence of adenocarcinoma among White men older than 60 years. The cause for the rising incidence and changing demographics is unknown, although part of the rise is due to the increasing incidence of Barrett esophagus and resulting adenocarcinoma in the distal esophagus.

13. What are the risk factors of esophageal cancer?

Risk factors for squamous cell carcinoma include tobacco use and excessive alcohol consumption, which appear to have a synergistic effect in its pathogenesis. Additionally, *N*-nitroso food compounds, achalasia, caustic injury, low socioeconomic status, prior thoracic irradiation, and human papillomavirus have been associated with an increased risk of the disease. Risk factors for the development of distal esophageal adenocarcinoma are less clear. The presence of Barrett esophagus and chronic GERD are both risk factors for developing adenocarcinoma.

14. Describe the relationship of Barrett esophagus to esophageal cancer.

Barrett esophagus is an acquired condition occurring in 10%–15% of individuals with chronic GERD and in 6.8% of the general population in which metaplastic columnar epithelium replaces the stratified squamous epithelium that normally lines the distal esophagus. It is generally believed that the disease progresses from Barrett metaplasia to low-grade dysplasia (LGD) to high-grade dysplasia (HGD) to adenocarcinoma. The incidence of adenocarcinoma increases nearly 40-fold in patients with Barrett esophagus. It is estimated that 5% of patients with Barrett esophagus will eventually develop invasive cancer, and patients with histologically proven Barrett esophagus require lifelong periodic surveillance with endoscopic four-quadrant biopsies every 2 cm (1 cm if known dysplasia) because of this risk.

15. Can Barrett esophagus regress after antireflux therapy?

Recent publications have suggested that curtailing reflux may decrease the tendency of patients with GERD without Barrett epithelium to develop Barrett esophagus. In addition, reflux control may diminish the tendency toward dysplastic or malignant degeneration of existing Barrett epithelium. That can be accomplished by either medical or surgical management, with the latter shown to be more effective. This effect is manifested by:
- Inducing actual regression of dysplastic to nondysplastic Barrett epithelium
- Stabilizing the Barrett epithelium in a nondysplastic state
- Allowing a return to normal squamous epithelium

The majority of regression occurs within 5 years after surgery. Though antireflux surgery does substantially reduce the risk of developing esophageal adenocarcinoma in those with Barrett esophagus, these patients remain at a 10-fold increased risk of developing esophageal adenocarcinoma compared with the general population.

16. Discuss the management of dysplasia in Barrett esophagus.

Many large surgical series document that following esophageal resection, 20%–40% of patients with Barrett esophagus who have HGD will be found to actually have invasive carcinoma in the specimen. Although this does not imply that the majority of the patients will have invasive carcinoma, the inability to reliably distinguish the two groups preoperatively means that every patient with HGD should be thought of as having a probable carcinoma. In addition, the likelihood of developing cancer in the first 3–5 years once HGD has been identified is 25%–50% and an 80% risk of adenocarcinoma development in 8 years. HGD in the setting of Barrett esophagus was traditionally treated with an esophagectomy, a procedure with an associated 50% morbidity and 6% mortality. In recent years, endoscopic eradication therapies (EET) such as radiofrequency ablation, photodynamic therapy, cryotherapy, and endoscopic mucosal resection have become the treatments of choice for both LGD and HGD, as well as for intramucosal cancers. These recommendations hinge on the fact that there is a very low rate of lymph node involvement in dysplasia and even intramucosal cancers (<2%), making the lymphadenectomy which can be achieved with a resection less beneficial. Esophagectomy is seldom used as the first-line treatment for HGD unless patients are willing or unable to undergo EET and lifelong endoscopic surveillance.

17. What are the surgical approaches for the patient with esophageal cancer?

Surgery is the primary treatment modality for esophageal cancer. In the United States, esophageal resection is most commonly performed, using one of the following approaches:
- *Transhiatal esophagectomy* involves both a midline laparotomy and left cervical incision. The short gastric and left gastric arteries are ligated, whereas the right gastric artery and right gastroepiploic arcade are carefully

preserved to allow a well-vascularized gastric conduit to reach the neck. The esophagus is resected through the abdominal and neck incisions. A cervical gastroesophageal (GE) anastomosis is performed through the cervical incision. The main advantage of this approach is avoidance of a thoracic anastomosis as a cervical leak carries much less morbidity than an intrathoracic leak.

- *Ivor-Lewis esophagectomy* requires a midline laparotomy and a right posterolateral thoracotomy. En bloc resection is performed from the hiatus to the apex of the chest just above the azygos vein. A GE anastomosis is performed in the right chest.
- *Three-hole esophagectomy* is performed less often and requires a midline laparotomy, right thoracotomy, and cervical incision.
- *Left thoracoabdominal esophagectomy* involves one incision extended across the abdomen and posterolateral chest for *en bloc* resection of the EGJ.
- *Minimally invasive esophagectomy* involves right thoracoscopic esophageal and lymph node–bearing tissue mobilization, laparoscopic mobilization of the stomach, and a high intrathoracic or cervical anastomosis.

Regardless of the approach, the same operative procedure is performed, that is, esophagogastrectomy with regional lymph node resection. For all of these approaches, portions of the operation can be done minimally invasively with a laparoscopic or robotic abdominal approach and/or a thoracoscopic or robotic thoracic approach which is associated with less pain and decreased length of stay. A recent analysis of the National Cancer Database showed that nearly half of esophagectomies in 2015 were performed minimally invasively with equivalent long-term survival and an increased lymph node yield.

18. **When is neoadjuvant therapy appropriate in the treatment of patients with esophageal carcinoma?**
The most recent guidelines from the American Society of Clinical Oncology recommend neoadjuvant chemoradiotherapy (CRT) for locally advanced squamous cell cancers and either neoadjuvant platinum-based chemotherapy or CRT for locally advanced adenocarcinomas. The benefit of neoadjuvant treatment for T2 tumors is less clear, so an individualized multidisciplinary approach should be used to decide between neoadjuvant treatment or a surgery-first approach.

19. **Describe nonsurgical options for the treatment of esophageal cancer.**
Nonsurgical options for the treatment of esophageal cancer can be divided into interventions for palliation and those for cure. Precancerous lesions or superficial cancers confined to the mucosa without evidence of metastatic spread can be cured with EET (see question 16). When curative treatment is not possible, in addition to systemic chemotherapy, palliative care measures have included external beam radiation, endoluminal brachytherapy, laser ablation, photodynamic therapy, endoluminal stenting, and surgical feeding access.

20. **What is the survival of patients with esophageal cancer?**
The overall 5-year survival in patients with esophageal cancer is 14%. Those patients with localized disease have a 5-year survival of approximately 47%. This drops off to 25% for regional disease and only 5% for metastatic disease with very few living beyond 18 months. Unfortunately, most esophageal cancers present at later stages with locally advanced disease or metastases, when a cure is not possible and palliation is the only treatment option.

GASTROESOPHAGEAL REFLUX AND PARAESOPHAGEAL HERNIAS

GASTROESOPHAGEAL REFLUX DISEASE

21. **Define GERD.**
GERD is defined as symptoms or mucosal injury caused by the abnormal reflux of gastric contents into the esophagus. It involves typical symptoms (Question 22) occurring two or more times weekly, or symptoms perceived as problematic to patients, or resulting in complications. One-third of the US population suffers from symptoms of GERD at least once monthly, 10%–20% once weekly, and 4%–7% daily. Although there is a high prevalence of heartburn, not everyone with heartburn has GERD.

22. **Describe the typical and atypical symptoms of GERD.**
The typical symptoms of GERD include heartburn, regurgitation, or water brash (in which the oral cavity suddenly fills with excessive amounts of saliva, sometimes mixed with stomach acids that have risen to the throat), and dysphagia (the blockage to the passage of food in the lower retrosternal area). Classic heartburn is defined as the retrosternal burning *rising from the stomach or lower chest toward the neckrising from the stomach or lower chest toward the neck* that lasts for a few moments to several minutes, that is relieved by antacids or food, and that occurs 30–60 minutes postprandially. Atypical or extraesophageal symptoms include cough, asthma, hoarseness, laryngitis, dental erosions, and noncardiac chest pain. Atypical symptoms are the primary complaint

in 20%–25% of patients with GERD and are secondarily associated with heartburn and regurgitation in many more. Nearly 50% of patients with chest pain and negative coronary angiograms, 75% with chronic hoarseness, and up to 80% with asthma have a positive 24-hour esophageal pH test, indicating abnormal acid reflux into the esophagus. Although many patients with atypical symptoms benefit from antireflux surgery, it is not as effective as for those patients with typical symptoms.

23. What factors play a role in altering the GE barrier?

The two most important are hypotension of the LES and loss of the angle of His as a result of paraesophageal hernia. Either may contribute to loss of competency of the sphincter and thus abnormal reflux. Physiologic reflux or reflux in early disease results from the transient loss of the high-pressure zone normally created by the tonic contraction of the smooth fibers of the LES. In severe GERD, the high-pressure zone is permanently reduced or nonexistent.

A large paraesophageal hernia alters the geometry of the EGJ and the angle of His is lost. There is a close relationship between the degree of gastric distention necessary to overcome the high-pressure zone and the morphologic characteristics of the gastric cardia. In patients with an intact angle of His, more gastric dilatation and higher intragastric pressure are necessary to overcome the sphincter than in patients with a paraesophageal hernia. Furthermore, a paraesophageal hernia may also result in hypotension of the LES. However, every patient with a paraesophageal hernia does not have GERD, and the presence of a small, sliding hiatal hernia without GERD is not an indication of medical or surgical intervention.

24. Describe the workup of patients with suspected GERD.

The four tests performed when GERD is suspected are barium swallow and upper gastrointestinal (GI) series, esophagogastroduodenoscopy (EGD), esophageal manometry, and 24-hour pH test, with the latter being the gold standard for a diagnosis of GERD.

- *Barium esophagram* provides both functional and structural information. It is most useful in assessing the size and reducibility of a paraesophageal hernia as well as the presence of esophageal shortening. A large, fixed hiatal hernia or paraesophageal hernia and a short esophagus are evidence of advanced disease and may predict a difficult operation.
- *EGD* helps to identify the presence of esophagitis and Barrett esophagus. It can also be used to evaluate response to treatment and to detect complications of GERD, including peptic stricture and foreshortened esophagus. Furthermore, endoscopy provides valuable information about the absence of other lesions in the upper GI tract that can produce symptoms identical to those of GERD.
- *Esophageal manometry* evaluates the peristaltic function of the esophagus as well as the pressure and relaxation of the LES. It is not a diagnostic test but provides information about the severity of the underlying physiologic defects of the LES and esophageal body. Furthermore, manometry helps rule out achalasia or other esophageal motility problems which may alter surgical planning. A normal manometric test includes a resting basal pressure at the LES of 10–45 mm Hg.
- *Esophageal 24-hour pH monitoring* is the most direct method for assessing the presence and severity of GERD and, because it has the highest sensitivity and specificity of all available tests, has become the gold standard for the diagnosis of GERD. It is very useful in the evaluation of patients with atypical symptoms and patients with typical symptoms but with no evidence of esophagitis on endoscopy. The test also measures the correlation between a patient's symptoms and documented episodes of reflux in the supine or erect position. It can also assess if there is adequate acid suppression when patients are on medical treatment. It should be performed in every patient before antireflux surgery and ideally with patients off acid suppression, though some patients may not tolerate this. pH monitoring is traditionally performed with a catheter that is placed transnasally through the esophagus and into the stomach. A newer alternative, Bravo pH capsule probe, is a miniaturized pH probe that is attached to the esophagus 5 cm above the LES (as determined by manometry) endoscopically. The Bravo capsule transmits pH data to a wearable recording device. It stays in the esophagus for 3–5 days and is then spontaneously excreted in the stool. The advantage of the Bravo is that it is tolerated much better than the standard nasoesophageal probes.

25. What is the significance of a defective LES?

The finding of a permanently defective LES (pressure <6 mm Hg) has several implications. First, it is almost always associated with esophageal mucosal injury and predicts that symptoms will be difficult to control with medical therapy alone. A defective LES results in an increased EGJ diameter and progressively leads to loss of the acute angle of His and therefore development of a paraesophageal hernia. It is a signal that surgical therapy is probably needed for consistent, long-term control as the condition is irreversible, even when the associated esophagitis has healed. The worse the esophageal injury, the more likely it is that the LES is defective. Approximately 40% of patients with pH-positive GERD and no mucosal injury have a mechanically defective LES, whereas nearly 100% of patients with long-segment Barrett esophagus have a defective LES.

26. What is the significance of abnormal esophageal motility in patients with GERD?

Long-standing, severe GERD can lead to deterioration of esophageal body function. Abnormalities of esophageal body function include ineffective esophageal motility (>70% ineffective swallows or ≥50% failed peristalsis) and absent contractility (100% failed peristalsis). Dysphagia is generally a prominent symptom in patients with defective peristalsis.

27. What are the indications for an antireflux operation?

The introduction of minimally invasive procedures to surgically treat GERD has increased the frequency of these operations. The ability to permanently stop gastroesophageal reflux and rid patients of dependence on medications has prompted gastroenterologists to refer patients for surgical therapy more readily. Indications for surgery include:

- Patient's wish to control symptoms without medication
- Persistent symptoms despite maximal medical therapy (most common)
- GERD with prominent regurgitation component
- Paraesophageal hernia
- Reflux complications (esophagitis, Barrett esophagus, bleeding, stricture, mucosal ulceration, and Cameron ulcer—chronic iron-deficiency anemia caused by slow bleeding from the point where the herniated stomach rubs against the diaphragm)

    Surgery may be the treatment of choice in patients who are at high risk of progression despite medical therapy. The risk factors for progression include the following:

- Nocturnal reflux on 24-hour esophageal pH study
- Structurally deficient LES (pressure less than 6 mm Hg)
- Mixed reflux of gastric and duodenal juice
- Mucosal injury at presentation

    Of note, Roux-en-Y gastric bypass is the preferred treatment for morbidly obese patients with GERD, with concomitant repair of a hiatal hernia if present. The gastric bypass both treats GERD and has the additional benefits of weight loss and improvement of obesity-related comorbidities.

28. What are the surgical options to relieve GERD?

All of the successful surgical procedures for GERD have certain characteristics in common. All create an intra-abdominal segment of esophagus, prevent recurrence of the paraesophageal hernia if present, and create an antireflux valve. Options include:

- Nissen fundoplication: total 360-degree fundoplication
- Toupet fundoplication: partial 270-degree posterior fundoplication
- Dor fundoplication: partial 180-degree anterior fundoplication
- Belsey Mark IV: partial 270-degree anterior fundoplication via thoracic approach
- Thal fundoplication: 90-degree anterior fundoplication
- Watson: 120-degree anterolateral fundoplication

    The approach to the repair can be abdominal (open, laparoscopic, or robotic), thoracic (open, thoracoscopic, or robotic), and even thoracoabdominal. None of the operations or approaches is perfect for all patients. If the esophagus is foreshortened from chronic inflammation, consider approaching from the chest and performing a Collis gastroplasty in which a portion of the lesser curvature is stapled and divided to create extra-esophageal length. If esophageal motility is an issue, consider a partial wrap so as not to produce severe dysphagia. Additionally, robot-assisted fundoplication has been widely performed with similar outcomes to laparoscopic fundoplication. A newer surgical technique is magnetic sphincter augmentation such as the LINX Reflux Management System. The LINX is a series of magnetic beads connected by a wire which are placed around the LES which apply pressure to the LES at baseline but can transiently open with a swallowing to allow the passage of ingested substances. Although there is good short-term relief of GERD symptoms, there are higher rates of dysphagia than seen with fundoplications. There are also nonoperative, endoscopic treatments such as transoral incisionless fixation (TIF) and radiofrequency treatment. TIF creates a full-thickness serosa-to-serosa partial fundoplication using small plastic fasteners. Stretta uses a specialized catheter to treat the esophagus with RF. Both of these options are only used in patients with small or no hiatal hernia. The long-term risk and benefit profiles of these newer therapies have not been well documented.

29. What are the important technical steps of a Nissen fundoplication?

Despite the caveats in Question 28, laparoscopic Nissen fundoplication is the procedure of choice for most patients requiring an antireflux operation. Four or five trocars are inserted in the upper abdomen to provide access to the laparoscope and instruments. Both the right and the left vagus nerves are identified and preserved. The short gastric vessels are divided in the proximal part of the stomach, thereby mobilizing the fundus so that it can be placed around the distal esophagus without tension (the *shoeshine* maneuver). Dissection is performed to identify the right and left crura of the diaphragm. The distal esophagus is mobilized so that at least 3 cm of the distal esophagus lies without tension in the abdomen. This often requires a high mediastinal dissection to

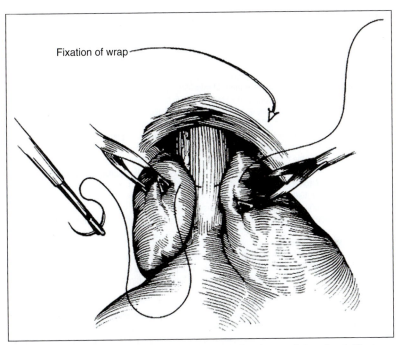

Fig. 72.1 Laparoscopic view of the placement of the first fundoplication stitch. (From Cameron JL. Current surgical therapy. Philadelphia, PA: Mosby; 2004.)

free the esophagus from surrounding structures 8–10 cm beyond the hiatus. The crura are approximated with nonabsorbable sutures (Fig. 72.1). A bougie (48–60 Fr depending on the size of the patient) is placed in the esophagus to prevent an excessively tight fundoplication. Some surgeons anchor the wrap to the crura and to the esophagus to help prevent it from herniating into the chest.

30. **What are the predictors of successful antireflux surgery?**
Predictors of successful antireflux surgery include typical symptoms of GERD (heartburn and regurgitation), an abnormal score on 24-hour esophageal pH monitor, and symptomatic improvement in response to acid suppression therapy before surgery.

31. **What are the predictors of poor outcomes after antireflux surgery?**
The presence of GI symptoms other than typical GERD symptoms, a large paraesophageal hernia, stricture with persistent dysphagia, and Barrett esophagus are characteristics of advanced GERD and may predict less-than-ideal results.

32. **Explain the benefits of surgical treatment of GERD.**
Antireflux procedures performed by experienced esophageal surgeons provide several benefits that cannot be accomplished with antacid medications. A successful operation augments the LES and repairs the hiatal hernia if present. It prevents the reflux of both gastric and duodenal juice, thus preventing aspiration. Antireflux operations also improve esophageal body motility and speed gastric emptying, which is often subclinically delayed in patients with GERD. More than 90% of patients are relieved of symptoms, eat unrestricted diets, and are satisfied with the surgical outcome.

33. **What are the complications of laparoscopic fundoplication?**
The overall incidence of complications after laparoscopic Nissen fundoplication is 2%–13%. Most complications are minor such as urinary retention, postoperative gastric distention, and superficial wound infections. Mild early dysphagia may be found in 15%–20% of patients, but the incidence of residual dysphagia after 3 months is less than 5%. Less than 1% of these patients need intervention to treat dysphagia. Splenectomy may be required in rare circumstances. Conversion rate of laparoscopic to open fundoplication is 1%–2%. The rate of major morbidity

(esophageal injury, stomach injury, leak, and pneumothorax) is 2%–10% and mortality rate up to 0.5%, making it a relatively safe procedure for alleviating GERD.

PARAESOPHAGEAL HERNIAS

34. Define the four types of hernias occurring at the hiatus.
- *Type I* is a *sliding* hiatal hernia in which the EGJ migrates through the hiatus into the posterior mediastinum as a result of laxity of the phrenoesophageal ligament. This is the most common type of hiatal hernia.
- *Type II* is a true paraesophageal hernia, characterized by an upward dislocation of the fundus of the stomach alongside a normally positioned GE junction. This is the least common type of hiatal hernia.
- *Type III* is a combination of types I and II, characterized by cephalad displacement of both the GE junction and typically a large portion of the fundus and body of the stomach into the chest. Type III hernias probably start as a sliding hernia, and as the hiatus enlarges over time, a progressively greater portion of the fundus and body of the stomach herniate through the defect. When more than 30% of the stomach is herniated in the stomach, the term *giant paraesophageal hernia* is used. An *intrathoracic stomach* is used to describe the condition in which all of the stomach is within the chest.
- *Type IV* are type III hernias in which other viscera such as the colon or spleen are included in the hernia sac. These are quite uncommon and represent only 2%–5% of all paraesophageal hernias (Table 72.1).

35. What causes a hiatal hernia?
The precise cause of a hiatal hernia is unknown. Its pathogenesis is thought to involve at least two important factors, including increased intra-abdominal pressure and a progressive enlargement of the diaphragmatic hiatus. The increased incidence with age suggests that these hernias are acquired.

36. What are the signs and symptoms of a hiatal hernia?
Many hiatal hernias are asymptomatic and are first recognized on chest radiography. Type I is often associated with reflux but does not cause direct symptoms. Paraesophageal hernias classically cause symptoms of substernal chest pain, often thought to be cardiac in origin, and shortness of breath after eating. Shortness of breath is secondary to loss of vital capacity caused by impingement of hernia contents on the lung. Other symptoms, which may or may not be present, include dysphagia, early satiety, abdominal bloating, and GE reflux, as well as aspiration manifested by chronic cough, dyspnea, and wheezing. Cameron ulcers are often the cause of unexplained microcytic anemia in older adults with otherwise normal upper and lower endoscopy. Rarely, acute herniation or volvulus occurs, causing sudden pain and symptoms of gastric outlet obstruction. Strangulation can cause gastric necrosis, resulting in rapid decompensation, shock, and death.

37. How are hiatal and paraesophageal hernias diagnosed and evaluated?
Hiatal hernias are often first suspected because of a chest radiograph abnormality. Classically, a retrocardiac air bubble with or without an air-fluid level will be present. Confirmation can be obtained with a barium swallow, which shows the typical appearance of a large intrathoracic stomach and evaluates the motility of the esophagus simultaneously. Upper endoscopy is useful to evaluate the distal esophagus and stomach for ulcers, erosions, Barrett esophagus, or neoplasms in this generally older population. An esophageal motility study is recommended in patients being considered for elective surgical correction of a paraesophageal hernia both to determine the status of the LES and to assess the function of the esophageal body. This is particularly true in any patient with symptoms of dysphagia. A 24-hour pH test is usually not necessary because a fundoplication is recommended as part of the procedure to correct this defect.

Table 72.1 Types of Hernias Occurring at the Hiatus.

HERNIA TYPE	LOCATION OF ESOPHAGOGASTRIC JUNCTION	HERNIA CONTENTS	SPONTANEOUS REDUCIBILITY
Type I (sliding)	Intrathoracic	Fundus	Usually reducible
Type II (true paraesophageal)	Intra-abdominal	Fundus ± body	Often fixed
Type III (mixed)	Intrathoracic	Fundus + body	Fixed
Type IV (type III with other viscera included)	Intrathoracic	Fundus + body + other organ	Fixed

38. **What are the indications for surgical repair of paraesophageal hernias?**

In most patients with paraesophageal hernias, it is the hernia itself that is responsible for symptoms and imparts the risk of life-threatening complications. There is no medical treatment appropriate for treating a paraesophageal hernia. Medications such as proton pump inhibitors may treat its symptoms, but the only therapy for the hernia is surgical. There used to be a controversy about which patients should have an operation and which procedure and approach are most appropriate. A prophylactic paraesophageal hernia repair in an asymptomatic patient is now rarely performed as the mortality rate after elective hernia repair in an asymptomatic patient ranges from 0.5% to 1.4%, whereas the probability of developing acute symptoms that will require emergent surgery is estimated to be 1.1%. However, all patients with symptoms or signs associated with the paraesophageal hernia should undergo repair in the absence of prohibitive surgical risk. Also, patients with gastric volvulus, obstruction, strangulation, perforation, and bleeding should undergo emergent repair.

39. **What is the operative strategy of a paraesophageal hernia repair?**

The key steps of paraesophageal hernia repair are the following:
- Return stomach and esophagus to their normal intra-abdominal positions
- Remove the hernia sac
- Close the hiatus
- Anchor the stomach below the diaphragm

In most circumstances, a fundoplication is added to augment the LES and to aid in stabilizing the repair below the diaphragm. The stomach can also be anchored below the diaphragm with either an anterior suture gastropexy or gastrostomy tube. In addition to providing gastric fixation, a gastrostomy tube can also aid in postoperative care by allowing venting of the stomach in the setting of delayed gastric emptying or for enteral nutrition. In the unfortunate situation when patients are acutely too sick and/or are too frail at baseline to undergo a formal paraesophageal hernia repair, a hybrid laparoscopic-endoscopic approach can be used to reduce the stomach into the abdomen with the placement of two percutaneous endoscopic gastrostomy (PEG) tubes without actually repairing the hernia. These PEGs act as a gastropexy to prevent recurrent herniation, provide gastric access for feeding or venting, and reduce the risk of volvulus compared to the placement of a single PEG. If the patient recovers or rehabilitates and develops a recurrence, a future formal repair can then be undertaken.

If the crural closure appears to be under tension, reinforcing the crural sutures with absorbable mesh reduces the short-term rates of herniation. A randomized trial of mesh reinforcement of hiatal repair versus suture repair only showed no difference in the rate of hernia recurrence but was associated with more symptomatic complaints among those repaired with mesh. Therefore the routine use of mesh in repair is not indicated.

Paraesophageal hernias can be approached either transabdominally or transthoracically. Traditionally, a transthoracic repair had been advocated because of the relative ease of mobilizing the esophagus and dissecting out the hernia sac and its contents. However, as the stomach is reduced blindly into the abdomen, an organoaxial rotation of the stomach could persist or redevelop and lead to an intra-abdominal gastric volvulus. The abdominal approach is now preferred with the main advantage being the ability to perform the surgery minimally invasively. Laparoscopic repair offers the advantages of decreased length of postoperative discomfort, earlier return to regular activities, and shorter hospital stay.

CLINICAL VIGNETTE

Available Online

BIBLIOGRAPHY

Available Online

SURGERY FOR PEPTIC ULCER DISEASE

Alex D. Michaels, MD and Theodore N. Pappas, MD

 Additional content available online.

1. **Describe the five types of gastric ulcers in terms of location, gastric acid secretory status, incidence, and complications.**

   Peptic ulcers are a common cause of upper gastrointestinal (GI) symptoms with peak incidence in middle-aged males (55–65 years). They arise at various locations, including the stomach (gastric ulcer), duodenum (duodenal ulcer), and esophagus (esophageal ulcer). Gastric ulcers are further divided into five types based on location, secretory status, and cause (Table 73.1 and Fig. 73.1).

2. **Describe the classic indications and goals for peptic ulcer surgery.**

   Since the introduction of H₂-receptor antagonists and proton pump inhibitors (PPIs) and the identification of *Helicobacter pylori* as an ulcerogenic cofactor, the frequency of elective operations for peptic ulcer disease (PUD) has decreased by more than 90%. Currently, surgery for duodenal and gastric ulcers is reserved for

Table 73.1 Five Types of Gastric Ulcers by Location, Gastric Acid Secretory Status, Complications, and Incidence.

TYPE	LOCATION	ACID HYPERSE-CRETION	COMPLICATIONS	INCIDENCE (%)
I	Gastric body, lesser curvature	No	Bleeding uncommon	55
II	Body of stomach + duodenal ulcer	Yes	Bleeding, perforation, obstruction	20
III	Prepyloric	Yes	Bleeding, perforation	20
IV	High on lesser curvature	No	Bleeding	<5
V	Anywhere (medication induced)	No	Bleeding, perforation	<5

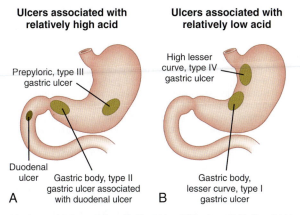

Fig. 73.1 Four types of gastric ulcers and their association with either high acid (A) or low acid (B). (From Sabiston DC Jr. Textbook of Surgery: The Biologic Basis of Modern Surgical Practice. Philadelphia, PA: WB Saunders; 1997.)

the management of complications of PUD, most commonly stricture and perforation (9% and 3% of patients, respectively).

The classic indications for peptic ulcer surgery are the following:
- Intractability of symptoms
- Suspicion of malignancy (peptic ulcer failed to heal after 12 weeks of PPI treatment, even with negative biopsies)
- Perforation
- Bleeding (after multiple endoscopic attempts and angiographic embolization fail to control hemorrhage or brisk hemorrhage leading to hemodynamic instability that requires control faster than nonoperative techniques would allow)
- Gastric outlet obstruction (GOO)

The main goals of surgery are to:
- Treat any complications of PUD
- Eliminate the factors that contribute to ulcer occurrence

3. What are the three classic operations used for PUD?

Truncal vagotomy and drainage
Truncal vagotomy and antrectomy
Highly selective vagotomy (parietal cell vagotomy or proximal gastric vagotomy)

4. Describe the truncal vagotomy, selective vagotomy, and highly selective vagotomy.

Truncal vagotomy involves the division of both the anterior and posterior vagal trunks at the esophageal hiatus above the origins of the hepatic and celiac branches. Periesophageal dissection must include the distal 6–8 cm of the esophagus to ensure the division of gastric vagal branches that arise from the trunks above the level of the hiatus. A drainage procedure such as a pyloroplasty must be concomitantly performed with a truncal vagotomy because denervation of the antrum and pylorus results in impaired gastric emptying.

Selective vagotomy involves division of the vagal trunks distal to the hepatic and celiac branches, thereby preserving vagal innervation to the gallbladder and celiac plexus. This reduces the incidence of gallbladder dysmotility, gallstones, and diarrhea. However, selective vagotomy also results in complete gastric vagotomy, necessitating a drainage procedure. Selective vagotomy is not the operation of choice, as it is needlessly complex and not superior to truncal vagotomy; it is rarely used and only of historic importance.

Highly selective vagotomy (parietal cell vagotomy or proximal gastric vagotomy) involves selective division of the vagal fibers to the acid-producing parietal cell mass of the gastric fundus while maintaining vagal fibers to the antrum and distal gut. The anterior and posterior neurovascular attachments are divided along the lesser curvature of the stomach, beginning approximately 7 cm from the pylorus and progressing to the gastroesophageal junction, with additional skeletonization of the distal 6–8 cm of the esophagus to ensure division of the *criminal nerve of Grassi*. Innervation of the antrum and pylorus is maintained because the two terminal branches of the anterior and posterior nerves of Latarjet are left intact, so no drainage procedure is necessary.

5. Why is an outlet or drainage procedure added to truncal vagotomy? What are the surgical options?

Truncal vagotomy involves division of both anterior and posterior vagal trunks at the esophageal hiatus. This procedure results in denervation of the acid-producing mucosa of the gastric fundus as well as to the pylorus and antrum, causing an alteration of normal pyloric coordination and impaired gastric emptying. Therefore a procedure to eliminate the function of the pyloric sphincter must be performed to allow gastric emptying. There are four primary options for an outlet procedure (Fig. 73.2):

Heineke-Mikulicz pyloroplasty: A longitudinal incision of the pyloric sphincter, extending onto the duodenum and antrum, is closed transversely. This is the most commonly performed technique.

Finney pyloroplasty: A U-shaped incision crossing the pylorus is made and a gastroduodenostomy is created; used in cases of extensive duodenal scarring to create a wider gastroduodenal opening.

Jaboulay gastroduodenostomy: A side-to-side gastroduodenostomy is created in which the incision does not cross the pyloric sphincter. Although rarely necessary, it is used when severe pyloric scarring precludes division of the pyloric channel.

Gastrojejunostomy: Billroth II or Roux-en-Y anastomosis is reserved for significant duodenal bulb scarring that makes pyloroplasty more challenging.

6. What are the relative indications and contraindications to highly selective vagotomy?

Highly selective vagotomy is indicated for the treatment of intractable duodenal ulcers because it does not require a drainage procedure. It has also been used in the emergent treatment of bleeding or perforated duodenal ulcers

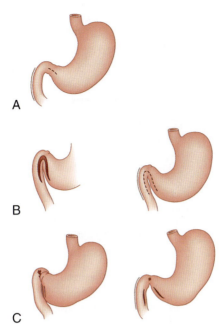

A

B

C

Fig. 73.2 (A) Heineke-Mikulicz pyloroplasty, (B) Finney pyloroplasty, and (C) Jaboulay gastroduodenostomy are the primary options for an outlet or *drainage* procedure after truncal vagotomy.

in stable patients. It reduces the basal and stimulated acid secretion by more than 75% and 50%, respectively. Highly selective vagotomy is contraindicated in patients with prepyloric ulcers or with GOO because they demonstrate high rates of recurrent ulceration. As most surgeons nowadays have very little experience with this procedure, and the fact that PPIs are so effective, this operation is rarely used today. In addition, patients with PUD who do not respond to high-dose PPI will be inadequately treated with a highly selective vagotomy. These patients required surgical therapy with a very low recurrence rate such as vagotomy and antrectomy.

7. **What are the surgical options for reconstruction after antrectomy?**
   Billroth I reconstruction consists of a gastroduodenostomy in which an end-to-end anastomosis is created between the gastric remnant and the duodenum (Fig. 73.3).
   Billroth II reconstruction consists of a gastrojejunostomy in which a side-to-side anastomosis is created between the gastric remnant and a loop of jejunum, with the closure of the duodenal stump (Fig. 73.4).
   Roux-en-Y reconstruction involves the creation of a jejunojejunostomy (forming a Y-shaped figure of small bowel) downstream from a side-to-side anastomosis of the free jejunal end to the gastric remnant (gastrojejunostomy). Unlike in gastric bypasses in which a long Roux limb is used, reconstruction after antrectomy should employ an approximately 40 cm Roux limb.

8. **How is the type of reconstruction determined for a given patient?**
   The decision of which type of reconstruction to perform is determined, in large part, by the extent of duodenal scarring caused by PUD and the ease with which the duodenum and the stomach can be brought together. Severely scarred duodenum cannot be used for a Billroth I anastomosis. The Billroth I reconstruction, however, offers the most physiologic anastomosis because it restores normal continuity of the GI tract. The Billroth II reconstruction may be complicated by afferent loop syndrome in which obstruction of the afferent limb results in the accumulation of bile and pancreatic secretions, causing right upper quadrant abdominal pain that is alleviated by bilious vomiting. Roux-en-Y reconstruction allows the diversion of bile and pancreatic secretions away from the gastric outlet, thereby reducing the risk of bile reflux gastritis. However, it can result in dumping syndrome and is associated with risks of internal hernias.

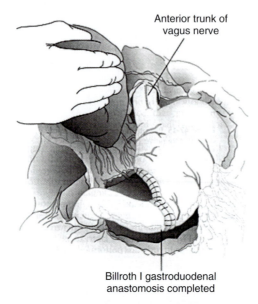

Anterior trunk of
vagus nerve

Billroth I gastroduodenal
anastomosis completed

Fig. 73.3 Hemigastrectomy with Billroth I anastomosis. (From Townsend CM. Sabiston Textbook of Surgery. 18th ed. Philadelphia, PA: WB Saunders; 2008.)

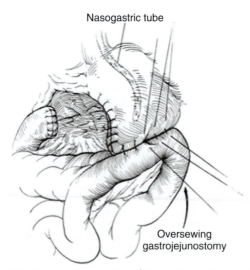

Nasogastric tube

Oversewing
gastrojejunostomy

Fig. 73.4 Hemigastrectomy with Billroth II anastomosis. (From Sabiston DC. Atlas of General Surgery. Philadelphia, PA: WB Saunders; 1994.)

9. Define intractability in terms of the medical treatment of PUD.

Intractability is defined as mucosal healing refractory to maximal medical therapy. The following two criteria define a refractory ulcer and are generally indications for operative intervention:

Ulcer persistence after 8–12 weeks of PPI treatment

Ulcer recurrence within 1 year, despite maintenance medical therapy (and ruling out *H. pylori*, aspirin use, nonsteroidal anti-inflammatory drug [NSAID] use, and hypersecretory states)

10. **Describe the most appropriate elective operative procedure for duodenal ulcers and each type of gastric ulcer.**

The choice of operation for gastric ulcers depends on several factors: ulcer location, acid secretory status, and presence of a coexistent duodenal ulcer. In general, gastric ulcers should be included with the resection while duodenal ulcers heal after acid suppression.

Type I: Antrectomy with inclusion of the ulcer and Billroth I or II reconstruction. Although type I gastric ulcers are associated with low to normal acid secretion, most surgeons include a truncal vagotomy, unless achlorhydria is demonstrated. It is associated with excellent symptomatic relief and low recurrence rates.

Type II and III: Truncal vagotomy, antrectomy with inclusion of the gastric ulcer and Billroth I reconstruction. Type II (gastric body) and III (prepyloric) gastric ulcers are associated with high rates of acid secretion, and therefore the goal of the surgery is removal of the gastric mucosa at risk for ulceration and reduction of acid secretion. Highly selective vagotomy has been associated with poor results and high recurrence rates.

Type IV: Distal gastrectomy with resection proximally to include the ulcer high on the lesser curvature and Billroth I anastomosis. Because type IV ulcers are located high on the lesser curvature, they are surgically challenging.

Type V: Surgery is reserved for the treatment of complications. Type V gastric ulcers generally heal rapidly with cessation of aspirin or an NSAID and institution of an H_2-receptor antagonist or PPI. An intractable type V gastric ulcer should raise suspicion for underlying malignancy.

Duodenal ulcer: Historically, the highly selective vagotomy has been the mainstay of treatment. However, the intractable duodenal ulcer is a rare entity in the PPI era and may represent a more resistant variant with a higher rate of recurrence. Therefore truncal vagotomy with pyloroplasty is predominantly used today. In cigarette smokers with PUD in the duodenum, recurrence rates are high after vagotomy and pyloroplasty so vagotomy and antrectomy as the primary surgical therapy is preferred.

11. **Describe the presentation of a patient with a perforated peptic ulcer.**

Patients usually describe a prodrome of gnawing localized pain in the epigastric region prior to perforation. With acute perforation, the epigastric pain becomes diffuse as a result of release of acidic fluid in the peritoneal cavity. The resulting release of vasoactive mediators is often associated with fever, tachycardia, tachypnea, and hypotension. Patients with a perforated posterior duodenal ulcer will often present with upper GI bleeding secondary to erosion into the gastroduodenal artery. On examination, the patient with peptic ulcer perforation lies immobile and the abdomen is diffusely tender and rigid. The white blood cell count is elevated, and in 70% of cases, free intraperitoneal air is found on upright abdominal radiographs. Although computed tomography (CT) scan is the most sensitive radiologic test for free intraperitoneal air, it is rarely indicated because patients with perforated peptic ulcers usually present with classic signs and symptoms, and CT scanning only serves to delay an operation.

12. **Why do almost all perforated gastric ulcers require an operation?**

Perforated gastric ulcers constitute 40% of perforated peptic ulcers and duodenal ulcers the remaining 60%.
- Unlike perforated duodenal ulcers, which may be treated nonoperatively if the ulcer has sealed itself as demonstrated on Gastrografin swallow, perforated gastric ulcers usually fail to heal spontaneously.
- They are associated with a risk of adenocarcinoma.
- Gastric ulcer disease due to *H. pylori* produces a hypoacidic environment with resultant bacterial overgrowth and abscess formation with perforation.

13. **What are the contraindications to medical management of perforated PUD?**
- Concurrent use of corticosteroids, which makes healing unlikely.
- Continued leak, as demonstrated by a contrast radiograph.
- Perforation in a patient taking an H_2-receptor antagonist or a PPI. A definitive ulcer operation is necessary to allow ulcer healing and to reduce the risk of recurrence.

14. **What are the three major goals of operation for perforated PUD?**

Repair of the perforation is usually performed by either plugging the defect with omental fat but not suturing the perforation closed (Graham patch) or by suturing the perforation closed and buttressing the repair with omental fat (modified Graham patch). The modified Graham patch is reserved for small defects without much inflammation as trying to bring together the two ends of a large defect or severely inflamed tissue will result in further tissue damage (Fig. 73.5).

The abdominal cavity is copiously irrigated.

Definitive ulcer operation is performed. A patient who has had a perforation for less than 24 hours and is hemodynamically stable without significant comorbidities should undergo a definitive ulcer operation if he or she has been receiving medical therapy for PUD or is taking medication that increases the risk of PUD. For the remainder of patients, definitive ulcer surgery is not indicated. Instead, treatment with PPI and *H. pylori* eradication, if applicable, are the mainstay of treatment.

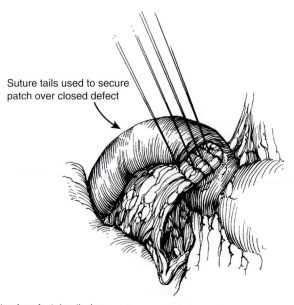

Suture tails used to secure
patch over closed defect

Fig. 73.5 Omental patching of a perforated peptic ulcer.

15. What are the roles of routine surgical drains and routine imaging after surgery for perforated PUD?

It is common practice to leave surgical drains adjacent to the site of repair. Two older, small randomized control trials with a combined 179 patients showed no benefit of routine drain placement. A more recent retrospective review of more than 4000 patients showed a lower incidence of postoperative interventions in patients who had surgical drains versus those who did not, though the overall rates were still low (1.9% vs. 5.6%).

While the classic teaching is to assess the repair a few days postoperatively with a contrasted upper GI imaging before allowing oral intake, this practice is associated with longer hospital stays without increased detection of clinically significant leaks. Therefore imaging should be saved when there is clinical suspicion of a leak.

16. What is the preferred operation for the treatment of perforated gastric ulcer?

Excision of the ulcer with or without vagotomy and drainage. The major distinction between surgical management of perforated duodenal and perforated gastric ulcers is that in all cases of perforated gastric ulcers, carcinoma must be excluded. Therefore all perforated gastric ulcers must undergo biopsy or resection. One option is to perform a wedge resection as diagnostic biopsy. Controversy exists as to whether a definitive ulcer operation should be added to this procedure, with most surgeons in favor of a definitive acid-reducing procedure in type II or III variant. An alternative for a perforated antral ulcer is antrectomy (with inclusion of the ulcer in the resection), to which truncal vagotomy may be added if the patient is an acid hypersecretor. The decision for the type of operation should be based on an individual patient, taking into account the patient's comorbidities, age, and severity at presentation.

17. What is the preferred operation for the treatment of a perforated duodenal ulcer?

The preferred operation is a simple patch (Graham patch) of the perforation, especially in the setting of shock or in patients with multiple comorbidities undergoing an emergent operation, when prolonged operative time can be detrimental. In patients who have undergone medical therapy to eradicate *H. pylori*, a reasonable approach for a perforated duodenal ulcer is truncal vagotomy and pyloroplasty, with incorporation of the perforation into the pyloroplasty closure. This relatively simple procedure requires a short operative time. In the ideal surgical candidate, highly selective vagotomy with patch closure of the perforation is recommended, although this procedure requires a high degree of surgical expertise. Patients who have not been treated for *H. pylori* prior to perforation should undergo repair and Graham patch of a perforated duodenal ulcer as stated previously with postoperative *H. pylori* eradication therapy, in lieu of a definitive ulcer operation.

18. **What are the major risk factors for mortality in the surgical treatment of perforated PUD?**
Patients with one of these risk factors have a mortality rate of approximately 10%; with two risk factors, the mortality rate increases to 46%. Patients with all three risk factors have a mortality rate of nearly 100%.
Severe comorbidities
Perforation present for longer than 24 hours
Hemodynamic instability on presentation

19. **Discuss the role for laparoscopy in the management of perforated PUD and the indications for conversion to an open operation.**
The surgical goals in the laparoscopic management of a perforated peptic ulcer are similar to those of open surgical management:
- Repair of the perforation.
- Copious irrigation of the abdominal cavity.
- Addition of a definitive ulcer operation is reserved for patients who have a history suggesting a high recurrence rate (cigarette smokers or chronic NSAID users). Adding a definitive ulcer operation will depend on the skill (experience) of the surgeon and may involve either laparoscopic truncal vagotomy and pyloroplasty or, on rare occasion, laparoscopic highly selective vagotomy.
    The relative indications for conversion to an open procedure include posterior location of the ulcer and inadequate localization. The presence of a perforated gastric ulcer with its suspicion for malignancy may necessitate conversion for definitive diagnosis.
    Laparoscopic repair of perforated PUD is associated with lower rates of complications, length of stay, and pain when compared with open operations. Of course, minimally invasive techniques should only be used when the patient's clinical status allow and the surgeon is comfortable with them.

20. **In patients with GI bleeding caused by PUD, what are the predictors for rebleeding in the hospital? What is the Forrest classification?**
- Hemodynamic instability (systolic blood pressure <100 mm Hg, heart rate >100–110 beats per minute)
- Large ulcer size (>1–2 cm)
- Ulcer location (posterior duodenal wall and high lesser curvature)
- Active bleeding during endoscopy
- Hematocrit less than 30
- Multiple comorbidities
- Coagulopathy
- Hematemesis
- Inability to clear the stomach with aggressive lavage
    The Forrest classification describes endoscopic risk factors for rebleeding (https://www.mdcalc.com/forrest-classification-upper-gi-bleeding; see Question 20 in Chapter 50).

21. **What is the preferred treatment for a bleeding peptic ulcer? What is the preferred treatment for rebleeding after endoscopic therapy? When is surgery indicated?**
Endoscopic therapy is the best first treatment for bleeding ulcers. If a patient rebleeds, repeated endoscopic therapy should be attempted. If bleeding either persists or recurs after two attempts at an endoscopic control, the next intervention would be either surgery or angioembolization. Operative intervention is indicated for continued bleeding after endoscopic therapy and angioembolization have failed, if they are not available, or massive hemorrhage with hemodynamic instability such that there is no time to attempt the less invasive options.

22. **What are the operative options for control of a bleeding gastric ulcer?**
The best option is excision. Bleeding gastric ulcers require excision and biopsy to rule out malignancy. Small gastric ulcers (less than 2 cm) can usually be excised easily and safely, with the addition of an acid-reducing operation for patients who are acid hypersecretors. Large gastric ulcers, lesser curvature ulcers, bleeding ulcers associated with gastritis, and gastric ulcers that penetrate into the pancreas often require a more radical and technically demanding operation (subtotal, 75% resection, or near-total [95% resection] gastrectomy) to control hemorrhage.

23. **What is the most appropriate surgical procedure for a bleeding duodenal ulcer?**
The best option is simple oversewing of the bleeding ulcer. Control of the ulcer bed is attained by performing an anterior duodenotomy with direct ligation of the bleeding vessel or complete plication of the ulcer bed. Three-point suture ligation takes place in the superior, inferior, and medial aspect of the vessel. If a posterior duodenal ulcer has eroded into the gastroduodenal artery, bleeding may be profuse. If a patient has ulcer disease refractory to medical management or is on chronic NSAID therapy, a definitive ulcer operation is then performed. This may consist of either truncal vagotomy and pyloroplasty or a truncal vagotomy and antrectomy. An alternative approach is to attain control of the bleeding duodenal ulcer through a pyloroplasty incision, in which case a

truncal vagotomy completes the definitive ulcer operation. Patients who have not been treated for *H. pylori* prior to bleeding should undergo ligation of the bleeder only, with postoperative *H. pylori* eradication therapy, in lieu of a definitive ulcer operation.

24. **How is GOO caused by PUD surgically managed?**
GOO can result from an acute exacerbation of PUD in the setting of chronic pyloric and duodenal scarring. Classically, patients with GOO will present with nausea, emesis, early satiety, and weight loss. Although radiologic contrast studies are useful in evaluation, upper endoscopy is critical to rule out a malignant cause of the obstruction. Although in patients who are positive a trial of medical management may be successful, operative intervention is necessary in more than 75% of patients presenting with GOO. The two main goals of surgery are to relieve the obstruction and to perform a definitive ulcer operation. Truncal vagotomy and antrectomy with Billroth II reconstruction are performed if the duodenal stump is healthy enough to be safely closed. If the stump cannot be closed, a tube duodenostomy is left in place for control of secretions until the stump closes by secondary intention. An alternative is to perform a truncal vagotomy and pyloroplasty, which often requires the Finney pyloroplasty or Jaboulay gastroduodenostomy due to severe scarring. Truncal vagotomy and gastrojejunostomy may be performed if the severe scarring precludes an adequate drainage procedure via the duodenum. In patients with a prolonged history of obstruction, postoperative gastric atony can be expected, so placement of a gastrostomy tube may be helpful in postoperative care. Also, the nutritional status of the patient should be taken into account and a feeding jejunostomy at the time of the operation may be deemed necessary as serum albumin <3 mg/dL is associated with higher rates of morbidity and mortality.

25. **Discuss the role for endoscopic and laparoscopic management of GOO secondary to PUD.**
Patients treated with balloon dilatation, without treatment of *H. pylori* infection have a higher rate of failure and recurrent obstruction. Patients who are negative for *H. pylori* do not respond favorably to balloon dilatation and should be considered for surgical treatment early in the process.
    Laparoscopic truncal vagotomy combined with either pyloroplasty or antrectomy with gastrojejunostomy has been described successfully with low morbidity. The choice of open or laparoscopic management depends on the skill and experience of the surgeon.

26. **What are the long-term outcomes and risks for complications after truncal vagotomy and drainage, truncal vagotomy and antrectomy, and highly selective vagotomy?**
Truncal vagotomy and antrectomy have the lowest recurrence rate but also have the highest morbidity and mortality (Table 73.2). Highly selective vagotomy has the lowest morbidity and mortality but has the highest recurrence rate. The surgeon must balance these issues, patient preference, and the pathophysiology of the ulcer type in question when choosing an operative plan.

27. **What are the Visick criteria?**
The Visick criteria are used to grade outcome after surgery for PUD:
Grades I and II are considered adequate results. Most poor outcomes fall into grade III.
Grade I—No symptoms
Grade II—Mild symptoms that do not affect daily life
Grade III—Moderate symptoms that affect daily life and require treatment but are not disabling
Grade IV—Recurrent ulceration or disabling symptoms

28. **How should postoperative gastroparesis be managed?**
Postoperative gastroparesis often occurs in patients who undergo surgery for GOO. Evaluation should begin with esophagogastroduodenoscopy, upper GI series with small bowel follow-through, and gastric emptying scan. Once mechanical obstruction has been ruled out, medical treatment is successful in most cases. Prokinetic agents such as erythromycin and metoclopramide may be helpful. The indications for reoperation are the following:

Table 73.2 Comparison of Surgical Options for Peptic Ulcer Disease.

	TRUNCAL VAGOTOMY AND ANTRECTOMY	TRUNCAL VAGOTOMY AND DRAINAGE	HIGHLY SELECTIVE VAGOTOMY
Mortality rate (%)	1–2	0.5–0.8	0.05
Recurrence rate	Low	Moderate	High
Dumping (%)	10–15	10	1–5
Diarrhea (%)	20	25	1–5

- Early marginal ulcers refractory to medical management
- Anatomic abnormalities of the gastric outlet
- Recurrent bezoar associated with weight loss

Intractable gastroparesis following vagotomy and drainage may be treated with subtotal gastrectomy and Roux-en-Y reconstruction. If the gastric remnant is large, a Billroth II reconstruction may be preferable to Roux-en-Y reconstruction because the latter option may be associated with persistent gastric emptying problems. Gastroparesis may be managed with preoperative nasogastric (NG) tube decompression for the severely dilated stomach.

29. Describe the management of duodenal stump disruption (blowout) after truncal vagotomy, antrectomy, and Billroth II reconstruction.

Patients presenting with postoperative localized right upper quadrant tenderness are managed by aggressive percutaneous drainage of the abscess under radiologic guidance. An acute abdomen with free perforation and leakage of duodenal contents into the peritoneal cavity may require reoperation including reclosure of the duodenal stump over a tube duodenostomy and wide external drainage. Mortality from stump blowout approaches 10%.

30. What is dumping syndrome? Describe the pathophysiologic findings and treatment.

Dumping syndrome occurs in 20% of patients after vagotomy and gastrectomy, consists of tachycardia, diaphoresis, hypotension, and abdominal pain after meals in patients who have undergone ulcer operations, such as truncal vagotomy. Its pathophysiologic characteristic is the loss of receptive relaxation of the fundus in response to a gastric load. Thus gastric pressure increases during a meal, and rapid decompression through the gastric outlet causes the release of vasoactive hormones (serotonin, vasoactive intestinal peptide) and the resulting classic signs and symptoms. This constellation of symptoms occurring hours after meals is described as late dumping syndrome and is due to hypoglycemia resulting from a postprandial insulin peak. Symptoms typically improve with time and can be alleviated in some patients by separation of solids and liquids during meals, as well as the introduction of smaller, more frequent meals high in protein and fat and low in carbohydrates. Conversion of a Billroth II to a Billroth I or a Billroth operation to a Roux-en-Y reconstruction can improve symptoms but is rarely necessary. Octreotide, a somatostatin analog administered on a monthly basis, can alleviate symptoms and improve quality of life but is only indicated if symptoms are severe.

31. Describe the pathophysiologic findings of bile reflux gastritis. How is it managed?

Bile reflux gastritis occurs when ablation or dysfunction of the pylorus results in stasis of bile in the stomach. The diagnosis is made with the following triad of findings:
Postprandial epigastric pain accompanied by nausea and bilious emesis
Evidence of bile reflux into the stomach or gastric remnant
Biopsy-proven gastritis

Bile reflux gastritis can occur after truncal vagotomy with either pyloroplasty or antrectomy with Billroth reconstruction. Although up to 20% of patients who undergo these operations may have transient bile reflux gastritis postoperatively, symptoms resolve in all but 1%–2%.

Treatment of bile reflux gastritis requires revision of the pyloroplasty or the Billroth reconstruction to a Roux-en-Y gastrojejunostomy with a 50- to 60 cm alimentary limb (Fig. 73.6). Bilious emesis resolves in nearly 100% of patients who undergo revision. The symptoms of bile reflux gastritis may be indistinguishable from those of gastroparesis. Because the Roux-en-Y gastrojejunostomy worsens the symptoms of gastroparesis, care must be taken to exclude the diagnosis of gastroparesis preoperatively.

32. What is the presentation of Zollinger-Ellison syndrome?

Most patients with Zollinger-Ellison syndrome (ZES) are between 20 and 50 years of age and present with PUD or diarrhea. Ulcers are typically duodenal. The diarrhea resembles steatorrhea. It results from a combination of high volumes of acid and neutralization of pancreatic enzymes. ZES is either sporadic or associated with multiple endocrine neoplasia type 1 (MEN1), which is associated with pancreatic islet cell tumors, hyperparathyroidism, and pituitary tumors.

33. How is Zollinger-Ellison syndrome diagnosed?

A high level of suspicion is required for the diagnosis of gastrinoma. Serum gastrin should be measured in all patients undergoing peptic ulcer surgery. A serum gastrin level >1000 pg/mL with a gastric pH <2 is diagnostic of gastrinoma. Most patients with ZES do not have gastrin levels elevated to that degree. These patients should undergo gastric pH analysis and a secretin test. The secretin test is performed by comparison of basal serum gastrin level with gastrin level after the administration of secretin. Gastrinoma is suspected in patients with an increase in the serum gastrin level of 120 pg/mL after secretin administration. Normal patients have no change or a reduction in serum gastrin after secretin administration. Because achlorhydria is more common than gastrinoma, an elevation in serum gastrin is more commonly due to the lack of gastric acid as opposed to ectopic

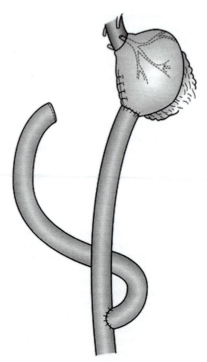

Fig. 73.6 Conversion of Billroth I or Billroth II reconstruction to a Roux-en-Y anastomosis. (From Cameron JL. Current Surgical Therapy. Philadelphia, PA: Mosby; 2004.)

gastrin production. Therefore measurement of acid production is also essential in making the correct diagnosis. Serum chromogranin A is a general marker for neuroendocrine tumors, and although it does not differentiate among the various types, it is also elevated in ZES.

34. For which patients with Zollinger-Ellison syndrome is operative intervention indicated?

Surgery is the treatment of choice for patients with nonmetastatic, sporadic gastrinoma. In addition, patients with metastatic gastrinoma who are unable to tolerate or are refractory to medical management should be considered for operative intervention. Sporadic gastrinomas are often solitary and located in the pancreas or duodenum, but not both, and are amenable to surgical resection and cure. Gastrinomas associated with MEN1 are usually multiple, virtually always in the duodenum, and often multicentric; they can also be found in the pancreas and are generally more difficult to cure surgically. Gastrinoma associated with hypercalcemia should suggest MEN1 complicated by hyperparathyroidism, and parathyroidectomy is essential for the management of gastric acid hypersecretion. Elevated serum gastrin levels postoperatively after gastrinoma surgery indicate residual gastrinoma(s) that should be treated medically. Medical management is also generally indicated for patients with metastatic gastrinoma. Medical management consists of high-dose PPIs with the goal of reducing gastric acid output to less than 10 mEq/hr for the hour that immediately precedes the next scheduled dose of antisecretory medication. Octreotide can be used as a second-line treatment when gastric acid secretion is not well controlled with PPIs alone.

35. Describe the preoperative evaluation for gastrinoma.

CT scan with intravenous and oral contrast is routine in the preoperative evaluation for gastrinoma resection to rule out metastatic disease, and its accuracy depends on the size of the gastrinoma. In some cases, magnetic resonance imaging (MRI) is used because it is more sensitive than CT scan for liver metastases. The addition of somatostatin receptor scintigraphy (octreotide) to traditional cross-sectional imaging has greatly improved the preoperative localization of gastrinomas. This study relies on the high density of somatostatin receptors on gastrinomas and uses the radiolabeled synthetic somatostatin analog, iodine-125—[^{125}I]octreotide—to identify primary and metastatic gastrinomas.

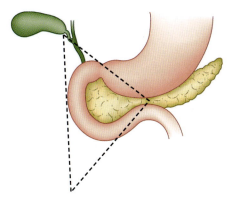

Fig. 73.7 The gastrinoma triangle.

Somatostatin receptor scintigraphy has high sensitivity and specificity for the detection of primary and metastatic gastrinomas. It also evaluates the extent of somatostatin receptors and addresses the need for somatostatin-based therapies. Endoscopic ultrasound has been used to localize gastrinomas; however, it is highly operator-dependent and does not reliably identify small tumors in the duodenum. Intraoperative upper endoscopy with transillumination or intraoperative ultrasound may also help to localize small duodenal gastrinomas.

36. **Where is the gastrinoma triangle? What percentage of tumors occur in this area?**
The apex of the gastrinoma triangle is at the cystic duct–common bile duct junction, and the triangle is bounded by the border of the second and third portions of the duodenum and the junction of the neck and body of the pancreas (Fig. 73.7). Approximately 60%–75% of gastrinomas are found within this triangle.

37. **Describe the operative scheme for exploration, localization, and removal of gastrinoma.**
If no tumor is apparent on preoperative imaging and other preoperative localization studies have failed, exploration begins with exposure of the anterior surface of the pancreas by mobilization of the transverse colon. A Kocher maneuver is then performed to mobilize the duodenum, allowing complete bimanual palpation of the pancreas. Intraoperative ultrasound is concentrated in the gastrinoma triangle. Biopsy of lymph nodes should be performed as gastrinoma can be localized to a solitary node. If an ultrasound of the pancreas does not reveal the tumor, duodenal gastrinoma should be suspected. A pyloroplasty incision is made, and the duodenal wall is visually inspected and manually palpated. An alternative method of localizing duodenal gastrinomas is to transilluminate the duodenal wall with intraoperative endoscopy. Gastrinomas in the duodenal wall or pancreas may be enucleated, but solitary lesions in the pancreatic tail are often treated by distal pancreatectomy.
If no lesion is found or if the disease is found to be multicentric or metastatic, an ulcer operation may be performed as palliation. This procedure often consists of a truncal vagotomy and pyloroplasty. Alternatively, the patient may be maintained on a PPI. In rare cases a total gastrectomy may be performed for control of acid production in patients who are refractory to medical therapy or unable to tolerate the side effects of the medication.

38. **Describe the risk of remnant gastric cancer after partial gastrectomy for duodenal and gastric ulcer.**
Remnant gastric cancer is defined as adenocarcinoma of the stomach that occurs after partial gastric resection for either benign or malignant disease. Even in patients who have had a partial distal gastrectomy for gastric ulcer, the relative risk is increased for up to 20 years following the index operation. Guidelines recommend annual surveillance endoscopy in patients who underwent gastric resection for 20 years followed by surveillance every 2–3 years thereafter.

CLINICAL VIGNETTE

Available Online

BIBLIOGRAPHY

Available Online

CHAPTER 74

SURGICAL APPROACH TO THE ACUTE ABDOMEN

William P. Hennrikus, MD and Matthew J. Bradley, MD

 Additional content available online.

1. **What is meant by the term acute abdomen?**
   The term acute abdomen refers to the sudden onset of severe abdominal pain of unclear cause. It implies a concern for an urgent pathology that requires prompt diagnosis and treatment. Peritonitis constitutes an acute abdomen but is not necessarily present in all acute abdomens. Many, but not all, of the diagnoses in the differential are surgical or potentially surgical in nature.

2. **What elements of a patient's history are most important?**
   - Age and sex
   - Abdominal quadrant of pain
   - Character (sharp, cramping, dull, and burning)
   - Onset and duration
   - Previous surgical history and medical comorbidities

3. **Which acute abdominal pathologies are associated with specific demographic groups?**
   - Neonates: intussusception, appendicitis, Meckel diverticulitis, mesenteric adenitis, midgut volvulus, malrotation, hypertrophic pyloric stenosis, and small bowel atresia
   - Females of childbearing age: ectopic pregnancy, ovarian torsion, pelvic inflammatory disease, and ruptured ovarian cyst
   - Adults: cholecystitis, diverticulitis, peptic ulcer disease (PUD), incarcerated hernia, ruptured spleen, renal or biliary stones, pancreatitis, and small bowel obstruction
   - Older adults: diverticulitis, colon cancer (perforation), appendicitis, aortic aneurysm, colonic and small bowel volvulus, and mesenteric ischemia

4. **Pain in each of these locations is often associated with which diagnoses?**
   - Right upper quadrant: biliary tract disease, hepatitis, PUD, and pneumonia
   - Right flank: hepatitis, pyelonephritis, and appendicitis
   - Right lower quadrant: appendicitis (late), incarcerated inguinal hernia, rectus sheath hematoma, ectopic pregnancy, ovarian torsion, pelvic inflammatory disease, ruptured ovarian cyst, Meckel diverticulitis, Crohn disease, and diverticulitis
   - Epigastrium: pancreatitis, PUD, gastritis, cardiac disease, and esophageal disease
   - Left upper quadrant: splenic rupture or infarct, PUD, pneumonia, and leaking abdominal aortic aneurysm
   - Left lower quadrant: diverticulitis, incarcerated inguinal hernia, rectus sheath hematoma, colon cancer (perforated), ectopic pregnancy, ovarian torsion, pelvic inflammatory disease, and ruptured ovarian cyst
   - Central abdomen/poorly localized/nonspecific: bowel obstruction, bowel ischemia, midgut volvulus, appendicitis (early), and ventral hernia

5. **What is peritonitis, and why does it manifest distinctly from visceral pain?**
   Peritonitis is inflammation of the parietal peritoneum, which shares its somatic innervation with the muscles of the abdominal wall it underlies. Parietal peritoneal inflammation manifests as sharp pain and tenderness that localizes to the specific area of the abdominal wall that is inflamed (or the entire abdominal wall, if diffuse peritonitis is present). In contrast, the visceral peritoneum lines the viscera and is not innervated itself, but its submesothelial tissue shares autonomic innervation with the viscera. This innervation can respond to various stimuli such as mechanical distension or hypoxia and produce vague, dull, crampy, or colicky, more central, poorly localized, nonspecific pain of insidious nature (a patient will often wave his or her hand over the umbilicus when asked to localize). Thus inflammation of a visceral organ will not manifest as peritonitis until the inflammation reaches the parietal peritoneum of the abdominal wall.

6. **What are peritoneal signs, and how do you elicit them on examination?**
Peritoneal signs are physical examination signs of parietal peritonitis. Focal tenderness is tenderness at the specific location being palpated. Rebound tenderness refers to tenderness upon undulation of the abdominal wall. A simple way to elicit rebound tenderness is to simply push and release the abdominal cavity at a location away from the patient's tenderness or jostle the patient at the hips to get the abdominal cavity to shake and observe the patient for signs of increased abdominal discomfort. *Involuntary guarding* refers to involuntary, reflexive contraction or spasm of the abdominal muscles on palpation due to localized peritoneal inflammation. This is in contrast to voluntary guarding, which is the conscious, voluntary contraction of the abdominal wall in anticipation of an examination maneuver that will cause discomfort. A tense abdomen in a patient lying perfectly still with involuntary guarding and rebound tenderness is foreboding and concerning for diffuse peritonitis. In contrast, the patient writhing around with voluntary guarding is not peritonitic. This is colicky pain, often the result of nephrolithiasis.

7. **To a surgeon, what do the adjectives "diffuse" and "nonspecific" imply when used to describe abdominal pain or tenderness?**
"Diffuse" abdominal pain or tenderness will likely suggest diffuse peritonitis to a surgeon and provoke concern and clarification. Use this adjective intentionally to raise a red flag. "Nonspecific" is a better description for vague, poorly localizing visceral discomfort.

8. **What is the difference between abdominal pain and abdominal tenderness?**
Pain is a component of the patient's history, reported by the patient. Tenderness is an examination finding—discomfort elicited by palpation on physical examination.

9. **What is Kehr sign, and what is meant by the term referred pain?**
Kehr sign describes pain in the left upper quadrant radiating to the left shoulder secondary to diaphragmatic irritation. It can be observed in the setting of perforated peptic ulcer, hematoma from splenic injury, or post laparoscopic surgery, in which it is believed that the carbon dioxide or mechanical stress of insufflation is the irritant. Kehr sign is an example of referred pain (felt at a location other than the site of painful stimulus). One theoretical explanation for this phenomenon is convergence projection, which hypothesizes that separate afferent axons converge on the same spinal neuron, producing the disturbed sensation.

10. **Define mittelschmerz.**
Mittelschmerz is lower abdominal pain that occurs during ovulation. The pain is usually ipsilateral to the side of ovulation.

11. **What is the significance of bowel sounds?**
There is little relevance in reporting the absence of bowel sounds to suggest an ileus or hyperactive, high-pitched, tinkling, or rushing bowel sounds to suggest an obstruction. Pain, constipation, obstipation, oral intolerance, distention, and tenderness are far more relevant to the consideration of these conditions.

12. **What are the most important components of the physical examination?**
Vital signs. An unstable patient with an acute abdomen could be dehydrated, acidotic, septic, or bleeding. Resuscitation should proceed without delay. Abdominal palpation may localize the abdominal quadrant of concern or peritonitis. Rectal examination may rule out gastrointestinal bleeding or distal obstruction. Pelvic examination can be invaluable in female patients of childbearing age with abdominal pain.

13. **What is Rovsing sign?**
Palpation of the left lower quadrant can elicit pain in the right lower quadrant, often seen in appendicitis. This is an example of focal peritonitis and rebound tenderness.

14. **What are the psoas and obturator signs?**
Inflammation of the psoas muscle causes pain in hip flexion or extension, whereas inflammation of the internal obturator muscle causes pain in internal rotation and flexion of the hip. A retrocecal appendicitis or, on occasion, diverticulitis may be responsible for these signs.

15. **Is acute abdomen ruled out by the absence of fever or leukocytosis?**
Not necessarily. Older and immunocompromised patients may not mount the expected inflammatory response even late in the course of the disease process.

16. **How does urinalysis help in the assessment?**
White blood cells in the urine may indicate urinary tract infection. Hematuria may suggest ureteral stones or tumor. Glucose or ketones may reveal diabetic ketoacidosis. An inflamed appendix abutting an adjacent ureter may lead to the finding of white or red blood cells in the analysis.

17. **What is the difference between an acute abdominal series (AAS) and a kidney ureter bladder (KUB) radiograph? What role do they play in the evaluation of an acute abdomen?**
AAS consists of three plain radiographs: upright chest, upright abdomen (or left lateral decubitus abdomen for patients who cannot stand), and supine abdomen. This series can identify free air under the diaphragm or over the liver, air-fluid levels suggesting bowel obstruction and lack of air in the colon and rectum suggesting complete obstruction. Air in the biliary tree may be seen with biliary-enteric fistula or pelvic pyelophlebitis. A KUB consists of a single plain radiograph: supine abdomen. The exposure technique in a KUB is optimized for the detection of stones. Only 10% of gallstones are radiopaque, but 90% of ureteral calculi are visualized. Appendiceal fecaliths are sometimes visualized.

18. **What is the role of ultrasound (US)?**
Right upper quadrant abdominal US evaluates for suspected liver or biliary pathology. US can also assess for free peritoneal fluid and can visualize the female adnexa. US examination is limited in the settings of obesity and bowel distention. US is often the preferred initial diagnostic imaging modality in children and pregnant females to avoid unnecessary radiation.

19. **What is the role of computed tomography (CT) scan?**
CT scan of the abdomen and pelvis can detect a wide range of inflammatory, obstructive, and vascular disease processes in the differential for acute abdomen (Fig. 74.1). Intravenous contrast is essential for the characterization of inflammation, tissue perfusion, and vascular integrity. Except in select cases such as suspicion of fistula or enteric leak, oral contrast can usually be deferred in the evaluation of the acute abdomen in the emergency department to benefit efficiency without significantly compromising diagnostic accuracy. A CT scan with intravenous contrast can, for example, diagnose small bowel obstruction and characterize relevant complications. This can be followed by a water-soluble oral contrast challenge if indicated.

20. **What is the role of magnetic resonance imaging (MRI)?**
In the workup of an acute abdomen, MRI is most frequently utilized in the form of magnetic resonance cholangiopancreatography to evaluate for choledocholithiasis or cholangitis when liver chemistries and US and/or CT demonstrate only intermediate risk and endoscopic retrograde cholangiopancreatography (ERCP) is not pursued immediately. MRI is a non-irradiating alternative to CT scan in the evaluation of pregnant patients and pediatric patients when appropriately resourced pediatric radiology capabilities are available.

21. **If the diagnosis remains uncertain, what else should be done?**
Surgical exploration of the abdomen is the next step if diagnostic studies are equivocal, and it is mandatory if the patient's condition worsens despite aggressive resuscitation.

22. **Is surgical exploration justified, even if a CT scan produces no significant findings?**
Yes. It is safer to undergo a surgical exploration than to miss an urgent diagnosis such as appendicitis or bowel infarction.

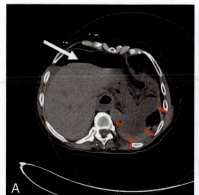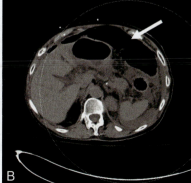

Fig. 74-1 (A) Axial cut of a computed tomography scan of the abdomen demonstrating massive pneumoperitoneum (*white arrow*) and free fluid (*red arrows*). The patient is a 70-year-old female who presented with 2 days of abdominal pain and peritonitis on examination. She underwent exploratory laparotomy and omental Graham patch repair of a perforated peptic ulcer. (B) Another axial cut of the same computed tomography scan demonstrating massive pneumoperitoneum (*white arrow*).

23. **When is surgery indicated for PUD?**
    - **Perforation**: Closure with an omental Graham patch is indicated for patients without previous history of PUD and for hemodynamically unstable patients. Definitive antiulcer surgery is indicated for hemodynamically stable patients with a prior history of chronic PUD. Resection of the ulcer with adequate margins should be performed for gastric ulcers. Definitive gastrectomy is undertaken after recovery if carcinoma is found in the specimen.
    - **Bleeding**: Surgery is indicated in the setting of hemodynamic instability or a transfusion of 6 units of blood within a 24-hour period. Esophagogastroduodenoscopy (EGD) as well as angiography can be very useful in this setting prior to these operative indications.
    - **Obstruction**: If duodenal obstruction from an ulcer is not relieved within 7 days, surgery is generally indicated. Balloon dilation and stenting are alternatives for patients who are poor surgical candidates.
    - **Intractability**: Despite benign biopsies, recurrent or nonhealing gastric ulcers should be resected because of the risk of underlying carcinoma.

24. **When should cholecystectomy be performed in the management of gallstone pancreatitis?**
    During the same index hospitalization, after pancreatic inflammation subsides. Compared to the historic approach of delaying cholecystectomy for weeks, same-admission cholecystectomy results in lower recurrence, complication, readmission, and mortality rates.

25. **When is surgery indicated for pancreatitis?**
    In the early phase of acute pancreatitis, decompressive laparotomy is indicated if abdominal compartment syndrome develops. Hemorrhagic pancreatitis is usually the result of splenic or gastroduodenal artery pseudoaneurysm and is managed with angioembolization, if possible, before open surgical control is attempted. Otherwise, operative debridement of pancreatic necrosis is deferred, if possible, for four weeks or more to avoid the high mortality of adding operative inflammation to the already physiologically overwhelmed patient. Indications for operative debridement include infected necrosis, persistent symptoms, and failure to thrive. Every attempt should be made within the 4-week window to manage infected or otherwise symptomatic peripancreatic collections with percutaneous drains. Such drains can serve as definitive management or as a temporizing bridge to a "step-up" approach to eventual video-assisted retroperitoneal debridement.

26. **What are omental infarction and epiploic appendagitis? What is the ideal treatment for these processes?**
    Spontaneous torsion or infarction of the omentum or epiploic appendages of the colon can mimic appendicitis and other acute abdominal diagnoses. Diagnosis is by CT. These processes are generally self-limiting and responsive to conservative (nonsurgical) care.

27. **What is the best method to diagnose pain secondary to mesenteric ischemia?**
    Despite multiple modalities (CT, US, and angiography) to assess intestinal vascular flow, high index of suspicion, a careful history, and physical examination remain the best methods to diagnose mesenteric ischemia. Pain out of proportion to physical examination is a classic finding. Atrial fibrillation, recent cardiac surgery, and any hypercoagulable state should arouse suspicion. Acidosis may reflect ischemia or necrosis, but a normal blood gas or lactate should not delay exploration. Laparoscopy can be helpful if there is no excessive bowel dilation.

28. **Describe the surgical strategy for the treatment of Crohn disease.**
    Because of the chronicity of the disease, any surgical strategy should preserve small bowel length. Stricturoplasty has been shown to be an effective measure with multiple Crohn strictures and maintains small bowel length. Surgery is reserved for obstructing strictures, inflammatory masses refractory to medical therapy, perforation, fistulae associated with recurrent infections or hygiene problems affecting quality of life, hemorrhage, and cancer.

29. **When should elective surgery be offered for uncomplicated acute diverticulitis?**
    The decision to pursue elective colectomy after recovery from nonoperatively managed uncomplicated acute diverticulitis should be individualized. Recurrence of symptomatic disease is common (13%–33%), but the lifetime risk of complicated disease recurrence requiring emergency colectomy is low (~5%). Factors to consider include frequency of attacks, smoldering symptoms, individualized perioperative risk assessment, and patient preference.

30. **Is there a role for laparoscopic peritoneal lavage in the management of diverticulitis?**
    No. This has been studied in the setting of Hinchey III diverticulitis (purulent peritonitis), and the accumulated data demonstrate an increased rate of major complications compared to colectomy.

31. **When is operative resection versus endoscopic detorsion recommended for colonic volvulus?**
    This depends on the presence of urgent complications (ischemia, perforation, peritonitis, or septic shock) and, if absent, the location of the volvulus. For *cecal* volvulus absent urgent surgical indication, resection is still

recommended, as endoscopic detorsion of the cecum is rarely successful. For *sigmoid* volvulus absent urgent surgical indication, endoscopy has initial success rates on the order of 60%–95% and is recommended to assess colonic viability, detorse, and decompress the colon. Urgent sigmoid resection is required if endoscopic detorsion is unsuccessful. If endoscopic detorsion is successful, elective sigmoid resection is still recommended, within the same hospitalization, after physiologic recovery from the acute phase of sigmoid volvulus to avoid the 42%–78% long-term risk of recurrence and associated mortality risk. Because resection has the lowest rate of recurrence, the roles of endoscopic sigmoidopexy and nonresectional operations (detorsion alone, with pexy, or with tube colostomy) are limited to settings of prohibitive surgical risk in patients unfit for resection.

32. **How should toxic megacolon in the setting of ulcerative colitis be managed?**
    Aggressive fluid resuscitation, bowel rest, broad-spectrum antibiotics, and intravenous corticosteroids. Serial abdominal examinations and plain films are mandatory to assess for colonic distention or impending perforation. Total abdominal colectomy with end-ileostomy is often required if there is no improvement in 48 hours.

33. **How should Ogilvie syndrome be managed?**
    Surgical resection is required for ischemia or perforation. In the absence of these or elevated risk of perforation (cecal diameter >12 cm), the vast majority of patients improve with the removal of narcotics and anticholinergics, treatment of any infection, bowel rest, resuscitation, and electrolyte repletion. Pharmacologic treatment with neostigmine is indicated if supportive therapy fails and has a success rate of up to 90%, although cardiac risk must be assessed prior to administration. Endoscopic decompression is indicated when neostigmine is ineffective or contraindicated. Colonoscopy carries a perforation rate of 1%–3% in this setting. Patients still refractory can have cecostomy performed via colonoscopy, interventional radiology, or surgery.

34. **After ERCP, a patient develops upper abdominal and back pain. What steps should be considered?**
    Serum lipase and CT scan or upper gastrointestinal (GI) series. Post–ERCP pancreatitis is the most frequent complication (2%–10%), and duodenal perforation is also possible (~0.5%). Pancreatitis is usually mild and can be treated expectantly. CT scan or upper GI series can usually pinpoint an injury to the duodenum after ERCP or polypectomy. Repeat EGD can provide the option of endoscopic repair but is less reliable for localization, especially of small injuries. The main focus should be on the location of the leak—is it the biliopancreatic system or the duodenum? Bile duct injury may be treated by endoscopic stent placement with percutaneous drainage of any biloma or surgical exploration if the injury is complex. A contained, small leak in the posterior duodenum (retroperitoneal) may be treated with bowel rest and gastric decompression. Exploration is indicated in the presence of ongoing pain or signs of diffuse peritonitis.

35. **What is the risk of colonic perforation after colonoscopy, and what is the management of this complication? Are there other potential surgical complications of colonoscopy?**
    The risk of perforation is ~0.5 per 1000 colonoscopies. In a well-prepped colon, bowel rest, antibiotics, and observation are often appropriate, provided there is no evidence of diffuse peritonitis. For small perforations, early (within 24 hours) laparoscopic repair is a viable alternative, with resection and primary anastomosis reserved for large injuries or devitalized tissue. Other complications such as operative bleeding or even splenic rupture are rarer.

36. **What are some other nonsurgical causes of acute abdomen?**
    The list of medical causes of acute abdominal pain is long. It includes diabetic ketoacidosis, hypercalcemia, myocardial infarction, pneumonia, ureteral calculi, and gastroenteritis. Careful history, repeat examinations, and judicious use of diagnostic imaging are paramount to avoid unnecessary surgery.

ACKNOWLEDGMENT
The authors acknowledge Kevin Rothchild, MD, and Jonathan A. Schoen, MD, who contributed to the previous version of this chapter.

CLINICAL VIGNETTE

Available Online

BIBLIOGRAPHY

Available Online

COLORECTAL SURGERY: POLYPOSIS SYNDROMES, COLORECTAL MALIGNANCIES, AND BENIGN DISEASES

CHAPTER 75

Amber M. Moyer, MD and Martin D. McCarter, MD

 Additional content available online

POLYPOSIS SYNDROMES

1. **Identify four different classes of intestinal polyps.**
   - Neoplastic (adenomatous, tubular, villous, tubulovillous, and serrated)
   - Hamartomatous
   - Inflammatory and lymphoid
   - Hyperplastic

2. **What is a hamartoma?**
   A hamartoma is an exuberant growth of normal tissue in an abnormal amount or location. An isolated hamartomatous polyp has no malignant potential.

3. **Which intestinal polyposis syndromes are associated with hamartomatous polyps?**
   - Peutz-Jeghers syndrome (PJS)
   - Juvenile polyposis (familial or generalized)
   - Cronkhite-Canada syndrome (hamartomatous polyps with alopecia, cutaneous pigmentation, and toenail and fingernail atrophy)
   - Intestinal ganglioneuromatosis (isolated or with von Recklinghausen disease or multiple endocrine neoplasia type 2)
   - Ruvalcaba-Myhre-Smith syndrome (polyps of colon and tongue, macrocephaly, intellectual disability, unique facies, and pigmented penile macules)
   - Cowden disease (gastrointestinal [GI] polyps with oral and cutaneous verrucous papules [trichilemmoma], associated with breast cancer, thyroid neoplasia, and ovarian cysts)

4. **How does PJS manifest?**
   This autosomal-dominant trait is often heralded by the presence of melanin spots on the lips and buccal mucosa. Hamartomas are almost always present in the small intestine and occasionally in the stomach and colon. Previously considered a benign process, patients with PJS are at increased risk for multiple extra-intestinal cancers: breast (50%), GI (50%), pancreatic (35%), gynecologic (10%–20%), and testicular (<10%). Cancer screening programs are recommended for persons with PJS.

5. **Describe the manifestation of familial adenomatous polyposis (FAP).**
   FAP is an autosomal-dominant, non–sex-linked disease in which more than 100 adenomatous polyps affect the colon and rectum. FAP is caused by mutation in the adenomatous polyposis coli (*APC*) gene on the long arm of chromosome 5 at the *5q21-q22* locus. The APC protein is a tumor suppressor that, when mutated, fails to bind beta-catenin and allows for unregulated cellular growth. One-third of patients present as the propositus case (presumed mutation) with no prior family history. The phenotype presents within the second and third decades of life. Extracolonic manifestations include upper gastrointestinal polyps (most commonly duodenal adenomas), desmoid tumors, thyroid cancer, congenital hypertrophy of the retinal pigment epithelium (CHRPE), fibromas, epidermoid cysts, osteomas, and dental abnormalities. FAP has a high penetrance and nearly 100% of patients will be diagnosed with colorectal cancer by age 50.

6. **What is attenuated FAP (AFAP)?**
   AFAP is a subset of FAP characterized by fewer than 100 adenomatous polyps (average of 30 polyps). Compared to classic FAP, people with AFAP develop polyps later in life and the polyps are more often located in the right

colon. Mutations in three specific areas of the *APC* gene have been associated with the AFAP phenotype, but not all patients with these mutations will develop polyps.

7. **What is MUTYH-associated polyposis (MAP)?**
MAP is an autosomal-recessive syndrome that mimics that of AFAP. This syndrome is caused by a germline mutation in both alleles of the *MUTYH* gene on chromosome 1.

8. **What is Gardner syndrome?**
Gardner syndrome is a phenotypic variant of FAP manifested by colonic polyposis plus fibromas of the skin, osteomas (typically of the mandible, maxilla, and skull), epidermoid cysts, desmoid tumors, and extra dentition.

9. **What is the screening for FAP?**
When family history is positive, children should undergo genetic testing and screening sigmoidoscopy at age 10–12 years. If no polyps are found on initial sigmoidoscopy, repeat screening should occur every 2 years. When polyps are identified, a full colonoscopy is recommended. Once multiple adenomas are documented, colectomy is recommended. Mutational analysis of the *APC* gene is the most accurate diagnosis. Ophthalmoscopic examination for CHRPE can detect involved patients as early as 3 months of age with a 97% positive predictive value for developing FAP. CHRPE is present in 55%–100% of patients with FAP.

10. **What surveillance is recommended for genetically confirmed FAP?**
In confirmed FAP, surveillance colonoscopy is recommended at 1- to 2-year intervals to reduce the risk of colorectal cancer.

11. **What are the elective surgical options for FAP?**
    - Total proctocolectomy with end (Brooke) ileostomy
    - Total proctocolectomy with continent ileostomy reservoir (Kock pouch)
    - Abdominal colectomy with ileorectal anastomosis
    - Near-total proctocolectomy ± rectal mucosectomy and ileal pouch-anal anastomosis (IPAA)

COLORECTAL MALIGNANCIES: COLON CANCER

12. **What are the fundamental principles of colon resection for cancer?**
    - A *5-cm margin* on either side of the tumor (Fig. 75.1)
    - Vascular supply taken at the origin of the closest named vessel (ileocolic, right colic, middle colic, left colic, and inferior mesenteric artery)
    - Adequate lymph node staging (minimum of 12 nodes evaluated)

13. **What are the pros and cons of minimally invasive surgery (laparoscopic or robotic) versus open colectomy?**
    Pros
    - Smaller incisions
    - Lower wound infection rate
    - Less postoperative pain

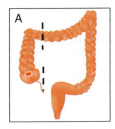 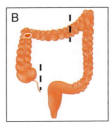 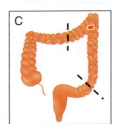 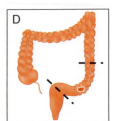

➤ Site of Colon Cancer   ‑ ‑ ‑ Demarcation of Surgical Resection

Fig. 75.1 (A) Right hemicolectomy, (B) extended right hemicolectomy, (C) splenic flexure resection, and (D) left hemicolectomy. (Adapted from Colon cancer treatment anastomosis. BioRender.com. Available at: https://app.biorender.com/biorender-templates. Published 2022.)

- Earlier return of bowel function
- Shorter postoperative hospital stay
- Quicker recovery and return to work

Cons
- Steep learning curve for technical proficiency
- Increased difficulty in reoperative settings or acute inflammation (diverticulitis)
- Increased cost

14. Which malignant polyps can be managed endoscopically?
Patients with a malignant polyp (T1 cancer arising in an adenomatous polyp) may be adequately treated by endoscopic excision if the polyp lacks high-risk features. Polyps with high-risk features harbor a higher risk of aggressive cancer or lymph node metastasis (Table 75.1).

15. How do you manage synchronous colon cancers?
Synchronous colon cancer means a second primary colon cancer is diagnosed at the same time, or up to 12 months after, as detection of the index colon cancer. These lesions can be treated by two segmental resections or subtotal colectomy, depending on the proximity of the two lesions.

16. What defines resectable stage IV colon cancer?
Management of resectable stage IV colon cancer is individualized with the help of a comprehensive multidisciplinary team. Patients with resectable stage IV disease limited to the liver should undergo resection of both the primary tumor and the metastatic foci in a single or staged operation. In patients with lung metastases, resection of metastases may be associated with prolonged survival. In selected patients with peritoneal metastases, cytoreductive surgery (CRS) with or without hyperthermic intraperitoneal chemotherapy can be considered.

17. What is Lynch syndrome?
Lynch syndrome (previously synonymous with hereditary nonpolyposis colorectal cancer) results from an autosomal-dominant mutation in one of the DNA mismatch repair (MMR) genes: *MLH1*, *MSH2*, *MSH6*, *PMS2*, and *EpCAM*. These genes are responsible for corrections during DNA replication. Lynch syndrome tumors are characterized by microsatellite instability (MSI), in which MMR deficiency leads to ubiquitous mutations at simple repetitive, noncoding sequences (microsatellites) that alter the DNA fingerprint. Lynch syndrome confers an increased lifetime risk of colorectal cancer: 70% for males and 40% for females. The mean age of diagnosis is 44–61 years of age. Colorectal cancer in Lynch syndrome typically occurs in the right colon, but left-sided colon cancer, rectal cancer, and synchronous lesions occur. Screening colonoscopy is recommended every 1–2 years beginning at age 20–25, or 2–5 years before the youngest age of diagnosis of colorectal cancer in the family.

The most common extracolonic cancer associated with Lynch syndrome is endometrial adenocarcinoma (30%–40% risk). Other associated cancers include ovarian (9%–12% risk), gastric (13% risk), urinary tract (4%–10% risk), small bowel (1%–3% risk), brain (1%–4% risk), and biliary (1%–5% risk).

18. What is the surgical treatment for colon cancer in the setting of Lynch syndrome?
There is no clear consensus on the surgical management of colon cancer in Lynch syndrome. Patients should be engaged in an informed decision-making process regarding the relative pros and cons of a total abdominal colectomy with ileorectal anastomosis versus a less-extensive operation. Less-extensive surgery should be considered in older individuals or patients with sphincter dysfunction.

19. How is appendiceal cancer managed?
Appendiceal neoplasms can be categorized as epithelial (adenoma or adenocarcinoma) or nonepithelial (neuroendocrine or lymphoma). Epithelial neoplasms are further subdivided into mucinous or nonmucinous. If an

Table 75.1 High-Risk Features of Colorectal Polyps.

HIGH-RISK POLYP FEATURES
• Poorly differentiated
• Lymphovascular invasion
• Perineural invasion
• Tumor budding
• Positive margin
• >1 mm depth

appendiceal neoplasm perforates and spreads throughout the peritoneal cavity with abundant mucin production, it is termed pseudomyxoma peritonei.

These neoplasms are more common in older males. Although appendiceal neoplasms are not appreciated on colonoscopy, colonoscopy is useful to detect synchronous lesions. Surgical treatment ranges from appendectomy (including mesoappendix) to right hemicolectomy, to cytoreductive surgery with or without intraperitoneal chemotherapy.

RECTAL CANCER

20. What is the best way to stage rectal cancer?
It has been said that an educated finger is the best instrument. After digital rectal examination (DRE), a rigid proctoscopic examination should be performed to evaluate the location of the tumor relative to the anal verge (assessment of height via flexible endoscopy is notoriously inaccurate). Rectal cancer protocol pelvic MRI is the preferred modality for locoregional clinical staging. Endorectal ultrasound may be considered if endoscopic mucosal resection (or endoscopic submucosal dissection) is feasible or if lymph node sampling would alter the treatment decisions. Clinical staging should also include contrast-enhanced computed tomography (CT) scan of the chest, abdomen, and $\pm$ pelvis to evaluate for metastatic disease.

21. When is local excision indicated?
Local excision with curative-intent is an appropriate treatment modality for carefully selected patients with cT1N0 tumors without high-risk features. Local excision involves full-thickness excision by either conventional transanal excision or endoscopically. The rate of local recurrence after local excision ranges from 7% to 21%.

22. What are the indications for neoadjuvant (before surgery) and adjuvant (after surgery) therapy?
Neoadjuvant therapy is recommended for patients with clinical stage II or III rectal cancer. The optimal timing and sequence of neoadjuvant chemotherapy and radiotherapy are still being debated. Neoadjuvant therapy decreases local recurrence rates and improves chances for sphincter preservation.

Adjuvant chemotherapy is recommended for patients with clinical or pathologic stage II (selected high risk) or III rectal cancer within 8 weeks of resection. The most common adjuvant regimen is FOLFOX (leucovorin, 5-fluorouracil, and oxaliplatin).

23. What is total neoadjuvant therapy (TNT)?
TNT employs both systemic chemotherapy and radiation therapy prior to surgical resection in select patients with clinical stage II or III rectal cancer. Proposed benefits include increased patient compliance and completion rates of chemotherapy, decreased treatment-related adverse effects and time with an ileostomy, and earlier treatment of undetected micrometastatic disease.

24. What is watch-and-wait management?
Select patients with a clinical complete response (cCR) to neoadjuvant therapy may be offered nonoperative, watch-and-wait management at some institutions. cCR is defined as (1) no palpable tumor on DRE, (2) no visible pathology other than flat scar on endoscopy, and (3) no evidence of disease on cross-sectional imaging.

25. Who is a good candidate for a sphincter preserving, low anterior resection (LAR)?
Patients with tumors that allow for at least a 2 cm distal mural margin (1 cm is acceptable for cancers located at or below the mesorectal margin for which radiation therapy was used) and that do not involve the external anal sphincter are candidates for LAR. Younger patients with good sphincter tone tend to adapt better to the physiologic changes associated with a LAR.

26. What are the pros and cons of a temporary diverting loop ileostomy following LAR?
Pros
- Reduces rate of *clinical* anastomotic leak
- Reduces rate of reoperation
- Promotes salvage of rectal function if a leak occurs
- Protects anastomosis in radiated or low surgical fields

Cons
- Risk of high stoma output and dehydration
- Decreased quality of life
- Additional operation for ileostomy reversal

27. What is LAR syndrome?

LAR syndrome is a constellation of symptoms including fecal incontinence, frequency, urgency, feelings of incomplete emptying, and clustering of bowel movements. These symptoms can severely impact quality of life with some patients requesting permanent ostomy.

28. What is an abdominoperineal resection (APR), and when is it indicated?

APR is the removal of the entire anus and rectum with an end colostomy. It is generally indicated for total anal incontinence or tumors that invade the anal sphincter. Low rectal cancers that do not directly invade the anal sphincter can, in certain situations, be managed with sphincter preservation and restorative coloanal anastomosis.

29. What is enhanced recovery after colon and rectal surgery (ERAS)?

ERAS encompasses a set of standardized perioperative procedures and practices for elective surgery to fast-track patients. This pathway includes components such as preadmission optimization, intraoperative colon bundle to limit surgical site infection, limited use of intra-abdominal drains and nasogastric tubes (NGTs), postoperative multimodal pain control, antiemetic prophylaxis, and early mobilization.

BENIGN COLON AND SMALL BOWEL DISEASE

30. What are the findings of sigmoid volvulus on plain abdominal film and contrast enema?

The plain film demonstrates a bent inner tube or coffee-bean sign of massively dilated, air-filled sigmoid colon arising out of the pelvis. The contrast enema shows a bird's beak appearance as the colon narrows at the twist at the rectosigmoid junction.

31. How is a nonstrangulated sigmoid volvulus treated?

Treatment is with rigid or flexible sigmoidoscopic or colonoscopic detorsion, followed by elective sigmoid resection.

32. Why should elective surgery be performed after a successful endoscopic detorsion and decompression of a sigmoid volvulus?

Recurrence is the rule with sigmoid volvulus. Elective sigmoid resection of prepped and decompressed bowel generally can be accomplished with very low mortality. Emergency operation for a sigmoid volvulus involves a higher mortality rate.

33. Do colon perforations from colonoscopy mandate surgical repair?

Not all perforations require surgery. Sound clinical judgment is critical. Limited controlled perforations with minimal contamination generally seal spontaneously. Signs of systemic illness (tachycardia, fever, hypotension, and increasing abdominal pain) generally require surgery (Fig. 75.2).

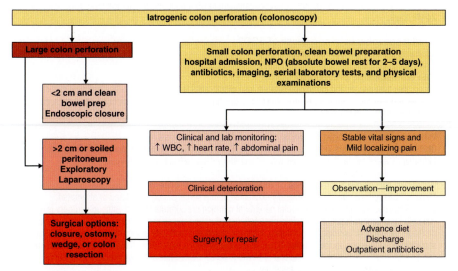

Fig. 75.2 Algorithm for managing colonoscopic perforation. *NPO,* Nothing by mouth; *WBC,* white blood cell. (Adapted from Flow chart (5 levels, vertical) 5. BioRender.com. Available at: https://app.biorender.com/biorender-templates. Published 2022.)

34. **What is Ogilvie syndrome?**
Colonic pseudo-obstruction, or Ogilvie syndrome, presents with signs, symptoms, and radiologic findings suggestive of obstruction without a mechanical source. It is most often seen in hospitalized patients with other underlying medical conditions found to have marked colonic air on abdominal radiographs. Treatments include managing underlying medical issues, colonoscopic decompression, and neostigmine.

35. **What does plain radiographic study of the abdomen reveal in large bowel obstruction (LBO)?**
An LBO demonstrates differential air-fluid levels (stair steps) of the small intestine or a massively dilated colon. The colon is identified by the presence of haustral folds, compared with the valvulae conniventes of the small intestine. The rectum is usually gasless, although gas distal to a colonic obstruction may not have completely cleared the distal colon. A picture resembling small bowel obstruction (SBO) alone may appear in a very proximal colon obstruction. Radiographic findings in colonic pseudo-obstruction may mimic a true obstruction.

36. **What radiologic findings are associated with gallstone ileus?**
Air in the gallbladder or biliary tree, SBO at the level of the ileocecal valve, LBO at the sigmoid colon, and, occasionally, a calcified mass at the point of obstruction are associated with gallstone ileus.

37. **What does endometriosis have to do with the alimentary system?**
Endometriosis is the presence of functioning endometrial tissue outside the uterus. When this hormonally active tissue implants on intestinal surfaces, it can cause pain, cyclical bleeding, and obstructive symptoms.

38. **What is a primary bowel obstruction?**
Primary bowel obstruction refers to an intestinal obstruction without a known cause, such as adhesions, or a prior cancer diagnosis. Primary bowel obstructions generally require an operation at some point.

39. **How is postoperative ileus differentiated from postoperative SBO?**
This distinction can be extremely difficult to determine. Postoperative ileus generally occurs up to 1 week after operation, whereas postoperative SBO may last 7 days or longer. SBO is associated with nausea, vomiting, distention, and abdominal pain, whereas an ileus may be associated with painless failure to pass bowel movements. The radiographic picture may or may not include differential air-fluid levels in each disorder.

40. **Is treatment of postoperative SBO different from the treatment of SBO remote from surgery?**
Yes. While NGT decompression is the mainstay of treatment for both postoperative SBO and remote SBO, the time course differs. Generally, if there is no evidence of strangulation or impending perforation, one waits out an early postoperative obstruction for a prolonged period of time. Approximately 80% resolve without surgery. Conversely, mechanical SBO remote from surgery in stable patients is often initially managed nonoperatively via NGT decompression with subsequent contrast administration, but patients who fail will progress to surgery within 24–48 hours.

41. **What is the most common cause of SBO?**
Adhesions are the most common cause of SBO.

42. **Can adhesions be prevented?**
Absorbable hyaluronate and carboxymethylcellulose membranes lead to a statistically significant reduction in the number and severity of intra-abdominal adhesions, although it is unclear if this translates into a reduced future need for operative intervention.

43. **What are the pathologic findings of late radiation enteritis?**
Obliterative arteritis occurs in late radiation enteritis. Severe fibrosis is commonly accompanied by telangiectasia formation. The pelvis may be *frozen* because of incredibly dense adhesions and fibrosis.

44. **What are the general principles of managing radiation enteritis?**
Medical management options are generally exhausted before surgery is contemplated or attempted. Cholestyramine, elemental diets, and total parenteral nutrition are commonly used. Although surgery is not withheld for urgent indications (complete obstruction, perforation, abscess not amenable to percutaneous drainage, bleeding, or unresponsive fistulas), it carries significant morbidity and mortality rates. Enterolysis, or separating of adhesions, in the radiated bowel is associated with a high rate of fistula formation. Anastomosis can be performed safely if at least one end of bowel to be connected has not been irradiated. Intestinal bypass procedures without resection may be necessary.

45. **What treatments are available for bleeding radiation proctitis?**
    Treatments include topical anti-inflammatory drugs (steroids, mesalamine enemas, or suppositories), targeted endoscopic application of thermal, bipolar, argon plasma coagulation or laser ablation of telangiectasias, and, lastly, application of 4% formaldehyde solutions (under controlled situations in the operating room).

CLINICAL VIGNETTE

Available Online

BIBLIOGRAPHY

Available Online

CHAPTER 76

GASTROINTESTINAL SECRETS: BARIATRIC SURGERY

Tamara J. Worlton, MD, FACS, FASMBS and Zachary A. Taylor, DO, FACS

 Additional content available online.

1. **What is obesity?**
   Obesity is defined by a body mass index (BMI) of $\geq$30 kg/m^2 ($\geq$27 kg/m^2 in Asians). Severe obesity is a BMI of $\geq$40 kg/m^2.

2. **Why is obesity something we need to be concerned about?**
   Obesity increases the risk of developing type 2 diabetes mellitus, heart disease, and several cancers. Other obesity-related medical conditions include reflux disease, joint and spine issues, fertility problems, sleep apnea, fatty liver, and many others. Obesity has also been shown to increase the risk of dying from infection from SARS-CoV-2. Estimates of health care expenditure on obesity in the United States are between $150 and $200 billion per year.

3. **How common is obesity in the United States?**
   The prevalence of obesity in the United States has risen from 30.5% to 42.4% between 2000 and 2017. Severe obesity has risen from 4.7% to 9.2% during the same period.

4. **What are the current treatments for obesity?**
   The treatment for overweight and obesity depends on how much weight needs to be lost. For people who are overweight (BMI 25–29.9 or 23.3–26.9 kg/m^2 in Asians), education about healthy food choices combined with calorie restriction and increased physical activity can be very effective. For patients with class 1 obesity (BMI 30–34.9 kg/m^2), there are many options including medications and reversible endoscopic treatments. US Food and Drug Administration (FDA)–approved endoscopic treatment of obesity includes intragastric balloon (IGB) placement, which remains in the stomach for 6–8 months, or endoscopic sleeve gastroplasty (ESG). For patients with a BMI of $\geq$35 kg/m^2 and a medical condition related to obesity or a BMI of $\geq$40 kg/m^2, the best treatment is bariatric surgery.

5. **What are the criteria that patients have to meet to qualify for bariatric surgery?**
   Individual insurance companies may have different criteria, but in general, patients must meet certain weight requirements such as a BMI of $\geq$40 or BMI of $\geq$35 kg/m^2 with a medical condition related to their obesity. Patients must be otherwise medically and psychologically stable and undergo dietary counseling. Often there are requirements for an exercise therapy consultation and attendance of bariatric surgery support groups.

6. **How many bariatric surgeries are performed per year in the United States?**
   In 2019 there were 256,000 bariatric surgeries performed. This means only 1% of patients who meet the criteria for bariatric surgery are being treated with surgery.

7. **What is the most common bariatric surgery performed in the United States?**
   The most common bariatric surgery is the sleeve gastrectomy (SG) which makes up more than half of all the bariatric procedures performed in the United States (Fig. 76.1). Roux-en-Y gastric bypass (RYGB) is the next most common bariatric surgery, comprising almost 18% of all bariatric surgeries (Fig. 76.2). The surgical anatomy and mechanisms for SG and RYGB-induced weight loss are illustrated in Fig. 76.3.

8. **What are the other bariatric surgeries and their frequencies?**
   The gastric band, which comprised 35% of surgeries in 2011, now is only 0.9% of bariatric surgeries. The conversion of gastric band to another bariatric procedure is likely why during the same time revisional surgery went from 6 % to 16.7%. The biliopancreatic diversion with duodenal switch has remained steady at about 1% of procedures over the last decade (Fig. 76.4). More recently, there has been interest in decreasing the number of surgical anastomoses in the biliopancreatic diversion with duodenal switch and RYGB leading to the single anastomosis duodenal ileal bypass and mini-gastric bypass.

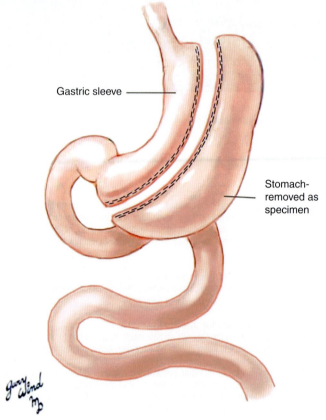

Gastric sleeve

Stomach-removed as specimen

Fig. 76.1 Surgical anatomy of gastric sleeve. (Courtesy Gary Wind, MD, FACS.)

9. **What is the efficacy of bariatric surgery?**
   On average, patients maintain 50% of their postbariatric surgical weight loss at 5 years. Patients who undergo bariatric surgery have a 30%–50% reduction in the risk of death when compared to obese patients who do not have bariatric surgery. Bariatric surgery is highly effective in treating type 2 diabetes mellitus with the majority of patients experiencing improvement in their diabetes control and many patients achieving remission of their diabetes altogether. Patients also see improvement in their hypertension, obstructive sleep apnea, dyslipidemia, infertility, and joint issues. Bariatric surgery reduces the risk of all cancers by 17%, major adverse cardiovascular events by 70%, and major adverse liver outcomes by 88%.

10. **What are some of the short-term complications related to bariatric surgery?**
    With any surgery, there is a risk of bleeding and leakage. In RYGB, there is a possibility of the gastrojejunal anastomosis developing a stricture. Patients undergoing bariatric surgery are at high risk for venous thromboembolic disease as well. The most common complication is dehydration, most often due to nausea after surgery. Patients can also experience dumping syndrome (bloating, diaphoresis, facial flushing, cramping, diarrhea, and vomiting) if they eat foods with a high concentration of fats and/or carbohydrates.

11. **What are some of the long-term complications related to bariatric surgery?**
    With the RYGB, patients are at risk for developing marginal ulcers (MUs) in the gastric pouch or the roux limb. Long-term MU can predispose to developing an abnormal connection between the gastric pouch and remnant stomach called a gastro-gastric (GG) fistula. Bypass anatomy also predisposes patients to internal hernias. Vitamin and mineral deficiencies can develop with any bariatric surgery at any time but are more common in the long term. SG anatomy is at higher risk for developing gastroesophageal reflux disease and potentially Barrett

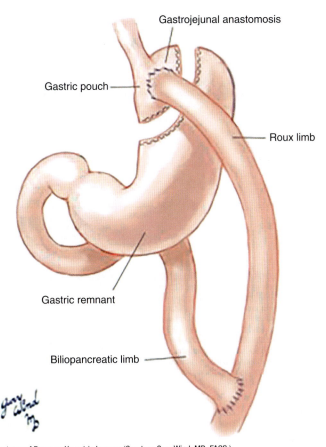

Fig. 76.2 Surgical anatomy of Roux-en-Y gastric bypass. (Courtesy Gary Wind, MD, FACS.)

esophagus. Patients with adjustable gastric bands are prone to having the band slip, which can cause acute intolerance of oral intake. Older model bands can erode into the stomach.

12. **What is the most serious nutritional deficiency after bariatric surgery?**
Patients can develop thiamine deficiency very rapidly. Patients with prolonged nausea and oral intolerance after surgery should be screened for thiamine deficiency. If thiamine deficiency is not addressed, they can develop Wernicke encephalopathy, which has a classic triad of confusion, ocular findings (nystagmus and double vision), and cerebellar dysfunction (ataxia).

13. **What is the most common reversible endoscopic therapy for weight loss in the United States?**
Placement of an IGB is an endoscopic alternative for weight loss in patients who do not meet the criteria for bariatric surgery. It can also be placed as an adjunct for preoperative weight loss before elective bariatric surgery in patients with high BMI. It is an expandable silastic balloon instilled with sterile water occupying space and partially distending the stomach helping to both limit intake and cause fullness. Percent excess weight loss (EWL) at 6 months of 36.2% ± 6.3% versus total body weight loss (TWL) of 15% at 8 months depending on balloon type. However, recidivism can be seen once the IGB is removed.

14. **Are there other approved endoscopic therapies for weight loss in the United States?**
ESG is a less-invasive primary weight loss procedure. It entails using advanced endoscopic suturing techniques to plicate the stomach along the greater curvature, reducing the volume by approximately 70% using a full-thickness endoscopic suturing device creating a tubularized stomach. Outcomes demonstrate significant, durable

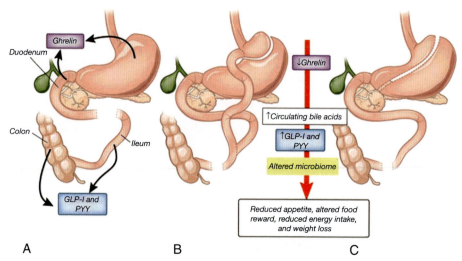

Fig. 76.3 Illustrations of the (A) normal gastrointestinal (GI) tract, (B) Roux-en-Y gastric bypass (RYGB), and (C) sleeve gastrectomy (SG). (A) Multiple regulatory enteric hormones are secreted by the GI tract. Ghrelin (hunger hormone) is secreted from the P/D1 cells of the gastric fundus, whereas glucagon-like peptide-1 (GLP-1) and peptide YY (PYY) acutely suppress appetite and stimulate insulin secretion from pancreatic β cells, both peptides are secreted from L cells located predominantly in the ileum and colon. (B) RYGB: nutrients bypass a significant portion of the small intestine (50–80 cm biliopancreatic limb and 125–150 cm alimentary/roux limb) and flow directly into the mid-jejunum. Anastomosis of the biliopancreatic limb with the jejunum allows the drainage of bile acids and digestive enzymes into the common channel, where ingested nutrients and digestive enzymes mix. (C) SG: nutrients pass rapidly from the gastric sleeve into the duodenum with unaltered flow of bile acids and digestive enzymes. Following RYGB and SG, circulating ghrelin levels are reduced, and meal-stimulated PYY and GLP-1 are increased. Bile acid secretion is enhanced and the microbiome is altered. (From Makaronidis JM, Batterham RL. Potential mechanisms mediating sustained weight loss following Roux-en-Y gastric bypass and sleeve gastrectomy. Endocrinol Metab Clin. 2016;45:539-552.)

weight loss with a mean TWL of 15.1% at 6 months and a sustained TWL of 16.5% and 17.2% at 12 and 18–24 months, respectively.

15. What endoscopic interventions exist for weight regain following bariatric surgery?

Transoral outlet reduction endoscopy can be performed in patients with weight regain after RYGB. The procedure incorporates the argon plasma coagulator to cauterize the gastric outlet creating scar tissue formation. This is coupled with the full-thickness endoscopic suturing device placing a purse-string suture around the gastric outlet and synched down over a 6 mm balloon placed through the gastric outlet. This creates a narrowed gastric outlet providing improved restriction. Plication of a dilated gastric pouch can be performed to reduce pouch size using the full-thickness endoscopic suturing device. Outcomes demonstrate significant, durable weight loss with percentages of EWL of 24.9% ± 2.6%, 20.0% ± 6.4%, and 19.2% ± 4.6% at 1, 2, and 3 years, respectively.

16. What endoscopic therapies are available to treat complications (bleeding, leak, band erosion, GG fistula, or stricture) following bariatric surgery?

There are numerous endoscopic options that vary based on the type of complication. Endoscopic clipping can be used for bleeding or GG fistula closure. Full-thickness suturing can be used for the closure of a leak, band erosion, or GG fistula. Endoscopic vacuum therapy can be used to place a wound vac sponge sutured to the end of a nasogastric tube through a gastric or esophageal defect into an abscess cavity following a leak to promote wound healing and obtain source control. Stent placement either across a gastric leak with the proximal end terminating in the distal esophagus excluding the gastric defect or across the gastric outlet in gastrojejunal leak with the proximal cuff either clipped or sutured in place to prevent migration. Balloon dilatation can be used to treat anastomotic stricture.

Biliopancreatic Diversion With Duodenal Switch

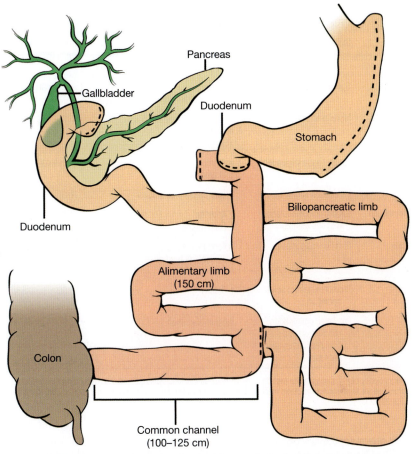

Fig. 76.4 Illustration of the alimentary and common channel length in biliopancreatic diversion with duodenal switch. (From Antanavicius G, Halawani HM. Single-docking robotic biliopancreatic diversion with duodenal switch technique. Surg Obes Relat Dis. 2017;13:1922-1926.)

17. **What gastrointestinal (GI) hormones are affected by weight loss surgery and help promote weight loss?**

There are numerous GI hormones directly affected by bariatric surgery (Table 76.1). Glucagon-like peptide-1 (GLP-1) is a well-studied and key hormone following bariatric surgery involved in regulating insulin secretion as well as appetite suppression, inhibition of glucagon secretion, and slowing gastric emptying. It is found to be elevated postbariatric surgery and likely contributes to rapid glycemic improvement. Ghrelin is a hormone produced by the gastric fundus responsible for increased hunger drive, which declines postbariatric surgery thereby lessening hunger and cravings.

Table 76.1 Gut - and Postmetabolic/Bariatric Surgery.

Impact of Hormonal Changes After Bariatric Surgery			
HORMONE	PRIMARY EFFECT	IMPACT OBESITY/DIABETES	POSTBARIATRIC Δ
Ghrelin	Stimulates hunger	↑ Hunger/appetite ↑ Insulin sensitivity ↑ Lipogenesis	↓ Short term and ↑ long term in RYGB ↓ after SG
Leptin	Suppresses hunger	↓ Hunger ↑ Energy expenditure	↓ Both RYGB and SG
GLP-1	Incretin effect	↑ Glucose-dependent insulin secretion ↓ Glucagon secretion	↑ Both RYGB and SG
Adiponectin	Target tissue dependent	Anti-inflammatory ↑ Insulin sensitivity	↑ Both RYGB and SG
Secretin	Pancreatic secretion	Brown adipose activation	↑ RYGB
Oxyntomodulin	Gastric acid modulation (oxyntic glands) ↓	↓ Appetite ↓ Food intake	↑ RYGB in response to oral glucose
Obestatin	Ghrelin antagonism	↓ Food intake ↓ Jejunal contraction ↓ Body weight	Inconclusive
Gastrin	Promotes gastric acid secretion	↑ Satiety	↓ RYGB ↑ SG
CCK	Promotes gallbladder contraction and pancreatic enzyme secretion	↑ Insulin secretion	↑ Both RYGB and SG

CCK, Cholecystokinin; *GLP-1*, glucagon-like peptide-1; *RYGB*, Roux-en-y gastric bypass; *SG*, sleeve gastrectomy.
Adapted from Luo JN, Tavakkoli A. Physiologic mechanisms of weight loss following metabolic/bariatric surgery. Surg Clin N Am. 2021;101(2):223-237.

18. **What pharmacotherapy options are available for patients not meeting National Institutes of Health criteria, assist in preoperative weight loss, and/or assist in weight regain following bariatric surgery?**

   GLP-1 agonists and combination medications are FDA approved for patients with a BMI of >27% and weight-related comorbidities or a BMI of >30% kg/m². GLP-1 agonists semaglutide (Wegovy) and liraglutide (Saxenda) improve glycemic control, suppress appetite, and slow gastric transit leading to early satiety impacting hunger drive. Average TWL is 12%–15%. Combination medications such as phentermine/Topamax (Qsymia) and naltrexone/bupropione (Contrave) target the hunger and craving centers in the brain to reduce hunger and decrease cravings. Average TWL is 5%–10%.

CLINICAL VIGNETTE

Available Online.

BIBLIOGRAPHY

Available Online.

CHAPTER 77

MINIMALLY INVASIVE SURGERY

Holly V. Spitzer, DO and Anthony J. LaPorta, MD, FACS

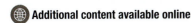 **Additional content available online**

1. **What does the field of minimally invasive surgery include?**

   Minimally invasive surgery is a field that has developed in recognition of increased risk, pain, and wound complications associated with traditional open surgery and large incisions. The field encompasses a broad range of surgical approaches including miniature incisions for procedures (like keyhole and port access coronary artery bypass graft procedures, which avoid sternotomy), laparoscopy/thoracoscopy for abdominal/thoracic procedures, endoscopic natural orifice and transluminal therapies, arthroscopy, percutaneous/endovascular procedures, and robotic surgery. The field of minimally invasive surgery is rapidly advancing with ongoing improvements in videoscopic platforms, haptic feedback, telecommunication, and adjuncts to standard techniques, including fluorescence and targeting. With improvements in training and resource availability, almost any abdominal procedure that can be done in an open fashion can now be performed via laparoscopic approach, with appropriate patient selection.

2. **When did laparoscopic surgery become an accepted surgical option?**

   Laparoscopic surgery has been explored since the early 1900s, initially as a diagnostic option. Dr. Kurt Semm, a German gynecologist, performed the first laparoscopic appendectomy in 1982. George Berci was one of the first general surgeons to champion laparoscopic surgery, but initially, he met resistance from the surgery community. In the 1980s general surgeons in Germany, France, and the United States independently developed techniques for laparoscopic cholecystectomy. Barry McKenna and William Say are credited with performing the first laparoscopic cholecystectomy in the United States in 1988. Although initially denounced, this procedure quickly became the standard of care, and by 1992 it was considered the treatment of choice for symptomatic cholelithiasis, despite higher rates of common bile duct injury with this approach.

3. **What are the advantages of laparoscopic surgery compared with open procedures?**

   Major advantages of laparoscopic surgery include reduction of abdominal wall trauma, with associated rapid recovery, reduction in pain, and reduced wound infections. Since the adoption of laparoscopic surgery, efficiency and affordability of this approach have improved substantially. As a result, laparoscopic surgery has become the standard of care for many operations, including cholecystectomy and adrenalectomy.

4. **What are contraindications for laparoscopic surgery?**

   Absolute contraindications include the patient's inability to tolerate general anesthesia or pneumoperitoneum, usually related to advanced cardiopulmonary disease. Although gasless laparoscopy is used in resource-compromised regions, this has not been widely adopted. Relative contraindications include coagulopathy and portal hypertension. The most important contraindication is lack of surgeon experience, as the ability to safely create working space is paramount. Additionally, the judgment to convert to an open procedure or incorporate adjuncts to the laparoscopic approach is key to the utility of laparoscopy and the maintenance of patient safety.

5. **What are the respiratory effects of pneumoperitoneum?**

   Pneumoperitoneum results in elevation of the diaphragm, leading to decreased functional residual capacity and total lung volume, contributing to ventilation-perfusion inequalities and atelectasis. Increased peak inspiratory pressure may be required to compensate for decreased compliance secondary to intra-abdominal hypertension. For healthy patients, no significant change in arterial oxygenation occurs with pneumoperitoneum. However, for patients with cardiopulmonary compromise, arterial oxygen reductions have been reported with pneumoperitoneum.

6. **What are the hemodynamic effects of pneumoperitoneum?**

   Intra-abdominal hypertension $\geq 15\,mm$ Hg can result in significant changes in central hemodynamics and splanchnic circulation. Mean arterial blood pressure and systemic peripheral resistance are increased (up to 35% and 160%, respectively) at operative levels of pneumoperitoneum (12–15 mm Hg), presumably from sympathetic vasoconstriction from hypercarbia. With further increases in intra-abdominal pressure, cardiac output falls and abdominal venous compliance decreases, which can cause hemodynamic compromise, especially in patients with preexisting cardiopulmonary disease.

7. **Summarize the key strategies for safe laparoscopic cholecystectomy.**

Cholecystectomy is one of the most common surgeries performed, with 750,000 cholecystectomies annually in the United States. The most feared complication of cholecystectomy is injury to the common bile duct, which occurs in approximately 3/1000 laparoscopic cholecystectomies. Surgeons can avoid this complication by following guidelines for safe cholecystectomy, including:

1. Use of the critical view of safety in identifying the cystic duct and cystic artery.
2. Understanding potential aberrant anatomies.
3. Liberal use of intraoperative cholangiography.
4. Use of adjuncts or conversion to open if conditions are unsafe. Request assistance when needed.

8. **What is the critical view of safety?**

First defined by Dr. Steven Strasberg, the critical view of safety is a method of approaching the cystic triangle that allows for a safe dissection and identification of critical structures (Fig. 77.1). Achieving the critical view of safety requires clearance of fat and fibrous tissue from the cystic triangle to expose only two structures that enter the gallbladder (cystic artery and cystic duct) with exposure of at least one-third of the cystic plate.

9. **When should an intraoperative cholangiogram (IOC) be performed?**

IOC is a method of imaging the common bile duct using contrast and x-ray to identify common bile duct obstruction, guiding further clearance of the duct. The procedure can also be used to elucidate difficult anatomy and confirm correct ligation. Although some surgeons endorse universal IOC, most surgeons employ selective IOC. Indications for IOC include findings suggestive of common duct obstruction, including history of jaundice, biliary pancreatitis, elevated laboratory tests (bilirubin, liver enzymes, or amylase/lipase), dilation of common bile duct on preoperative ultrasonography, visible stone obstructing the common bile duct on ultrasound, magnetic resonance cholangiopancreatography or other imaging, dilated common bile duct (>5–7 mm in diameter), and multiple small gallstones. Other indications include unclear intraoperative anatomy, concern for bile duct injury or leak, and short cystic duct.

10. **What are the benefits and drawbacks of laparoscopic inguinal hernia repair versus open inguinal hernia repair?**

The decision to perform laparoscopic versus open inguinal hernia repair should be made on a case-by-case basis with consideration of patient-specific factors (including age, history of prior hernias and repairs, hernia size, comorbidities, history of pelvic radiation or extensive pelvic surgery, and activity level) and surgeon expertise. Some studies have demonstrated an earlier return to activity and decreased pain with the laparoscopic approach. Many surgeons endorse the laparoscopic approach when multiple hernias are present, as additional repairs can be performed without additional incisions. Additionally, many surgeons utilize the laparoscopic approach for recurrent hernias to allow dissection in a *virgin* plane. Like any laparoscopic procedure, the ability to visualize and safely dissect is paramount. Therefore prior history of pelvic radiation or pelvic surgery may contraindicate a laparoscopic approach.

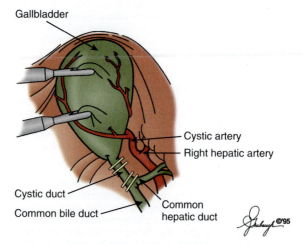

Fig. 77.1 The triangle of Calot is formed by the cystic duct, cystic artery, and common hepatic duct. The hepatocystic triangle is the area between the cystic duct, the common hepatic duct, and the border of the liver. These areas should be familiar to surgeons performing laparoscopic cholecystectomies as they are fundamental to safe cholecystectomy.

11. **Which laparoscopic inguinal hernia repair is preferred: transabdominal preperitoneal (TAPP) hernia repair or totally extraperitoneal patch plasty (TEP)?**
In general, TAPP (that requires peritoneal insufflation and incision of the peritoneum to gain access to the myopectineal orifice) and TEP (access to the myopectineal orifice by a preperitoneal approach) are reasonable approaches for most patients. The major indications for each are surgeon familiarity and the pursuit of the virgin plane to facilitate safe surgery. However, the major contraindication of TEP is a concern for bowel compromise from incarceration or strangulation. These cases should be approached via TAPP or open approach to facilitate inspection of the bowel. In general, conversion to open may be preferred if the bowel is found to be nonviable on inspection, as the laparoscopic approach relies on the placement of synthetic mesh, which may not be preferred in the contaminated repair. (It should be noted that recent studies indicate that synthetic mesh is safe in contaminated hernia repairs, these data are primarily describing ventral hernia repairs and this practice has not yet been widely adopted.)

12. **Is there a clearly defined benefit to laparoscopic appendectomy?**
Laparoscopic appendectomy has been shown to have a number of benefits compared to open appendectomy in adults, including reduced pain in the postoperative period, decreased wound infection risk, abbreviated length of stay, and faster return to normal activity.

13. **Is gangrenous or perforated appendicitis a contraindication to laparoscopic appendectomy?**
No. Laparoscopic appendectomy has been shown to be noninferior and, in some cases, superior to open appendectomy for reduced postoperative pain, shorter operative time and length of stay, and fewer surgical site infections and postoperative ileus, among other complications.

14. **Can laparoscopic cholecystectomy or laparoscopic appendectomy be performed safely in a pregnant patient? What are some technical considerations specific to operating laparoscopically on the pregnant patient?**
Yes. Laparoscopic cholecystectomy and appendectomy can be safely performed at any trimester of pregnancy without increased risk of fetal demise or preterm labor. Postponing cholecystectomy and appendectomy have been shown to increase complications in pregnant patients, including preterm labor and fetal demise. Positioning on the operative table should be adjusted in all second- and third-trimester patients to avoid uterine compression of the inferior vena cava. The approach to intra-abdominal access should be adjusted superiorly based on fundal height and insufflation pressure kept at <15 mm Hg.

15. **What is the role of laparoscopic surgery for curable colon cancer?**
Laparoscopic colon resection for curable colon cancer has been shown to be safe and effective as long as oncologic principles can be followed, including proximal ligation of the primary vascular supply with adequate lymphadenectomy and en bloc resection to appropriate proximal and distal margins. If the procedure cannot be performed to oncologic standards, an open approach should be utilized.

16. **Does laparoscopy have a role in acute trauma care?**
Yes! Laparoscopic surgery can be safely performed in trauma patients and has been shown to reduce laparotomy rates. It is also associated with reduced blood loss and shortened length of stay compared to laparotomy in blunt trauma patients. The primary benefit of laparoscopy in trauma is seen in patients with blunt trauma and concern for hollow viscous injury.

17. **What percentage of patients have free intra-abdominal air on upright radiograph 24 hours after laparoscopic procedure?**
In the non postoperative state the presence of subdiaphragmatic free air on an upright radiograph is diagnostic of intra-abdominal perforation. After an open abdominal or laparoscopic procedure, the significance of intra-abdominal free air is less clear. Nonpathologic subdiaphragmatic air may be seen in 24%–39% of patients after laparoscopic surgery and in 60% of patients after open surgery (CO_2 used for laparoscopic pneumoperitoneum is absorbed more quickly than room air introduced with open surgery). However, if postoperative free air is observed on x-ray, clinicians should consider pathologic causes of free air prior to considering nonpathologic causes.

18. **What role does endoscopic intervention play in the management of gastroesophageal reflux disease (GERD)? How has minimally invasive surgery been incorporated in the surgical management of esophageal cancer?**
The field of endoscopic management of GERD has exploded in recent years, with numerous approaches, including submucosal injection and plication. Although these approaches have been shown to be superior to medical therapy alone, they have not been shown to be superior to fundoplication. The reader is referred to Chapters 5, 7, and 72 for new endoscopic treatments of Barrett esophagus and low-stage esophageal malignancy.

19. **How are minimally invasive approaches incorporated in the surgical management of rectal pathology?**
   Transanal minimally invasive surgery combines transanal endoscopic microsurgery and single-site laparoscopy for resection of low rectal lesions. It has been shown to be an effective method of resecting both benign and malignant diseases in the distal rectum and may represent an alternative to major procedures such as abdominoperineal resection for well-selected patients.

20. **Is laparoscopic/robotic surgery safe in the era of coronavirus disease 2019 (COVID-19)?**
   Although concerns exist regarding the possibility of transmission of COVID-19 by aerosolization during laparoscopic surgery, there is no evidence to support that this occurs. Given the benefits of laparoscopy over open surgery for many common procedures, the current guidelines recommend the use of laparoscopy with precautions in patients with COVID-19. Patients should only be treated nonoperatively as an alternative to laparoscopic surgery if it is safe for the patient.

CLINICAL VIGNETTE

Available Online

BIBLIOGRAPHY

Available Online

Note: Page numbers followed by *b* indicate boxes, e indicate online contents, *f* indicate figures, and *t* indicate tables.

Contents

Columbia University Press
Publishers Since 1893
New York   Chichester, West Sussex
cup.columbia.edu

Library of Congress Cataloging-in-Publication Data
Names: Solider, Dave, 1956– author.
Title: Music, math, and mind : the physics and neuroscience of music /
David Sulzer.
Description: New York : Columbia University Press, 2021. |
Includes bibliographical references and index.
Identifiers: LCCN 2020045865 (print) | LCCN 2020045866 (ebook) |
ISBN 9780231193788 (hardback) | ISBN 9780231193795 (trade paperback) |
ISBN 9780231550505 (ebook)
Subjects: LCSH: Music—Acoustics and physics. | Musical perception. |
Music—Physiological aspects. | Neurobiology. | Hearing.
Classification: LCC ML3805 .S62 2021 (print) | LCC ML3805 (ebook) |
DDC 781.1—dc23
LC record available at https://lccn.loc.gov/2020045865
LC ebook record available at https://lccn.loc.gov/2020045866

Cover design: Noah Arlow

MUSIC, MATH, AND MIND

The Physics and Neuroscience of Music

• • • • • • • • • • • • •

DAVID SULZER

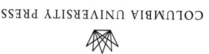

COLUMBIA UNIVERSITY PRESS
New York